Adult Telephone Protocols 4th Edition

Office Version

David A. Thompson, MD, FACEP

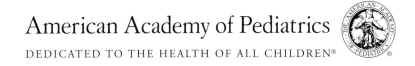

American Academy of Pediatrics

DEDICATED TO THE HEALTH OF ALL CHILDREN®

American Academy of Pediatrics Publishing Staff
Mary Lou White, *Chief Product and Services Officer/SVP, Membership, Marketing, and Publishing*
Mark Grimes, *Vice President, Publishing*
Peter Lynch, *Senior Manager, Digital Strategy and Product Development*
Evonne Acevedo, *Editor, Digital Publishing*
Shannan Martin, *Production Manager, Consumer Publications*
Jason Crase, *Manager, Editorial Services*
Linda Diamond, *Art Direction and Production*
Mary Jo Reynolds, *Marketing Manager, Practice Publications*

Published by the American Academy of Pediatrics
345 Park Blvd
Itasca, IL 60143
Telephone: 630/626-6000
Facsimile: 847/434-8000
www.aap.org

The American Academy of Pediatrics is an organization of 67,000 primary care pediatricians, pediatric medical subspecialists, and pediatric surgical specialists dedicated to the health, safety, and well-being of infants, children, adolescents, and young adults.

User's Responsibility: Author and Publisher Disclaimer Notice

- These protocols are clinical guidelines that must be used in conjunction with critical thinking and clinical judgment. Therefore, these protocols are most suitable for use by physicians and clinically experienced nurses, nurse practitioners, and physician assistants. All licensed health professionals should receive special training before using these protocols (with training and ongoing quality assurance audits). Non-licensed and non-health professionals (e.g., secretaries) should not use these protocols.

- These protocols should not be used unless they have been reviewed, amended as necessary, and approved by a supervising physician or medical director responsible for overseeing their use.

- These protocols are as up-to-date as is reasonably possible at the time of publication. However, medical knowledge is constantly changing and expanding. It is the responsibility of the supervising physician or medical director to review and update these protocols on a yearly basis.

- The contents of these protocols have been reviewed and tested for accuracy, but they are not, and cannot be, perfect. Therefore, the author, publisher, and distributors disclaim responsibility for any harmful consequence, loss, injury, or damage associated with the use and application of information or advice contained in these protocols.

- The author, publisher, and distributors do not warrant or guarantee the accuracy, safety, efficacy, or completeness of any of these protocols.

- Any person, institution, or organization using these protocols assumes full responsibility for acts or omissions arising out of their use or misuse. The user assumes all risks associated with using these protocols.

- Using this product means the user has read and accepts this disclaimer.

Alphabetic Listing—*Adult Telephone Protocols*

Anatomic Listing—*Adult Telephone Protocols*

Category Listing—*Adult Telephone Protocols*

Appendix Table of Contents—*Adult Telephone Protocols*

ABDOMINAL PAIN (FEMALE)

Definition
- Pain or discomfort located between the bottom of the rib cage and the groin crease
- Female

Pain Severity Scale
- **Mild (1-3):** Doesn't interfere with normal activities, abdomen soft and not tender to touch.
- **Moderate (4-7):** Interferes with normal activities or awakens from sleep, tender to touch.
- **Severe (8-10):** Excruciating pain, doubled over, unable to do any normal activities.

TRIAGE ASSESSMENT QUESTIONS

Call EMS 911 Now
- Passed out (i.e., fainted, collapsed and was not responding)
  R/O: shock
  First Aid: Lie down with the feet elevated.
- Shock suspected (e.g., cold/pale/clammy skin, too weak to stand)
  R/O: shock
  First Aid: Lie down with the feet elevated.
- Sounds like a life-threatening emergency to the triager

See More Appropriate Protocol
- Chest pain
  Go to Protocol: Chest Pain on page 73 first; then use appropriate Abdominal Pain protocol
- Pain is mainly in upper abdomen (if needed, ask: "Is it mainly above the belly button?")
  Go to Protocol: Abdominal Pain (Upper) on page 9

Go to ED Now
- SEVERE abdominal pain (e.g., excruciating)
  R/O: acute abdomen
- Vomiting red blood or black (coffee-ground) material
  R/O: gastritis, peptic ulcer disease, Mallory-Weiss tear
- Bloody, black, or tarry bowel movements
  R/O: GI bleed
  (Exception: chronic-unchanged black-gray bowel movements and is taking iron pills or Pepto-Bismol)

Go to ED/UCC Now
(or to Office With PCP Approval)
- Constant abdominal pain lasting > 2 hours
  R/O: acute abdomen
- Vomiting bile (green color)
  R/O: intestinal obstruction
- Patient sounds very sick or weak to the triager
  Reason: severe acute illness or serious complication suspected

Go to Office Now
- Vomiting and abdomen looks much more swollen than usual
- White of the eyes have turned yellow (i.e., jaundice)
  R/O: cholelithiasis, hepatitis
- Blood in urine (red, pink, or tea-colored)
  R/O: kidney stone
- Fever > 103° F (39.4° C)
- Fever > 100.5° F (38.1° C) and > 60 years of age
- Fever > 100.0° F (37.8° C) and has diabetes mellitus or a weak immune system (e.g., HIV positive, cancer chemotherapy, organ transplant, splenectomy, chronic steroids)
- Fever > 100.0° F (37.8° C) and bedridden (e.g., nursing home patient, stroke, chronic illness, recovering from surgery)
  Reason: higher risk of bacterial infection
  Note: May need ambulance transport to ED.
- Pregnant or could be pregnant (i.e., missed last menstrual period)
  R/O: spontaneous abortion or ectopic pregnancy

See Today in Office
- MODERATE or MILD pain that comes and goes (cramps) lasts > 24 hours
- Unusual vaginal discharge
  R/O: vaginitis, PID
- Age > 60 years
  Reason: higher risk of serious cause of abdominal pain
- Patient wants to be seen

See Within 2 Weeks in Office
- Abdominal pain is a chronic symptom (recurrent or ongoing AND lasting > 4 weeks)
- Pain with sexual intercourse (dyspareunia)

Home Care
- Mild abdominal pain

HOME CARE ADVICE

❶ **Reassurance:**
- A mild stomachache can be caused by indigestion, gas pains, or overeating. Sometimes a stomachache signals the onset of a vomiting illness due to a viral gastroenteritis ("stomach flu").
- *Here is some care advice that should help.*

❷ **Rest:** Lie down and rest until you feel better.

❸ **Fluids:** Sip clear fluids only (e.g., water, flat soft drinks, half-strength fruit juice) until the pain has been gone for > 2 hours. Then slowly return to a regular diet.

❹ **Diet:**
- Slowly advance diet from clear liquids to a bland diet.
- Avoid alcohol or caffeinated beverages.
- Avoid greasy or fatty foods.

❺ **Pass a BM:** Sit on the toilet and try to pass a bowel movement (BM). Do not strain. This may relieve the pain if it is due to constipation or impending diarrhea.

❻ **Avoid NSAIDs and Aspirin:** Avoid any drug that can irritate the stomach lining and make the pain worse (especially aspirin and NSAIDs like ibuprofen).

❼ **Expected Course:** With harmless causes, the pain is usually better or goes away within 2 hours. With viral gastroenteritis ("stomach flu"), belly cramps may precede each bout of vomiting or diarrhea and may last 2-3 days. With serious causes (e.g., appendicitis) the pain becomes constant and more severe.

❽ **Pregnancy Test, When in Doubt:**
- If there is a chance that you might be pregnant, use a urine pregnancy test.
- You can buy a pregnancy test at the drugstore.
- It works best if you test your first urine in the morning.
- *Follow the instructions included in the package.*
- Call back if you are pregnant.

❾ **Call Back If:**
- Abdominal pain is constant and present for > 2 hours.
- Abdominal pains come and go and are present for > 24 hours.
- You are pregnant.
- You become worse.

FIRST AID

First Aid Advice for Shock:
Lie down with the feet elevated.

BACKGROUND

Key Points
- Abdominal pain is a very common symptom. Sometimes it may be a symptom of a benign gastrointestinal disorder like gas, overeating, or gastroenteritis. At times, abdominal pain is a symptom of a moderately serious problem like appendicitis or biliary colic (gallstones). Abdominal pain may also be the warning symptom of life-threatening conditions like perforated peptic ulcer disease, mesenteric ischemia, and ruptured abdominal aortic aneurysm.
- There are multiple causes of abdominal pain in women. In women, the range of diagnoses needs to be broadened to include problems related to pregnancy and the female genitourinary organs.
- Pain in the elderly carries with it a higher risk of serious illness. In one study of elderly patients presenting to an ED with abdominal pain, 40% had surgical illness.

Top Causes of Abdominal Pain in Women < 50 Years of Age
- Nonspecific abdominal pain
- Appendicitis
- Peptic ulcer disease
- Gallbladder disease
- Ectopic pregnancy
- Spontaneous abortion
- Pelvic inflammatory disease (PID)
- Ovarian cysts
- Endometriosis

Top Causes of Abdominal Pain in Women > 50 Years of Age
- Appendicitis
- Bowel obstruction
- Diverticulitis
- Gallbladder disease
- Pancreatitis
- Peptic ulcer disease

Location of Pain and Possible Etiologies
- **RUQ:** Liver and gallbladder
- **Epigastric:** Heart, stomach, duodenum, esophagus
- **LUQ:** Spleen, stomach
- **Periumbilical:** Pancreas, early appendicitis, small bowel
- **RLQ:** Ileum, appendix, ovary, kidney
- **Suprapubic:** Uterus, bladder, rectum
- **LLQ:** Sigmoid colon, ovary, kidney

ABDOMINAL PAIN (MALE)

Definition
- Pain or discomfort located between the bottom of the rib cage and the groin crease
- Male

Pain Severity Scale
- **Mild (1-3):** Doesn't interfere with normal activities, abdomen soft and not tender to touch.
- **Moderate (4-7):** Interferes with normal activities or awakens from sleep, tender to touch.
- **Severe (8-10):** Excruciating pain, doubled over, unable to do any normal activities.

TRIAGE ASSESSMENT QUESTIONS

Call EMS 911 Now
- Passed out (i.e., fainted, collapsed and was not responding)
  R/O: shock
  First Aid: Lie down with the feet elevated.
- Shock suspected (e.g., cold/pale/clammy skin, too weak to stand)
  R/O: shock
  First Aid: Lie down with the feet elevated.
- Sounds like a life-threatening emergency to the triager

See More Appropriate Protocol
- Chest pain
  Go to Protocol: Chest Pain first on page 73; then use appropriate Abdominal Pain protocol.
- Pain is mainly in upper abdomen (if needed, ask: "Is it mainly above the belly button?")
  Go to Protocol: Abdominal Pain (Upper) on page 9

Go to ED Now
- SEVERE abdominal pain (e.g., excruciating)
  R/O: acute abdomen
- Vomiting red blood or black (coffee-ground) material
  R/O: gastritis, peptic ulcer disease
- Bloody, black, or tarry bowel movements
  R/O: GI bleed
  (Exception: chronic-unchanged black-gray bowel movements and is taking iron pills or Pepto-Bismol)

- Unable to urinate (or only a few drops) and bladder feels very full
  R/O: urinary retention
- Pain in scrotum persists > 1 hour
  R/O: kidney stone

Go to ED/UCC Now
(or to Office With PCP Approval)
- Constant abdominal pain lasting > 2 hours
  R/O: acute abdomen
- Vomiting bile (green color)
  R/O: intestinal obstruction
- Patient sounds very sick or weak to the triager
  Reason: severe acute illness or serious complication suspected

Go to Office Now
- Vomiting and abdomen looks much more swollen than usual
- White of the eyes have turned yellow (i.e., jaundice)
  R/O: cholelithiasis, hepatitis
- Blood in urine (red, pink, or tea-colored)
  R/O: kidney stone
- Fever > 103° F (39.4° C)
- Fever > 100.5° F (38.1° C) and > 60 years of age
- Fever > 100.0° F (37.8° C) and has diabetes mellitus or a weak immune system (e.g., HIV positive, cancer chemotherapy, organ transplant, splenectomy, chronic steroids)
- Fever > 100.0° F (37.8° C) and bedridden (e.g., nursing home patient, stroke, chronic illness, recovering from surgery)
  Reason: higher risk of bacterial infection
  Note: May need ambulance transport to ED.

See Today in Office
- MILD pain that comes and goes (cramps) lasts > 24 hours
- Age > 60 years
  Reason: higher risk of serious cause of abdominal pain
- Patient wants to be seen

See Within 2 Weeks in Office
- Abdominal pain is a chronic symptom (recurrent or ongoing AND lasting > 4 weeks)

Home Care
○ Mild abdominal pain

HOME CARE ADVICE

❶ Reassurance:
- A mild stomachache can be caused by indigestion, gas pains, or overeating. Sometimes a stomachache signals the onset of a vomiting illness due to a viral gastroenteritis ("stomach flu").
- *Here is some care advice that should help.*

❷ Rest: Lie down and rest until you feel better.

❸ Fluids: Sip clear fluids only (e.g., water, flat soft drinks, half-strength fruit juice) until the pain has been gone for > 2 hours. Then slowly return to a regular diet.

❹ Diet:
- Slowly advance diet from clear liquids to a bland diet.
- Avoid alcohol or caffeinated beverages.
- Avoid greasy or fatty foods.

❺ Pass a BM: Sit on the toilet and try to pass a bowel movement (BM). Do not strain. This may relieve pain if it is due to constipation or impending diarrhea.

❻ Avoid NSAIDs and Aspirin: Avoid any drug that can irritate the stomach lining and make the pain worse (especially aspirin and NSAIDs like ibuprofen).

❼ Expected Course: With harmless causes, the pain is usually better or goes away within 2 hours. With viral gastroenteritis ("stomach flu"), belly cramps may precede each bout of vomiting or diarrhea and may last 2-3 days. With serious causes (e.g., appendicitis) the pain becomes constant and more severe.

❽ Call Back If:
- Abdominal pain is constant and present for > 2 hours.
- Abdominal pains come and go and are present for > 24 hours.
- You become worse.

FIRST AID

First Aid Advice for Shock:
Lie down with the feet elevated.

BACKGROUND

Key Points
- Abdominal pain is a very common symptom. Sometimes it may be a symptom of a benign gastrointestinal disorder like gas, overeating, or gastroenteritis. At times, abdominal pain is a symptom of a moderately serious problem like appendicitis or biliary colic (gallstones). Abdominal pain may also be the warning symptom of life-threatening conditions like perforated peptic ulcer disease, mesenteric ischemia, and ruptured abdominal aortic aneurysm.
- Pain in the elderly carries with it a higher risk of serious illness. In one study of elderly patients presenting to an ED with abdominal pain, 40% had surgical illness.

Top Causes of Abdominal Pain in Men < 50 Years of Age
- Appendicitis
- Gallbladder disease
- Nonspecific abdominal pain
- Peptic ulcer disease

Top Causes of Abdominal Pain in Men > 50 Years of Age
- Appendicitis
- Bowel obstruction
- Diverticulitis
- Gallbladder disease
- Pancreatitis
- Peptic ulcer disease

Location of Pain and Possible Etiologies
- **RUQ:** Liver and gallbladder
- **Epigastric:** Heart, stomach, duodenum, esophagus, gallbladder, pancreas
- **LUQ:** Spleen, stomach
- **Periumbilical:** Pancreas, early appendicitis, small bowel
- **RLQ:** Ileum, appendix, kidney
- **Suprapubic:** Bladder, rectum, colon
- **LLQ:** Sigmoid colon, kidney

ABDOMINAL PAIN (MENSTRUAL CRAMPS)

Definition
- Pain in lower abdomen, commencing at onset of a menstrual period
- Crampy or constant pain, may radiate into back or upper thighs
- Has experienced similar menstrual cramps in the past

Pain Severity Scale
- **Mild (1-3):** Doesn't interfere with normal activities, lasting 1-2 days.
- **Moderate (4-7):** Interferes with normal activities (missing work or school), lasting 2-3 days, some associated GI symptoms.
- **Severe (8-10):** Excruciating pain, lasting 2-7 days, associated GI symptoms, pain radiating into thighs and back.

TRIAGE ASSESSMENT QUESTIONS

Call EMS 911 Now
- ● Sounds like a life-threatening emergency to the triager

See More Appropriate Protocol
- ● Abdominal cramps unrelated to menstrual period
  Go to Protocol: Abdominal Pain (Female) on page 1

Go to ED Now
- ● SEVERE pain and pain clearly increases with coughing
  Reason: possible peritonitis

Go to ED/UCC Now
(or to Office With PCP Approval)
- ● Patient sounds very sick or weak to the triager
  Reason: severe acute illness or serious complication suspected

Go to Office Now
- ● SEVERE vaginal bleeding (i.e., 2 pads/hour x 2 hours OR 1 pad/hour x 6 hours) and worse than ever before
  Reason: significant vaginal bleeding

- ● Fever > 100.5° F (38.1° C)
  R/O: PID
- ● Could be pregnant (e.g., missed last menstrual period)
  R/O: spontaneous abortion, ectopic pregnancy

Call Transferred to PCP Now
- ● SEVERE pain (e.g., excruciating cramps) and worse than ever before and not improved with ibuprofen or naproxen

See Today in Office
- ● Pain present > 3 days and normally menstrual cramps last 1-3 days
  R/O: PID
- ● Pain only on one side
  R/O: PID or corpus luteum cyst
- ● Unusual vaginal discharge before period began
  R/O: vaginitis, PID
- ● Patient wants to be seen

See Within 2 Weeks in Office
- ● MODERATE pain (e.g., cramps interfere with normal activities) and not relieved by ibuprofen or naproxen used per Home Care Advice
  Reason: inadequate treatment
- ● Pain present > 3 days and occurs with every menstrual period
  R/O: endometriosis
- ● Pain during sexual intercourse
  R/O: endometriosis
- ● Symptoms began at age > 21
  Reason: may be secondary dysmenorrhea, patient needs physician evaluation
- ● Vomiting or diarrhea is also present
  R/O: inadequate treatment of dysmenorrhea

Home Care
- ○ Normal menstrual cramps

HOME CARE ADVICE

❶ Reassurance:
- Cramps occur in 50% of women during their menstrual period. Treatment with ibuprofen or naproxen usually helps reduce the pain.
- *Here is some care advice that should help.*

❷ General Health:
- Try to exercise regularly. This improves blood flow and may help reduce cramps. However, avoid strenuous exercise during your period.
- Get enough sleep, at least 7-8 hours per night.

❸ Heat:
- Apply a heating pad or warm washcloth to the lower abdomen for 20 minutes twice a day. This may help reduce pain.
- Another option is to try sitting in a tub filled with warm water.
- Never sleep on a heating pad.

❹ Ibuprofen for Pain:
- Ibuprofen is a very effective drug for menstrual cramps.
- **Dosage:** Take 2 or 3 ibuprofen 200 mg tablets 3 or 4 times a day.
- **Available OTC:** Advil, Medipren, Motrin, and Nuprin are some of the over-the-counter brand names.
- **Women With Regular Periods:** Some women report a benefit from starting the ibuprofen the day before their periods start. If your periods are regular, you might consider trying this.

Extra Notes:
- CAUTION: Do not take ibuprofen if you have stomach problems, have kidney disease, are pregnant, or have been told by your doctor to avoid this type of anti-inflammatory drug. Do not take ibuprofen for > 7 days without consulting your doctor.
- Use the lowest amount of medicine that makes your pain feel better.
- *Before taking any medicine, read all the instructions on the package.*

❺ Naproxen for Pain:
- If the patient has tried ibuprofen without adequate pain relief, recommend switching to naproxen (Aleve, Anaprox).
- **Dosage:** Take 220 mg (1 tablet) every 8 hours for 2 or 3 days. Take with food. The first dosage should be 2 tablets (440 mg).
- **Available OTC in the U.S.:** Anaprox, Aleve
- **Women With Regular Periods:** Some women report a benefit from starting the naproxen the day before periods start. If your periods are regular, you might consider trying this.

Extra Notes:
- CAUTION: Do not take naproxen if you have stomach problems, have kidney disease, are pregnant, or have been told by your doctor to avoid this type of anti-inflammatory drug. Do not take naproxen for > 7 days without consulting your doctor.
- Use the lowest amount of medicine that makes your pain feel better.
- Before taking any medicine, read all the instructions on the package.

❻ Pregnancy Test, When in Doubt:
- If there is a chance that you might be pregnant, use a urine pregnancy test.
- You can buy a pregnancy test at the drugstore.
- It works best if you test your first urine in the morning.
- *Follow the instructions included in the package.*
- Call back if you are pregnant.

❼ Call Back If:
- Severe pain and not adequately relieved by ibuprofen or naproxen.
- Your cramps cause you to miss work, school, or other important activities.
- Your cramps last > 3 days.
- You become worse.

BACKGROUND

Key Points

- Painful menstruation is a very common problem. Approximately 50% of women experience it. The medical term for it is *dysmenorrhea*.
- There are 2 types of dysmenorrhea: primary and secondary.

Primary Dysmenorrhea

- **Definition:** Painful menstrual cramps and no demonstrable pelvic pathology.
- **Onset:** Begins within a year or two of the onset of first menses (menarche); usually disappears after 5-10 years or after the first pregnancy.
- **Epidemiology:** The prevalence of primary dysmenorrhea is highest in the 20- to 24-year-old age group (approximately 50% of women) and becomes less common with increasing age.
- **Symptoms:** Crampy or sustained lower abdominal pain ("menstrual cramps") beginning just before or after onset of menstrual flow. The pain is usually most unpleasant during the first 2 days of the menstrual period. Pain usually subsides by day 3 of the menstrual period.
- **Associated Symptoms:** Nausea, vomiting, diarrhea, abdominal bloating.
- **Treatment—NSAIDs:** NSAIDs like ibuprofen (Motrin, Advil) or naproxen (Aleve) are quite effective in reducing the pain of dysmenorrhea. NSAIDs are superior to acetaminophen (Tylenol) in the treatment of dysmenorrhea.
- **Treatment—Birth Control Pills:** Birth control pills and other hormonal contraceptives (e.g., patch, vaginal ring, Depo-Provera, hormonal intrauterine device [IUD]) may be effective in treating the pain of dysmenorrhea. Of course, they cannot be used in a woman who is trying to get pregnant.

Secondary Dysmenorrhea

- **Definition:** Painful menses as the result of pelvic pathology.
- **Causes:** Uterine fibroids, adenomyosis, endometriosis, pelvic inflammatory disease (PID), or an IUD.
- **Onset:** Painful menstruation that appears for the first time in females > 21 years of age.
- **Symptoms:** Crampy or constant lower abdominal pain during menstrual period. Pain usually lasts 5-7 days, each menstrual period. Some report worsening symptoms over time.
- **Associated Symptoms:** Dyspareunia (painful intercourse).
- **Treatment:** NSAIDs like ibuprofen (Motrin, Advil) or naproxen (Aleve) are effective in reducing the pain of dysmenorrhea. Identifying and treating the underlying pathology is key.

ABDOMINAL PAIN (UPPER)

Definition
- Pain is primarily centered in the upper abdomen (if needed, ask: "Is it just below the rib cage and above the belly button?").
- Pain may radiate into chest, back, or other location.

Pain Severity Scale
- **Mild (1-3):** Doesn't interfere with normal activities, abdomen soft and not tender to touch.
- **Moderate (4-7):** Interferes with normal activities or awakens from sleep, tender to touch.
- **Severe (8-10):** Excruciating pain, doubled over, unable to do any normal activities.

TRIAGE ASSESSMENT QUESTIONS

Call EMS 911 Now
- Passed out (i.e., fainted, collapsed and was not responding)
  R/O: shock
  First Aid: Lie down with the feet elevated.
- Shock suspected (e.g., cold/pale/clammy skin, too weak to stand)
  R/O: shock
  First Aid: Lie down with the feet elevated.
- Visible sweat on face or sweat is dripping down

See More Appropriate Protocol
- Chest pain
  Go to Protocol: Chest Pain on page 73

Go to ED Now
- SEVERE abdominal pain (e.g., excruciating)
  R/O: acute abdomen
- Pain lasting > 10 minutes and > 50 years old
  Reason: higher risk of cardiac ischemia or surgical cause of abdominal pain
- Pain lasting > 10 minutes and > 40 years old and associated chest, arm, neck, upper back, or jaw pain
  Reason: higher risk of cardiac ischemia as cause of pain
- Pain lasting > 10 minutes and > 35 years old and at least one cardiac risk factor (Risks include: hypertension, diabetes, high cholesterol, obesity, family history of heart disease, smoking)

- Pain lasting > 10 minutes and history of heart disease (i.e., heart attack, bypass surgery, angina, angioplasty, CHF)
  Reason: higher risk of cardiac ischemia as cause of pain
- Recent injury to the abdomen
- Vomiting red blood or black (coffee-ground) material
  R/O: gastritis, peptic ulcer disease
- Bloody, black, or tarry bowel movements
  R/O: GI bleed
  (Exception: chronic-unchanged black-gray bowel movements and is taking iron pills or Pepto-Bismol)

Go to L&D Now
- Pregnant > 24 weeks and hand or face swelling
  R/O: preeclampsia

Go to ED/UCC Now (or to Office With PCP Approval)
- Constant abdominal pain lasting > 2 hours
  R/O: acute abdomen
- Vomiting bile (green color)
  R/O: intestinal obstruction
- Patient sounds very sick or weak to the triager
  Reason: severe acute illness or serious complication suspected

Go to Office Now
- Vomiting and abdomen looks much more swollen than usual
- White of the eyes have turned yellow (i.e., jaundice)
  R/O: cholelithiasis, hepatitis
- Fever > 103° F (39.4° C)
- Fever > 100.5° F (38.1° C) and > 60 years of age
- Fever > 100.0° F (37.8° C) and has diabetes mellitus or a weak immune system (e.g., HIV positive, cancer chemotherapy, organ transplant, splenectomy, chronic steroids)
- Fever > 100.0° F (37.8° C) and bedridden (e.g., nursing home patient, stroke, chronic illness, recovering from surgery)
  Reason: higher risk of bacterial infection
  Note: May need ambulance transport to ED.

See Today in Office
- Age > 60 years
  Reason: risk of serious cause
- Patient wants to be seen

See Today or Tomorrow in Office
- MILD pain that comes and goes (cramps) lasts > 24 hours
- Alcohol abuse known or suspected

See Within 2 Weeks in Office
- Abdominal pain is a chronic symptom (recurrent or ongoing AND lasting > 4 weeks)
- Intermittent burning pains radiating into chest or sour taste in mouth
  R/O: possible reflux esophagitis

Home Care
- ◯ Mild abdominal pain

HOME CARE ADVICE

❶ **Reassurance:**
  - A mild stomachache can be from indigestion, stomach irritation, or overeating. Sometimes a stomachache signals the onset of a vomiting illness from a viral infection.
  - *Here is some care advice that should help.*

❷ **Fluids:** Sip clear fluids only (e.g., water, flat soft drinks, half-strength fruit juice) until the pain is gone for 2 hours. Then slowly return to a regular diet.

❸ **Diet:**
  - Slowly advance diet from clear liquids to a bland diet.
  - Avoid alcohol or caffeinated beverages.
  - Avoid greasy or fatty foods.

❹ **Antacid:** If having pain now, try taking an antacid (e.g., Mylanta, Maalox). Dose: 2 tablespoons (30 mL) of liquid by mouth.

❺ **Avoid NSAIDs and Aspirin:** Avoid any drug that can irritate the stomach lining and make the pain worse (especially aspirin and NSAIDs like ibuprofen).

❻ **Stop Smoking:** Smoking can aggravate heartburn and stomach problems.

❼ **Reducing Reflux Symptoms (GERD):** Eat smaller meals and avoid snacks for 2 hours before sleeping. Avoid the following foods, which tend to aggravate heartburn and stomach problems: fatty/greasy foods, spicy foods, caffeinated beverages, mints, and chocolate.

❽ **Expected Course:** With harmless causes, the pain usually lessens or is resolved in 2 hours. With gastroenteritis, stomach cramps may precede each bout of vomiting or diarrhea. With serious causes (e.g., appendicitis), the pain becomes constant and severe.

❾ **Call Back If:**
  - Abdominal pain is constant and present for > 2 hours.
  - You become worse.

FIRST AID

First Aid Advice for Shock:
Lie down with the feet elevated.

BACKGROUND

Key Points
- There are multiple causes of upper abdominal pain.
- Gastritis and peptic ulcer disease are common and typically cause pain in the epigastrium, sometimes accompanied by vomiting.
- Gastroesophageal reflux disease (GERD) causes a burning pain that radiates into chest. Patients with GERD frequently state that their symptoms are aggravated by laying down and that they frequently get a sour or bitter taste in their mouth.
- Pain in the elderly carries with it a higher risk of serious illness. In one study of elderly patients presenting to an ED with abdominal pain, 40% had surgical illness. In patients > 50, gallbladder disease is the number one cause of upper abdominal pain.
- The possibility of a heart attack needs to be considered in anybody > 40 years of age or anybody who has cardiac risk factors. Cardiac risk factors include: diabetes, hypertension, hyperlipidemia, smoking, and a family history of heart attack at an age < 60.

Top Causes in Patients < 50 Years of Age

- Gastritis and peptic ulcer disease
- GERD
- Gallbladder disease
- Nonspecific abdominal pain, irritable bowel syndrome

Top Causes in Patients > 50 Years of Age

- Gallbladder disease (cholecystitis, cholelithiasis)
- Peptic ulcer disease and gastritis
- Bowel obstruction

Other Causes

- Cardiac disease: angina, MI, pericarditis
- Pancreatitis
- Pneumonia
- Hepatitis
- Abdominal aortic aneurysm
- Renal colic
- Herpes zoster

Caution: Cardiac Ischemia

- The most life-threatening cause of acute upper abdominal pain is cardiac ischemia.
- Rarely patients may present with upper abdominal pain as the sole symptom of a myocardial infarction. Usually there will be other associated symptoms of cardiac ischemia: chest pain, shortness of breath, nausea, and/or diaphoresis.
- Cardiac ischemia should be suspected in any patients with risk factors for cardiac disease. These include: hypertension, smoking, diabetes, hyperlipidemia, a strong family history of heart disease, and age > 50.
- Consider cardiac ischemia in patients who complain of indigestion.

ALCOHOL ABUSE AND DEPENDENCE

Definition
- Known or suspected alcohol abuse
- Questions or concerns related to alcohol intoxication, withdrawal, dependence, or abuse

TRIAGE ASSESSMENT QUESTIONS

Call EMS 911 Now
- Coma (e.g., not moving, not talking, not responding to stimuli)
  R/O: severe alcohol intoxication, overdose, occult head trauma, hepatic encephalopathy, hypoglycemia
- Difficult to awaken or acting confused (e.g., disoriented, slurred speech)
  R/O: Delirium tremens (DTs), severe alcohol intoxication, overdose, occult head trauma, hepatic encephalopathy, hypoglycemia
- Seeing, hearing, or feeling things that are not there (i.e., visual, auditory, or tactile hallucinations)
  R/O: alcohol withdrawal, alcoholic hallucinosis
- Slow, shallow, and weak breathing
  R/O: impending respiratory arrest
- Seizure
  R/O: alcohol withdrawal seizure
- Violent behavior or threatening to kill someone
  R/O: alcohol intoxication, DTs, homicidal ideation
- Patient attempted suicide
  R/O: physical injury or overdosage
- Threatening suicide
  Reason: suicidal ideation
- Sounds like a life-threatening emergency to the triager

See More Appropriate Protocol
- Substance abuse or dependence, question or problem related to
  Go to Protocol: Substance Abuse and Dependence on page 382
- Depression is main problem or symptom (e.g., feelings of sadness or hopelessness)
  Go to Protocol: Depression on page 103

Go to ED Now
- SEVERE abdominal pain (e.g., excruciating)
  R/O: pancreatitis or other acute abdomen
- Constant abdominal pain lasting > 2 hours
  R/O: pancreatitis or other acute abdomen
- Bloody, black, or tarry bowel movements
  R/O: gastritis, peptic ulcer disease, esophageal varices, lower GI bleed
  (Exception: chronic-unchanged black-gray bowel movements and is taking iron pills or Pepto-Bismol)
- Vomiting red blood or black (coffee-ground) material
  (Exception: few red streaks in vomit that only happened once)
  R/O: gastritis, esophageal varices, Mallory-Weiss tear
- Multiple episodes of vomiting and lasting > 2 hours
  R/O: alcoholic ketoacidosis
- Feeling very shaky (i.e., visible tremors of hands)
  R/O: alcohol dependence, alcohol withdrawal

Go to ED/UCC Now (or to Office With PCP Approval)
- Patient sounds very sick or weak to the triager
  Reason: severe acute illness or serious complication suspected

See Today in Office
- White of the eyes have turned yellow (i.e., jaundice)
  R/O: alcoholic hepatitis, cirrhosis of the liver
- Fever > 101° F (38.3° C)
  R/O: bacterial illness

See Today or Tomorrow in Office
- Drinks alcohol daily and prior alcohol withdrawal seizures
  Reason: higher risk of alcohol withdrawal; counseling needed
  R/O: alcohol dependence
- Drinks alcohol daily and prior DTs
  Reason: higher risk of alcohol withdrawal; counseling needed
  R/O: alcohol dependence
- Patient wants to be seen

Callback by PCP Today

- Pregnant and intoxicated or admits to drinking problem
  Reason: risk to fetus (fetal alcohol syndrome)

Call Local Agency Today

- Alcohol or drug abuse, known or suspected
  Note: The CAGE questionnaire is a simple screening tool for alcohol abuse and dependence (see Background).
- Requesting admission for alcohol abuse
- Requesting to talk with a counselor (mental health worker, psychiatrist, etc.)
- Alcohol use interferes with work or school
- Male and ≥ 14 drinks/week, or > 4 drinks on single occasion
  Reason: at-risk drinking, further evaluation and counseling needed
- Female or elderly and ≥ 7 drinks/week, or > 3 drinks on single occasion
  Reason: at-risk drinking, further evaluation and counseling needed

Home Care

- ○ Alcohol use, abuse, and dependence, questions about
- ○ Blood alcohol level, question about
- ○ Sobering up from alcohol intoxication, questions about
  Reason: caller wants to know "how to help a friend/family member sober up"
- ○ Pregnancy and alcohol, questions about

HOME CARE ADVICE

General Information

❶ Reassurance:
- People with a drinking problem should cut back or quit drinking alcohol. They may need help to do this. Support groups and treatment programs can help a person to recover.
- *Here is some care advice that should help.*

❷ Do NOT Drink and Drive:
- Do not drive a car after you drink alcohol.
- If you and your friends are drinking, pick a designated driver. This is a driver who will not be drinking.

❸ Do NOT Drink Alcohol if You Are Pregnant:
- Drinking alcohol while you are pregnant can harm the baby. It may cause birth defects. It may cause fetal alcohol syndrome.
- Drinking small amounts (1 drink) every once in a while may be OK. Research has not yet shown if this will harm the baby.
- The **safest** thing is **not to drink** any alcohol while you are pregnant.

❹ What Is the Effect of Drinking Alcohol on the Blood Alcohol Level?
- For an average-sized person, each of the following will raise the blood alcohol level approximately 25 mg/dL: 1 oz (one shot; 30 mL) of alcohol, 4 oz (half cup; 120 mL) of wine, or 12 oz (one can; 360 mL) of beer.
- An average adult will break down (metabolize) alcohol at a rate of 15-25 mg/dL per hour.
- **Example:** Drinking 3-4 beers will raise your alcohol level from 0 to 100 mg/dL and it will take 4-7 hours before your alcohol level is back to 0 (zero).

❺ At What Blood Alcohol Level Are You Considered Legally Drunk?
- The normal blood alcohol level is 0 (zero).
- There are various different terminologies for reporting a blood alcohol level. Each of the following has the same meaning: 80 milligrams/dL, 80 grams per cent, 80 mg/100 mL, or 0.08.
- Drinking 3-4 drinks is sufficient to make an average-sized person legally drunk.
- **In the U.S. the legal definition of alcohol intoxication varies from state to state: 80 mg/dL–100 mg/dL.**
- **In Canada it is a criminal offense to drive a car while having a blood alcohol level > 80 mg/dL (0.08).** Some Canadian provinces have sanctions (suspensions) for levels > 50 mg/dL (0.05).

❻ **What Does Your Blood Alcohol Level Do to Your Behavior?**
- **50 mg/dL:** You may feel flushed. Your skin may be red and feel warm. You may get emotional and talk a lot. You may lack normal judgment.
- **100 mg/dL:** You may have slowed reactions and thinking. You may be less coordinated. You may laugh and slur your speech.
- **200 mg/dL:** You may have trouble walking or feel shaky. You may feel sleepy. You may have trouble sitting up straight. Your speech may be very slurred.
- **300 mg/dL:** You may be unable to wake up unless slapped or pinched. You may snore loudly.
- **400 mg/dL:** This can lead to coma. You may be unable to control your urine.
- **500 mg/dL:** You could die.
- Alcoholics build up tolerance. The above effects at any alcohol level may be less.

❼ **Call Back If:**
- You have more questions about alcohol or alcohol abuse.
- You become worse.

Caring for the Adult Who Is Intoxicated (Drunk)
❶ **Reassurance:**
- The body will break down the alcohol in your body. Alcohol intoxication does go away.
- However, no medicines speed up the sobering process (e.g., drinking coffee does not help). Taking a cold shower may temporarily make someone more alert, but it will not speed up the sobering process.
- *Here is some care advice that should help.*

❷ **Treatment for Alcohol Intoxication (Drunkenness):**
- Do not allow the patient to drive.
- Watch and protect the person from harm (e.g., dangerous activities, high places).
- Keep alcohol away from the person (e.g., take patient away from bar/party, remove any nearby alcohol).
- If the person wants to sleep, lay the patient on his or her side. This is important in case of vomiting.

❸ **Expected Course:**
- An average adult will break down (metabolize) alcohol at a rate of 15-25 mg/dL per hour.
- The more alcohol a person drank, the longer it takes to become sober.
- For example, drinking 3-4 beers can raise the blood alcohol level from 0 to 100 mg/dL. It then will take 4-7 hours before the alcohol level is back to 0 (zero).

❹ **Call 911 If:**
- Violent behavior.
- Difficulty breathing occurs.
- You cannot wake the drunk person.

Caring for the Adult With a Hangover
❶ **Reassurance:**
- If a person drinks too much alcohol, he or she can have a hangover the next day. Even small amounts of alcohol can sometimes do this.
- Symptoms of a hangover include feeling extremely thirsty/dehydrated, feeling more tired than usual, and headache.
- The symptoms do get better over 12 to 24 hours.
- *Here is some care advice that should help.*

❷ **Treatment for a Hangover:**
- Drink more liquids than normal. Some of the symptoms of a hangover are due to mild dehydration.
- Take acetaminophen (Tylenol) for headache pain.
- Make certain that you have had plenty of sleep.
- Do not drink alcohol for the next 2 days.

❸ **Pain Medicines:**
- For pain relief, you can take either acetaminophen, ibuprofen, or naproxen.
- They are over-the-counter (OTC) pain drugs. You can buy them at the drugstore.

Acetaminophen (e.g., Tylenol):
- **Regular Strength Tylenol:** Take 650 mg (two 325 mg pills) by mouth every 4-6 hours as needed. Each Regular Strength Tylenol pill has 325 mg of acetaminophen.
- **Extra Strength Tylenol:** Take 1,000 mg (two 500 mg pills) every 8 hours as needed. Each Extra Strength Tylenol pill has 500 mg of acetaminophen.
- The most you should take each day is 3,000 mg (10 Regular Strength or 6 Extra Strength pills a day).

Ibuprofen (e.g., Motrin, Advil):
- Take 400 mg (two 200 mg pills) by mouth every 6 hours.
- Another choice is to take 600 mg (three 200 mg pills) by mouth every 8 hours.
- The most you should take each day is 1,200 mg (six 200 mg pills), unless your doctor has told you to take more.

Naproxen (e.g., Aleve):
- Take 220 mg (one 220 mg pill) by mouth every 8 hours as needed. You may take 440 mg (two 220 mg pills) for your first dose.
- The most you should take each day is 660 mg (three 220 mg pills a day), unless your doctor has told you to take more.

❹ **Pain Medicines—Extra Notes:**
- Use the lowest amount of medicine that makes your pain better.
- Acetaminophen is thought to be safer than ibuprofen or naproxen in people > 65 years old. Acetaminophen is in many OTC and prescription medicines. It might be in more than one medicine that you are taking. You need to be careful and not take an overdose. An acetaminophen overdose can hurt the liver.
- McNeil, the company that makes Tylenol, has different dosage instructions for Tylenol in Canada and the United States. In Canada, the maximum recommended dose per day is 4,000 mg or 12 Regular Strength (325 mg) pills. In the United States, McNeil recommends a maximum dose of 10 Regular Strength (325 mg) pills.
- CAUTION: Do not take acetaminophen if you have liver disease.
- CAUTION: Do not take ibuprofen or naproxen if you have stomach problems, have kidney disease, are pregnant, or have been told by your doctor to avoid this type of anti-inflammatory drug. Do not take ibuprofen or naproxen for > 7 days without consulting your doctor.
- *Before taking any medicine, read all the instructions on the package.*

❺ **Call Back If:**
- You have more questions about alcohol or alcohol abuse.
- You become worse.

Referral and Additional Resources
- **Local Alcohol Treatment Program:**
  - If available, local alcohol treatment program:

    __ __ __ - __ __ __ - __ __ __ __
  - If available, local psychiatric crisis service at _____hospital:

    __ __ __ - __ __ __ - __ __ __ __
- **Alcoholics Anonymous (AA):**
  - The Alcoholics Anonymous organization is a *"fellowship of men and women who share their experience, strength and hope with each other that they may solve their common problem and help others to recover from alcoholism. The only requirement for membership is a desire to stop drinking."*
  - If available, local phone number:

    __ __ __ - __ __ __ - __ __ __ __.
  - National phone number: 212/870-3400.
  - Web site: www.aa.org.
- **Al-Anon/Alateen:**
  - The goal of Al-Anon is *"to help families and friends of alcoholics recover from the effects of living with the problem drinking of a relative or friend."*
  - If available, local phone number:

    __ __ __ - __ __ __ - __ __ __ __.
  - National phone number: 888/425-2666.
  - Web site: www.al-anon.org
  - Web site: https://al-anon.org/for-members/group-resources/alateen
- **Canada—Hotlines and Helplines:**
  - The Canadian Centre on Substance Use and Addiction provides a list of addiction treatment helplines at: www.ccsa.ca/Eng/Pages/Addictions-Treatment-Helplines-Canada.aspx.
  - Alberta: Addiction Helpline—866/332-2322, 780/427-7164.
  - New Brunswick: Department of Health and Wellness Addiction Services. Offered by region.
  - Newfoundland and Labrador: Newfoundland and Labrador Addictions Services. Services are offered by region. See Web site (www.health.gov.nl.ca/health/addictions/services.html) for listing.
  - Northwest Territories: Nats'ejée K'éh Treatment Centre crisis line—800/661-0846.
  - Ontario: ConnexOntario: Provides access to addiction, mental health, and problem gambling services. Available at: http://www.connexontario.ca. The phone number for the helpline is 866-531-2600.
  - Ontario: Centre for Addiction and Mental Health (CAMH)—800/463-6273.

- **United States—Substance Abuse and Mental Health Services Administration (SAMHSA):**
  - This governmental agency works to improve the quality and availability of substance abuse prevention, alcohol and drug addiction treatment, and mental health services.
  - More information is available at www.samhsa.gov.
- **United States—SAMHSA National Helpline:**
  - The SAMHSA National Helpline (http://samhsa.gov/treatment) is a *"confidential, free, 24-hour-a-day, 365-day-a-year, information service, in English and Spanish, for individuals and family members facing substance abuse and mental health issues. This service provides referrals to local treatment facilities, support groups, and community-based organizations. Callers can also order free publications and other information in print on substance abuse and mental health issues."*
  - The phone number is 800/662-HELP (4357).
- **United States—SAMHSA Substance Abuse Treatment Facility Locator:**
  - SAMHSA has an Internet tool for finding local drug abuse treatment programs.
  - This locator is available at http://findtreatment.samhsa.gov.

BACKGROUND

Key Points
- Approximately 6% of the population in the United States and Canada meets diagnostic criteria for alcohol abuse or dependence.
- Women and the elderly will have a higher blood alcohol level in comparison with men for the same amount of alcohol consumption.

Definitions and Patterns of Alcohol Use
- **A Drink:** 1.5 oz hard liquor (one shot or jigger; 45 mL), 5 oz wine (small glass; 150 mL), 12 oz beer (one can; 360 mL).
- **Moderate Drinking** (social drinking): Men who have ≤ 2 drinks per day. Women/elderly who have ≤ 1 drinks per day.
- **At-Risk Drinking:** Individuals have no apparent medical, social, or legal problems related to alcohol but drink excessively. Men who have > 14 drinks per week or > 4 drinks on occasion. Women/elderly who have > 7 drinks per week or > 3 drinks on occasion. Drinking alcohol during pregnancy.

- **Alcohol Abuse** (problem drinking, harmful drinking): Individuals with alcohol abuse have patterns of alcohol drinking that lead to health, occupational, legal, or social problems. This can range from minor problems like waking up with a hangover to more serious consequences such as motor vehicle accidents and missing work.
- **Alcohol Dependence** (alcoholism): Alcoholism is a disease. Alcoholics are physically addicted to alcohol and demonstrate withdrawal symptoms when they stop drinking. Alcoholics also develop tolerance, which means that they have to drink more alcohol to achieve the same level of intoxication. Alcoholics feel compelled to drink and continue to drink in the face of adverse consequences.

CAGE Questionnaire: These 4 questions are a simple way to screen for alcohol abuse and dependence. One or 2 positive answers suggest at-risk alcohol drinking and the individual should see PCP for further evaluation. Three or 4 positive answers indicate a high likelihood of alcohol abuse and/or dependency.
1. Have you ever felt you should CUT down on your drinking?
2. Have people ever ANNOYED you by criticizing your drinking?
3. Have you ever felt bad or GUILTY about your drinking?
4. Have you ever had a drink first thing in the morning to steady your nerves or to get rid of a hangover (EYE-OPENER)?

Effect of Drinking on Blood Alcohol Level
- For an average-sized person, each of the following will raise the blood alcohol level approximately 25 mg/dL (0.025): 1 oz (one shot; 30 mL) of alcohol, 4 oz (half cup; 120 mL) of wine, or 12 oz (one can; 360 mL) of beer.
- An average adult will break down (metabolize) alcohol at a rate of 15-25 mg/dL (0.015-0.025) per hour.
- **Example:** Drinking 3-4 beers will raise your alcohol level from 0 to 100 mg/dL and it will take 4-7 hours before your alcohol level is back to 0 (zero).

Effect of Alcohol Level on Behavior

- **50 mg/dL (0.05):** Flushed skin, more talkative, loss of emotional restraint, feeling of warmth, mild impairment of judgment.
- **100 mg/dL (0.10):** Reduced reaction time and coordination (e.g., writing, driving), slowed thinking, inappropriate laughter, mildly slurred speech.
- **200 mg/dL (0.20):** Unsteady or staggering gait, sleepy but arousable by voice, difficulty sitting up straight in a chair, very slurred speech.
- **300 mg/dL (0.30):** Stuporous and arousable only by physical means (e.g., slapping face, forceful pinching), loud snoring.
- **400 mg/dL (0.40):** Coma, incontinence of urine.
- **500 mg/dL (0.50):** Death.
- Alcoholics develop tolerance and may show less physical effects at any alcohol level.

Definition of Legally Drunk

- The normal blood alcohol level is 0 (zero).
- **Blood Alcohol Level Terminology, With Same Meaning:** A level of 80 milligrams/dL, 80 mg/100 mL, or 0.08.
- **In the U.S. the legal definition of alcohol intoxication varies from state to state:** 80 mg/dL–100 mg/dL (0.08-0.10).
- **In Canada it is a criminal offense to operate a car while having a blood alcohol level > 80 mg/dL (0.08).** Some Canadian provinces have sanctions (suspensions) for levels > 50 mg/dL (0.05).
- Drinking 3-4 drinks is sufficient to make an average-sized person legally drunk.

Conversion of Alcohol Level to SI Units

- mg/dL ethanol X 0.2171 = mmol/L
- mmol/L ethanol X 4.61 = mg/dL

Caution: Always Consider the Following Associated Conditions in Individuals With Alcohol-Related Problems:

- Depression and other psychiatric illnesses
- **Gastrointestinal Complications:** Pancreatitis, gastritis, gastrointestinal bleeding
- **Liver Disease:** Hepatitis, cirrhosis
- **Infectious Diseases:** Tuberculosis, pneumonia
- **Injury:** From fights, accidents
- Malnutrition and vitamin deficiency
- **Neurologic Complications:** Seizures
- Polydrug abuse
- Suicidal ideation and attempt

ANAPHYLAXIS

Definition
- Anaphylaxis is a serious allergic reaction that is rapid in onset and may cause death.
- Most anaphylactic reactions start within 10-20 minutes (and always within 2 hours) of exposure to a medication, food, sting, or other allergic substance.
- Death may result from either respiratory compromise (bronchospasm and upper airway obstruction) or from cardiovascular collapse (shock).
- *Use this protocol only if the patient has symptoms that match Anaphylaxis.*

Symptoms of Anaphylaxis
- **Oral:** Difficulty swallowing, drooling, swollen tongue
- **Respiratory:** Difficulty breathing, hoarseness, stridor (laryngeal edema), wheezing (bronchospasm)
- **Cardiovascular:** Fainting, profound weakness
- **CNS:** Confusion

Accompanying Symptoms of Anaphylaxis
- Sense of impending doom
- **Oral:** Itching (pruritus) and swelling (edema) of lips and mouth
- **Skin:** Urticaria (hives), swelling of the deeper dermis (angioedema), itching, flushing
- **Gastrointestinal:** Nausea, vomiting, diarrhea, crampy abdominal pain

TRIAGE ASSESSMENT QUESTIONS

Call EMS 911 Now
- ● Life-threatening reaction in the past to similar substance (e.g., food, insect bite/sting, medication, etc.) and < 2 hours since exposure
- ● Wheezing, stridor, hoarseness, or difficulty breathing
- ● Tightness in the chest or throat and begins within 2 hours of exposure to allergic substance
- ● Difficulty swallowing, drooling, or slurred speech
  R/O: swollen tongue
- ● Difficult to awaken or acting confused (e.g., disoriented, slurred speech)
- ● Unresponsive, passed out, or very weak
- ● Other symptom of severe allergic reaction
  (Exception: hives or facial swelling alone)

- ● Sounds like a life-threatening emergency to the triager
  Note: patient may describe a sense of impending doom

See More Appropriate Protocol
- ● Widespread hives and onset > 2 hours after exposure to high-risk allergen (e.g., sting, nuts, first dose of antibiotic)
  Go to Protocol: Hives on page 226

Go to ED Now
- ● Widespread hives, itching, or facial swelling and onset < 2 hours of exposure to high-risk allergen (e.g., sting, nuts, first dose of antibiotic)
  R/O: allergic reaction
  Note: No history of life-threatening reaction and no anaphylactic symptoms.
- ● Vomiting or abdominal cramps and onset < 2 hours of exposure to high-risk allergen (e.g., sting, nuts, first dose of antibiotic)
  R/O: allergic reaction
  Note: No history of life-threatening reaction and no anaphylactic symptoms.
- ● Gave epinephrine shot and no symptoms now
  R/O: biphasic reaction
  Reason: may need oral steroids
- ● Gave asthma inhaler or neb and no symptoms now
  R/O: biphasic reaction
  Reason: may need oral steroids

See Today in Office
- ● Patient wants to be seen

See Within 3 Days in Office
- ● Took antihistamine (e.g., Benadryl) by mouth and no symptoms now
  R/O: mild allergic reaction

HOME CARE ADVICE

Life-threatening Allergic Reaction Suspected—Anaphylaxis (Call 911)

❶ **Note to Triager:**
- Give brief **First Aid Advice** and then they should **call 911.**
  (Reason: lifesaving advice)

❷ **First Aid Advice for Anaphylaxis—Epinephrine:**
- If the patient has an epinephrine autoinjector, **give it now.** Do not delay.
- Use the autoinjector on the upper outer thigh. You may give it through clothing if necessary.
- Give epinephrine first, then call 911.
- Epinephrine is available in autoinjectors under trade names: EpiPen, EpiPen Jr, and Auvi-Q (Allerject in Canada). Auvi-Q has an audio chip and talks patients and caregivers through injection process.
- You may give a second (repeat) dose of epinephrine 10-15 minutes later, IF the person with anaphylaxis does not respond to the first dose AND ambulance arrival takes > 10 minutes.

❸ **First Aid Advice for Anaphylaxis—Benadryl:**
- Give antihistamine by mouth **NOW** if able to swallow.
- Use Benadryl (diphenhydramine; adult dose: 50 mg) or any other available antihistamine medicine.

Moderate-Severe Allergic Reaction (Go to ED)

❶ **Take an Antihistamine (e.g., Benadryl) NOW:**
- If you have it readily available, take a dose of Benadryl (OTC diphenhydramine, 50 mg by mouth).
- If you do not have Benadryl, you can use any antihistamine cold medicine that you might have.

❷ **Call 911 if you become worse.**

Mild Allergic Reaction (Office Visit)

❶ **Observe:** Watch out for any new symptoms during the next 2 hours.

❷ **Avoid Allergens:** If you think your symptoms were triggered by a particular substance (e.g., food, cat, medications, weeds), avoid it until you have seen or talked with your doctor.

❸ **Call Back If:**
- Difficulty breathing occurs.
- Difficulty swallowing occurs.
- Allergic symptoms come back.
- You become worse.

FIRST AID

First Aid Advice for Anaphylaxis—Epinephrine:
- If the patient has an epinephrine autoinjector, **give it now.** Do not delay.
- Use the autoinjector on the upper outer thigh. You may give it through clothing if necessary.
- Give epinephrine first, then call 911.
- Epinephrine is available in autoinjectors under trade names: EpiPen, EpiPen Jr, and Auvi-Q (Allerject in Canada). Auvi-Q has an audio chip and talks patients and caregivers through injection process.
- You may give a second (repeat) dose of epinephrine 10-15 minutes later, IF the person with anaphylaxis does not respond to the first dose AND ambulance arrival takes > 10 minutes.

First Aid Advice for Anaphylaxis—Benadryl:
- Give antihistamine by mouth **NOW** if able to swallow.
- Use Benadryl (diphenhydramine; adult dose: 50 mg) or any other available antihistamine medicine.

First Aid Advice for Anaphylactic Shock
(pending EMS arrival):
Lie down with the feet elevated.

BACKGROUND

Key Points

- Some people are allergic to various substances. People can be allergic to foods like peanuts, antibiotics like penicillin, or insect venom from a bee sting.
- An allergic reaction can range from mild to severe. Mild allergic reaction symptoms include rashes and hives. Symptoms of a more moderate allergic reaction are angioedema (large areas of swelling) and wheezing. *Anaphylaxis is a severe and potentially life-threatening allergic reaction.*
- It is not clear why some people are more prone to allergies than others. It is also not clear why some people are so severely allergic to a substance that it triggers an anaphylactic reaction.

Triggers of an Anaphylactic Reaction

- **Drugs:** Antibiotics (e.g., especially penicillins).
- **Drugs:** Other (e.g., aspirin, NSAIDs).
- Exercise-induced.
- Foods (e.g., peanuts, fish and shellfish, milk, soy, egg, tree nuts).
- Insect bites.
- Latex (e.g., gloves, medical supplies, balloons).
- **Radiocontrast Materials** (e.g., CT scan dye): This is not a true anaphylactic reaction. However, the symptoms and treatment are identical.
- Stings (e.g., bee, yellow jacket, wasp).

Risk Factors for Anaphylaxis

- **Age:** Adults are more likely to develop anaphylactic reactions than children.
- **Asthma:** Individuals who have asthma are more likely to have severe allergic reactions.
- **Prior History:** Once a person has had an anaphylactic reaction to a substance, it is likely that they will have a severe reaction again if exposed to it.

Complications of Anaphylaxis

- Anaphylaxis is a life-threatening event.
- Death may result from either cardiovascular collapse (shock) or from respiratory compromise (bronchospasm and upper airway obstruction).

Treatment of Anaphylaxis

- Epinephrine
- Antihistamines
- Corticosteroids

When to Give an Epinephrine Injection

Epinephrine is the best and first treatment for an anaphylactic reaction.

- **Indications:** (1) Symptoms of an anaphylactic reaction, and (2) prior life-threatening reaction in the past and now has been reexposed to the same allergic substance (e.g., medication, food, bee sting).
- **Availability:** Epinephrine is available in autoinjectors under trade names: EpiPen, EpiPen Jr, and Auvi-Q. Auvi-Q has an audio chip and talks patients and caregivers through injection process. You may give a second (repeat) dose of epinephrine 10-15 minutes later, IF the person with anaphylaxis does not respond to the first dose AND ambulance arrival takes > 10 minutes.
- **Education:** Instructional materials and an educational video are available online for both EpiPen and for Auvi-Q.

Prevention of Anaphylaxis

- Avoid substances to which you are allergic.
- Carry an emergency kit containing injectable epinephrine (EpiPen) and chewable antihistamine.
- Wear a medical necklace/bracelet indicating the allergy.
- For known allergies to certain drugs, antihistamines and corticosteroids may be given in advance to minimize allergic reaction to the drug when the drug is absolutely needed.

Biphasic Anaphylactic Reaction

A biphasic reaction means a patient develops a classic anaphylactic reaction, seems to recover (for 1 to 3 hours), and then experiences a recurrence of anaphylactic symptoms. Although initial symptoms tend to be more severe, occasionally the second phase is more severe or even fatal. Biphasic reactions are the main reason that adults with anaphylactic reactions (even with apparent recovery after receiving epinephrine) are referred to the ED for observation. It's also a reason for initiating treatment with corticosteroids.

Hives Alone: Guideline Management

- The onset of cutaneous symptoms (hives or facial swelling) may be a precursor to anaphylaxis. However, if they don't progress to respiratory symptoms or hypotension, these isolated symptoms usually represent a harmless allergic reaction (not anaphylaxis).
- **Hives Starting > 2 Hours After Exposure:** If the onset of hives is > 2 hours after exposure to the allergen, they definitely don't represent anaphylaxis.
- **Hives Starting < 2 Hours After Exposure:** If onset is < 2 hours after exposure, they may represent the precursor to anaphylaxis. The following are considered higher risk exposures (triggers): high-risk foods (e.g., peanuts, tree nuts, fish, shellfish), prescription medications (e.g., antibiotics; especially if the hives begin after the first dose), *Hymenoptera* stings (e.g., bee, hornet, wasp).

ANIMAL BITE

Definition
- Bite or claw wound from a pet, farm, or wild animal
- Includes follow-up calls about receiving an antibiotic for an animal bite infection

Wild Animals at Risk for Rabies:
- Bat, skunk, raccoon, fox, coyote
- Any other large wild animal

Pet Animals at Risk for Rabies:
- Outdoor pets who are stray, sick, or unvaccinated AND living in communities where rabies occurs in pets. Triagers should check with the local public health department about the risk for rabies in their community.
- Dogs and cats in developing countries.
- Unprovoked bite.

TRIAGE ASSESSMENT QUESTIONS

Call EMS 911 Now
- ● Major bleeding (actively dripping or spurting) that can't be stopped
  First Aid: Apply direct pressure to the entire wound with a clean cloth.
- ● Sounds like a life-threatening emergency to the triager

Go to ED Now
- ● Any break in skin (e.g., cut, puncture, or scratch) and wild animal at risk for RABIES (e.g., bat, raccoon, fox, skunk, coyote, other carnivores)
  Reason: needs irrigation AND may need rabies vaccine and human rabies immunoglobulin (HRIG)
- ● Any break in skin (e.g., cut, puncture, or scratch) and dog, cat, or ferret at risk for RABIES (e.g., sick, stray, unprovoked bite, developing country)
  Reason: needs irrigation AND may need rabies vaccine and human rabies immunoglobulin (HRIG)
- ● Any break in skin (e.g., cut, puncture, or scratch) and monkey
  Reason: needs irrigation and evaluation for possible herpesvirus simiae exposure

Go to ED/UCC Now
(or to Office With PCP Approval)
- ● Cut (length > 1/8" or 3 mm) or skin tear and any animal
  Reason: cuts may need irrigation; larger cuts may need sutures
- ● Bleeding won't stop after 10 minutes of direct pressure (using correct technique)
- ● Sounds like a serious bite injury to the triager

Go to Office Now
- ● SEVERE pain (e.g., excruciating)
- ● Non-bite body fluid contact (e.g., saliva, brain) and animal at high risk for RABIES (e.g., bat, raccoon, skunk, fox, coyote, other carnivores)
  Reason: postexposure rabies prophylaxis may be indicated
- ● Puncture wound (holes through the skin) from cat (teeth or claws)
  Reason: 50% risk of wound infection; antibiotics are often indicated
- ● Puncture wound or small cut on face
  Reason: cosmetic risk and may need prophylactic antibiotics
- ● Puncture wound or small cut on hands or genitals
  Reason: increased infection risk and may need prophylactic antibiotics (Exception: puncture from small pet [e.g., gerbil, mouse, hamster, puppy])
- ● Bite looks infected (e.g., red area, red streak, pus, or fever)
  R/O: cellulitis, lymphangitis

See Today in Office
- ● No bite mark and suspected bat exposure (e.g., bat found in same room as sleeping adult)
  Reason: postexposure rabies prophylaxis may be indicated
- ● Wound and no tetanus booster in > 5 years (All animal bites are dirty.)
  Reason: may need a tetanus booster shot (vaccine)
- ● Patient wants to be seen

Home Care
○ Minor animal bite or claw wound, too small to irrigate
○ Small puncture wound (e.g., from gerbil, mouse, hamster, puppy)
○ Superficial scratch (didn't go through the dermis)
○ Bite that didn't break the skin
  R/O: bruise

HOME CARE ADVICE

Treatment of Minor Cuts, Scratches, and Puncture Wounds

❶ **Bleeding:** For any bleeding, apply continuous pressure for 10 minutes.

❷ **Cleaning:**
- Wash all wounds immediately with soap and water for 5 minutes. Scrub the wound enough to make it rebleed a little.
- Also, flush vigorously under a faucet for a few minutes.
- Cleaning the wound helps prevent infection.

❸ **Antibiotic Ointment:** Apply an antibiotic ointment (e.g., Neosporin, bacitracin) to the bite 3 times a day for 3 days.

❹ **Expected Course:** Most scratches, scrapes, and other minor bites heal up fine in 3 to 5 days.

❺ **Call Back If:**
- Wound begins to look infected (redness, swelling, warmth, tender to touch, or red streaks).
- You become worse.

Treating Minor Bruises

❶ **Treating Bruises:**
- **Cold Pack for First 48 Hours:** For bruises or swelling, apply a cold pack or an ice bag (wrapped in a moist towel) to the area for 20 minutes. Repeat in 1 hour, then as needed for the first 48 hours after the injury.
  (Reason: to reduce the bruising, swelling, and pain)
- **Local Heat After 48 Hours:** After 48 hours apply a warm, moist washcloth or heating pad for 10 minutes 3 times a day to help the body absorb the blood.

❷ **Pain Medicines:**
- For pain relief, you can take either acetaminophen, ibuprofen, or naproxen.
- They are over-the-counter (OTC) pain drugs. You can buy them at the drugstore.

Acetaminophen (e.g., Tylenol):
- **Regular Strength Tylenol:** Take 650 mg (two 325 mg pills) by mouth every 4-6 hours as needed. Each Regular Strength Tylenol pill has 325 mg of acetaminophen.
- **Extra Strength Tylenol:** Take 1,000 mg (two 500 mg pills) every 8 hours as needed. Each Extra Strength Tylenol pill has 500 mg of acetaminophen.
- The most you should take each day is 3,000 mg (10 Regular Strength or 6 Extra Strength pills a day).

Ibuprofen (e.g., Motrin, Advil):
- Take 400 mg (two 200 mg pills) by mouth every 6 hours.
- Another choice is to take 600 mg (three 200 mg pills) by mouth every 8 hours.
- The most you should take each day is 1,200 mg (six 200 mg pills), unless your doctor has told you to take more.

Naproxen (e.g., Aleve):
- Take 220 mg (one 220 mg pill) by mouth every 8 hours as needed. You may take 440 mg (two 220 mg pills) for your first dose.
- The most you should take each day is 660 mg (three 220 mg pills a day), unless your doctor has told you to take more.

❸ **Pain Medicines—Extra Notes:**
- Use the lowest amount of medicine that makes your pain better.
- Acetaminophen is thought to be safer than ibuprofen or naproxen in people > 65 years old. Acetaminophen is in many OTC and prescription medicines. It might be in more than one medicine that you are taking. You need to be careful and not take an overdose. An acetaminophen overdose can hurt the liver.
- McNeil, the company that makes Tylenol, has different dosage instructions for Tylenol in Canada and the United States. In Canada, the maximum recommended dose per day is 4,000 mg or 12 Regular Strength (325 mg) pills. In the United States, McNeil recommends a maximum dose of 10 Regular Strength (325 mg) pills.
- CAUTION: Do not take acetaminophen if you have liver disease.
- CAUTION: Do not take ibuprofen or naproxen if you have stomach problems, have kidney disease, are pregnant, or have been told by your doctor to avoid this type of anti-inflammatory drug. Do not take ibuprofen or naproxen for > 7 days without consulting your doctor.
- *Before taking any medicine, read all the instructions on the package.*

❹ **Expected Course:** Bruises should fade away over 7-14 days.

Who Should Call Animal Control
❶ **United States—Contacting Animal Control:**
- For patients referred in for evaluation, the ED or PCP will call the animal control center.
- For patients not referred in, the patient should call the animal control center in the county where the bite occurred if a rabies-prone wild animal or stray pet animal attempted to bite an adult but was unsuccessful (i.e., the adult does not need to be seen). The animal control center will initiate a search for the animal. If located, any rabies-prone animals will be observed 10 days for rabies or sacrificed and tested for rabies. Dangerous strays will be taken to the local animal shelter.

❷ **Canada—Contacting the Public Health Department:**
- For adults referred into ED, the ED will call the local public health department.
- For adults not referred into the ED, the triager needs to instruct the caller to report the bite by contacting the local public health department in the area where the bite occurred (provide service referral).
- Public health should be notified of any animal bite (or other animal contact) that might result in rabies.

Reporting Wild Animals and Strays
❶ **Canada:** You can report the animal to the local medical officer of health and to the nearest Canadian Food Inspection Agency veterinarian.
❷ **United States:** You can report the animal to the animal control center for your county.

FIRST AID

First Aid Advice for Bleeding:
Apply direct pressure to the entire wound with a clean cloth.

First Aid Advice for All Bites and Scratches:
Wash all bite wounds and scratches with soap and warm water.

BACKGROUND

Key Points
- Animal bites usually need to be seen by a physician because all bites are contaminated with saliva and are prone to wound infection.
- Bites on the hands are at increased risk of complications.
- **Wound Infection:** Any redness (regardless of size) that develops at the site of an animal bite that happened 24-96 hours previously—most likely (high specificity) indicates the onset of infection (e.g., cellulitis, lymphangitis).

Types of Wounds

- **Bruising:** There is no break in the skin. No risk of infection.
- **Abrasion or Scratch:** These are superficial wounds that don't go all the way through the skin. The risk of infection is low. Prophylactic antibiotic therapy is not indicated.
- **Laceration or Cut:** These are wounds that go through the skin (dermis) into the fat or muscle tissue. There is an intermediate risk of infection. Wound cleansing and irrigation can help prevent infection by washing out the bacteria from the wound. Sometimes debridement of the wound edges is needed. Prophylactic antibiotic therapy may be required.
- **Puncture Wound:** Intermediate risk of infection. Puncture wounds from cat bites are especially prone to getting infected; many physicians will prescribe prophylactic antibiotics for cat bites.

Rabies

- Rabies is very rare in humans but is nearly always fatal.
- **Exposure:** Bites or scratches from a bat, skunk, raccoon, fox, coyote, or other carnivores are more likely to transmit rabies than pets or other animals. These animals can transmit rabies even if they have no symptoms. Bats have transmitted rabies without a detectable bite mark. In the United States and Canada, approximately 90% of cases of rabies in humans are attributed to bats.
- **Postexposure Treatment:** Postexposure prophylaxis consists of an injection of one dose of immunoglobulin (IG) and 4 injections of rabies vaccine over a 14-day period. Rabies IG and the first dose of rabies vaccine should be given as soon as possible after an exposure. The subsequent injections of rabies vaccine should be given on days 3, 7, and 14 after the first vaccination.
- **Incubation Period:** The incubation period for rabies in humans can be days, months, and even possibly longer than a year. Therefore, if there has been a definite or likely exposure, then postexposure prophylaxis (e.g., rabies vaccine, rabies IG) should be given regardless of the interval since the exposure.
- **Risk of Transmission—Type of Animal Bite:** The risk of transmission depends on the type of animal bite. See the next section.

- **Risk of Transmission—Type of Body Fluid:** The rabies virus is transmitted through saliva and brain/nervous system tissue from infected animals. Only these specific body fluids and tissues can transmit the rabies virus. The Centers for Disease Control and Prevention recommends that other contact, such as touching an animal or contact with blood, urine, or feces, is not considered an exposure; no postexposure prophylaxis is needed in these situations.

Types of Animal Bites

- **Puppy Teeth and Puncture Wounds:** This protocol does not refer in the tiny puncture wounds from puppy teeth for prophylactic antibiotics. The reason is that they barely puncture the skin (if at all) and can't be irrigated. Puppy teeth are tiny and sharp. They cause shallow punctures that look like "a dot." They occur commonly in the majority of children and adults who care for a puppy.
- **Small Indoor Pet Animal Bites:** Small indoor pets (gerbils, hamsters, guinea pigs, domesticated mice, rats, etc.) are at no risk for rabies. Puncture wounds from these small animals also don't need to be seen. There is only a small risk for developing a wound infection. *(Reason: The wound infection rate is low because the bites often don't penetrate the dermis.)*
- **Large Pet Animal Bites:** Most bites from pets are from dogs or cats. Bites from domestic animals such as horses can be handled using these protocols. The main risk from pet bites is serious wound infection. Cat bites become infected more often than dog bites. Claw wounds from cats are treated the same as bite wounds, since the claws may be contaminated with saliva. Bites from pet pigs or primates also have a high rate of wound infection. Bites on the hands or feet have a higher risk of infection than bites to other parts of the body.
- **Small Wild Animal Bites:** Rabbits and small rodents (e.g., squirrels, mice, rats, and chipmunks) rarely become infected with rabies and have not been known to transmit it to humans. These bites can sometimes get infected.
- **Bites From Rabies-Prone Wild Animals:** Bites or scratches from a bat, skunk, raccoon, fox, coyote, or other carnivores are more dangerous than other animals. These animals can transmit rabies even if they have no symptoms. There are cases where bats have transmitted rabies without a detectable bite mark (*MMWR Recomm Rep.* 2008;57[RR-3]:1–28).

Dogs and Cats and the Risk of Rabies

- **Indoor Versus Outdoor Pets:** Dogs and cats that are never allowed to roam freely outdoors are considered free of rabies. Outdoor pets who are (1) stray, sick, or unvaccinated AND (2) living in communities where rabies occurs in pets are considered at risk for rabies in the United States and Canada.
- **Metropolitan Versus Rural Location:** Dogs and cats in most metropolitan areas in the U.S. and Canada are free of rabies.
  (Exception: lower Texas, Northwest Territories)
  Dogs and cats in rural areas have a higher risk of rabies.
- **Provoked Versus Unprovoked Bite:** An unprovoked attack by a domestic animal increases the likelihood that an animal is rabid. Note that bites inflicted while a person is attempting to feed or handle a healthy animal are considered provoked.
- **Developing Countries Versus United States and Canada:** Dogs and cats in developing countries have a higher risk of rabies; rabies postexposure prophylaxis is indicated if a bite occurs in a developing country.
- *Nurses and physicians must check with the local public health department about the risk for rabies in their community.*

Bat Bites and Rabies

- All bat bites are considered rabies-prone. During the past 2 decades, nearly all cases of human rabies in the United States and Canada were caused by bats.
- Bat bites are painless and difficult to see. A bat bite is about the same size as a puncture wound from a 27-gauge needle.
- Rabies postexposure prophylaxis should be considered when direct contact between a human and a bat has occurred, unless the exposed person can be certain a bite, scratch, or mucous membrane exposure did not occur (ACIP 1999). Exposure that occurs during sleep, involving unattended preverbal children, or involving intellectually disabled individuals is included.
- Rabies postexposure prophylaxis should also be considered for persons who were in the same room as the bat and who might be unaware that a bite or direct contact had occurred (e.g., a sleeping person awakens to find a bat in the room) (ACIP 1999).
- State or provincial health departments can test bats for rabies only if human contact has occurred.

Coyote Bites and Rabies

- All coyote bites are considered rabies-prone.
- Coyotes are found throughout the United States and Canada. Parents who see a coyote often worry about the safety of their children. Parents can be reassured that in general coyotes are afraid of humans.
- Coyote bites occur < 10 times per year in the United States. Most of them are in children < 5 years old while unattended. The last recorded death due to a coyote attack in the United States was in 1980 in California.

Wound Irrigation—Why It's Important

- Careful wound irrigation and debridement in the ED or office are more effective at preventing infection than prophylactic antibiotics.
- The following wounds need vigorous irrigation: cuts deep enough to see fat or bloody tissue inside or cuts > 1/8" (3 mm). Puncture wounds can't be irrigated, and superficial scratches don't need to be irrigated.
- All bites should be washed at home immediately for 3 minutes under running water before going in to the ED or office.

Suturing Animal Bites

1. **Delayed primary closure** is suturing a wound on day 4 or 5, after we're sure it's not infected. This approach is used for many animal bites and other contaminated wounds that are brought in after 12 to 24 hours. All of these adults need to be seen initially, however, for wound irrigation, debridement, and possibly antibiotics.
2. **Primary closure** is the suturing of a new wound. The sooner a wound is closed, the lower the infection rate. A laceration should be sutured within 12 hours on most of the body and generally within 24 hours on the face and scalp.
   (Reason: highly vascular area)
   Clean wounds can wait longer than dirty wounds.
3. **Secondary closure** is having a wound heal over without suturing. It may leave a wider scar. This approach is often used for infected wounds and abscesses.

ANKLE AND FOOT INJURY

Definition

- Injuries to a bone, muscle, joint, or ligament of the ankle and foot.
- Associated skin and soft tissue injuries are also included.

TRIAGE ASSESSMENT QUESTIONS

Call EMS 911 Now

- Major bleeding (actively dripping or spurting) that can't be stopped
  First Aid: Apply direct pressure to the entire wound with a clean cloth.
- Amputation or bone sticking through the skin
  First Aid: Apply direct pressure to the entire wound with a clean cloth.
- Looks like a dislocated joint (crooked or deformed)
  R/O: dislocation, fracture
- Sounds like a life-threatening emergency to the triager

See More Appropriate Protocol

- Wound looks infected
  Go to Protocol: Wound Infection on page 443
- Caused by an animal bite
  Go to Protocol: Animal Bite on page 22
- Puncture wound of foot
  Go to Protocol: Puncture Wound on page 319
- Toe injury is the main symptom
  Go to Protocol: Toe Injury on page 403

Go to ED Now

- Bullet, stabbed by knife or other serious penetrating wound
  First Aid: If penetrating object is still in place, don't remove it.

Go to ED/UCC Now
(or to Office With PCP Approval)

- Can't stand (bear weight) or walk (e.g., 4 steps)
  R/O: fracture, severe sprain
- Skin is split open or gaping (length > ½" or 12 mm)
  Reason: may need laceration repair (e.g., sutures)
- Bleeding won't stop after 10 minutes of direct pressure (using correct technique)

- Dirt in the wound and not removed after 15 minutes of scrubbing
  Reason: needs irrigation or debridement
- Numbness (new loss of sensation) of toe(s)
- Looks infected (e.g., spreading redness, pus, red streak)
  R/O: cellulitis, lymphangitis
- Sounds like a serious injury to the triager

See Today in Office

- SEVERE pain (e.g., excruciating)
  R/O: fracture, severe sprain
- A "snap" or "pop" was heard at the time of injury
  R/O: ligament tear
- Large swelling or bruise and size > palm of person's hand
  R/O: fracture, large contusion
- Patient wants to be seen

See Today or Tomorrow in Office

- Has diabetes (diabetes mellitus) and any bruising or wound
  Reason: diabetic neuropathy reduces pain of fracture and wound infection
- High-risk adult (e.g., age > 60, osteoporosis, chronic steroid use)
  Reason: greater risk of fracture in patients with osteoporosis
- Suspicious history for the injury
  R/O: domestic violence or elder abuse
- Wound and no tetanus booster in > 5 years (or > 10 years for clean cuts)
  Reason: may need a tetanus booster shot (vaccine)

See Within 3 Days in Office

- Injury and pain has not improved after 3 days
- Injury is still painful or swollen after 2 weeks

Home Care

- ○ Minor ankle or foot injury
  R/O: bruise, strain, or sprain

HOME CARE ADVICE

Treatment of a Minor Bruise, Sprain, or Strain

❶ Reassurance—Direct Blow (Contusion, Bruise):
- A direct blow to your ankle or foot can cause a contusion. Contusion is the medical term for bruise.
- Symptoms are mild pain, swelling, and/or bruising.
- *Here is some care advice that should help.*

❷ Reassurance—Bending or Twisting Injury (Strain, Sprain):
- Strain and sprain are the medical terms used to describe overstretching of the muscles and ligaments of the ankle or foot. A twisting or bending injury can cause a strain or sprain.
- The main symptom is pain that is worse with movement and walking. Swelling can occur. Rarely there may be slight bruising.
- *Here is some care advice that should help.*

❸ Apply a Cold Pack:
- Apply a cold pack or an ice bag (wrapped in a moist towel) to the area for 20 minutes. Repeat in 1 hour, then every 4 hours while awake.
- Continue this for the first 48 hours after an injury.
- This will help decrease pain and swelling.

❹ Apply Heat to the Area:
- Beginning 48 hours after an injury, apply a warm washcloth or heating pad for 10 minutes 3 times a day.
- This will help increase blood flow and improve healing.

❺ Wrap With an Elastic Bandage:
- Wrap the injured part with a snug, elastic bandage for 48 hours.
- The pressure from the bandage can make it feel better and help prevent swelling.
- If you start to get numbness or tingling of your foot or toes the bandage may be too tight. Loosen the bandage wrap.

❻ Elevate the Ankle and Foot:
- Lay down and put your ankle and foot on a pillow. This puts (elevates) the ankle and foot above the heart.
- Do this for 15-20 minutes, 2-3 times a day, for the first 2 days.
- This can also help decrease swelling, bruising, and pain.

❼ Rest Versus Movement:
- Movement is generally more healing in the long term than rest.
- Continue normal activities (like walking) as much as your pain permits.
- Avoid running and active sports for 1-2 weeks or until the pain and swelling are gone.
- Complete rest should only be used for the first day or two after an injury. If it really hurts too much to walk, you will need to see the doctor.

❽ Expected Course:
- Pain, swelling, and bruising usually start to get better 2-3 days after an injury.
- Swelling most often is gone after 1 week.
- Bruises fade away slowly over 1-2 weeks.
- It may take 2 weeks for pain and tenderness of the injured area to go away.

❾ Call Back If:
- Pain becomes severe.
- Pain does not improve after 3 days.
- Pain or swelling lasts > 2 weeks.
- You become worse.

Treatment of a Small Cut or Scrape

❶ Reassurance—Superficial Laceration (Cut or Scratch) or Abrasion (Scrape):
- This sounds like a small cut or scrape that we can treat at home.
- *Here is some care advice that should help.*

❷ Bleeding: Apply direct pressure for 10 minutes with a sterile gauze to stop any bleeding.

❸ Cleaning the Wound:
- Wash the wound with soap and water for 5 minutes.
- For any dirt, scrub gently with a washcloth.
- For any bleeding, apply direct pressure with a sterile gauze or clean cloth for 10 minutes.

❹ Antibiotic Ointment:
- Apply an antibiotic ointment (e.g., over-the-counter bacitracin), covered by a Band-Aid or dressing. Change daily or if it becomes wet.
- Option: A Telfa dressing won't stick to the wound when it is removed.
- Option: Another option is to use a liquid skin bandage that only needs to be applied once. Don't use antibiotic ointment if you use a liquid skin bandage.

❺ **Liquid Skin Bandage:**
- You can use a liquid skin bandage instead of antibiotic ointment and a dressing or a Band-Aid.
- **Benefits:** Liquid skin bandage has several benefits when compared with a regular bandage (e.g., a dressing, a Band-Aid). You only need to put a liquid bandage on once to minor cuts and scrapes. It helps stop minor bleeding. It seals the wound and may promote faster healing and lower infection rates. However, it also costs more.
- **How to Use It:** First, clean and dry the wound. You put on the liquid as spray or with a swab. It dries in < 1 minute and usually lasts a week. You can get it wet.
- **Examples:** Liquid skin bandage is available over the counter. Examples are Band-Aid Liquid Bandage, New Skin, Curad Spray Bandage, and 3M No Sting Liquid Bandage Spray.

❻ **Call Back If:**
- Looks infected (pus, redness, increasing tenderness).
- Doesn't heal within 10 days.
- You become worse.

Over-the-counter Pain Medicines

❶ **Pain Medicines:**
- For pain relief, you can take either acetaminophen, ibuprofen, or naproxen.
- They are over-the-counter (OTC) pain drugs. You can buy them at the drugstore.

Acetaminophen (e.g., Tylenol):
- **Regular Strength Tylenol:** Take 650 mg (two 325 mg pills) by mouth every 4-6 hours as needed. Each Regular Strength Tylenol pill has 325 mg of acetaminophen.
- **Extra Strength Tylenol:** Take 1,000 mg (two 500 mg pills) every 8 hours as needed. Each Extra Strength Tylenol pill has 500 mg of acetaminophen.
- The most you should take each day is 3,000 mg (10 Regular Strength or 6 Extra Strength pills a day).

Ibuprofen (e.g., Motrin, Advil):
- Take 400 mg (two 200 mg pills) by mouth every 6 hours.
- Another choice is to take 600 mg (three 200 mg pills) by mouth every 8 hours.
- The most you should take each day is 1,200 mg (six 200 mg pills), unless your doctor has told you to take more.

Naproxen (e.g., Aleve):
- Take 220 mg (one 220 mg pill) by mouth every 8 hours as needed. You may take 440 mg (two 220 mg pills) for your first dose.
- The most you should take each day is 660 mg (three 220 mg pills a day), unless your doctor has told you to take more.

❷ **Pain Medicines—Extra Notes:**
- Use the lowest amount of medicine that makes your pain better.
- Acetaminophen is thought to be safer than ibuprofen or naproxen in people > 65 years old. Acetaminophen is in many OTC and prescription medicines. It might be in more than one medicine that you are taking. You need to be careful and not take an overdose. An acetaminophen overdose can hurt the liver.
- McNeil, the company that makes Tylenol, has different dosage instructions for Tylenol in Canada and the United States. In Canada, the maximum recommended dose per day is 4,000 mg or 12 Regular Strength (325 mg) pills. In the United States, McNeil recommends a maximum dose of 10 Regular Strength (325 mg) pills.
- CAUTION: Do not take acetaminophen if you have liver disease.
- CAUTION: Do not take ibuprofen or naproxen if you have stomach problems, have kidney disease, are pregnant, or have been told by your doctor to avoid this type of anti-inflammatory drug. Do not take ibuprofen or naproxen for > 7 days without consulting your doctor.
- *Before taking any medicine, read all the instructions on the package.*

❸ **Call Back If:**
- You have more questions.
- You become worse.

FIRST AID

First Aid Advice for Bleeding:
Apply direct pressure to the entire wound with a clean cloth.

First Aid Advice for Penetrating Object:
If penetrating object is still in place, don't remove it.

First Aid Advice for Shock:
Lie down with the feet elevated.

First Aid Advice for a Sprain or Twisting Injury of Ankle or Foot:
- Apply a cold pack or an ice bag (wrapped in a moist towel) to the area for 20 minutes.
- Wrap area with an elastic bandage.

First Aid Advice for Suspected Fracture or Dislocation of Ankle or Foot:
- Do not remove the shoe.
- Immobilize the ankle and foot by wrapping them with a soft splint (e.g., a pillow, a rolled-up blanket, a towel).
- Use tape to keep this splint in place.

Transport of an Amputated Body Part:
- Briefly rinse amputated part with water (to remove any dirt).
- Place amputated part in plastic bag (to protect and keep clean).
- Place plastic bag containing part in a container of ice (to keep cool and preserve tissue).

BACKGROUND

Types of Foot and Ankle Injuries
- **Achilles Tendon Rupture:** There is pain in the Achilles tendon (area above heel and behind ankle). There is weakness or inability to extend the foot (e.g., can't stand on tiptoes).
- **Contusion:** A direct blow or crushing injury results in bruising of the skin, muscle, and underlying bone.
- Cuts, abrasions.
- Dislocations (bone out of joint).
- Fractures (broken bones).
- **Sprains:** Stretches and tears of ligaments.
- **Strains:** Stretches and tears of muscles (e.g., pulled muscle).

What Cuts Need to Be Sutured?
- Any cut that is split open or gaping probably needs sutures (or staples or skin glue).
- Cuts > ½" (1 cm) usually need sutures.
- Any open wound that may need sutures should be evaluated by a physician regardless of the time that has passed since the initial injury.

When Does an Adult Need a Tetanus Booster (Tetanus Shot)?
- **Clean Cuts and Scrapes—Tetanus Booster Needed Every 10 Years:** Patients with clean minor wounds AND who have previously had ≥ 3 tetanus shots (full series) need a booster every 10 years. Examples of minor wounds include a superficial abrasion or a shallow cut from a clean knife blade. Obtain booster within 72 hours.
- **Dirty Wounds—Tetanus Booster Needed Every 5 Years:** Patients with dirty wounds need a booster if it has been > 5 years since the last booster. Examples of dirty wounds include those contaminated with soil, feces, and/or saliva and more serious wounds from deep punctures, crushing, and burns. Obtain booster within 72 hours.

ANKLE PAIN

Definition
- Pain in the ankle
- Not due to a traumatic injury

Pain Severity Scale
- **Mild (1-3):** Doesn't interfere with normal activities.
- **Moderate (4-7):** Interferes with normal activities (e.g., work or school), awakens from sleep, or limping.
- **Severe (8-10):** Excruciating pain, unable to do any normal activities, unable to walk.

TRIAGE ASSESSMENT QUESTIONS

See More Appropriate Protocol
- Followed an injury
  Go to Protocol: Ankle and Foot Injury on page 27
- Thigh or calf pain is the main symptom
  Go to Protocol: Leg Pain on page 273
- Thigh or calf swelling is the main symptom
  Go to Protocol: Leg Swelling and Edema on page 279
- Foot pain is the main symptom
  Go to Protocol: Foot Pain on page 182

Go to ED Now
- Entire foot is cool or blue in comparison with other side
  R/O: iliofemoral arterial occlusion (ischemic foot)

Go to ED/UCC Now
(or to Office With PCP Approval)
- Fever and red area (or area very tender to touch)
  R/O: cellulitis, lymphangitis
  Note: It may be difficult to determine the rash color in people with darker-colored skin.
- Fever and swollen joint
  R/O: septic arthritis, cellulitis
- Thigh or calf pain and only 1 side and present > 1 hour
  R/O: DVT
- Thigh or calf swelling and only 1 side
  R/O: DVT
- Patient sounds very sick or weak to the triager
  Reason: severe acute illness or serious complication suspected

Go to Office Now
- SEVERE pain (e.g., excruciating, unable to walk) and not improved after 2 hours of pain medicine
  R/O: forgotten trauma, severe joint effusion, severe arthritis, gout
- Looks infected (spreading redness, pus) and large red area (> 2" or 5 cm)
  R/O: cellulitis, erysipelas

See Today in Office
- Looks like a boil, infected sore, deep ulcer, or other infected rash (spreading redness, pus)
- Redness of the skin and no fever
  R/O: early cellulitis, inflammatory arthritis

See Within 3 Days in Office
- MODERATE pain (e.g., interferes with normal activities, limping) and present > 3 days
  R/O: sciatica, arthritis
- Swollen joint with no fever or redness
  R/O: degenerative arthritis
- Patient wants to be seen

See Within 2 Weeks in Office
- MILD pain (e.g., does not interfere with normal activities) and present > 7 days
  R/O: muscle strain, sciatica, arthritis, bursitis
- Ankle pain is a chronic symptom (recurrent or ongoing AND present > 4 weeks)
  R/O: arthritis

Home Care
- Caused by overuse from recent vigorous activity (e.g., running, sports)
  R/O: muscle strain, overuse
- Ankle pain

HOME CARE ADVICE

Ankle Pain—General Care Advice

❶ **Reassurance:**
- The symptoms you describe do not sound serious. You have told me that there is no redness, swelling, or fever. You have also told me that there has been no recent major injury.
- Ankle pain can be caused be mild arthritis and other minor problems.
- *Here is some care advice that should help.*

❷ **Pain Medicines:**
- For pain relief, you can take either acetaminophen, ibuprofen, or naproxen.
- They are over-the-counter (OTC) pain drugs. You can buy them at the drugstore.

Acetaminophen (e.g., Tylenol):
- **Regular Strength Tylenol:** Take 650 mg (two 325 mg pills) by mouth every 4-6 hours as needed. Each Regular Strength Tylenol pill has 325 mg of acetaminophen.
- **Extra Strength Tylenol:** Take 1,000 mg (two 500 mg pills) every 8 hours as needed. Each Extra Strength Tylenol pill has 500 mg of acetaminophen.
- The most you should take each day is 3,000 mg (10 Regular Strength or 6 Extra Strength pills a day).

Ibuprofen (e.g., Motrin, Advil):
- Take 400 mg (two 200 mg pills) by mouth every 6 hours.
- Another choice is to take 600 mg (three 200 mg pills) by mouth every 8 hours.
- The most you should take each day is 1,200 mg (six 200 mg pills), unless your doctor has told you to take more.

Naproxen (e.g., Aleve):
- Take 220 mg (one 220 mg pill) by mouth every 8 hours as needed. You may take 440 mg (two 220 mg pills) for your first dose.
- The most you should take each day is 660 mg (three 220 mg pills a day), unless your doctor has told you to take more.

❸ **Pain Medicines—Extra Notes:**
- Use the lowest amount of medicine that makes your pain better.
- Acetaminophen is thought to be safer than ibuprofen or naproxen in people > 65 years old.

- Acetaminophen is in many OTC and prescription medicines. It might be in more than one medicine that you are taking. You need to be careful and not take an overdose. An acetaminophen overdose can hurt the liver.
- McNeil, the company that makes Tylenol, has different dosage instructions for Tylenol in Canada and the United States. In Canada, the maximum recommended dose per day is 4,000 mg or 12 Regular Strength (325 mg) pills. In the United States, McNeil recommends a maximum dose of 10 Regular Strength (325 mg) pills.
- CAUTION: Do not take acetaminophen if you have liver disease.
- CAUTION: Do not take ibuprofen or naproxen if you have stomach problems, have kidney disease, are pregnant, or have been told by your doctor to avoid this type of anti-inflammatory drug. Do not take ibuprofen or naproxen for > 7 days without consulting your doctor.
- *Before taking any medicine, read all the instructions on the package.*

❹ **Expected Course:**
- Pain from a mild strain or joint irritation usually gets better within a week.
- If this does not get better during the next week, you should make an appointment to see your doctor.

❺ **Call Back If:**
- Moderate pain (e.g., limping) lasts > 3 days.
- Mild pain lasts > 7 days.
- You become worse.

Overuse Injury

❶ **Reassurance—Overuse:**
- **Definition:** Muscle strain and joint irritation are very common following vigorous activity. Such activities include sports like tennis and basketball, jogging, and certain types of work.
- **Symptoms:** People often describe a widespread soreness and aching in the overused muscles and joints.
- *Here is some care advice that should help.*

❷ **Apply Cold to the Area:**
- Apply a cold pack or an ice bag (wrapped in a moist towel) to the area for 20 minutes. Repeat in 1 hour, then every 4 hours while awake.
- Continue this for the first 48 hours after an injury. *(Reason: to reduce the swelling and pain)*

❸ **Apply Heat to the Area:**
- Beginning 48 hours after an injury, apply a warm washcloth or heating pad for 10 minutes 3 times a day.
- This will help increase blood flow and improve healing.

❹ **Pain Medicines:**
- For pain relief, you can take either acetaminophen, ibuprofen, or naproxen.
- They are over-the-counter (OTC) pain drugs. You can buy them at the drugstore.

Acetaminophen (e.g., Tylenol):
- **Regular Strength Tylenol:** Take 650 mg (two 325 mg pills) by mouth every 4-6 hours as needed. Each Regular Strength Tylenol pill has 325 mg of acetaminophen.
- **Extra Strength Tylenol:** Take 1,000 mg (two 500 mg pills) every 8 hours as needed. Each Extra Strength Tylenol pill has 500 mg of acetaminophen.
- The most you should take each day is 3,000 mg (10 Regular Strength or 6 Extra Strength pills a day).

Ibuprofen (e.g., Motrin, Advil):
- Take 400 mg (two 200 mg pills) by mouth every 6 hours.
- Another choice is to take 600 mg (three 200 mg pills) by mouth every 8 hours.
- The most you should take each day is 1,200 mg (six 200 mg pills), unless your doctor has told you to take more.

Naproxen (e.g., Aleve):
- Take 220 mg (one 220 mg pill) by mouth every 8 hours as needed. You may take 440 mg (two 220 mg pills) for your first dose.
- The most you should take each day is 660 mg (three 220 mg pills a day), unless your doctor has told you to take more.

❺ **Pain Medicines—Extra Notes:**
- Use the lowest amount of medicine that makes your pain better.
- Acetaminophen is thought to be safer than ibuprofen or naproxen in people > 65 years old. Acetaminophen is in many OTC and prescription medicines. It might be in more than one medicine that you are taking. You need to be careful and not take an overdose. An acetaminophen overdose can hurt the liver.
- McNeil, the company that makes Tylenol, has different dosage instructions for Tylenol in Canada and the United States. In Canada, the maximum recommended dose per day is 4,000 mg or 12 Regular Strength (325 mg) pills. In the United States, McNeil recommends a maximum dose of 10 Regular Strength (325 mg) pills.
- CAUTION: Do not take acetaminophen if you have liver disease.
- CAUTION: Do not take ibuprofen or naproxen if you have stomach problems, have kidney disease, are pregnant, or have been told by your doctor to avoid this type of anti-inflammatory drug. Do not take ibuprofen or naproxen for > 7 days without consulting your doctor.
- *Before taking any medicine, read all the instructions on the package.*

❻ **Rest:** You should try to avoid any exercise or activity that makes the pain worse for the next 3 days.

❼ **Call Back If:**
- Fever occurs.
- Redness or swelling occurs.
- Pain lasts > 7 days.
- You become worse.

BACKGROUND

Causes
- Achilles tendinitis
- Arthritis (e.g., degenerative, gouty, infectious, inflammatory, traumatic)
- Bursitis
- Cellulitis
- Trauma (e.g., contusion, dislocation, fracture, sprain, strain)

Serious Signs and Symptoms
- Severe pain, unable to walk
- Ankle swelling with fever
  R/O: septic arthritis
- Unilateral calf pain and/or swelling
  R/O: DVT

Caution: Deep Vein Thrombosis (DVT)
- Consider the possibility of DVT in anyone with unexplained calf swelling and pain, especially if symptoms are predominantly unilateral.
- **Risk Factors:** Include venous stasis (e.g., casting, long-distance travel, prolonged bed rest), leg/venous injury (e.g., fracture, prior DVT, leg surgery), and hypercoagulable states (e.g., pregnancy, cancer).

ARM PAIN

Definition
- Pain in the arm.
- Not due to a traumatic injury.
- Minor muscle strain and overuse are covered in this protocol.

Pain Severity Scale
- **Mild (1-3):** Doesn't interfere with normal activities.
- **Moderate (4-7):** Interferes with normal activities (e.g., work or school) or awakens from sleep.
- **Severe (8-10):** Excruciating pain, unable to do any normal activities, unable to hold a cup of water.

TRIAGE ASSESSMENT QUESTIONS

Call EMS 911 Now
- Shock suspected (e.g., cold/pale/clammy skin, too weak to stand)
  R/O: shock
  First Aid: Lie down with the feet elevated.
- Similar pain previously and it was from "heart attack"
  R/O: cardiac ischemia, myocardial infarction
- Similar pain previously from "angina" and not relieved by nitroglycerin
  R/O: cardiac ischemia
- Sounds like a life-threatening emergency to the triager

See More Appropriate Protocol
- Chest pain
  Go to Protocol: Chest Pain on page 73
- Wound looks infected
  Go to Protocol: Wound Infection on page 443
- Elbow pain is the main symptom
  Go to Protocol: Elbow Pain on page 146
- Hand or wrist pain is the main symptom
  Go to Protocol: Hand and Wrist Pain on page 193

Go to ED Now
- Difficulty breathing or unusual sweating (e.g., sweating without exertion)
  R/O: cardiac ischemia
- Chest pain lasting > 5 minutes
  R/O: cardiac ischemia
- Age > 40 and no obvious cause for pain, pain still present even when not moving the arm
  R/O: cardiac ischemia

Go to ED/UCC Now
(or to Office With PCP Approval)
- Fever and red area (area very tender to touch)
  R/O: cellulitis, lymphangitis
- Fever and swollen joint
  R/O: septic arthritis
- Entire arm is swollen
  R/O: DVT of upper extremity
- Patient sounds very sick or weak to the triager
  Reason: severe acute illness or serious complication suspected

Go to Office Now
- SEVERE pain (e.g., excruciating, unable to do any normal activities)
  Reason: inadequate analgesia
  R/O: herniated cervical disk
- Red area or streak and large (> 2" or 5 cm)
  R/O: cellulitis, erysipelas, lymphangitis
  Note: It may be difficult to determine the rash color in people with darker-colored skin.
- Cast on wrist or arm and now increasing pain
  R/O: swelling (cast may need to be bivalved)
- Weakness (i.e., loss of strength) in hand or fingers
  R/O: herniated cervical disk
- Arm pains with exertion (e.g., occurs with walking; goes away on resting)
  R/O: angina

See Today in Office
- Painful rash with multiple small blisters grouped together (i.e., dermatomal distribution or "band" or "stripe")
  R/O: herpes zoster (shingles)
- Looks like a boil, infected sore, deep ulcer, or other infected rash (spreading redness, pus)
  R/O: abscess, cellulitis
- Localized rash is very painful (no fever)
  R/O: cellulitis, spider bite, bee sting, herpes zoster (shingles)

See Today or Tomorrow in Office

● Numbness (i.e., loss of sensation) in hand or fingers
R/O: neuropathy, cervical radiculopathy, herniated cervical disk, carpal tunnel syndrome
● Localized pain, redness, or hard lump along vein
R/O: superficial thrombophlebitis
● Patient wants to be seen

See Within 3 Days in Office

● MODERATE pain (e.g., interferes with normal activities) and present > 3 days
R/O: arthritis, tendonitis, carpal tunnel syndrome
● Pain is worsened or caused by bending the neck
R/O: cervical radiculopathy

See Within 2 Weeks in Office

● MILD pain and present > 7 days
● Arm pain is a chronic symptom (recurrent or ongoing AND lasting > 4 weeks)

Home Care

○ Arm pain
R/O: muscle strain, arthritis
○ Caused by strained muscle
R/O: muscle strain (pulled muscle)
○ Caused by overuse from recent vigorous activity (e.g., sports, lifting, physical work)
R/O: muscle strain, overuse (sore muscles from overuse)
○ Caused by phantom arm pain
R/O: phantom limb pain after amputation

HOME CARE ADVICE

Arm Pain—General Care Advice

❶ **Pain Medicines:**
  • For pain relief, you can take either acetaminophen, ibuprofen, or naproxen.
  • They are over-the-counter (OTC) pain drugs. You can buy them at the drugstore.

  Acetaminophen (e.g., Tylenol):
  • **Regular Strength Tylenol:** Take 650 mg (two 325 mg pills) by mouth every 4-6 hours as needed. Each Regular Strength Tylenol pill has 325 mg of acetaminophen.
  • **Extra Strength Tylenol:** Take 1,000 mg (two 500 mg pills) every 8 hours as needed. Each Extra Strength Tylenol pill has 500 mg of acetaminophen.
  • The most you should take each day is 3,000 mg (10 Regular Strength or 6 Extra Strength pills a day).

Ibuprofen (e.g., Motrin, Advil):
  • Take 400 mg (two 200 mg pills) by mouth every 6 hours.
  • Another choice is to take 600 mg (three 200 mg pills) by mouth every 8 hours.
  • The most you should take each day is 1,200 mg (six 200 mg pills), unless your doctor has told you to take more.

Naproxen (e.g., Aleve):
  • Take 220 mg (one 220 mg pill) by mouth every 8 hours as needed. You may take 440 mg (two 220 mg pills) for your first dose.
  • The most you should take each day is 660 mg (three 220 mg pills a day), unless your doctor has told you to take more.

❷ **Pain Medicines—Extra Notes:**
  • Use the lowest amount of medicine that makes your pain better.
  • Acetaminophen is thought to be safer than ibuprofen or naproxen in people > 65 years old. Acetaminophen is in many OTC and prescription medicines. It might be in more than one medicine that you are taking. You need to be careful and not take an overdose. An acetaminophen overdose can hurt the liver.
  • McNeil, the company that makes Tylenol, has different dosage instructions for Tylenol in Canada and the United States. In Canada, the maximum recommended dose per day is 4,000 mg or 12 Regular Strength (325 mg) pills. In the United States, McNeil recommends a maximum dose of 10 Regular Strength (325 mg) pills.
  • CAUTION: Do not take acetaminophen if you have liver disease.
  • CAUTION: Do not take ibuprofen or naproxen if you have stomach problems, have kidney disease, are pregnant, or have been told by your doctor to avoid this type of anti-inflammatory drug. Do not take ibuprofen or naproxen for > 7 days without consulting your doctor.
  • *Before taking any medicine, read all the instructions on the package.*

❸ **Call Back If:**
  • Moderate pain (e.g., interferes with normal activities) lasts > 3 days.
  • Mild pain lasts > 7 days.
  • Arm swelling occurs.
  • Signs of infection occur (e.g., spreading redness, warmth, fever).
  • You become worse.

Muscle Strain or Overuse

❶ Reassurance—Muscle Strain:
- **Definition:** A muscle strain occurs from over-stretching or tearing a muscle. People often call this a "pulled muscle." This muscle injury can occur while exercising, while lifting something, or sometimes during normal activities.
- **Symptoms:** People often describe a sharp pain or popping when the muscle strain occurs. The muscle pain worsens with movement of the arm.
- *Here is some care advice that should help.*

❷ Reassurance—Overuse:
- **Definition:** Sore muscles are common following vigorous activity (overuse injury), especially when your body is not used to this amount of activity (e.g., sports, weight lifting, moving furniture).
- **Symptoms:** People often describe a diffuse soreness and aching in the overused muscles.
- *Here is some care advice that should help.*

❸ Apply Cold to the Area for First 48 Hours:
- Apply a cold pack or an ice bag (wrapped in a moist towel) to the area for 20 minutes. Repeat in 1 hour, then every 4 hours while awake.
- Continue this for the first 48 hours after an injury. *(Reason: to reduce the swelling and pain)*

❹ Apply Heat to the Area:
- Beginning 48 hours after an injury, apply a warm wash-cloth or heating pad for 10 minutes 3 times a day.
- This will help increase blood flow and improve healing.

❺ Local Heat (shower option): If stiffness lasts > 48 hours, relax in a hot shower twice a day and gently exercise the involved part under the falling water.

❻ Rest: You should try to avoid any exercise or activity that caused this pain for the next 3 days.

❼ Pain Medicines:
- For pain relief, you can take either acetaminophen, ibuprofen, or naproxen.
- They are over-the-counter (OTC) pain drugs. You can buy them at the drugstore.

Acetaminophen (e.g., Tylenol):
- **Regular Strength Tylenol:** Take 650 mg (two 325 mg pills) by mouth every 4-6 hours as needed. Each Regular Strength Tylenol pill has 325 mg of acetaminophen.
- **Extra Strength Tylenol:** Take 1,000 mg (two 500 mg pills) every 8 hours as needed. Each Extra Strength Tylenol pill has 500 mg of acetaminophen.
- The most you should take each day is 3,000 mg (10 Regular Strength or 6 Extra Strength pills a day).

Ibuprofen (e.g., Motrin, Advil):
- Take 400 mg (two 200 mg pills) by mouth every 6 hours.
- Another choice is to take 600 mg (three 200 mg pills) by mouth every 8 hours.
- The most you should take each day is 1,200 mg (six 200 mg pills), unless your doctor has told you to take more.

Naproxen (e.g., Aleve):
- Take 220 mg (one 220 mg pill) by mouth every 8 hours as needed. You may take 440 mg (two 220 mg pills) for your first dose.
- The most you should take each day is 660 mg (three 220 mg pills a day), unless your doctor has told you to take more.

❽ Pain Medicines—Extra Notes:
- Use the lowest amount of medicine that makes your pain better.
- Acetaminophen is thought to be safer than ibuprofen or naproxen in people > 65 years old. Acetaminophen is in many OTC and prescription medicines. It might be in more than one medicine that you are taking. You need to be careful and not take an overdose. An acetaminophen over-dose can hurt the liver.
- McNeil, the company that makes Tylenol, has different dosage instructions for Tylenol in Canada and the United States. In Canada, the maximum recommended dose per day is 4,000 mg or 12 Regular Strength (325 mg) pills. In the United States, McNeil recommends a maximum dose of 10 Regular Strength (325 mg) pills.
- CAUTION: Do not take acetaminophen if you have liver disease.
- CAUTION: Do not take ibuprofen or naproxen if you have stomach problems, have kidney disease, are pregnant, or have been told by your doctor to avoid this type of anti-inflammatory drug. Do not take ibuprofen or naproxen for > 7 days without consulting your doctor.
- *Before taking any medicine, read all the instructions on the package.*

❾ Expected Course:
- **Muscle Strain:** A minor muscle strain usually hurts for 2-3 days. The pain often peaks on day 2. A more severe muscle strain can hurt for 2-4 weeks.
- **Muscle Overuse:** Sore muscles from overuse usually hurt for 2-4 days. The pain often peaks on day 2.

⑩ Call Back If:
- Moderate pain (e.g., interferes with normal activities) lasts > 3 days.
- Mild pain lasts > 7 days.
- You become worse.

Phantom Arm Pain

❶ Reassurance—Phantom Pain and Phantom Sensations:
- **Phantom Pain:** Phantom pain is pain that occurs in the part of the limb that is left after amputation. The pain can be aching, cramping, burning, sharp, or shooting. Most people experience phantom pain in the arm after an amputation. It seems that the worse the pain was in the arm prior to amputation, the more phantom pain a person will have.
- **Phantom Sensation:** There are a number of other phantom sensations that amputees can experience in the amputated part of the arm. These include tingling, numbness, cramping, cold, and warmth.
- Research has not shown a single best treatment for these pains and sensations.
- *Here is some care advice that may help.*

❷ Treatment—Phantom Pain:
- Try gently rubbing (massaging) or touching (tapping) your stump.
- Move or exercise other parts of your body.
- Do something to take your mind off the pain. Listen to music, read a book, watch a TV show.

❸ Treatment—Phantom Hand or Fingers Feel Twisted or Cramped:
- Move the normal arm into a position of comfort.
- By doing this it may help the phantom arm feel better.

❹ Expected Course:
- Usually, phantom pain and phantom sensation slowly get better over time.
- You should speak with your doctor if you have more questions about this.

❺ Call Back If:
- You become worse.

FIRST AID

First Aid Advice for Shock:
Lie down with the feet elevated.

BACKGROUND

Causes of Arm Pain
- **Cervical Radiculopathy:** This is caused by pressure on the spinal nerve roots from a herniated disk or from spinal arthritis.
- **Deep Vein Thrombosis (DVT):** DVT of the arm is rare. Symptoms include arm pain and swelling.
- **Muscle Cramps:** Brief pains (1-15 minutes) may be due to muscle spasms. The pain should resolve completely after an episode of muscle spasm.
- **Muscle Strain** (pulled muscle): A muscle strain occurs from overstretching or tearing a muscle. This muscle injury can occur while exercising, while lifting something, and sometimes during normal activities. This is also referred to as a "pulled muscle."
- **Muscle Strain** (sore muscles from overuse): Continuous acute pains (hours to 3 days) are often due to overly strenuous activities or forgotten muscle injuries from recent exercise or work-related activities.
- **Phantom Limb Pain:** Phantom pain is pain that occurs in the part of the limb that is left after amputation. The pain can be aching, cramping, burning, sharp, or shooting. Most people experience phantom pain in the arm after an amputation.
- **Viral Illness:** Mild bilateral diffuse muscle aches also occur with many viral illnesses.

Other causes include unwitnessed fracture, arthritis, skin infection (cellulitis, erysipelas), bursitis.

Serious Signs and Symptoms
- Severe pain.
- Red area with streak.
  R/O: cellulitis with lymphangitis; common
- Joint swelling with fever.
  R/O: septic arthritis; rare
- Entire arm is swollen.
  R/O: DVT of upper extremity; rare

Caution: Cardiac Ischemia
- Rarely, patients may present with arm pain as the sole symptom of a myocardial infarction. Usually there will be other associated symptoms of cardiac ischemia: chest pain, shortness of breath, nausea, and/or diaphoresis.
- Cardiac ischemia should be suspected in any patients with risk factors for cardiac disease. These include hypertension, smoking, diabetes, hyperlipidemia, a strong family history of heart disease, and age > 50.

ASTHMA ATTACK

Definition
- Adult is having an asthma attack.
- Previously diagnosed as having asthma, asthmatic bronchitis, or reactive airway disease by a physician, or treated in the past with asthma medications by inhaler or nebulizer.
- *Use this protocol only if the patient has symptoms that match Asthma Attack.*

Symptoms
- Recurring episodes of wheezing, cough, chest tightness, and difficulty breathing.
- Wheezing is a high-pitched or whistling sound heard on expiration.

Asthma Attack Severity
- **Mild:** No shortness of breath (SOB) at rest, mild SOB with walking, speaks normally in sentences, can lie down, no retractions, pulse < 100 (GREEN Zone: peak expiratory flow rate [PEFR] 80%-100%).
- **Moderate:** SOB at rest, SOB with exertion and prefers to sit, cannot lie down flat, speaks in phrases, mild retractions, audible wheezing, pulse 100-120 (YELLOW Zone: PEFR 50%-80%).
- **Severe:** Very SOB at rest, speaks in single words, agitated, sitting hunched forward, cannot lie down flat, retractions, usually loud wheezing, sometimes minimal wheezing because of decreased air movement, pulse >120 (RED Zone: PEFR < 50%).
- **Respiratory Arrest Imminent:** Struggling to breathe, unable to speak, drowsy or confused.

TRIAGE ASSESSMENT QUESTIONS

Call EMS 911 Now
- ● SEVERE difficulty breathing (e.g., struggling for each breath, speaks in single words)
  R/O: respiratory failure, hypoxia
  First Aid: Take 4 puffs from your quick-relief inhaler (e.g., albuterol).
- ● Bluish (or gray) lips or face
  First Aid: Take 4 puffs from your quick-relief inhaler (e.g., albuterol).

- ● Wheezing started suddenly after medicine, an allergic food, or bee sting
  R/O: anaphylaxis
  First Aid: Take 4 puffs from your quick-relief inhaler (e.g., albuterol).
- ● Passed out (i.e., fainted, collapsed and was not responding)
- ● Sounds like a life-threatening emergency to the triager

Go to ED Now
- ● SEVERE asthma attack (e.g., very SOB at rest, speaks in single words, loud wheezes)
  First Aid: Take 4 puffs from your quick-relief inhaler (e.g., albuterol).

Go to ED/UCC Now
(or to Office With PCP Approval)
- ● SEVERE wheezing or coughing and doesn't have nebulizer or inhaler available
  Reason: needs immediate nebulizer or inhaler treatment
- ● PEFR < 50% of baseline level (RED Zone)
- ● Hospitalized before with asthma; now feels same
- ● Chest pain
  R/O: pneumothorax
- ● Patient sounds very sick or weak to the triager
  Reason: severe acute illness or serious complication suspected

Go to Office Now
- ● MODERATE asthma attack (e.g., SOB at rest, speaks in phrases, audible wheezes) and not resolved after 2 nebulizer or inhaler treatments given 20 minutes apart
  Reason: may need oral corticosteroid burst
- ● PEFR 50%-80% of baseline level (YELLOW Zone) after using 2 nebulizer or inhaler treatments given 20 minutes apart

See Today in Office
- ● Fever > 103° F (39.4° C)
  R/O: bacterial pneumonia
- ● Fever > 100.5° F (38.1° C) and > 60 years of age
- ● Continuous (nonstop) coughing that keeps patient from working or sleeping, and not improved after inhaler or nebulizer
  Reason: may need for oral corticosteroid burst

- Asthma medicine (nebulizer or inhaler) is needed more frequently than every 4 hours to keep you comfortable
- Fever present > 3 days (72 hours)
- Patient wants to be seen

See Today or Tomorrow in Office

- MILD asthma attack (e.g., no SOB at rest, mild SOB with walking, speaks normally in sentences, mild wheezing) and persists > 24 hours on appropriate treatment
  Reason: may need oral corticosteroid burst
- Intermittent mild wheezing persists > 5 days
- Nasal discharge present > 10 days
- Sinus pain (around cheekbone or eye)

Discuss With PCP and Callback by Nurse Today

- Influenza prevalent in community (or household) and has flu symptoms (e.g., cough WITH fever, etc) with onset < 48 hours ago
  Reason: antiviral treatment may be indicated

See Within 2 Weeks in Office

- No asthma checkup in > 6 months
  Reason: review treatment program
- Missing > 1 day of work or school per month because of asthma

Home Care

○ MILD asthma attack (e.g., no SOB at rest, mild SOB with walking, speaks normally in sentences, mild wheezing)

HOME CARE ADVICE

❶ **Quick-Relief Asthma Medicine:**
  - Start your quick-relief medicine (e.g., albuterol, salbutamol) at the first sign of any coughing or shortness of breath (don't wait for wheezing). Use your inhaler (2 puffs each time) or nebulizer every 4 hours. Continue the quick-relief medicine until you have not wheezed or coughed for 48 hours.
  - The best "cough medicine" for an adult with asthma is always the asthma medicine.
    Note: Don't use cough suppressants, but cough drops may help a tickly cough.

❷ **Long-term–Control Asthma Medicine:** If you are using a controller medicine (e.g., inhaled steroids or cromolyn), continue to take it as directed.

❸ **Drinking Liquids:** Try to drink normal amount of liquids (e.g., water). Being adequately hydrated makes it easier to cough up the sticky lung mucus.

❹ **Humidifier:** If the air is dry, use a cool mist humidifier to prevent drying of the upper airway.

❺ **Hay Fever:** If you have nasal symptoms from hay fever, it's OK to take antihistamines.
  (Reason: Poor control of allergic rhinitis makes asthma worse, whereas antihistamines don't make asthma worse.)

❻ **Remove Allergens:** Take a shower to remove pollens, animal dander, or other allergens from the body and hair.

❼ **Avoid Triggers:** Avoid known triggers of asthma attacks (e.g., tobacco smoke, cats, other pets, feather pillows, exercise).

❽ **Work With Your Doctor:** There is no cure for asthma, but you can take charge and learn to control it. The best way to take charge of asthma is to work with your doctor (over many months) to find the right controller (preventive) medicine so your asthma is under control. If you keep having asthma attacks, then the asthma is not under control. People can die from asthma if they do not take it seriously and work with a doctor to control it.

❾ **Expected Course:** If treatment is started early, most asthma attacks are quickly brought under control. All wheezing should be gone by 5 days.

❿ **Call Back If:**
  - Inhaled asthma medicine (nebulizer or inhaler) is needed more often than every 4 hours.
  - Wheezing has not completely cleared after 5 days.
  - You become worse.

How to Use an Inhaler or Spacer

❶ **How to Use a Metered Dose Inhaler (MDI):**
  - **Step 1:** Remove the cap and shake the inhaler.
  - **Step 2:** Hold the inhaler about 1-2" (2-5 cm) in front of the mouth. Breathe out—completely.
  - **Step 3:** Press down on the inhaler to release the medicine as you start to breathe in slowly.
  - **Step 4:** Breathe in slowly for 3-5 seconds.
  - **Step 5:** Hold your breath for 10 seconds to allow the medicine to reach deeply into your lungs.
  - If your doctor has prescribed 2 puffs, wait 1 minute and then repeat steps 2-5.

❷ How to Use an MDI With a Spacer:
- **Step 1:** Shake the inhaler and then attach it to the spacer or holding chamber.
- **Step 2:** Breathe out completely.
- **Step 3:** Place the mouthpiece of the spacer in your mouth.
- **Step 4:** Press down on the inhaler. This will put one puff of the medicine in the holding chamber or spacer.
- **Step 5:** Breathe in slowly for 5 seconds.
- **Step 6:** Hold your breath for 10 seconds and then exhale.
- If your doctor has prescribed 2 or more puffs, wait 1 minute between each puff and then repeat steps 2-6.

❸ How to Use a Dry Powder Inhaler:
- **Step 1:** Remove the cap and follow manufacturer's instructions to load a dose of medicine.
- **Step 2:** Breathe out completely.
- **Step 3:** Put the mouthpiece of the inhaler in the mouth.
- **Step 4:** Breathe in quickly and deeply.
- **Step 5:** Hold your breath for 10 seconds to allow the medicine to reach deeply into your lungs.
- If your doctor has prescribed 2 or more inhalations, wait 1 minute and then repeat steps 2-5.

❹ How to Tell if Your MDI Is Empty:
- An empty MDI can sometimes be the reason that an asthma attack is not getting better.
- **Shaking Inhaler Not Helpful:** Shaking the inhaler and hearing fluid in it is not very helpful. When the medicine is gone, extra propellant still remains.
- **"Float Test" Not Recommended:** The float test involves putting your MDI in a sink or pan of water and seeing if it will float. An empty inhaler lies horizontal on top of the water. A full inhaler usually is vertical and sinks under the top of the water. Unfortunately, this test is NOT very accurate.
- **Best Way:** Most MDIs hold around 200 puffs of albuterol or other medicine. However, every type of inhaler is different. It should say on the side of the inhaler. This information is usually quite accurate. Thus, the best way is to keep track of how many puffs you use each day and then do the math. For example, 4 puffs a day for 30 days equals 120 puffs.
- The Ventolin HFA inhaler contains a dose counter that makes it easier to keep track of your puffs.

Your Peak Flow Meter

❶ Peak Flow Meter:
- Every adult with asthma should have a peak flow meter.
- A peak flow meter is a device that measures how well air moves out of your lungs.
- The number that is obtained is called the peak expiratory flow rate (PEFR).
- The "personal best" value is the highest PEFR number that a person obtains when they are feeling well.

❷ How to Use a Peak Flow Meter:
- **Step 1:** Move the indicator to the bottom of the numbered scale. Stand up.
- **Step 2:** Take a deep breath, filling your lungs completely.
- **Step 3:** Place the mouthpiece in your mouth and close your lips around it. Do not put your tongue inside the hole.
- **Step 4:** Blow out as hard and fast as you can.
- **Step 5:** Repeat the process 2 more times.
- **Step 6:** Write down the highest of the 3 numbers.

❸ Using a Peak Flow Meter to Determine the Severity of an Asthma Attack:
- **GREEN Zone**—MILD Attack: PEFR 80%-100% of personal best
- **YELLOW Zone**—MODERATE Attack: PEFR 50%-80%
- **RED Zone**—SEVERE Attack: PEFR < 50%.

FIRST AID

First Aid Advice for Asthma Attack:
Take 4 puffs on your quick-relief inhaler (e.g., albuterol, salbutamol, Xopenex) right now.

BACKGROUND

Asthma Triggers
Different things can cause an asthma attack. These are called asthma triggers.
- Allergens (pollen, house dust, mold, animals)
- Irritants (cigarette smoke, dirt, pollution)
- Exercise
- Respiratory infections (cold or flu)
- Sudden changes in the weather (generally cold weather)

Asthma Medications
There are 2 main types of asthma medications, long-term control and quick relief.

- **A long-term–control** (preventive, controller) medicine keeps asthma attacks from starting. It works slowly over many weeks to stop the swelling in the airways. Adults must take it every day, even when they feel fine and can breathe well. Examples of preventive medicines include inhaled steroids (e.g., AeroBid, Azmacort, Beclovent, Flovent, Pulmicort, Vanceril) and cromolyn.
- **A quick-relief** (rescue, reliever) medicine helps stop an asthma attack that has already started. It can keep the attack from getting serious. It works fast to stop the tightness and opens the airways in the lungs during an asthma attack. An adult should take it at the first sign of a wheeze, cough, or drop in peak flow measurement. Sometimes doctors will tell an adult to take it every day for a week or two after an asthma attack, but quick-relief medicines are not meant to be used to stop attacks every day for weeks and weeks. Examples of quick-relief medicines include inhaled or nebulized beta-agonists (e.g., Proventil, Alupent, Albuterol, Ventolin, Salbutamol).

Albuterol (Salbutamol) Quick-Relief Treatments for Asthma Attacks and the NAEPP Guidelines

- **Quick-Relief (Rescue) Treatment:** Bronchodilator treatment with albuterol is indicated for asthma attack symptoms. The patient should take up to 2 treatments 20 minutes apart using an inhaler (2-6 puffs) or a nebulizer.
- **Response to Treatment Is PEFR < 50%:** Adults having an asthma attack with a PEFR < 50% should start oral steroid and either go to the ED or call EMS 911.
- **Response to Treatment Is PEFR 50%-80%:** Adults with an asthma attack who have an incomplete response (PEFR 50%-80%) to quick-relief treatment need to be started on a steroid burst. If they do not have access to prednisone through their on-call PCP, they need to be seen in the ED.
- Reference: National Asthma Education and Prevention Program *Expert Panel Report 3: Guidelines for the Diagnosis and Management of Asthma—Summary Report 2007.* This report is available online at: www.nhlbi.nih.gov/guidelines/asthma/asthgdln.htm.

Levalbuterol (Xopenex)

- Levalbuterol is a newer bronchodilator that is related chemically to albuterol (it is the L stereoisomer of albuterol).
- Levalbuterol costs more than albuterol.
- Generally, patients will not be using both of these medications together.

Peak Flow Meters

Peak flow meters measure how fast an adult can move air out of the lungs. Every adult with asthma should have a peak flow meter. These measurements are very useful for grading the severity of an asthma attack. The normal peak expiratory flow rate (PEFR) for a healthy adult female is 400-500 and the normal value is 500-650 for a healthy adult male. Peak flow rates decrease during an asthma attack. In general, medications should be increased when the PEFR is < 80% of baseline and an adult should be seen immediately in the ED if the PEFR is < 50%.

- **Mild Attack:** PEFR 80%-100% of baseline (personal best/GREEN Zone)
- **Moderate Attack:** PEFR 50%-80% (YELLOW Zone)
- **Severe Attack:** PEFR < 50% (RED Zone)

Using a Spacer (Holding Chamber) with a Metered Dose Inhaler (MDI)

- Many individuals can benefit from using a spacer (holding chamber), especially individuals who have difficulty coordinating taking a breath and activating the MDI. For such individuals, adding a spacer to their inhaler may double the delivery of albuterol to the lungs.
- Metered dose inhalers with a spacer work as well as a nebulizer treatment.

Internet Resources

- **Asthma Action Plan:** The National Heart, Lung, and Blood Institute has developed this asthma action plan template: www.nhlbi.nih.gov/health/public/lung/asthma/asthma_actplan.pdf.
- **Learn About Asthma:** This Web page is from the Chest Foundation. It has general information on asthma. It also has specific information on how to take medicines, how to use a peak flow meter, and how to use inhalers. Available at: https://foundation.chestnet.org/patient-education-resources/asthma.

Caution: Asthma-Related Death

Asthma patients are at risk for asthma-related death. Risk factors include:

- Current use of, or recent withdrawal from, systemic corticosteroids
- Prior intubation for asthma or admission to an intensive care unit
- Hospitalizations or multiple emergency visits for asthma within the past year
- History of psychosocial problems or denial of asthma or its severity
- History of noncompliance with asthma medication plan

ATHLETE'S FOOT

Definition
- Fungus infection of the feet.
- Causes itchy rash between the toes.
- *Use this protocol only if the patient has symptoms that match Athlete's Foot.*

Symptoms
- Rash with redness, maceration, and fissuring between the toes, especially in the web space between the third/fourth and fourth/fifth toes.
- Often involves the insteps of the feet.
- The rash itches and burns.

TRIAGE ASSESSMENT QUESTIONS

See More Appropriate Protocol
- ● Doesn't match the SYMPTOMS for athlete's foot
  Go to Protocol: Rash or Redness, Localized on page 326

Go to ED/UCC Now
(or to Office With PCP Approval)
- ● Patient sounds very sick or weak to the triager
  Reason: severe acute illness or serious complication suspected; feeling unwell is not typical of athlete's foot

Go to Office Now
- ● Fever and bright red area or streak
  R/O: cellulitis, lymphangitis

See Today in Office
- ● Rash looks infected (e.g., spreading redness, pus)
  R/O: cellulitis
- ● Rash is very painful
  R/O: cellulitis
- ● Diabetes
  Reason: diabetic foot care

See Today or Tomorrow in Office
- ● After week on treatment and rash continues to spread
  R/O: wrong diagnosis
- ● Rash has spread beyond the instep and toes
  R/O: contact dermatitis from sneakers, "moccasin-type" tinea pedis
- ● Patient wants to be seen

See Within 3 Days in Office
- ● After 4 weeks on treatment and rash has not cleared completely
  R/O: wrong diagnosis

Home Care
- ○ Athlete's foot with no complications

HOME CARE ADVICE

General Care Advice for Athlete's Foot
❶ Antifungal Cream: Apply the antifungal cream 2 times a day to the affected areas of the feet. Continue the cream for at least 7 days after the rash is cleared.
- Available over the counter in United States as terbinafine (Lamisil AT), clotrimazole (Lotrimin AF), or miconazole (Micatin, Monistat Derm).
- Available over the counter in Canada as clotrimazole (clotrimazole cream, Canesten, Clotrimaderm) or miconazole (Micatin Cream, Micozole, Monistat Derm).
- Terbinafine (Lamisil AT) is most recommended but is not available in Canada.
- *Before taking any medicine, read all the instructions on the package.*

❷ Keep the Feet Clean and Dry: Wash the feet 2 times every day. Dry the feet completely, especially between the toes. Then apply the cream. Wear clean socks and change them twice daily.

❸ Avoid Scratching: Scratching infected feet will delay healing. Rinse the itchy feet in cool water for relief.

❹ Contagiousness:
- The condition is not very contagious.
- The fungus can't grow on dry, normal skin.
- Adults with athlete's foot do not need to miss any school or work. You can continue to play sports.
- The socks can be washed with regular laundry. They don't need to be boiled.

❺ Expected Course: With proper treatment, athlete's foot should decrease substantially within 1 week and disappear within 2 weeks.

❻ Call Back If:
- Rash looks infected (e.g., spreading redness, streaks, pus).
- Rash continues to spread after 1 week of treatment.
- Rash has not cleared after 2 weeks of treatment.
- You become worse.

Prevention

❶ Avoid Being Barefoot in Public Areas

(e.g., showers, bathrooms, swimming pools): You can get athlete's foot from walking barefoot in these areas. Wear sandals.

❷ Keep the Feet Clean and Dry:
- Wash your feet with warm, soapy water once a day. Rinse the feet and dry thoroughly, especially between the toes.
- Wear clean cotton socks and change daily.

BACKGROUND

Key Points
- Athlete's foot is an infection caused by a fungus that grows best on the warm, damp skin of the foot and toes.
- It is a common malady, with up to 70% of the adult population having it at some point in their lives.
- The medical term for athlete's foot is tinea pedis.
- Lack of involvement of the web space between the third/fourth or fourth/fifth toes should make the triager hesitate in attributing the rash to athlete's foot.

Treatment
- There are both topical and oral medications that work well in treating this infection.
- Most healthy individuals will be able to treat athlete's foot effectively using a topical agent.
- Oral medications must be prescribed by a physician and have a greater risk of side effects (e.g., hepatotoxicity).

BACK INJURY

Definition
- Injury to the upper, mid, or lower back

Excluded:
- Pain in the back from overuse (repetitive movements) from work, gardening, sports, etc., should be triaged using the Back Pain procotol on page 48.
- Pain in the back from a self-induced twisting, lifting, or bending injury should be triaged using the Back Pain protocol on page 48.

TRIAGE ASSESSMENT QUESTIONS

Call EMS 911 Now
- Dangerous mechanism of injury (e.g., MVA, contact sports, trampoline, diving, fall > 10 feet or 3 m)
  (Exception: back pain began > 1 hour after injury)
  First Aid: Do not move until a spine board is applied.
- Weakness (i.e., paralysis, loss of muscle strength) of the leg(s) or foot and sudden onset after back injury
  R/O: fracture, spinal cord injury, nerve root compression
  First Aid: Do not move until a spine board is applied.
- Numbness (i.e., loss of sensation) of the leg(s) or foot and sudden onset after back injury
  R/O: fracture, spinal cord injury, nerve root compression
  First Aid: Do not move until a spine board is applied.
- Major bleeding (actively dripping or spurting) that can't be stopped
  First Aid: Apply direct pressure to the entire wound with a clean cloth.
- Bullet, knife, or other serious penetrating wound
  First Aid: If penetrating object is still in place, don't remove it.
  Reason: removal could increase bleeding.
- Shock suspected (e.g., cold/pale/clammy skin, too weak to stand)
  R/O: shock
  First Aid: Lie down with the feet elevated.
- Sounds like a life-threatening emergency to the triager

See More Appropriate Protocol
- Back pain not from an injury
  Go to Protocol: Back Pain on page 48
- Back pain from overuse (work, exercise, gardening) OR from twisting, lifting, or bending injury
  Go to Protocol: Back Pain on page 48

Go to ED Now
- SEVERE pain in kidney area (flank) that follows a direct blow to that site
  R/O: renal injury
- Blood in urine (red, pink, or tea-colored)
  R/O: renal injury
- Unable to urinate (or only a few drops) > 4 hours and bladder feels very full (e.g., palpable bladder or strong urge to urinate)
  R/O: cauda equina syndrome, conus medullaris syndrome
- Urinary or bowel incontinence (i.e., loss of bladder or bowel control) and new onset
  R/O: urinary retention with overflow incontinence, cauda equina syndrome, conus medullaris syndrome
- Numbness (loss of sensation) in groin or rectal area
  R/O: cauda equina syndrome, conus medullaris syndrome
- Skin is split open or gaping (length > ½" or 12 mm)
  Reason: may need laceration repair (e.g., sutures)
- Puncture wound of back
  R/O: injury to deeper back structures
- Bleeding and won't stop after 10 minutes of direct pressure (using correct technique)
  R/O: need for sutures
- Sounds like a serious injury to the triager

Go to ED/UCC Now
(or to Office With PCP Approval)
- Weakness of a leg or foot (e.g., unable to bear weight, dragging foot)
  R/O: nerve root compression, herniated disk
- Numbness of a leg or foot (i.e., loss of sensation)
  R/O: nerve root compression, herniated disk

Go to Office Now

- SEVERE pain (e.g., excruciating, unable to do any normal activities)
  R/O: fracture
- Pain radiates into the thigh or further down the leg now
  R/O: sciatica from nerve root compression or herniated disc
- Landed hard on feet or buttocks and pain over spine
  R/O: compression fracture of vertebrae, muscle strain

See Today in Office

- Large swelling or bruise and size > palm of person's hand
  R/O: rib fracture, spinous process fracture, large contusion
- Patient is confused or is an unreliable provider of information (e.g., dementia, profound intellectual disability, alcohol intoxication)
- Patient wants to be seen

See Today or Tomorrow in Office

- Wound and no tetanus booster in > 5 years (or > 10 years for clean cuts)
  Reason: may need a tetanus booster shot (vaccine)
- High-risk adult (e.g., age > 60, osteoporosis, chronic steroid use)
  Reason: greater risk of fracture in patients with osteoporosis
- Suspicious history for the injury
  R/O: domestic violence or elder abuse

See Within 3 Days in Office

- Injury and pain has not improved after 3 days
- Injury is still painful or swollen after 2 weeks

Home Care

- Back swelling, bruise, or pain from direct blow to the back
  R/O: minor back contusion
- Back pain or stiffness from bending or twisting injury
  R/O: minor back strain or sprain

HOME CARE ADVICE

Treatment of a Minor Bruise, Sprain, or Strain

❶ **Reassurance—Bending or Twisting Injury (Strain, Sprain):**
- Strain and sprain are the medical terms used to describe overstretching of the muscles and ligaments of the back. A twisting or bending injury can cause back strain and sprain.
- The main symptom is pain that gets worse with movement.
- *Here is some care advice that should help.*

❷ **Reassurance—Direct Blow (Contusion, Bruise):**
- A direct blow to your back can cause a contusion. Contusion is the medical term for bruise.
- Symptoms are mild pain, swelling, and/or bruising.
- *Here is some care advice that should help.*

❸ **Apply a Cold Pack:**
- Apply a cold pack or an ice bag (wrapped in a moist towel) to the area for 20 minutes. Repeat in 1 hour, then every 4 hours while awake.
- Continue this for the first 48 hours after an injury. *(Reason: to reduce the swelling and pain)*

❹ **Apply Heat to the Area:**
- Beginning 48 hours after an injury, apply a warm washcloth or heating pad for 10 minutes 3 times a day.
- This will help increase blood flow and improve healing.

❺ **Avoid:** Avoid heavy lifting and any sports activities for the first week after an injury.

❻ **Rest Versus Movement:**
- Movement of the back is generally more healing in the long term than rest. Continue normal activities as much as your pain permits.
- Rest should only be used for the first couple days after an injury.

❼ **Call Back If:**
- Severe pain lasts > 2 hours after pain medicine and ice.
- Swelling or bruise becomes > 5" (> size of palm).
- Pain not improving after 3 days.
- Pain or swelling lasts > 7 days.
- You become worse.

Treatment of a Small Cut or Scrape

❶ **Reassurance—Superficial Laceration (Cut or Scratch) or Abrasion (Scrape):**
- This sounds like a small cut or scrape that we can treat at home.
- *Here is some care advice that should help.*

❷ **Bleeding:** Apply direct pressure for 10 minutes with a sterile gauze to stop any bleeding.

❸ **Cleaning the Wound:**
- Wash the wound with soap and water for 5 minutes.
- For any dirt, scrub gently with a washcloth.
- For any bleeding, apply direct pressure with a sterile gauze or clean cloth for 10 minutes.

❹ **Antibiotic Ointment:**
- Apply an antibiotic ointment (e.g., over-the-counter bacitracin), covered by a Band-Aid or dressing. Change daily or if it becomes wet.
- Option: A Telfa dressing won't stick to the wound when it is removed.
- Option: Another option is to use a liquid skin bandage that only needs to be applied once. Don't use antibiotic ointment if you use a liquid skin bandage.

❺ **Liquid Skin Bandage:**
- You can use a liquid skin bandage instead of antibiotic ointment and a dressing or a Band-Aid.
- **Benefits:** Liquid skin bandage has several benefits when compared with a regular bandage (e.g., a dressing or a Band-Aid). You only need to put a liquid bandage on once to minor cuts and scrapes. It helps stop minor bleeding. It seals the wound and may promote faster healing and lower infection rates. However, it also costs more.
- **How to Use It:** First clean and dry the wound. You put on the liquid as spray or with a swab. It dries in < 1 minute and usually lasts a week. You can get it wet.
- **Examples:** Liquid skin bandage is available over the counter. Examples are Band-Aid Liquid Bandage, New Skin, Curad Spray Bandage, and 3M No Sting Liquid Bandage Spray.

❻ **Call Back If:**
- Dirt is still present in the wound after scrubbing.
- Looks infected (pus, redness).
- Doesn't heal within 10 days.
- You become worse.

Over-the-counter Pain Medicines

❶ **Pain Medicines:**
- For pain relief, you can take either acetaminophen, ibuprofen, or naproxen.
- They are over-the-counter (OTC) pain drugs. You can buy them at the drugstore.

Acetaminophen (e.g., Tylenol):
- **Regular Strength Tylenol:** Take 650 mg (two 325 mg pills) by mouth every 4-6 hours as needed. Each Regular Strength Tylenol pill has 325 mg of acetaminophen.
- **Extra Strength Tylenol:** Take 1,000 mg (two 500 mg pills) every 8 hours as needed. Each Extra Strength Tylenol pill has 500 mg of acetaminophen.
- The most you should take each day is 3,000 mg (10 Regular Strength or 6 Extra Strength pills a day).

Ibuprofen (e.g., Motrin, Advil):
- Take 400 mg (two 200 mg pills) by mouth every 6 hours.
- Another choice is to take 600 mg (three 200 mg pills) by mouth every 8 hours.
- The most you should take each day is 1,200 mg (six 200 mg pills), unless your doctor has told you to take more.

Naproxen (e.g., Aleve):
- Take 220 mg (one 220 mg pill) by mouth every 8 hours as needed. You may take 440 mg (two 220 mg pills) for your first dose.
- The most you should take each day is 660 mg (three 220 mg pills a day), unless your doctor has told you to take more.

❷ **Pain Medicines—Extra Notes:**
- Use the lowest amount of medicine that makes your pain better.
- Acetaminophen is thought to be safer than ibuprofen or naproxen in people > 65 years old. Acetaminophen is in many OTC and prescription medicines. It might be in more than one medicine that you are taking. You need to be careful and not take an overdose. An acetaminophen overdose can hurt the liver.

- McNeil, the company that makes Tylenol, has different dosage instructions for Tylenol in Canada and the United States. In Canada, the maximum recommended dose per day is 4,000 mg or 12 Regular Strength (325 mg) pills. In the United States, McNeil recommends a maximum dose of 10 Regular Strength (325 mg) pills.
- CAUTION: Do not take acetaminophen if you have liver disease.
- CAUTION: Do not take ibuprofen or naproxen if you have stomach problems, have kidney disease, are pregnant, or have been told by your doctor to avoid this type of anti-inflammatory drug. Do not take ibuprofen or naproxen for > 7 days without consulting your doctor.
- *Before taking any medicine, read all the instructions on the package.*

❸ **Call Back If:**
  - You have more questions.
  - You become worse.

FIRST AID

First Aid Advice for Bleeding:
Apply direct pressure to the entire wound with a clean cloth.

First Aid Advice for Penetrating Object:
If penetrating object is still in place, don't remove it. *Reason: Removal could increase bleeding.*

First Aid Advice for Shock:
Lie down with the feet elevated.

First Aid Advice for Suspected Spinal Cord Injury:
Do not move until a spine board is applied.

BACKGROUND

Types of Back Injuries
- **Muscle Injuries:** Muscular back injuries are the most commonly seen back injury. Most of these injuries are the result of either muscle bruising (contusion) from a fall or a direct blow to the back or pulled muscles (strain) from sudden twisting, heavy lifting, or overuse.
- **Renal Injuries:** Blows to the lower back, especially if noted in the flank area, can cause kidney injuries.

- **Spinal Cord (T1-S4) Injuries:** Spinal cord injuries from trauma to the thoracolumbar spine are uncommon. This is in contrast to the much larger number of cord injuries seen with neck trauma (C1-C7). Spinal cord compromise in the thoracic and lumbar spine areas is usually incurred when an excessive amount of force results in a vertebral fracture/dislocation or burst fracture.
- **Thoracolumbar Vertebral Fractures:** Most vertebral injuries are compression fractures that heal without intervention and do not cause spinal cord compression.

Use the Back Pain Protocol Instead for Self-induced Back Strain
- Self-induced strained or pulled back muscles is a common cause of back pain in adults.
- The triggering event is carrying something too heavy, lifting from an awkward position, bending too far backward or sideways, or overuse (e.g., gardening, sports, work).
- Self-induced back strain is best handled by the Back Pain protocol on page 48, since there isn't any direct blow, collision, fall, accident, or external force.

What Cuts Need Sutures?
- Any cut that is split open or gaping probably needs sutures (or staples or skin glue).
- Cuts > ½" (1 cm) usually need sutures.
- Any open wound that may need sutures should be evaluated by a physician regardless of the time that has passed since the initial injury.

When Does an Adult Need a Tetanus Booster (Tetanus Shot)?
- **Clean Cuts and Scrapes—Tetanus Booster Needed Every 10 Years:** Patients with clean minor wounds AND who have previously had ≥ 3 tetanus shots (full series) need a booster every 10 years. Examples of minor wounds include a superficial abrasion or a shallow cut from a clean knife blade. Obtain booster within 72 hours.
- **Dirty Wounds—Tetanus Booster Needed Every 5 Years:** Patients with dirty wounds need a booster if it has been > 5 years since the last booster. Examples of dirty wounds include those contaminated with soil, feces, and/or saliva and more serious wounds from deep punctures, crushing, and burns. Obtain booster within 72 hours.

BACK PAIN

Definition
- Complains of upper, mid, or lower back pain that occurs mainly in the midline.
- Not due to a traumatic injury.
- Minor muscle strain and overuse are covered in this protocol. Sciatic pain is also covered.

Pain Severity Scale
- **Mild (1-3):** Doesn't interfere with normal activities.
- **Moderate (4-7):** Interferes with normal activities or awakens from sleep.
- **Severe (8-10):** Excruciating pain, unable to do any normal activities.

Excluded:
- Pain in the back from significant blunt or penetrating trauma should be triaged using the Back Injury protocol on page 44.
- **Pain in the Lower Back in Pregnant Women:** Consider labor.

TRIAGE ASSESSMENT QUESTIONS

Call EMS 911 Now
- Passed out (i.e., fainted, collapsed and was not responding)
  R/O: Ruptured abdominal aortic aneurysm
  First Aid: Lie down with the feet elevated.
- Shock suspected (e.g., cold/pale/clammy skin, too weak to stand)
  R/O: Ruptured abdominal aortic aneurysm
  First Aid: Lie down with the feet elevated.
- Sounds like a life-threatening emergency to the triager

See More Appropriate Protocol
- Major injury to the back (e.g., MVA, fall > 10 feet or 3 m, penetrating injury, etc.)
  Go to Protocol: Back Injury on page 44
- Pain in the upper back over the ribs (rib cage) that radiates (travels) into the chest
  Go to Protocol: Chest Pain on page 73
- Pain in the upper back over the ribs (rib cage) and worsened by coughing (or clearly increases with breathing)
  Go to Protocol: Chest Pain on page 73

Go to ED Now
- SEVERE abdominal pain (e.g., excruciating)
- Abdominal pain and age > 60
  R/O: compression fracture, aortic aneurysm
- Unable to urinate (or only a few drops) and bladder feels very full
  R/O: urinary retention, cauda equina syndrome
- Numbness (loss of sensation) in groin or rectal area

Go to ED/UCC Now
(or to Office With PCP Approval)
- Sudden onset of severe back pain and age > 60
  R/O: compression fracture, aortic aneurysm
- Pain radiates into groin, scrotum
  R/O: kidney stones
- Blood in urine (red, pink, or tea-colored)
- Vomiting and pain over lower ribs of back (i.e., flank—kidney area)
- Weakness of a leg or foot (e.g., unable to bear weight, dragging foot)
  R/O: nerve root impingement or cord compression
- Patient sounds very sick or weak to the triager
  Reason: severe acute illness or serious complication suspected

Go to Office Now
- SEVERE back pain
- Fever > 100.5° F (38.1° C) and flank pain
  R/O: pyelonephritis
- Pain or burning with urination
  R/O: pyelonephritis

See Today in Office
- Can't walk or can barely walk
  R/O: severe back strain, cord compression
- Tingling or numbness in the legs or feet
  R/O: severe back strain, cord compression
- High-risk adult (e.g., history of cancer, history of HIV, or history of IV drug abuse)
  R/O: metastasis, epidural abscess
- Painful rash with multiple small blisters grouped together (i.e., dermatomal distribution or "band" or "stripe")
  R/O: herpes zoster (shingles)
- Pain radiates into the thigh or further down the leg, and in both legs
  Reason: bilateral sciatica carries higher risk

See Today or Tomorrow in Office

- Pain radiates into the thigh or further down the leg
  R/O: sciatica
- Age > 50 and no history of prior similar back pain
  Reason: higher risk of serious medical cause
- Patient wants to be seen

See Within 2 Weeks in Office

- Back pain persists > 2 weeks
- Back pain is a chronic symptom (recurrent or ongoing AND lasting > 4 weeks)

Home Care

- ○ Back pain
  R/O: muscle strain, overuse
- ○ Caused by a twisting, bending, or lifting injury
  R/O: muscle strain, overuse
- ○ Caused by overuse from recent vigorous activity (e.g., exercise, gardening, lifting and carrying, sports)
  R/O: muscle strain, overuse
- ○ Preventing back strain, questions about

HOME CARE ADVICE

Back Pain

❶ Reassurance:
- Twisting or heavy lifting can cause back pain. It can also occur after unnoticed minor back injuries
- With treatment, the pain most often goes away in 1-2 weeks.
- You can treat most back pain at home.
- *Here is some care advice that should help.*

❷ Cold or Heat:
- **Cold Pack:** For pain or swelling, use a cold pack or ice wrapped in a wet cloth. Put it on the sore area for 20 minutes. Repeat 4 times on the first day, then as needed.
- **Heat Pack:** If pain lasts > 2 days, apply heat to the sore area. Use a heat pack, heating pad, or warm, wet washcloth. Do this for 10 minutes, then as needed. For widespread stiffness, take a hot bath or hot shower instead. Move the sore area under the warm water.

❸ Sleep:
- Sleep on your side with a pillow between your knees. If you sleep on your back, put a pillow under your knees.
- Avoid sleeping on your stomach.
- Your mattress should be firm. Avoid waterbeds.

❹ Activity:
- Keep doing your day-to-day activities if it is not too painful. Staying active is better than resting.
- Avoid anything that makes your pain worse. Avoid heavy lifting, twisting, and too much exercise until your back heals.
- You do not need to stay in bed.

❺ Pain Medicines:
- For pain relief, you can take either acetaminophen, ibuprofen, or naproxen.
- They are over-the-counter (OTC) pain drugs. You can buy them at the drugstore.

Acetaminophen (e.g., Tylenol):
- **Regular Strength Tylenol:** Take 650 mg (two 325 mg pills) by mouth every 4-6 hours as needed. Each Regular Strength Tylenol pill has 325 mg of acetaminophen.
- **Extra Strength Tylenol:** Take 1,000 mg (two 500 mg pills) every 8 hours as needed. Each Extra Strength Tylenol pill has 500 mg of acetaminophen.
- The most you should take each day is 3,000 mg (10 Regular Strength or 6 Extra Strength pills a day).

Ibuprofen (e.g., Motrin, Advil):
- Take 400 mg (two 200 mg pills) by mouth every 6 hours.
- Another choice is to take 600 mg (three 200 mg pills) by mouth every 8 hours.
- The most you should take each day is 1,200 mg (six 200 mg pills), unless your doctor has told you to take more.

Naproxen (e.g., Aleve):
- Take 220 mg (one 220 mg pill) by mouth every 8 hours as needed. You may take 440 mg (two 220 mg pills) for your first dose.
- The most you should take each day is 660 mg (three 220 mg pills a day), unless your doctor has told you to take more.

❻ **Pain Medicines—Extra Notes:**
- Use the lowest amount of medicine that makes your pain better.
- Acetaminophen is thought to be safer than ibuprofen or naproxen in people > 65 years old. Acetaminophen is in many OTC and prescription medicines. It might be in more than one medicine that you are taking. You need to be careful and not take an overdose. An acetaminophen overdose can hurt the liver.
- McNeil, the company that makes Tylenol, has different dosage instructions for Tylenol in Canada and the United States. In Canada, the maximum recommended dose per day is 4,000 mg or 12 Regular Strength (325 mg) pills. In the United States, McNeil recommends a maximum dose of 10 Regular Strength (325 mg) pills.
- CAUTION: Do not take acetaminophen if you have liver disease.
- CAUTION: Do not take ibuprofen or naproxen if you have stomach problems, have kidney disease, are pregnant, or have been told by your doctor to avoid this type of anti-inflammatory drug. Do not take ibuprofen or naproxen for > 7 days without consulting your doctor.
- *Before taking any medicine, read all the instructions on the package.*

❼ **Call Back If:**
- Numbness or weakness occur.
- Bowel/bladder problems occur.
- Pain lasts for > 2 weeks.
- You become worse.

Preventing Back Strain

❶ **Prevention:**
- The only way to prevent future backaches is to keep your back muscles in excellent physical condition.
- A sedentary lifestyle (lack of exercise) is a risk factor for developing back pain.
- Walking, stationary biking, and swimming provide good aerobic conditioning as well as exercise for your back.
- Being overweight puts more weight on the spine and thus increases the risk of back pain. If you are overweight, work with your doctor to develop a weight-loss program.

❷ **Good Body Mechanics:**
- **Lifting:** Stand close to the object to be lifted. Keep your back straight and lift by bending your legs. Ask for lifting help if needed.
- **Sleeping:** Sleep on a firm mattress.
- **Sitting:** Avoid sitting for long periods without a break. Avoid slouching. Place a pillow or towel behind your lower back for support.
- **Posture:** Maintain good posture.

❸ **Strengthening Exercises:**
- During the first couple days after an injury, strengthening exercises should be avoided. The following exercises can help strengthen the back. Perform the following exercises 3-10 times each day, for 5-10 seconds each time:
- **Bent Knee Sit-ups:** Lay on back, curl forward lifting shoulders about 6" (15 cm) off the floor.
- **Leg Lifts:** Lay on back, lift foot 6" (15 cm) off floor (one leg at a time).
- **Pelvic Tilt:** Lay on back with knees bent, push lower back against floor.
- **Chest Lift:** Lie face down on ground, place arms by your sides, lift shoulders off the floor.

❹ **Call Back If:**
- You have more questions.
- You become worse.

FIRST AID

First Aid Advice for Shock:

Lie down with the feet elevated.

BACKGROUND

Key Points

- Lower back pain is a cause of countless visits to physicians' offices and EDs. It is the second most common cause of lost workdays, after cold and flu symptoms. More than 80% of people at some point in their lives have lower back pain.
- However, there is some good news. In most cases, the back pain is not serious and it has a self-limited course. Pain subsides within 4-6 weeks in 90% of individuals experiencing acute low back pain.

Four Categories of Back Pain

- **Potentially Serious:** Examples include abdominal aortic aneurysm, neoplasm, osteomyelitis, epidural abscess, vertebral fracture, and neurologic emergencies (e.g., cauda equina syndrome).
- **Sciatica** (back pain with neurologic symptoms): There is radiation of the back pain (or buttock pain) into a lower extremity suggesting lumbosacral nerve root compression. There may be associated leg weakness, numbness, or paresthesia.
- **Nonspecific Back Pain:** No neurologic symptoms. Examples include lumbar strain/sprain, degenerative osteoarthritis, lumbar disc disease, and fibromyalgia.
- **Referred Back Pain:** There are gastrointestinal causes like pancreatitis, biliary colic, and posterior gastric ulcer; genitourinary causes like renal colic, pyelonephritis, endometriosis, and ovarian cyst.

Lumbar Strain

- Acute lower back pain in the 18- to 50-year-old age group is usually a symptom of strain of some of the 200 muscles in the back that allow us to stand upright.
- Often the triggering event is carrying something too heavy, lifting from an awkward position, bending too far backward or sideways, or overuse.
- Individuals with strained back muscles often note that the pain is increased by bending or twisting movements, relieved by assuming certain positions, and that the back muscles are tender.

Degenerative Osteoarthritis

- Degenerative osteoarthritis is a common cause of back pain in the elderly population.
- In uncomplicated osteoarthritis, individuals will complain of chronic midline back discomfort. Frequently, there is morning stiffness that improves as the day progresses.

Bed Rest and Overtreatment

- Complete bed rest is inconvenient and unnecessary in the majority of patients, including those who need to be examined by the physician. Complete bed rest should never be recommended over the telephone.
- Research has demonstrated that continuing ordinary activities within the limits permitted by pain results in a speedier recovery than rest (Malmivaara).

BEE STING

Definition
- Stung by a honeybee, bumblebee, hornet, wasp, or yellow jacket

Three Types of Reactions
- **Local Reaction:** Localized pain, swelling, itching, and mild redness at stinger site.
- **Toxic Reaction:** History of multiple stings; larger venom dose; systemic symptoms include light-headedness, vomiting, diarrhea.
- **Anaphylactic Reaction:** Severe life-threatening allergic reaction to sting.

TRIAGE ASSESSMENT QUESTIONS

Call EMS 911 Now
- Passed out (i.e., fainted, collapsed and was not responding)
  R/O: anaphylaxis
  Use First Aid Advice for anaphylaxis.
- Wheezing or difficulty breathing
  R/O: anaphylaxis
  Use First Aid Advice for anaphylaxis.
- Hoarseness, cough, or tightness in the throat or chest
  R/O: anaphylaxis
  Use First Aid Advice for anaphylaxis.
- Swollen tongue or difficulty swallowing
  R/O: anaphylaxis
  Use First Aid Advice for anaphylaxis.
- Life-threatening reaction in past to sting (anaphylaxis) and < 2 hours since sting
  Note: Anaphylaxis usually starts within 20 minutes and always by 2 hours following a sting.
- Sounds like a life-threatening emergency to the triager

See More Appropriate Protocol
- Not a bee, wasp, hornet, or yellow jacket sting
  Go to Protocol: Insect Bite on page 257

Go to ED/UCC Now
(or to Office With PCP Approval)
- Widespread hives, itching, or facial swelling and started within 2 hours of sting
  R/O: allergic reaction
  Note: No history of life-threatening reaction and no current anaphylactic symptoms.
- Vomiting or abdominal cramps and started within 2 hours of sting
  R/O: allergic reaction
  Note: No history of life-threatening reaction and no current anaphylactic symptoms.
- Gave epinephrine shot and no symptoms now
  R/O: biphasic reaction; may need oral steroids
- Patient sounds very sick or weak to the triager
  Reason: severe acute illness or serious complication suspected

Go to Office Now
- Sting inside the mouth
  R/O: swelling of the airway
- Sting on eyeball (e.g., cornea)
  R/O: corneal scar
- More than 50 stings
  Reason: risk for systemic toxic reaction from a large dose of venom
- Fever and area is red
  R/O: cellulitis, lymphangitis
  Reason: fever and looks infected
- Fever and area is very tender to touch
  R/O: cellulitis, lymphangitis
  Reason: fever and looks infected
  Note: Skin infection after a sting is uncommon.
- Red streak or red line and length > 2" (5 cm)
  R/O: lymphangitis
  Note: Lymphangitis looks like a red streak or line originating at the wound and ascending the arm or leg toward the heart. Skin infection is uncommon after a sting.

See Today in Office

- Red or very tender (to touch) area, and started
  > 24 hours after the sting
  R/O: cellulitis
  *Note: Cellulitis is uncommon after a sting. Any redness
  starting in the first 24 hours is just due to the sting venom.*
- Red or very tender (to touch) area, getting larger
  > 48 hours after the sting
  R/O: cellulitis, but probably due to venom
  Note: Cellulitis is uncommon after a sting.
- Swelling is huge (e.g., > 4" or 10 cm, spreads beyond
  wrist or ankle)
  *R/O: cellulitis, but more likely is large local reaction
  to venom*
- Patient wants to be seen

See Within 3 Days in Office

- Widespread hives, itching, or facial swelling and
  started > 2 hours after sting
  R/O: allergic reaction
  *Note: No history of life-threatening reaction and no
  anaphylactic symptoms.*
- Scab drains pus or increases in size, and not improved
  after applying antibiotic ointment for 2 days
  R/O: infected sore, impetigo

Home Care

- ○ Normal local reaction to bee, wasp, or yellow
  jacket sting
- ○ Scab drains pus or increases in size
  R/O: infected sore, impetigo

HOME CARE ADVICE

General Care Advice for Bee, Wasp, or Yellow Jacket Sting

❶ **Try to Remove the Stinger** (if present):
- The stinger looks like a tiny black dot in the sting.
- There are several different methods of removal.
  Removing the stinger quickly is more important
  than how you remove it.
- Use a fingernail, credit card edge, or knife-edge
  to scrape it off. Don't pull it out.
  (Reason: squeezes out more venom)
  If the stinger is below the skin surface, leave it alone.
  It will be shed with normal skin healing.
- In many cases no stinger will be present. Only bees
  leave their stingers. Wasps, yellow jackets, and
  hornets do not.

❷ **Apply Cold to the Area for Pain—
Cold Pack Method:**
- Wrap a bag of ice in a towel (or use a bag of
  frozen vegetables such as peas).
- Apply this cold pack to the area of the sting for
  10-20 minutes.
- You may repeat this as needed, to relieve
  symptoms of pain and swelling.

❸ **Pain Medicines:**
- For pain relief, you can take either acetaminophen,
  ibuprofen, or naproxen.
- They are over-the-counter (OTC) pain drugs.
  You can buy them at the drugstore.

Acetaminophen (e.g., Tylenol):
- **Regular Strength Tylenol:** Take 650 mg
  (two 325 mg pills) by mouth every 4-6 hours
  as needed. Each Regular Strength Tylenol pill
  has 325 mg of acetaminophen.
- **Extra Strength Tylenol:** Take 1,000 mg (two 500 mg
  pills) every 8 hours as needed. Each Extra Strength
  Tylenol pill has 500 mg of acetaminophen.
- The most you should take each day is 3,000 mg
  (10 Regular Strength or 6 Extra Strength pills a day).

Ibuprofen (e.g., Motrin, Advil):
- Take 400 mg (two 200 mg pills) by mouth every
  6 hours.
- Another choice is to take 600 mg (three 200 mg
  pills) by mouth every 8 hours.
- The most you should take each day is 1,200 mg
  (six 200 mg pills), unless your doctor has told
  you to take more.

Naproxen (e.g., Aleve):
- Take 220 mg (one 220 mg pill) by mouth every
  8 hours as needed. You may take 440 mg
  (two 220 mg pills) for your first dose.
- The most you should take each day is 660 mg
  (three 220 mg pills a day), unless your doctor
  has told you to take more.

❹ **Pain Medicines—Extra Notes:**
- Use the lowest amount of medicine that makes
  your pain better.
- Acetaminophen is thought to be safer than
  ibuprofen or naproxen in people > 65 years old.
  Acetaminophen is in many OTC and prescription
  medicines. It might be in more than one medicine
  that you are taking. You need to be careful and
  not take an overdose. An acetaminophen
  overdose can hurt the liver.

- McNeil, the company that makes Tylenol, has different dosage instructions for Tylenol in Canada and the United States. In Canada, the maximum recommended dose per day is 4,000 mg or 12 Regular Strength (325 mg) pills. In the United States, McNeil recommends a maximum dose of 10 Regular Strength (325 mg) pills.
- CAUTION: Do not take acetaminophen if you have liver disease.
- CAUTION: Do not take ibuprofen or naproxen if you have stomach problems, have kidney disease, are pregnant, or have been told by your doctor to avoid this type of anti-inflammatory drug. Do not take ibuprofen or naproxen for > 7 days without consulting your doctor.
- *Before taking any medicine, read all the instructions on the package.*

❺ **Hydrocortisone Cream for Itching:**
- Put 1% hydrocortisone cream on the sting 3 times a day. Use it for a couple days, until it feels better. This will help decrease the itching.
- This is an over-the-counter (OTC) drug. You can buy it at the drugstore.
- Some people like to keep the cream in the refrigerator. It feels even better if the cream is used when it is cold.
- CAUTION: Do not use hydrocortisone cream for > 1 week without talking to your doctor.
- *Read the instructions and warnings on the package insert for all medicines you take.*

❻ **Antihistamine Medicines for Itching:**
- If the sting becomes very itchy, you can take **diphenhydramine** (e.g., Benadryl). The adult dosage is 25-50 mg by mouth every 6 hours on an as-needed basis.
- **Loratadine** is a newer (second-generation) antihistamine. The dosage of loratadine (e.g., OTC Claritin, Alavert) is 10 mg once a day.
- **Cetirizine** is a newer (second-generation) antihistamine. The dosage of cetirizine (e.g., OTC Zyrtec) is 10 mg once a day.
- CAUTION: Antihistamines may cause sleepiness. Do not drink, drive, or operate dangerous machinery while taking antihistamines. Do not take antihistamines if you have prostate problems.

- Loratadine and cetirizine cause less sleepiness than diphenhydramine (Benadryl) or chlorpheniramine (Chlor-Trimeton, Chlor-Tripolon).
- *Before taking any medicine, read all the instructions on the package.*

❼ **Expected Course:**
- **Pain:** Severe pain or burning at the site lasts 1-2 hours. Pain after this period is usually minimal. Itching often follows the pain.
- **Redness and Swelling:** Normal redness and swelling from the venom can increase for 24 hours following the sting. Redness at the sting site is normal. It doesn't mean that it is infected. The redness can last 3 days and the swelling 7 days.
- Stings only rarely get infected.

❽ **Call Back If:**
- Difficulty breathing or swallowing (generally develops within the first 2 hours after the sting; call EMS 911).
- Swelling becomes huge.
- Sting begins to look infected.
- You become worse.

Preventing Stings
❶ **Some Outdoor Activity Tips**
- Wear long-sleeved shirts, long pants, and shoes when you are in grassy areas or outdoors and exposed to stinging insects.
- Avoid using perfumes and hair sprays; these attract insects.
- Wear dark or drab-colored clothes rather than bright colors.
- Take special care when eating or preparing food outdoors. These odors can attract insects (especially yellow jackets).

Tetanus Vaccination and Stings
❶ **Getting a Tetanus Booster:**
- Tetanus vaccination (booster) after a bee sting is not necessary.
- However, if it has been > 10 years since your last tetanus vaccination, it is appropriate from a preventive health care standpoint to obtain a vaccination (i.e., Td or Tdap) sometime in the next couple weeks.

Infected Sore or Scab

❶ Reassurance:
- Sometimes a small infected sore can develop at the site of a cut, scratch, insect bite, or sting.
- The typical appearance is a sore < 1" (2.5 cm) in diameter. It is often covered by a soft, "honey-yellow" or yellow-brown crust or scab. Sometimes the scab may drain a tiny amount of pus or yellow fluid. Usually there is minimal to no pain.
- Small infected sores usually get better with regular cleansing and use of an antibiotic ointment.
- *Here is some care advice that should help.*

❷ Cleaning:
- Wash the area 2-3 times daily with an antibacterial soap and warm water.
- Gently remove any scab. The bacteria live underneath the scab. You may need to soak the scab off by placing a warm, wet washcloth (or gauze) on the sore for 10 minutes.

❸ Antibiotic Ointment:
- Apply an antibiotic ointment 3 times per day.
- Cover the sore with a Band-Aid to prevent scratching and spread.
- Use bacitracin ointment (over the counter in United States) or Polysporin ointment (over the counter in Canada) or one that you already have.

❹ Avoid Picking: Avoid scratching and picking. This can spread a skin infection.

❺ Contagiousness:
- Infected sores can be contagious by skin-to-skin contact.
- Wash your hands frequently and avoid touching the sore.
- **Work and School:** You can attend school or work if the sore is covered.
- **Contact Sports:** Generally, you need to receive antibiotic treatment for 3 days before you can return to the sport. There can be no pus or drainage. You should check with your trainer, if there is one for your sports team.

❻ Expected Course:
- The sore should stop growing in 1-2 days and it should begin improving within 2-3 days.
- The sore should be completely healed in 7-10 days.

❼ Call Back If:
- Fever occurs.
- Spreading redness or a red streak occurs.
- Sore increases in size.
- Sore not improving after 2 days using antibiotic ointment.
- Sore not completely healed in 7 days (1 week).
- New sore appears.
- You become worse.

FIRST AID

First Aid Advice for Minor Bee Sting
(localized symptoms only):
Apply a cold pack to the area of the sting for 10-20 minutes.

First Aid Advice for Anaphylaxis—Epinephrine:
- If the patient has an epinephrine autoinjector, **give it now.** Do not delay.
- Use the autoinjector on the upper outer thigh. You may give it through clothing if necessary.
- Give epinephrine first, then call 911.
- Epinephrine is available in autoinjectors under trade names: EpiPen, EpiPen Jr, and Auvi-Q (Allerject in Canada). Auvi-Q has an audio chip and talks patients and caregivers through injection process.
- You may give a second (repeat) dose of epinephrine 10-15 minutes later, IF the person with anaphylaxis does not respond to the first dose AND ambulance arrival takes > 10 minutes.

First Aid Advice for Anaphylaxis—Benadryl:
- Give antihistamine by mouth **NOW** if able to swallow.
- Use Benadryl (diphenhydramine; adult dose: 50 mg) or any other available antihistamine medicine.

First Aid Advice for Anaphylactic Shock
(pending EMS arrival):
Lie down with the feet elevated.

BACKGROUND

Key Points
- *Hymenoptera* is the scientific name for the class/order of venomous insects that includes bees, wasps, hornets, and yellow jackets.
- More than 95% of stings are from honeybees or yellow jackets.
- Tetanus vaccination after a bee sting is not necessary.
- A person who accidentally injects epinephrine (eg, an EpiPen) into the hand, finger, foot, or toe should be directed to call the Poison Center. Most cases do not need treatment. Still, there is a potential concern for ischemia of the finger or toe.

Types

There are 3 types of reactions:
- Local reaction
- Systemic (toxic) reaction
- Anaphylactic reaction

Local Reaction

- The stinger injects venom into the skin; it is the venom that causes the pain and other symptoms. The main symptoms are localized pain, swelling, itching, and mild redness at the sting site.
- **Pain:** Severe pain or burning at the site lasts 1-2 hours. Itching often follows the pain.
- **Swelling:** Normal swelling can increase for 24 hours following the sting. Stings of the upper face can cause marked swelling around the eye, but this is harmless.
- **Redness:** Bee stings can normally become red. That doesn't mean they are infected. Infections rarely occur in stings.
- **Expected Course:** The redness can last 3 days and the swelling 7 days.

Systemic (Toxic) Reaction From a Large Number of Stings

- Nonallergic systemic reactions occur with a minimum of 50 stings in adults. Betten 2005 recommends that any adult with > 50 stings be observed in a medical setting for 24 hours for signs of delayed venom toxicity. He suggests a rule of 1 sting per kg for children.
- Symptoms of a large number of stings include vomiting and diarrhea developing within 8 hours of the stings. This venom reaction can progress over 24 hours to hemolysis, rhabdomyolysis (muscle breakdown), and renal failure.
- Death from massive envenomation occurs mainly in adults with > 500 stings. It has been estimated that the median lethal dose of honeybee venom is 500-1,400 stings in an adult (who is not allergic to bee stings).

Anaphylactic Reaction

- Anaphylactic reactions to *Hymenoptera* stings occur in 0.4% of patients.
- Generally, the shorter the interval between the sting and the first onset of systemic symptom, the more serious the reaction will be. Anaphylaxis usually starts within 20 minutes and almost always by 2 hours. If no symptoms occur by 2 hours, the risk for anaphylaxis is minimal.

- Systemic symptoms include: wheezing, hypotension, shock, generalized urticaria, and abdominal cramping.

Preventing Stings: Some Outdoor Activity Tips

- Wear long-sleeved shirts, long pants, and shoes when you are in grassy areas or outdoors and exposed to stinging insects.
- Avoid using perfumes and hair sprays; these attract insects.
- Wear dark or drab-colored clothes rather than bright colors.
- Take special care when eating or preparing food outdoors. These odors can attract insects (especially yellow jackets).

Removing the Stinger

- The stingers on wasps, hornets, and yellow jackets do not detach, and, thus, they are able to sting multiple times.
- Honeybees are capable of stinging only once because they have tiny barbs on their stingers that get embedded in the skin. After stinging, the stinger apparatus detaches from the bee's body and the bee dies.
  Therefore, it is only with honeybee stings that there is a stinger that sometimes needs to be removed.
- There are several different methods of removal. Removing the stinger quickly is more important than the type of removal used (Visscher). The patient can grab it with his fingers, scrape it out with a credit card, or use adhesive tape (e.g., Scotch tape).

Home Remedy—Meat Tenderizer Solution

- **Background:** Meat tenderizer is a home remedy that some people use to treat a bee sting. There is no research that has shown that it works or does not work. Many Web sites list it as a possible treatment.
- **Why It Might Work:** Meat tenderizer contains papain. Papain is an enzyme that can break down (deactivate) proteins. Theoretically, it might be able to break down bee and wasp venom.
- **How to Use It:** Make a paste with meat tenderizer and water. Put it on the sting. Wipe it off after a few minutes.
- **Avoid:** Do not use it near the eye.

BREATHING DIFFICULTY

Definition
- Difficult or labored breathing
- Also known as respiratory distress or shortness of breath (SOB)

Severity
- **Mild:** No SOB at rest, mild SOB with walking, speaks normally in sentences, can lie down, no retractions, pulse < 100.
- **Moderate:** SOB at rest, SOB with minimal exertion and prefers to sit, cannot lie down flat, speaks in phrases, mild retractions, audible wheezing, pulse 100-120.
- **Severe:** Very SOB at rest, speaks in single words, struggling to breathe, sitting hunched forward, retractions, pulse > 120.

Excluded:
- Difficulty breathing because of a stuffy nose should be triaged using the Common Cold protocol on page 79 or the Sinus Pain and Congestion protocol on page 352.

TRIAGE ASSESSMENT QUESTIONS

Call EMS 911 Now
- Breathing stopped and hasn't returned
  First Aid: Begin mouth-to-mouth breathing.
- Choking on something
  First Aid: If breathing stopped, quickly discuss the abdominal thrust maneuver (Heimlich).
- SEVERE difficulty breathing (e.g., struggling for each breath, speaks in single words, pulse > 120)
  R/O: respiratory failure, hypoxia
- Bluish (or gray) lips or face
  R/O: cyanosis and need for oxygen
- Difficult to awaken or acting confused (e.g., disoriented, slurred speech)
  R/O: hypoxia, hypercapnia
- Passed out (i.e., fainted, collapsed and was not responding)
  R/O: anaphylaxis, severe hypoxia or cough syncope
- Wheezing started suddenly after medicine, an allergic food, or bee sting
  R/O: anaphylaxis
- Stridor
  R/O: upper airway obstruction

- Slow, shallow, and weak breathing
  R/O: impending respiratory arrest
- Sounds like a life-threatening emergency to the triager

See More Appropriate Protocol
- Chest pain
  Go to Protocol: Chest Pain on page 73
- Wheezing (high-pitched whistling sound) and previous asthma attacks or use of asthma medicines
  Go to Protocol: Asthma Attack on page 38
- Difficulty breathing and only present when coughing
  Go to Protocol: Cough on page 95
- Difficulty breathing and only from stuffy or runny nose
  Go to Protocol: Common Cold on page 79

Go to ED Now
- MODERATE difficulty breathing (e.g., speaks in phrases, SOB even at rest, pulse 100-120) of new onset or worse than normal
- Wheezing can be heard across the room
- Drooling or spitting out saliva (because can't swallow)
  R/O: epiglottitis, severe tonsillopharyngitis
- Any history of prior "blood clot" in leg or lungs
  Note: A "blood clot" typically would have required treatment with heparin or coumadin.
  Reason: increased risk of thromboembolism
  R/O: deep vein thrombosis
- Recent illness requiring prolonged bed rest (i.e., immobilization)
  R/O: pulmonary embolus
- Hip or leg fracture in past 2 months (e.g., had cast on leg or ankle)
  R/O: pulmonary embolus
- Major surgery in the past month
  R/O: pulmonary embolus
- Recent long-distance travel with prolonged time in car, bus, plane, or train (i.e., within past 2 weeks; ≥ 6 hours' duration)
  Reason: immobilization during prolonged travel increases risk of pulmonary embolus
- Extra heartbeats OR irregular heart beating (i.e., "palpitations")
  R/O: dysrhythmia

Go to ED/UCC Now
(or to Office With PCP Approval)

- Fever > 103° F (39.4° C)
  R/O: pneumonia
- Fever > 100.5° F (38.1° C) and > 60 years of age
  R/O: pneumonia
- Fever > 100.0° F (37.8° C) and bedridden
  (e.g., nursing home patient, stroke, chronic
  illness, recovering from surgery)
  R/O: pneumonia
  Note: May need ambulance transport to ED.
- Fever > 100.0° F (37.8° C) and diabetes mellitus or
  weak immune system (e.g., HIV positive, cancer
  chemotherapy, splenectomy, organ transplant,
  chronic steroids)
  R/O: pneumonia
- Periods where breathing stops and then resumes
  normally and bedridden (e.g., nursing home
  patient, CVA)
  R/O: Cheyne-Stokes
- Pregnant or postpartum (< 1 month since delivery)
  R/O: pulmonary embolus
- Patient sounds very sick or weak to the triager
  *Reason: severe acute illness or serious complication
  suspected*

Go to Office Now

- MILD difficulty breathing (e.g., minimal/no SOB at
  rest, SOB with walking, pulse < 100) of new onset
  or worse than normal
- Long-standing difficulty breathing (e.g., CHF, COPD,
  emphysema) and worse than normal
  R/O: worsening CHF or COPD
- Long-standing difficulty breathing and not
  responding to usual therapy
  R/O: worsening CHF or COPD
- Continuous (nonstop) coughing
- Patient wants to be seen

See Within 3 Days in Office

- MODERATE long-standing difficulty breathing
  (e.g., speaks in phrases, SOB even at rest, pulse
  100-120) and same as normal
  *R/O: stable COPD, emphysema, CHF, or other chronic
  lung disease*

See Within 2 Weeks in Office

- MILD long-standing difficulty breathing (e.g., speaks
  in phrases, SOB even at rest, pulse 100-120) and
  same as normal
  *R/O: stable COPD, emphysema, CHF, or other chronic
  lung disease*

HOME CARE ADVICE

❶ **General Care Advice for Breathing Difficulty:**
- Find position of greatest comfort. For most
  patients the best position is semi-upright
  (e.g., sitting up in a comfortable chair or
  lying back against pillows).
- Elevate head of bed (e.g., use pillows or place
  blocks under bed).
- Avoid smoke or fume exposure.
- Create a draft (e.g., use a fan directed at the face,
  open a window).
- Keep room temperature slightly on the cool side.
- Limit activities or space activities apart during the
  day. Prioritize activities.
- Use a humidifier.

❷ **Fever Medicines:**
- For fevers > 101° F (38.3° C) take either
  acetaminophen or ibuprofen.
- They are over-the-counter (OTC) drugs that help
  treat both fever and pain. You can buy them at
  the drugstore.
- The goal of fever therapy is to bring the fever
  down to a comfortable level. Remember that fever
  medicine usually lowers fever 2° F (1–1½° C).

Acetaminophen (e.g., Tylenol):
- **Regular Strength Tylenol:** Take 650 mg
  (two 325 mg pills) by mouth every 4-6 hours
  as needed. Each Regular Strength Tylenol pill
  has 325 mg of acetaminophen.
- **Extra Strength Tylenol:** Take 1,000 mg
  (two 500 mg pills) every 8 hours as needed.
  Each Extra Strength Tylenol pill has 500 mg
  of acetaminophen.
- The most you should take each day is 3,000 mg
  (10 Regular Strength or 6 Extra Strength pills
  a day).

Ibuprofen (e.g., Motrin, Advil):
- Take 400 mg (two 200 mg pills) by mouth every 6 hours.
- Another choice is to take 600 mg (three 200 mg pills) by mouth every 8 hours.
- The most you should take each day is 1,200 mg (six 200 mg pills), unless your doctor has told you to take more.

❸ **Fever Medicines—Extra Notes:**
- Use the lowest amount of medicine that makes your fever better.
- Acetaminophen is thought to be safer than ibuprofen or naproxen in people > 65 years old. Acetaminophen is in many OTC and prescription medicines. It might be in more than one medicine that you are taking. You need to be careful and not take an overdose. An acetaminophen overdose can hurt the liver.
- McNeil, the company that makes Tylenol, has different dosage instructions for Tylenol in Canada and the United States. In Canada, the maximum recommended dose per day is 4,000 mg or 12 Regular Strength (325 mg) pills. In the United States, McNeil recommends a maximum dose of 10 Regular Strength (325 mg) pills.
- CAUTION: Do not take acetaminophen if you have liver disease.
- CAUTION: Do not take ibuprofen if you have stomach problems, have kidney disease, are pregnant, or have been told by your doctor to avoid this type of anti-inflammatory drug. Do not take ibuprofen for > 7 days without consulting your doctor.
- *Before taking any medicine, read all the instructions on the package.*

❹ **Call Back If:**
- Severe difficulty breathing occurs.
- Fever > 100.5° F (38.1° C).
- You become worse.

FIRST AID

First Aid Advice for Breathing Stopped or Cardiac Arrest

Hands-Only CPR
- Call 911.
- Push hard and fast on the center of the chest.

Special Notes:
- **High-quality CPR:** Rescuers should push hard to a depth of at least 2" (5 cm), at a rate of at least 100 compressions per minute; allow full chest recoil; and minimize interruptions in chest compressions. The disco song "Stayin' Alive" has the right beat for CPR.
- The American Heart Association (AHA) provides a 1-minute instructional video on Hands-Only CPR at: http://handsonlycpr.org. Be prepared. Watch it now, before you need it!
- Answers to frequently asked questions about Hands-Only CPR are available at: www.heart.org/HEARTORG/CPRAndECC/HandsOnlyCPR/LearnMore/Learn-More_UCM_440810_FAQ.jsp.
- You are strongly encouraged to get training in CPR from the American Red Cross or the AHA.
- Hands-Only CPR is a trademark of the AHA.

"All rescuers, regardless of training, should provide chest compressions to all cardiac arrest victims. Because of their importance, chest compressions should be the initial CPR action for all victims regardless of age. Rescuers who are able should add ventilations to chest compressions. Highly trained rescuers working together should coordinate their care and perform chest compressions as well as ventilations in a team-based approach." Source: 2010 AHA Guidelines for Cardiopulmonary Resuscitation and Emergency Cardiovascular Care

CPR by Trained Rescuers
Trained (confident) rescuers should add ventilations to chest compressions while waiting for paramedics to arrive:
- Call 911.
- Perform chest compressions and mouth-to-mouth breathing in cycles of 30 compressions and then 2 breaths.

Special Notes:
- Rescuers should push hard to a depth of at least 2" (5 cm), at a rate of at least 100 compressions per minute; allow full chest recoil; and minimize interruptions in chest compressions.

First Aid Advice for Anaphylaxis—Epinephrine:
- If the patient has an epinephrine autoinjector, **give it now.** Do not delay.
- Use the autoinjector on the upper outer thigh. You may give it through clothing if necessary.
- Give epinephrine first, then call 911.
- Epinephrine is available in autoinjectors under trade names: EpiPen, EpiPen Jr, and Auvi-Q (Allerject in Canada). Auvi-Q has an audio chip and talks patients and caregivers through injection process.
- You may give a second (repeat) dose of epinephrine 10-15 minutes later, IF the person with anaphylaxis does not respond to the first dose AND ambulance arrival takes > 10 minutes.

First Aid Advice for Anaphylaxis—Benadryl:
- Give antihistamine by mouth **NOW** if able to swallow.
- Use Benadryl (diphenhydramine; adult dose: 50 mg) or any other available antihistamine medicine.

First Aid Advice for Choking
IF COUGHING AND BREATHING, encourage coughing.
❶ As long as the adult is breathing and coughing, just encourage him/her to cough the material up by himself/herself.
   (Reason: The cough reflex can usually clear the windpipe.)
❷ Don't offer anything to drink.
   (Reason: Fluids take up space needed for air passage.)

IF BREATHING STOPS, perform ABDOMINAL THRUST (Heimlich) maneuver.
❶ If the adult can't breathe, cough, or make a sound, proceed with high abdominal thrusts.
❷ Grasp the adult from behind, just below the lower ribs but above the navel, in bear hug fashion. Make a fist with one hand and fold the other hand over it.
❸ Give a sudden upward and backward jerk (at a 45° angle) to try to squeeze all the air out of the chest and pop the lodged object out of the windpipe.

❹ Repeat this upward abdominal thrust 10 times in rapid succession, until the object comes out. If the adult is too heavy for you to suspend from your arms, lay him on his back on the floor. Put your hands on both sides of the abdomen, just below the ribs, and apply sudden, strong bursts of upward pressure.

IF THE ADULT PASSES OUT, give mouth-to-mouth breathing.
❶ Quickly open the mouth and look inside to see if there is any object that can be removed with a sweep of your finger (usually there is not). Avoid "blind" sweeps.
❷ Then begin resuscitation. Air can usually be forced past the foreign object temporarily until help arrives.
❸ If mouth-to-mouth breathing doesn't move the chest, repeat the abdominal thrusts or chest compressions.

BACKGROUND

Key Points
- Some adults with long-standing cardiopulmonary disorders have chronic dyspnea. Such patients generally can be evaluated in the office setting on a nonurgent basis, if current symptoms are unchanged from their baseline.
- Patients with new onset or worsening shortness of breath require more urgent follow-up.

Causes
- Anaphylaxis
- Anemia
- Anxiety states, hyperventilation syndrome
- Asthma—bronchospasm
- Congestive heart failure
- Chronic obstructive pulmonary disease
- Diabetic ketoacidosis
- Pneumonia
- Pulmonary embolism
- Spontaneous pneumothorax
- Upper respiratory infection, acute bronchitis

BURNS

Definition
- Thermal burns are skin injuries from heat.
- Thermal burns include explosions, fireworks.

Pain Severity Scale
- **Mild (1-3):** Doesn't interfere with normal activities.
- **Moderate (4-7):** Interferes with normal activities (e.g., work or school) or awakens from sleep.
- **Severe (8-10):** Excruciating pain, unable to do any normal activities, unable to move limb at all due to pain.

Excluded:
- Sunburn is covered in a separate protocol (page 392).

TRIAGE ASSESSMENT QUESTIONS

Call EMS 911 Now
- Difficulty breathing after exposure to fire, smoke, or fumes
  R/O: inhalation injury
- Difficult to awaken or acting confused (e.g., disoriented, slurred speech)
  R/O: inhalation injury, carbon monoxide poisoning
  First Aid: Move to fresh air.
- Burn area larger than 10 palms of hand (> 10% BSA) with blisters
  Reason: large second-degree burn; risk of shock
- Sounds like a life-threatening emergency to the triager

See More Appropriate Protocol
- Chemical gets into the eye from fingers, contaminated object, spray, or splash
  Go to Protocol: Eye, Chemical In on page 150
- Sunburn
  Go to Protocol: Sunburn on page 392

Go to ED Now
- Burn area larger than 4 palms of hand (> 4% BSA)
- Burn completely circles an arm or leg
  Reason: circumferential burn
- Caused by explosion or gunpowder
  R/O: other injuries and need for debridement
- Headache or nausea after exposure to fire and smoke
  R/O: smoke inhalation, carbon monoxide poisoning

Go to ED/UCC Now
(or to Office With PCP Approval)
- Hoarseness or cough after exposure to fire and smoke
  R/O: smoke inhalation
- Blister (intact or ruptured) and > 2" (5 cm)
  Reason: may need debridement
- Blister (intact or ruptured) on the hand and > 1" (2.5 cm)
  R/O: risk of contracture
- Blisters (intact or ruptured) on the face, neck, or genitals
  Reason: cosmetic concerns, possible partner abuse
- Caused by very hot substance and center of burn is white (or charred)
  R/O: full thickness third-degree burn
- Sounds like a serious burn to the triager

Go to Office Now
- SEVERE pain (e.g., excruciating)
  R/O: need for narcotic analgesia
- Acid or alkali (lye) burn
- Chemical on skin that causes a blister
- Looks infected (e.g., fever, red streaks, spreading red area, pus)
  R/O: cellulitis

See Today in Office
- Broken (ruptured) blister and caller doesn't want to trim the dead skin
- Suspicious history for the burn
  R/O: domestic violence or elder abuse
- Patient wants to be seen

See Today or Tomorrow in Office
- No tetanus booster in > 5 years
  Reason: minor thermal burn, may need a tetanus booster shot (vaccine)
- No prior tetanus shot
  Reason: minor thermal burn, needs to get full tetanus vaccination (a series of 3 shots)

See Within 3 Days in Office
- After 10 days and burn isn't healed
- Has diabetes and minor burn of lower leg or foot
  Reason: diabetic neuropathy and decreased resistance to infection

Home Care
○ Minor thermal or chemical burn
○ Mouth or lip pain from hot food or drink

HOME CARE ADVICE

First-degree Burns or Small Blisters

❶ **Reassurance:**
- A minor thermal or chemical burn can be treated at home.
- *Here is some care advice that should help.*

❷ **Cleaning:** Wash the area gently with an antibacterial liquid soap and water once a day.

❸ **Ruptured (Broken or Open) Blisters:**
- You should remove the dead blister skin for any ruptured blisters.
- **Method 1:** The easiest way to do this is gently wipe away the dead skin with some wet gauze or a wet washcloth.
- **Method 2:** If that fails, trim off the dead skin with a fine scissors.

❹ **Antibiotic Ointment for Ruptured Blisters:**
- Apply an antibiotic ointment (e.g., over-the-counter bacitracin) directly to a Band-Aid or dressing.
  (Reason: Prevent unnecessary pain of applying it directly to burn.)
- Then apply the Band-Aid or dressing over the burn.
- Change the dressing every other day. Use warm water and 1 or 2 wipes with a wet washcloth to remove any surface debris.
- Be gentle with burns.

❺ **Intact (Closed) Blisters:**
- **First 7 Days After a Burn:** Leave intact blisters alone.
- **After 7 Days:** You can gently remove the blisters. The easiest way to do this is gently wipe away the dead skin with some wet gauze or a wet washcloth.

❻ **Expected Course:**
- Burns usually hurt for 2-3 days.
- **First-degree Burns:** Usually peel like a sunburn in about a week. The skin should look nearly normal after 2 weeks.
- **Second-degree Burns:** Blisters usually rupture within 7 days. Second-degree burns take 14-21 days to heal (longer than first-degree burns). Sometimes the skin looks a little darker or lighter than before after it has healed.
- **Scarring:** Fortunately, first- and second-degree burns don't leave scars.

❼ **Pain Medicines:**
- For pain relief, you can take either acetaminophen, ibuprofen, or naproxen.
- They are over-the-counter (OTC) pain drugs. You can buy them at the drugstore.

Acetaminophen (e.g., Tylenol):
- **Regular Strength Tylenol:** Take 650 mg (two 325 mg pills) by mouth every 4-6 hours as needed. Each Regular Strength Tylenol pill has 325 mg of acetaminophen.
- **Extra Strength Tylenol:** Take 1,000 mg (two 500 mg pills) every 8 hours as needed. Each Extra Strength Tylenol pill has 500 mg of acetaminophen.
- The most you should take each day is 3,000 mg (10 Regular Strength or 6 Extra Strength pills a day).

Ibuprofen (e.g., Motrin, Advil):
- Take 400 mg (two 200 mg pills) by mouth every 6 hours.
- Another choice is to take 600 mg (three 200 mg pills) by mouth every 8 hours.
- The most you should take each day is 1,200 mg (six 200 mg pills), unless your doctor has told you to take more.

Naproxen (e.g., Aleve):
- Take 220 mg (one 220 mg pill) by mouth every 8 hours as needed. You may take 440 mg (two 220 mg pills) for your first dose.
- The most you should take each day is 660 mg (three 220 mg pills a day), unless your doctor has told you to take more.

❽ Pain Medicines—Extra Notes:
- Use the lowest amount of medicine that makes your pain better.
- Acetaminophen is thought to be safer than ibuprofen or naproxen in people > 65 years old. Acetaminophen is in many OTC and prescription medicines. It might be in more than one medicine that you are taking. You need to be careful and not take an overdose. An acetaminophen overdose can hurt the liver.
- McNeil, the company that makes Tylenol, has different dosage instructions for Tylenol in Canada and the United States. In Canada, the maximum recommended dose per day is 4,000 mg or 12 Regular Strength (325 mg) pills. In the United States, McNeil recommends a maximum dose of 10 Regular Strength (325 mg) pills.
- CAUTION: Do not take acetaminophen if you have liver disease.
- CAUTION: Do not take ibuprofen or naproxen if you have stomach problems, have kidney disease, are pregnant, or have been told by your doctor to avoid this type of anti-inflammatory drug. Do not take ibuprofen or naproxen for > 7 days without consulting your doctor.
- *Before taking any medicine, read all the instructions on the package.*

❾ Call Back If:
- Severe pain lasts > 2 hours after taking pain medicine.
- Burn starts to look infected (pus, red streaks, increased tenderness).
- You become worse.

Mouth or Lip Pain From Hot Food or Drink

❶ Reassurance:
- Minor burns of the mouth from hot food usually are painful for 2 days.
- They heal quickly because the lining of the mouth heals twice as fast as the skin.
- *Here is some care advice that should help.*

❷ Local Ice:
- Put a piece of ice in the mouth immediately for 10 minutes.
  (Reason: Reduce swelling and pain.)
- Rinse the mouth with ice water every hour for 4 hours.

❸ Expected Course:
- The pain usually resolves after 2 days.
- Second-degree burns can cause some blisters that quickly turn into shallow ulcers. These take 3 or 4 days to heal. They normally have a white surface.

❹ Call Back If:
- Difficulty with swallowing occurs.
- Difficulty with breathing occurs.
- Pain becomes severe.
- You become worse.

When Does an Adult Need a Tetanus Booster?

❶ Tetanus Booster Needed Every 5 Years:
- For a burn, a tetanus booster is recommended if it has been > 5 years since the prior tetanus shot.
- Try to get the tetanus booster as soon as possible.
- Make certain to get the booster within 3 days of the injury.

❷ Call Back If:
- You have more questions.
- You become worse.

Internet Resources

❶ American Burn Association, Including Burn Center Search: http://ameriburn.org

❷ Burn Center Referral Criteria, From the American Burn Association: http://ameriburn.org/public-resources/burn-center-referral-criteria

FIRST AID

First Aid Advice for Thermal Burns:
- Immediately (don't take time to remove clothing) put the burned part in cold tap water or pour cold water over it for 10 minutes.
- For burns on the face, apply a cold, wet washcloth. *Reason: lessens the depth of the burn and relieves pain*

BACKGROUND

Key Points

- The triager should first determine burn severity (i.e., first, second, third degree). Sometimes it may be a mixture.
- The triager should then estimate the size of the burn in terms of total body surface area (BSA). The victim's palm represents approximately 1% of the BSA. The Rule of 9s can also be used to estimate burn size.
- The triager should confirm that there is no inhalation injury from hot or toxic fumes. Symptoms of inhalation injury include coughing and difficulty breathing.
- The triager should also be suspicious of carbon monoxide (CO) poisoning in situations of smoke inhalation, especially house fires. Mild symptoms of CO poisoning include headache and nausea. More severe poisoning can cause confusion and coma.

Causes

- **Household Burns:** Most burns are scalds from hot water or hot drinks. Others are from hot ovens, stoves, electric or kerosene space heaters, exhaust pipes, grease, hair-curling irons, clothes irons, heating grates, and cigarettes.
- **Workplace Burns:** Common sources of injury are cooking oils and hot water/steam, usually in workers involved with food preparation.

Degrees of Burns (Severity)

- **First Degree** (superficial burns): Reddened skin without blisters (does not need to be seen).
- **Second Degree** (partial thickness burns): Reddened skin with blisters (heals from bottom up, takes 2-3 weeks).
  - **Small intact blisters (< 2" [< 5 cm])** can usually be left alone; initial debridement is not needed. An intact blister serves as a physiologic dressing, decreases the risk of infection, and reduces pain. However, most blisters > 1" (2.5 cm) will go on to rupture.
  - **Large intact blisters (> 2" [> 5 cm])** almost always rupture within a couple days of the burn. They should be debrided (remove dead blister skin). Generally, this is best done by a physician or other health care professional.
  - **All ruptured blisters** need debridement (removal) of the dead skin; this can be done by the caller, a physician, or other health care professional. Most ruptured blisters are empty of fluid. A blister with a small opening and slow fluid leak can be recognized by the appearance of wrinkled skin.
- **Third Degree** (full thickness burns): Deep burns with white or charred skin. The area also loses sensation to pain and touch (i.e., numb). Usually needs a skin graft to prevent bad scarring if it is larger than a quarter (1" or 2.5 cm) in size. If a third-degree burn is < 1" (2.5 cm) in size, usually it will heal from the margins.

Rule of 9s for Estimating Burn Size: Each part of the body contributes a predictable portion of the total BSA.

- Head and neck: 9%
- Each arm: 9%
- Anterior chest and abdomen: 18%
- Entire back: 18%
- Each leg: 18%
- Genital region: 1%

Rule of Palms for Estimating Burn Size

- A person's palm (not including the fingers) represents 1% of the total BSA.
- For example, if a person had blistering of the left shoulder the size of 2 palms, the total area of blistering would be 2% of the BSA.

CAST SYMPTOMS AND QUESTIONS

Definition
- Symptoms occurring in arm or leg after cast placement
- Other questions about cast care

A CAST is made of a hard material (plaster or fiberglass) and it goes all the way around the injured part (e.g., hand, arm, foot, leg).

In contrast, a SPLINT is placed on only one side of the injured part and then held in place with a soft material, like a cotton gauze wrapping or an elastic bandage. Callers can use their fingers to tell the difference.

TRIAGE ASSESSMENT QUESTIONS

Go to ED Now
- ● Chest pain
  R/O: DVT, pulmonary embolus
- ● Difficulty breathing
  R/O: DVT, pulmonary embolus

Go to ED/UCC Now
(or to Office With PCP Approval)
- ● Patient sounds very sick or weak to the triager
  Reason: severe acute illness or serious complication suspected

Go to Office Now
- ● SEVERE pain of fingers or toes, and not improved after pain medications and elevation
  R/O: tight cast, compartment syndrome
  Note: Most follow-up cast care should be handled by doctor (e.g., orthopedist) who put on the cast.
- ● Numbness or tingling of fingers or toes, and not improved after elevation
  R/O: tight cast, compartment syndrome
- ● Blueness or pallor of fingers or toes (compared to non-injured side)
  R/O: tight cast, compartment syndrome, or simple bruising
- ● Increasing pain under cast and cast put on > 24 hours ago, and not improved after elevation
  R/O: cast too tight, DVT, wound infection
  Note: Most follow-up cast care should be handled by doctor (e.g., orthopedist) who put on the cast.
  Elevation instructions are in Home Care Advice.

See Today in Office
- ◐ Swelling of fingers or toes, and not improved after elevation
  Reason: cast check
  Note: Most follow-up cast care should be handled by doctor (e.g., orthopedist) who put on the cast.
- ◐ Coolness or tingling of fingers or toes, and not improved after elevation
  Reason: cast check
- ◐ Can't wiggle fingers or toes
  Reason: cast check
- ◐ Foreign body gets stuck under the cast
- ◐ Bad odor comes from underneath the cast
  R/O: wound infection, pressure sore, poor cast hygiene
- ◐ Drainage comes through cast or out of end of cast
  R/O: wound infection, pressure sore
- ◐ Unexplained fever occurs
  R/O: wound infection, pressure sore, osteomyelitis
- ◐ Plaster cast gets wet and is soft after attempted drying
- ◐ Plaster or fiberglass cast gets wet and patient has metal pins sticking out of skin
  Reason: evaluate cast, possible replacement
  Note: Most follow-up cast care should be handled by doctor (e.g., orthopedist) who put on the cast.
- ◐ Skin becomes red or raw at edge of cast
- ◐ Cast breaks, cracks, or falls off

Discuss With PCP and Callback by Nurse Today
- ○ SEVERE pain (e.g., excruciating) under the cast and not improved after pain medicines and elevation
  Reason: need new analgesic medication or dosage adjustment
  Note: Most follow-up cast care should be handled by doctor (e.g., orthopedist) who put on the cast.
- ○ Cast feels too loose
  Note: Most follow-up cast care should be handled by doctor (e.g., orthopedist) who put on the cast.
- ○ Cast feels too tight
  Note: No severe pain; normal color and sensation for fingers/toes. Most follow-up cast care should be handled by doctor (e.g., orthopedist) who put on the cast.
- ○ Cast removal date, questions about
  Note: Most follow-up cast care should be handled by doctor (e.g., orthopedist) who put on the cast.
- ○ Triager unable to answer question

See Within 3 Days in Office
● Patient wants to be seen

Home Care
○ Pain under the cast
Reason: expected pain from injury
○ Itchy skin under the cast
○ Numbness or tingling of fingers or toes and has not tried elevation
R/O: mild swelling
○ Normal cast care, questions about
○ Wet cast, questions about
○ Sharp edges on cast, questions about

HOME CARE ADVICE

Normal Cast Care

❶ **Elevation for Arm-Wrist Cast:**
• Elevate the arm above your heart; this will help reduce swelling and pain.
• Elevation is especially important during the first 3 days after putting on the cast.
• Occasional wiggling of fingers will also prevent some swelling.

❷ **Elevation for Leg-Ankle Cast:**
• Elevate the leg by propping it up on pillows. Ideally, your leg should be above your heart. This will limit the amount of swelling that occurs and reduce the pain.
• Elevation is especially important during the first 3 days after putting on the cast.
• Occasional wiggling of the toes will also prevent some swelling.

❸ **Keep Cast Dry:**
• Don't get the cast wet.
• **Plaster Cast:** Wet plaster can become soft and crumble.
• **Fiberglass:** Wet padding under a fiberglass cast can cause skin rashes.
• **Fiberglass With Gore-Tex Liner:** Patients with this special type of water-resistant cast may have been given permission to get the cast wet. Follow the doctor's instructions.

❹ **How to Bathe With a Cast:**
• To avoid getting the cast wet, enclose it in a plastic bag for bathing. Close the upper part of the plastic with tape or an elastic strap. You can also buy a waterproof sleeve at some drugstores.
• Use a bathtub, because it's harder to keep a cast dry in a shower. Don't submerge the cast in bathwater even though it's covered.

❺ **Activities:**
• Adults with casts can usually go to school and work (unless the doctor specifically gave patient other instructions).
• Mild exercise of the unaffected parts of the body is fine.
• Avoid contact or dangerous sports.
(Reason: fall and reinjury)
• Avoid exercise that causes excessive sweating.
(Reason: Cast will become damp.)
• Avoid swimming.
(Reason: Cast will often get wet even if using a plastic bag to cover it.)

❻ **Walking:**
• If the cast is on a leg, don't walk on it unless you have your physician's approval. Never walk on it the first 48 hours because it takes that long for plaster to completely dry and become strong.
• If you were given crutches or a walker, you should not put any body weight on the cast when walking.

❼ **Call Back If:**
• Finger or toes develop numbness, tingling, or pain.
• Can't wiggle fingers or toes.
• Fingers or toes become bluish or pale.
• You become worse.

Pain and Itching

❶ Pain From Fracture(s):

- Fractures can be quite painful. The pain is worst the first 1-4 days after the injury and slowly decreases over the next couple weeks. A fracture takes 4-6 weeks to heal completely.
- Many patients find that the most effective way to reduce pain is elevation.
- Patients also find that using ice reduces pain.
- Pain medications are also important.

❷ Prescription Pain Medication:

- The doctor who put on the cast has probably recommended or prescribed a pain medication. Take this as directed.
- There are also over-the-counter pain medications that you can take: acetaminophen (e.g., Tylenol) and ibuprofen (e.g., Motrin).

❸ Pain Medicines:

- For pain relief, you can take either acetaminophen, ibuprofen, or naproxen.
- They are over-the-counter (OTC) pain drugs. You can buy them at the drugstore.

Acetaminophen (e.g., Tylenol):

- **Regular Strength Tylenol:** Take 650 mg (two 325 mg pills) by mouth every 4-6 hours as needed. Each Regular Strength Tylenol pill has 325 mg of acetaminophen.
- **Extra Strength Tylenol:** Take 1,000 mg (two 500 mg pills) every 8 hours as needed. Each Extra Strength Tylenol pill has 500 mg of acetaminophen.
- The most you should take each day is 3,000 mg (10 Regular Strength or 6 Extra Strength pills a day).

Ibuprofen (e.g., Motrin, Advil):

- Take 400 mg (two 200 mg pills) by mouth every 6 hours.
- Another choice is to take 600 mg (three 200 mg pills) by mouth every 8 hours.
- The most you should take each day is 1,200 mg (six 200 mg pills), unless your doctor has told you to take more.

Naproxen (e.g., Aleve):

- Take 220 mg (one 220 mg pill) by mouth every 8 hours as needed. You may take 440 mg (two 220 mg pills) for your first dose.
- The most you should take each day is 660 mg (three 220 mg pills a day), unless your doctor has told you to take more.

❹ Pain Medicines—Extra Notes:

- Use the lowest amount of medicine that makes your pain better.
- Acetaminophen is thought to be safer than ibuprofen or naproxen in people > 65 years old. Acetaminophen is in many OTC and prescription medicines. It might be in more than one medicine that you are taking. You need to be careful and not take an overdose. An acetaminophen overdose can hurt the liver.
- McNeil, the company that makes Tylenol, has different dosage instructions for Tylenol in Canada and the United States. In Canada, the maximum recommended dose per day is 4,000 mg or 12 Regular Strength (325 mg) pills. In the United States, McNeil recommends a maximum dose of 10 Regular Strength (325 mg) pills.
- CAUTION: Do not take acetaminophen if you have liver disease.
- CAUTION: Do not take ibuprofen or naproxen if you have stomach problems, have kidney disease, are pregnant, or have been told by your doctor to avoid this type of anti-inflammatory drug. Do not take ibuprofen or naproxen for > 7 days without consulting your doctor.
- *Before taking any medicine, read all the instructions on the package.*

❺ Itching:

- Use a hair dryer to blow some COOL air into the cast.
- Do NOT stick anything down into the cast, such as a coat hanger or pencil, to scratch an itch. It might injure the skin and lead to infection or get stuck inside the cast.

❻ Call Back If:

- Pain under cast increases.
- Pain under cast becomes severe.
- You become worse.

Numbness and Tingling

❶ Expected Course With Elevation:

- Numbness and tingling can sometimes occur because of swelling and from pressure from the cast.
- It should go away with elevation. If it does not, you will need to be examined.

❷ Call Back If:

- Numbness or tingling persist after 1-2 hours of elevation.
- You become worse.

Wet Cast

❶ Drying a Plaster Cast:
- A small wet spot can be blow-dried with a hair dryer. Try to dry it with the hair dryer set at a low setting.
  (Caution: Hot air can cause burns.)
- If a larger area of the cast becomes wet, you can also use a hair dryer to dry the cast. Unfortunately, even if dried, a plaster cast will usually stay soft and need to be replaced.

❷ Drying a Fiberglass Cast:
- The outside (fiberglass portion) of a fiberglass cast is waterproof. However, the inside lining that is next to your skin is cotton and is not waterproof.
- You usually dry the inner cotton lining with a hair dryer. Try to dry the lining with the hair dryer set at a low setting.
  (Caution: Hot air can cause burns.)
- If you can't dry it, the wet lining will cause itching or rashes under the cast.

❸ Call Back If:
- Cast becomes very soft.
- Cast cracks.
- You become worse.

Sharp Edges on Cast

❶ Sharp Edge on a Cast:
- If an edge is sharp you can carefully file it down with an emery board (nail file).
- Another option is to cover the area with tape, or you can pad it with a cotton ball and some tape.

❷ Call Back If:
- This care advice does not help.
- Redness or drainage occurs.
- You become worse.

BACKGROUND

Casts

- A cast is a hard splint that completely encloses part of an injured arm or leg in the best position for healing.
- The purpose of a cast is to keep fractures (broken bones) from moving (immobilization) until they heal. Casts for fractures are usually applied for 4-6 weeks. Casts help reduce pain because when fractures move, they hurt. Casts can also be used to help treat severe sprains (torn ligaments).
- The cast itself can be made out of fiberglass or plaster. Generally, fiberglass is better than plaster. Fiberglass casts are lighter, less bulky, and stronger than plaster casts. Fiberglass casts are more durable, and the outside of a fiberglass cast is waterproof. Fiberglass casts are strong within 30 minutes of application. It takes plaster casts 48 hours to become completely dry and strong.
- The innermost layer of a cast is usually cotton padding to protect the skin. Gore-Tex liners are also available for use with fiberglass casts and have the advantage of being waterproof.

Common Cast Problems and Questions

- **Compartment Syndrome:** See below.
- **Pressure Sores:** A pressure sore can develop over an area of bony prominence as a result of pressure of the cast. This can usually be avoided with adequate padding at the time of casting.
- **Tight Casts:** Most questions are about tight casts. A tight cast can decrease circulation to the fingers and toes. The main symptoms are numbness, tingling, or increased pain in the fingers or toes. Other symptoms are color changes (bluish or pale) or swelling of the fingers or toes.
- **Wound Infection:** Sometimes a cast is placed over a wound. The wound can be a surgical incision from an operation or a traumatic wound from a compound fracture (bone poke through skin). These hidden wounds can become infected.

Compartment Syndrome

- **Definition:** Severely compromised capillary blood flow due to severe swelling inside a cast. This is an orthopedic emergency.
- **Complications:** Permanent muscle or nerve damage.
- **Symptoms:** Severe pain with passive stretching (flexion or extension) of fingers or toes is the most reliable sign. Other symptoms include moderate pain at rest, increasing pain, tingling, numbness, or pale fingers or toes.

CHEST INJURY

Definition

- Injuries to the chest, the area from the lower neck to the bottom of the rib cage

TRIAGE ASSESSMENT QUESTIONS

Call EMS 911 Now

- Major injury from dangerous force or speed (e.g., MVA, fall > 10 feet or 3 m)
- Bullet wound, knife wound, or other penetrating object
  First Aid: If penetrating object is still in place, don't remove it.
  Reason: removal could increase internal bleeding
- Puncture wound that sounds life-threatening to the triager
  R/O: serious internal injury
- Severe difficulty breathing (e.g., struggling for each breath, speaks in single words)
  R/O: pneumothorax/hemothorax
- Major bleeding (actively dripping or spurting) that can't be stopped
  First Aid: Apply direct pressure to the entire wound with a clean cloth.
- Open wound of the chest with sound of moving air (sucking wound) or visible air bubbles
  First Aid: Cover the opening with a square piece of plastic taped down on 3 sides to chest wall.
- Shock suspected (e.g., cold/pale/clammy skin, too weak to stand)
  R/O: shock
  First Aid: Lie down with the feet elevated.
- Coughing or spitting up blood
  R/O: pulmonary laceration
- Bluish (or gray) lips or face
  R/O: cyanosis and need for oxygen
- Unconscious or was unconscious
  R/O: cardiac arrhythmia, cardiac contusion, serious injury
- Sounds like a life-threatening emergency to the triager

See More Appropriate Protocol

- Chest pain not from an injury
  Go to Protocol: Chest Pain on page 73
- Wound looks infected
  Go to Protocol: Wound Infection on page 443

Go to ED Now

- SEVERE chest pain
  R/O: pneumothorax, rib fracture(s)
- Difficulty breathing and not severe
  R/O: lung injury
- Skin is split open or gaping (or length > ½" or 12 mm)
  Reason: may need laceration repair (e.g., sutures)
  R/O: deeper injury
- Bleeding and won't stop after 10 minutes of direct pressure (using correct technique)
  R/O: need for sutures
- Sounds like a serious injury to the triager

Go to ED/UCC Now
(or to Office With PCP Approval)

- Can't take a deep breath but no respiratory distress (e.g., hurts to take a deep breath)
  R/O: rib fracture
- Shallow puncture wound
  R/O: deeper injury

Go to Office Now

- Collarbone is painful and difficulty raising arm
  R/O: clavicle fracture

See Today in Office

- Patient is confused or is an unreliable provider of information (e.g., dementia, profound intellectual disability, alcohol intoxication)
- Patient wants to be seen

See Today or Tomorrow in Office

- Wound and no tetanus booster in > 5 years (or > 10 years for clean cuts)
  Reason: may need a tetanus booster shot (vaccine)
- High-risk adult (e.g., age > 60, osteoporosis, chronic steroid use)
  Reason: greater risk of fracture in patients with osteoporosis
- Suspicious history for the injury
  R/O: domestic violence or elder abuse

See Within 3 Days in Office

● Large swelling or bruise and size > palm of
person's hand
R/O: rib fracture, large contusion
● Injury and pain has not improved after 3 days
● Injury is still painful or swollen after 2 weeks

Home Care

○ Chest wall swelling, bruise, or pain from direct
blow to chest
R/O: minor contusion of chest wall
○ Superficial cut (scratch) or abrasion (scrape)

HOME CARE ADVICE

Treatment of a Minor Bruise or Strain

❶ **Reassurance—Bending or Twisting Injury (Strain):**
• Strain and sprain are the medical terms used
to describe overstretching of the muscles of
the chest. A twisting or bending injury can
cause rib strain.
• The main symptom is pain that gets worse
with movement.
• *Here is some care advice that should help.*

❷ **Reassurance—Direct Blow (Contusion, Bruise):**
• A direct blow to your chest can cause a
contusion. Contusion is the medical term
for bruise.
• Symptoms are mild pain, swelling, and/or
bruising.
• *Here is some care advice that should help.*

❸ **Apply a Cold Pack:**
• Apply a cold pack or an ice bag (wrapped in a
moist towel) to the area for 20 minutes. Repeat
in 1 hour, then every 4 hours while awake.
• Continue this for the first 48 hours after an injury.
(Reason: to reduce the swelling and pain)

❹ **Apply Heat to the Area:**
• Beginning 48 hours after an injury, apply a warm
washcloth or heating pad for 10 minutes 3 times
a day.
• This will help increase blood flow and improve
healing.

❺ **Breathing Exercises:**
• Take 2 deep breaths and then cough once each
hour while awake. Use a pillow over the injured
area to reduce the pain of this activity.
• This help you get good air movement to all parts
of your lungs and help prevent lung infection.

❻ **Limit Activities:**
• Avoid strenuous activities or contact sports until
the pain is gone.

❼ **Call Back If:**
• Swelling or bruise becomes > 2" (5 cm).
• Pain not improved after 72 hours.
• Pain or swelling lasts > 7 days.
• You become worse.

Treatment of a Small Cut or Scrape

❶ **Reassurance—Superficial Laceration
(Cut or Scratch) or Abrasion (Scrape):**
• This sounds like a small cut or scrape that we
can treat at home.
• *Here is some care advice that should help.*

❷ **Bleeding:** Apply direct pressure for 10 minutes
with a sterile gauze to stop any bleeding.

❸ **Cleaning the Wound:**
• Wash the wound with soap and water for
5 minutes.
• For any dirt, scrub gently with a washcloth.
• For any bleeding, apply direct pressure with a
sterile gauze or clean cloth for 10 minutes.

❹ **Antibiotic Ointment:**
• Apply an antibiotic ointment (e.g., over-the-
counter bacitracin), covered by a Band-Aid or
dressing. Change daily or if it becomes wet.
• Option: A Telfa dressing won't stick to the
wound when it is removed.
• Option: Another option is to use a liquid skin
bandage that only needs to be applied once.
Don't use antibiotic ointment if you use a liquid
skin bandage.

❺ **Liquid Skin Bandage:**
- You can use a liquid skin bandage instead of antibiotic ointment and a dressing or a Band-Aid.
- **Benefits:** Liquid skin bandage has several benefits when compared with a regular bandage (e.g., a dressing or a Band-Aid). You only need to put a liquid bandage on once to minor cuts and scrapes. It helps stop minor bleeding. It seals the wound and may promote faster healing and lower infection rates. However, it also costs more.
- **How to Use It:** First, clean and dry the wound. You put on the liquid as spray or with a swab. It dries in < 1 minute and usually lasts a week. You can get it wet.
- **Examples:** Liquid skin bandage is available over the counter. Examples are Band-Aid Liquid Bandage, New Skin, Curad Spray Bandage, and 3M No Sting Liquid Bandage Spray.

❻ **Call Back If:**
- Looks infected (pus, redness, increasing tenderness).
- Doesn't heal within 10 days.
- You become worse.

Over-the-counter Pain Medicines

❶ **Pain Medicines:**
- For pain relief, you can take either acetaminophen, ibuprofen, or naproxen.
- They are over-the-counter (OTC) pain drugs. You can buy them at the drugstore.

Acetaminophen (e.g., Tylenol):
- **Regular Strength Tylenol:** Take 650 mg (two 325 mg pills) by mouth every 4-6 hours as needed. Each Regular Strength Tylenol pill has 325 mg of acetaminophen.
- **Extra Strength Tylenol:** Take 1,000 mg (two 500 mg pills) every 8 hours as needed. Each Extra Strength Tylenol pill has 500 mg of acetaminophen.
- The most you should take each day is 3,000 mg (10 Regular Strength or 6 Extra Strength pills a day).

Ibuprofen (e.g., Motrin, Advil):
- Take 400 mg (two 200 mg pills) by mouth every 6 hours.
- Another choice is to take 600 mg (three 200 mg pills) by mouth every 8 hours.
- The most you should take each day is 1,200 mg (six 200 mg pills), unless your doctor has told you to take more.

Naproxen (e.g., Aleve):
- Take 220 mg (one 220 mg pill) by mouth every 8 hours as needed. You may take 440 mg (two 220 mg pills) for your first dose.
- The most you should take each day is 660 mg (three 220 mg pills a day), unless your doctor has told you to take more.

❷ **Pain Medicines—Extra Notes:**
- Use the lowest amount of medicine that makes your pain better.
- Acetaminophen is thought to be safer than ibuprofen or naproxen in people > 65 years old. Acetaminophen is in many OTC and prescription medicines. It might be in more than one medicine that you are taking. You need to be careful and not take an overdose. An acetaminophen overdose can hurt the liver.
- McNeil, the company that makes Tylenol, has different dosage instructions for Tylenol in Canada and the United States. In Canada, the maximum recommended dose per day is 4,000 mg or 12 Regular Strength (325 mg) pills. In the United States, McNeil recommends a maximum dose of 10 Regular Strength (325 mg) pills.
- CAUTION: Do not take acetaminophen if you have liver disease.
- CAUTION: Do not take ibuprofen or naproxen if you have stomach problems, have kidney disease, are pregnant, or have been told by your doctor to avoid this type of anti-inflammatory drug. Do not take ibuprofen or naproxen for > 7 days without consulting your doctor.
- *Before taking any medicine, read all the instructions on the package.*

❸ **Call Back If:**
- You have more questions.
- You become worse.

FIRST AID

First Aid Advice for Bleeding:
Apply direct pressure to the entire wound with a clean cloth.

First Aid Advice for Penetrating Object:
If penetrating object is still in place, don't remove it. *Reason: Removal could increase bleeding.*

First Aid Advice for Shock:
Lie down with the feet elevated.

First Aid Advice for Sucking (Open) Chest Wound:
- Completely cover the wound with a square piece of plastic (e.g., plastic wrap).
- Tape 3 sides of this plastic covering to the chest wall, leaving the fourth side un-taped. *Reason: taping fourth side could cause tension pneumothorax*
- If these materials are not available, instead loosely cover with a cloth dressing or gauze.

BACKGROUND

Types of Chest Injuries:
Chest injuries include
- Muscle bruise (e.g., pectoralis muscle in front).
- Bone bruise.
- **Fractures:** Broken ribs, clavicle, sternum, or scapula.
- **Flail Chest:** Multiple adjacent fractured ribs. This gives a nonattached area of the chest wall that is sucked in during inspiration and bulges out during expiration.
- **Open Wound of Chest** (sucking wound): A sucking wound of the chest is one that goes through to the pleural space or lung. It is evident by the sound of air being sucked into the chest with each effort to breathe in.
- **Lung Injury:** Pulmonary contusion, pulmonary laceration, secondary pneumothorax (air leak), or hemothorax (blood leak) from rib fracture.
- **Heart Injury:** Pericardial tamponade, cardiac contusion, arrhythmia.

What Cuts Need to Be Sutured?
- Any cut that is split open or gaping probably needs sutures (or staples or skin glue).
- Cuts > ½" (1 cm) usually need sutures.
- Any open wound that may need sutures should be evaluated by a physician regardless of the time that has passed since the initial injury.

When Does an Adult Need a Tetanus Booster (Tetanus Shot)?
- **Clean Cuts and Scrapes—Tetanus Booster Needed Every 10 Years:** Patients with clean minor wounds AND who have previously had ≥ 3 tetanus shots (full series) need a booster every 10 years. Examples of minor wounds include a superficial abrasion or a shallow cut from a clean knife blade. Obtain booster within 72 hours.
- **Dirty Wounds—Tetanus Booster Needed Every 5 Years:** Patients with dirty wounds need a booster if it has been > 5 years since the last booster. Examples of dirty wounds include those contaminated with soil, feces, and/or saliva and more serious wounds from deep punctures, crushing, and burns. Obtain booster within 72 hours.

CHEST PAIN

Definition
- Uncomfortable pressure, fullness, squeezing, or other pain in the chest.
- This includes the area from the clavicles to the bottom of the rib cage.
- Not due to a traumatic injury.

TRIAGE ASSESSMENT QUESTIONS

Call EMS 911 Now
- SEVERE difficulty breathing (e.g., struggling for each breath, speaks in single words)
  R/O: respiratory failure, hypoxia, acute pulmonary edema
- Passed out (i.e., fainted, collapsed and was not responding)
  R/O: shock
- Chest pain lasting > 5 minutes and ANY of the following:
  - > 50 years old
  - > 30 years old and at least one cardiac risk factor (i.e., high blood pressure, diabetes, high cholesterol, obesity, smoker, or strong family history of heart disease)
  - Pain is crushing, pressure-like, or heavy
  - Took nitroglycerin and chest pain was not relieved
  - History of heart disease (i.e., angina, heart attack, bypass surgery, angioplasty, CHF)
    R/O: myocardial infarction, acute coronary syndrome
- Visible sweat on face or sweat dripping down face
  R/O: myocardial infarction, acute coronary syndrome
- Sounds like a life-threatening emergency to the triager

See More Appropriate Protocol
- Followed an injury to chest
  Go to Protocol: Chest Injury on page 69

Go to ED Now
- SEVERE chest pain
- Pain also present in shoulder(s) or arm(s) or jaw
  R/O: acute coronary syndrome
- Difficulty breathing
- Cocaine use within last 3 days
  Reason: cocaine can precipitate acute coronary syndrome
- History of prior "blood clot" in leg or lungs (i.e., deep vein thrombosis, pulmonary embolism)
  Note: A "blood clot" typically would have required treatment with heparin or coumadin.
  Reason: increased risk of thromboembolism
  R/O: DVT
- Recent illness requiring prolonged bed rest (i.e., immobilization)
  R/O: pulmonary embolism
- Hip or leg fracture in past 2 months (e.g., had cast on leg or ankle)
  R/O: pulmonary embolism
- Major surgery in the past month
  R/O: pulmonary embolism
- Recent long-distance travel with prolonged time in car, bus, plane, or train (i.e., within past 2 weeks; ≥ 6 hours' duration)
  Reason: immobilization during prolonged travel increases risk of pulmonary embolus
- Heart beating irregularly or very rapidly
  R/O: SVT, tachyarrhythmia

Go to ED/UCC Now (or to Office With PCP Approval)
- Chest pain lasting > 5 minutes
  Reason: chest pain is a high-risk complaint; referral for evaluation
- Intermittent chest pain and pain has been increasing in severity or frequency
  R/O: unstable angina
- Dizziness or light-headedness
- Coughing up blood
- Patient sounds very sick or weak to the triager
  Reason: severe acute illness or serious complication suspected

See Today in Office
- Fever > 100.5° F (38.1° C)
- Intermittent chest pains persist > 3 days
- All other patients with chest pain
  Alternate Disposition: Have physician speak directly with patient.
- Patient wants to be seen

Home Care
○ Intermittent mild chest pain lasting a few seconds each time

HOME CARE ADVICE

❶ **Fleeting Chest Pain:** Fleeting chest pains that last only a few seconds and then go away are generally not serious. They may be from pinched muscles or nerves in your chest wall.

❷ **Chest Pain Only When Coughing:** Chest pains that occur with coughing generally come from the chest wall and from irritation of the airways. They are usually not serious.

❸ **Cough Medicines:**
- **OTC Cough Syrups:** The most common cough suppressant in OTC cough medications is dextromethorphan. Often, the letters DM appear in the name.
- **OTC Cough Drops:** Cough drops can help a lot, especially for mild coughs. They reduce coughing by soothing your irritated throat and removing that tickle sensation in the back of the throat. Cough drops also have the advantage of portability—you can carry them with you.
- **Home Remedy—Hard Candy:** Hard candy works just as well as medicine-flavored OTC cough drops. People who have diabetes should use sugar-free candy.
- **Home Remedy—Honey:** This old home remedy has been shown to help decrease coughing at night. The adult dosage is 2 teaspoons (10 mL) at bedtime. Honey should not be given to infants < 1 year of age.

❹ **Expected Course:** These mild chest pains usually disappear within 3 days.

❺ **Call Back If:**
- Severe chest pain.
- Constant chest pain lasting > 5 minutes.
- Difficulty breathing.
- Fever.
- You become worse.

FIRST AID

First Aid Advice for Shock:
Lie down with the feet elevated.

First Aid Advice for Breathing Stopped or Cardiac Arrest

Hands-Only CPR
- Call 911.
- Push hard and fast on the center of the chest.

Special Notes:
- **High-quality CPR:** Rescuers should push hard to a depth of at least 2" (5 cm), at a rate of at least 100 compressions per minute; allow full chest recoil; and minimize interruptions in chest compressions. The disco song "Stayin' Alive" has the right beat for CPR.
- The American Heart Association (AHA) provides a 1-minute instructional video on Hands-Only CPR at: http://handsonlycpr.org. Be prepared. Watch it now, before you need it!
- You are strongly encouraged to get training in CPR from the American Red Cross or the AHA.
- Hands-Only CPR is a trademark of the AHA.

"All rescuers, regardless of training, should provide chest compressions to all cardiac arrest victims. Because of their importance, chest compressions should be the initial CPR action for all victims regardless of age. Rescuers who are able should add ventilations to chest compressions. Highly trained rescuers working together should coordinate their care and perform chest compressions as well as ventilations in a team-based approach." Source: 2010 AHA Guidelines for Cardiopulmonary Resuscitation and Emergency Cardiovascular Care

CPR by Trained Rescuers

Trained (confident) rescuers should add ventilations to chest compressions while waiting for paramedics to arrive:

• Call 911.
• Perform chest compressions and mouth-to-mouth breathing in cycles of 30 compressions and then 2 breaths.

Special Notes:

• Rescuers should push hard to a depth of at least 2" (5 cm), at a rate of at least 100 compressions per minute; allow full chest recoil; and minimize interruptions in chest compressions.

BACKGROUND

Key Points

• Chest pain is a challenging symptom from a triage perspective, as there are a number of potentially life-threatening causes of pain and no combination of symptoms that sufficiently discriminate serious from nonserious pain.
• A conservative stance in triaging patients with chest pain is recommended.

Serious Causes of Chest Pain

• **Acute Coronary Syndromes (Angina, Myocardial Infarction):** Chest pain caused by atherosclerotic blockages in the coronary arteries is the most common cause of acute coronary syndromes. This chest pain syndrome is typically seen with exertion, unless the blockage in a particular coronary artery is complete, and then pain occurs at rest. Acute myocardial infarctions result from a complete loss of blood supply to the blocked coronary artery involved, often the result of an acute thrombus formation in the diseased vessel or disruption of an atherosclerotic plaque. Atherosclerotic heart disease, also referred to as ischemic heart disease, remains the leading cause of death in adults in the United States. See the Caution statement on page 76 for further symptom description.

• **Pulmonary Embolus:** This potentially life-threatening process occurs when a clot, usually from a source in the lower extremities, dislodges and causes mechanical obstruction in the pulmonary arterial system of the lungs. The classic clinical picture is pleuritic chest pain, dyspnea, and hemoptysis. Some or all of these symptoms may be present. Risk factors include immobilization (e.g., bedbound, recent surgery, prolonged travel); trauma, especially to the pelvis or lower extremities; and peripartum and hypercoagulable states (e.g., birth control pills, estrogen use, malignancy).
• **Pneumothorax:** Lung collapse can occur spontaneously or with trauma. The symptoms typically include pleuritic chest pain and dyspnea.
• **Thoracic Aortic Dissection:** A tear in the thoracic aorta usually presents with acute severe chest pain, often described as sharp and tearing in nature. This pain can be referred to the interscapular area. This disease entity is typically seen in the elderly.
• **Pericarditis:** Inflammation of the sac surrounding the heart or pericardium can result in positional chest pain, often pleuritic, and dyspnea.

Other Less Serious Causes of Chest Pain

• **Pneumonia:** Some patients with pneumonia will complain of a sharp localized pleuritic pain. In general, any patient with pneumonia who is hypoxemic, has multilobe involvement, is unable to keep down liquids or medications, or is of advanced age or immunocompromised will require hospitalization.
• **Herpes Zoster:** Usually pain precedes the typical rash of grouped vesicles on a red base in a nerve root distribution.
• **Cholecystitis, Cholelithiasis:** The typical pain of gallstone disease is in the epigastrium and right upper quadrant, is crampy in nature, but can be confused with chest pain. Gallstone abdominal pain can radiate to the upper back in the region of the shoulder blade.
• **Costochondritis:** Caused by inflammation of the rib cartilages where they attach to the sternum in the front of the chest. The pain is usually sharp. The pain often is worsened by breathing in, and it usually hurts when one touches the area. Costochondritis is a diagnosis of exclusion in those with risk factors for the more serious and life-threatening causes of chest pain.

- **Rib-Muscle Strain:** Typically the pain is positional, localized, intermittent, and sharp. This pain is often worse with breathing, and it usually hurts when one touches the area.
- **Reflux Esophagitis:** Patients will often describe an acid or sour taste from the reflux of stomach contents and acid into the throat and mouth.

Myocardial Infarction—Should a Telephone Triage Nurse Recommend Aspirin?

- **Background:** Research has shown that early administration of aspirin reduces mortality from myocardial infarction. EMS 911 dispatchers sometimes instruct patients to take aspirin after an ambulance has been dispatched. Aspirin for cardiac chest pain is a standing medical order for all EMS providers across the United States and Canada. Aspirin is also the standard of care for treating cardiac chest pain, once the patient reaches the ED. There is no evidence that taking aspirin at home provides any additional benefit over taking aspirin during paramedic transport or on arrival in the ED.
- **Telephone Triage and an EMS 911 Disposition:** Generally, these should be very short calls, with the goal being to have the caller speak with the EMS 911 dispatcher as soon as possible. *The triager should deliver and the caller should hear one piece of information: CALL 911 NOW.* One can imagine a scenario in which the nurse triager spends too long on the phone with a caller clarifying allergies or whether the caller already took aspirin, or explaining the difference between true aspirin and nonaspirin pain relievers (e.g., Tylenol).
- **If the Caller Asks About Aspirin:** Emphasize the importance of calling EMS 911 first. If there is no aspirin allergy, the patient may chew an aspirin (160-325 mg) while waiting for the paramedics to arrive.

Caution—Cardiac Ischemia

- Cardiac ischemia is the most common life-threatening cause of acute chest pain.
- Sometimes adults may present with chest pain as the sole symptom of a myocardial infarction. Often there will be other associated symptoms of cardiac ischemia: shortness of breath, nausea, and/or diaphoresis.
- Some adults can have cardiac ischemia without chest discomfort; for example, a diabetic with diaphoresis and shortness of breath.
- Women are less likely to experience chest pain and are more likely to have atypical symptoms; this can lead to delays in evaluation and treatment.
- Cardiac ischemia should be suspected in any patients with risk factors for cardiac disease. These include: hypertension, smoking, diabetes, hyperlipidemia, a strong family history of heart disease, and age > 50.

COLD SORES (FEVER BLISTERS OF LIP)

Definition
- Recurrent sores on the outer lips caused by the herpes simplex virus.
- *Use this protocol only if the patient has symptoms that match Cold Sores.*

Symptoms
- Tingling or burning on the outer lip where cold sores previously occurred is an early warning sign of another episode of cold sores.
- A cold sore starts off as a cluster of painful 1-3 mm small bumps or blisters on the outer lip.
- The small blisters often rupture and form one big sore (i.e., cold sore).
- It is present only on one side of the mouth (i.e., doesn't cross the midline).
- Usually lasts 7-10 days.

TRIAGE ASSESSMENT QUESTIONS

Go to ED/UCC Now (or to Office With PCP Approval)
- Patient sounds very sick or weak to the triager
  Reason: severe acute illness or serious complication suspected

Go to Office Now
- Sores on the eye, eyelids, or tip of nose
  R/O: herpes of the cornea
- Red streak or red area spreading from the cold sore
  R/O: cellulitis

See Today in Office
- Weak immune system (e.g., HIV positive, cancer chemotherapy, splenectomy, organ transplant, chronic steroids)
  Reason: antiviral treatment indicated
- New sores occur in another area
  R/O: impetigo

See Today or Tomorrow in Office
- Sores last > 2 weeks
  R/O: wrong diagnosis, impetigo
- Patient wants to be seen

Callback by PCP Today
- Herpes sores are a recurrent problem, and caller wants a prescription medicine to take the next time they occur

Home Care
- Cold sores without complications

HOME CARE ADVICE

❶ General Information—Cold Sores:
- Fever blisters or cold sores occur on one side of the outer lip.
- Typically last 7-10 days.
- Treatment with a cold sore cream can reduce the pain and shorten the course by a day or 2.

❷ Docosanol 10% Cream:
- Apply over-the-counter docosanol cream (trade name Abreva) to the cold sore 5 times daily until healing occurs.
- Begin using this cream as soon as you first sense the beginning of an outbreak.
- Docosanol is not available in Canada.
- Read and follow the package instructions. Ask your physician's opinion.

❸ Contagiousness:
- Herpes from cold sores is contagious to other people. Discourage picking or rubbing the sore. Don't open the blisters. Wash your hands frequently. The cold sores are contagious until dry (approximately 5-7 days). Most cold sore sufferers note a tingling in the lip before the sore appears (prodromal phase). Patients are also contagious during this period.
- **Eyes:** Avoid spreading the virus to someone's eye by kissing or touching; an eye infection can be serious (herpes keratitis).
- **Mouth:** Since the blisters and mouth secretions are contagious, avoid kissing other people during this time. Avoid sharing drinking glasses, eating utensils, or razors.
- **Sex:** Avoid oral sex during this time. Herpes from sores on your mouth can spread to your partner's genital area.

- **Contact With Immunocompromised People:** Avoid contact with anyone who has eczema or a weakened immune system.
- ❹ **Expected Course:** The pain typically subsides over 4-5 days and the sores typically heal over a 7- to 10-day period. On average, patients note recurrences 2-3 times per year.
- ❺ **Prevention:** Since cold sores are often triggered by exposure to intense sunlight, use a lip balm containing a sunscreen (SPF 30 or higher).
- ❻ **Recurrence:** Tingling or burning on the outer lip where cold sores previously occurred is an early sign of the new onset of recurrent cold sores.
- ❼ **National Herpes Hotline:** 919/361-8488. Counselors provide information about transmission, treatment, prevention, and emotional issues. The hotline is open from 9:00 am to 7:00 pm, Eastern time, Monday through Friday.
- ❽ **Call Back If:**
  - Sores look infected (spreading redness).
  - Sores occur near or in the eye.
  - Sores last > 10 days.
  - You become worse.

BACKGROUND

Key Points

- Colds sores/blisters are recurrent, painful blisters on the outer lip caused by the herpes simplex virus (usually human herpesvirus type 1). They are also called fever blisters.
- **Primary Herpes Simplex:** Approximately 80% of the adult population has had herpes simplex at some point in their lives. The very first episode of infection (primary herpes simplex) can present as a gingivo-stomatitis (with fever and malaise) or, more commonly, is asymptomatic.
- **Recurrent Herpes Simplex Labialis (Fever Blisters):** The virus, which lies dormant in a sensory nerve, can be reactivated by sun exposure, fever, friction, trauma, menstrual periods, stress, or physical exhaustion. Such recurrences occur in 20% of the adult population. Typically, the symptoms are confined to the lip and there is no fever. The medical term for these recurring fever blisters of the lip is herpes simplex labialis. *Cold sores* is another term that people use.

Contagiousness

- Cold sores contain live herpesvirus that is contagious to other people.
- Most patients note a tingling in the lip before the sore appears (prodromal phase). Patients are also contagious during this period.

Treatment—Over the Counter With Docosanol Cream

- Docosanol cream (Abreva) has been demonstrated to reduce severity, pain, and duration of cold sores (Sacks 2001; Treister 2010).
- Docosanol is FDA approved. It is not available in Canada.

Treatment—Prescription Options

- Cold sores are a self-limiting illness that resolves without any treatment in 7-10 days.
- **Topical Prescription Treatment:** Penciclovir 1% cream 4 times a day has been shown to reduce the severity, pain, and duration of cold sores in immunocompetent adults (Spruance 1997). It is more expensive than docosanol.
- **Oral Prescription Treatment:** Available oral antiviral medications include acyclovir (Zovirax) and famciclovir (Famvir). There appears to be some modest benefit obtained from oral antiviral treatment if initiated early. A study demonstrated that a single 1,500 mg dose of famciclovir taken shortly after the onset of prodromal symptoms (i.e., lip tingling) healed cold sores 2 days faster than placebo (Spruance 2006).

COMMON COLD

Definition
- Viral respiratory infection of the nose and throat.
- *Use this protocol only if the patient has symptoms that match a cold.*

Definition—Severe Difficulty Breathing:
- Marked respiratory effort (struggling to breathe). Can only speak in single words. Cyanosis may occur. *(Response: Activate EMS.)*

Symptoms
- Runny or congested (stuffy) nose is the main symptom. The nasal discharge may be clear, cloudy, yellow, or green.
- Sneezing.
- Mild fever and muscle aches, feeling tired and sleepy, headache.
- Scratchy or sore throat.
- Postnasal drip, throat clearing, cough.
- Sometimes associated with hoarseness, tearing eyes, and swollen lymph nodes in the neck.

TRIAGE ASSESSMENT QUESTIONS

Call EMS 911 Now
- ● SEVERE difficulty breathing (e.g., struggling for each breath, speaks in single words)
  R/O: respiratory failure, hypoxia
- ● Very weak (can't stand)
- ● Sounds like a life-threatening emergency to the triager

See More Appropriate Protocol
- ● Runny nose is caused by pollen or other allergies
  Go to Protocol: Hay Fever (Nasal Allergies) on page 197
- ● Cough is the main symptom
  Go to Protocol: Cough on page 95
- ● Sore throat is the main symptom
  Go to Protocol: Sore Throat on page 369

Go to ED/UCC Now
(or to Office With PCP Approval)
- ● Patient sounds very sick or weak to the triager
  Reason: severe acute illness or serious complication suspected

Go to Office Now
- ● Fever > 103° F (39.4° C)
  R/O: pneumonia
- ● Fever > 100.5° F (38.1° C) and > 60 years of age
- ● Fever > 100.0° F (37.8° C) and has diabetes mellitus or a weak immune system (e.g., HIV positive, cancer chemotherapy, organ transplant, splenectomy, chronic steroids)
- ● Fever > 100.0° F (37.8° C) and bedridden (e.g., nursing home patient, stroke, chronic illness, recovering from surgery)
  Reason: higher risk of bacterial infection
  Note: May need ambulance transport to ED.

See Today in Office
- ◓ Fever present > 3 days (72 hours)
  R/O: bacterial sinusitis, bronchitis, pneumonia
- ◓ Fever returns after gone for > 24 hours and symptoms worse or not improved
  R/O: bacterial sinusitis, bronchitis, pneumonia
- ◓ Sinus pain (not just congestion) and fever
  R/O: bacterial sinusitis
- ◓ Earache
  R/O: otitis media

See Today or Tomorrow in Office
- ◓ Sinus congestion (pressure, fullness) present > 10 days
  R/O: bacterial sinusitis, allergic rhinitis
- ◓ Nasal discharge present > 10 days
  R/O: bacterial sinusitis, allergic rhinitis
- ◓ Using nasal washes and pain medicine > 24 hours and sinus pain (lower forehead, cheekbone, or eye) persists
  R/O: sinusitis
- ◓ Patient wants to be seen

Strep Test Only Visit Today or Tomorrow
- ◓ Sore throat present > 5 days
  R/O: strep pharyngitis

Home Care
- ○ Colds with no complications
- ○ Vitamin and herbal supplements for colds, questions about
- ○ Neti pot, questions about

HOME CARE ADVICE

General Care Advice for Treating a Cold

❶ Reassurance:
- It sounds like an uncomplicated cold that we can treat at home.
- Colds are very common and may make you feel uncomfortable.
- Colds are caused by viruses, and no medicine or "shot" will cure an uncomplicated cold.
- Colds are usually not serious.
- *Here is some care advice that should help.*

❷ For a Runny Nose With Profuse Discharge: Blow the Nose
- Nasal mucus and discharge helps to wash viruses and bacteria out of the nose and sinuses.
- Blowing the nose is all that is needed.
- If the skin around your nostrils gets irritated, apply a tiny amount of petroleum ointment to the nasal openings once or twice a day.

❸ Nasal Washes for a Stuffy Nose:
- **Introduction:** Saline (salt water) nasal irrigation (nasal wash) is an effective and simple home remedy for treating stuffy nose and sinus congestion. The nose can be irrigated by pouring, spraying, or squirting salt water into the nose and then letting it run back out.
- **How It Helps:** The salt water rinses out excess mucus and washes out any irritants (dust, allergens) that might be present. It also moistens the nasal cavity.
- **Methods:** There are several ways to irrigate the nose. You can use a saline nasal spray bottle (available over the counter), a rubber ear syringe, a medical syringe without the needle, or a neti pot.

❹ Nasal Washes—Step-by-step Instructions:
- **Step 1:** Lean over a sink.
- **Step 2:** Gently squirt or spray warm salt water into one of your nostrils.
- **Step 3:** Some of the water may run into the back of your throat. Spit this out. If you swallow the salt water it will not hurt you.
- **Step 4:** Blow your nose to clean out the water and mucus.
- **Step 5:** Repeat steps 1-4 for the other nostril. You can do this a couple times a day if it seems to help you.

❺ How to Make Saline (Salt Water) Nasal Wash:
- You can make your own saline nasal wash.
- Add ½ tsp of table salt to 1 cup (8 oz; 240 mL) of warm water.
- You should use sterile, distilled, or previously boiled water for nasal irrigation.

❻ Treatment for Associated Symptoms of Colds:
- **For Muscle Aches, Headaches, or Moderate Fever (> 101° F or 38.9° C):** Take acetaminophen every 4 hours.
- **Sore Throat:** Try throat lozenges, hard candy, or warm chicken broth.
- **Cough:** Use cough drops.
- **Hydrate:** Drink adequate liquids.

❼ Humidifier: If the air in your home is dry, use a cool-mist humidifier.

❽ Contagiousness:
- The cold virus is present in your nasal secretions.
- Cover your nose and mouth with a tissue when you sneeze or cough.
- Wash your hands frequently with soap and water.
- You can return to work or school after the fever is gone and you feel well enough to participate in normal activities.

❾ Expected Course:
- Fever may last 2-3 days.
- Nasal discharge 7-14 days.
- Cough up to 2-3 weeks.

❿ Call Back If:
- Difficulty breathing occurs.
- Fever lasts > 3 days.
- Nasal discharge lasts > 10 days.
- Cough lasts > 3 weeks.
- You become worse.

Over-the-counter Medicines for a Cold

❶ **Medicines for a Stuffy or Runny Nose:**
- Most cold medicines that are available over the counter (OTC) are not helpful.
- **Antihistamines:** Are only helpful if you also have nasal allergies.
- If you have a very runny nose and you really think you need a medicine, you can try using a nasal decongestant for a couple days.

❷ **Nasal Decongestants for a Very Stuffy or Runny Nose:**
- **Most people do not need to use these medicines.**
- If your nose feels blocked, you should try using nasal washes first.
- If you have a very stuffy nose, nasal decongestant medicines can shrink the swollen nasal mucosa and allow for easier breathing. If you have a very runny nose, these medicines can reduce the amount of drainage. They may be taken as pills by mouth or as a nasal spray.
- **Pseudoephedrine (Sudafed):** Available OTC in pill form. Typical adult dosage is two 30 mg tablets every 6 hours.
- **Oxymetazoline Nasal Drops (Afrin):** Available OTC. Clean out the nose before using. Spray each nostril once, wait 1 minute for absorption, and then spray a second time.
- **Phenylephrine Nasal Drops (Neo-Synephrine):** Available OTC. Clean out the nose before using. Spray each nostril once, wait 1 minute for absorption, and then spray a second time.
- *Before taking any medicine, read all the instructions on the package.*

❸ **Caution—Nasal Decongestants:**
- Do not take these medications if you have high blood pressure, heart disease, prostate problems, or an overactive thyroid.
- Do not take these medications if you are pregnant.
- Do not take these medications if you have used a monoamine oxidase (MAO) inhibitor, such as isocarboxazid (Marplan), phenelzine (Nardil), rasagiline (Azilect), selegiline (Eldepryl, Emsam, Zelapar), or tranylcypromine (Parnate), in the past 2 weeks. Life-threatening side effects can occur.
- Do not use these medications for > 3 days. *(Reason: rebound nasal congestion)*

❹ **Cough Medicines:**
- **OTC Cough Syrups:** The most common cough suppressant in OTC cough medications is dextromethorphan. Often the letters DM appear in the name.
- **OTC Cough Drops:** Cough drops can help a lot, especially for mild coughs. They reduce coughing by soothing your irritated throat and removing that tickle sensation in the back of the throat. Cough drops also have the advantage of portability—you can carry them with you.
- **Home Remedy—Hard Candy:** Hard candy works just as well as medicine-flavored OTC cough drops. People who have diabetes should use sugar-free candy.
- **Home Remedy—Honey:** This old home remedy has been shown to help decrease coughing at night. The adult dosage is 2 teaspoons (10 mL) at bedtime. Honey should not be given to infants < 1 year of age.

❺ **OTC Cough Syrup—Dextromethorphan:**
- Cough syrups containing the cough suppressant dextromethorphan (DM) may help decrease your cough. Cough syrups work best for coughs that keep you awake at night. They can also sometimes help in the late stages of a respiratory infection when the cough is dry and hacking. They can be used along with cough drops.
- **Examples:** Benylin, Robitussin DM, Vicks 44 Cough Relief.
- *Before taking any medicine, read all the instructions on the package.*

❻ **Caution—Dextromethorphan:**
- Do not try to completely suppress coughs that produce mucus and phlegm. Remember that coughing is helpful in bringing up mucus from the lungs and preventing pneumonia.
- **Research Notes:** Dextromethorphan in some research studies has been shown to reduce the frequency and severity of cough in adults (≥ 18 years) without significant adverse effects. However, other studies suggest that DM is no better than placebo at reducing a cough.
- **Drug Abuse Potential:** It should be noted that DM has become a drug of abuse. This problem is seen most often in adolescents. Overdose symptoms can range from giggling and euphoria to hallucinations and coma.

- **Contraindicated:** Do not take DM if you are taking an MAO inhibitor now or in the past 2 weeks. Examples of MAO inhibitors include isocarboxazid (Marplan), phenelzine (Nardil), rasagiline (Azilect), selegiline (Eldepryl, Emsam, Zelapar), and tranylcypromine (Parnate). Do not take DM if you are taking venlafaxine (Effexor).

❼ Pain and Fever Medicines:
- For pain or fever relief, take either acetaminophen or ibuprofen.
- They are OTC drugs that help treat both fever and pain. You can buy them at the drugstore.
- Treat fevers > 101° F (38.3° C). The goal of fever therapy is to bring the fever down to a comfortable level. Remember that fever medicine usually lowers fever 2° F (1-1½° C).

Acetaminophen (e.g., Tylenol):
- **Regular Strength Tylenol:** Take 650 mg (two 325 mg pills) by mouth every 4-6 hours as needed. Each Regular Strength Tylenol pill has 325 mg of acetaminophen.
- **Extra Strength Tylenol:** Take 1,000 mg (two 500 mg pills) every 8 hours as needed. Each Extra Strength Tylenol pill has 500 mg of acetaminophen.
- The most you should take each day is 3,000 mg (10 Regular Strength or 6 Extra Strength pills a day).

Ibuprofen (e.g., Motrin, Advil):
- Take 400 mg (two 200 mg pills) by mouth every 6 hours.
- Another choice is to take 600 mg (three 200 mg pills) by mouth every 8 hours.
- The most you should take each day is 1,200 mg (six 200 mg pills), unless your doctor has told you to take more.

❽ Pain and Fever Medicines—Extra Notes:
- Use the lowest amount of medicine that makes your pain or fever better.
- Acetaminophen is thought to be safer than ibuprofen or naproxen in people > 65 years old. Acetaminophen is in many OTC and prescription medicines. It might be in more than one medicine that you are taking. You need to be careful and not take an overdose. An acetaminophen overdose can hurt the liver.

- McNeil, the company that makes Tylenol, has different dosage instructions for Tylenol in Canada and the United States. In Canada, the maximum recommended dose per day is 4,000 mg or 12 Regular Strength (325 mg) pills. In the United States, McNeil recommends a maximum dose of 10 Regular Strength (325 mg) pills.
- CAUTION: Do not take acetaminophen if you have liver disease.
- CAUTION: Do not take ibuprofen if you have stomach problems, have kidney disease, are pregnant, or have been told by your doctor to avoid this type of anti-inflammatory drug. Do not take ibuprofen for > 7 days without consulting your doctor.
- *Before taking any medicine, read all the instructions on the package.*

Mineral, Vitamin, and Herbal Supplements
❶ Zinc:
- Some studies have reported that zinc gluconate lozenges (i.e., Cold-Eeze) may reduce the duration and severity of cold symptoms.
- **Dosage:** Taken by mouth. You should take this with food to minimize the chance of nausea. Follow package instructions.
- **Side Effects:** Some people complain of nausea and a bad taste in their mouth when they take zinc.
- **Important Note About Zicam:** A zinc nasal gel (i.e., Zicam) is also available OTC. There have been a number of lawsuits claiming that Zicam causes loss of smell (anosmia); it is uncertain whether this truly happens, but for now you should not use this medicine.

❷ Vitamin C:
- A number of experts, including Nobel Prize–winner Linus Pauling, have promoted taking high doses of this vitamin as a treatment for the common cold.
- Research to date shows that vitamin C has minimal (if any) effect on the duration or degree of cold symptoms. Thus, it cannot be recommended as a treatment.
- Vitamin C is probably harmless in standard doses (< 2 g daily).

❸ **Echinacea:** There is no proven benefit of using this herbal remedy in treating or preventing the common cold. In fact, current research suggests that it does not help.

❹ *Read the package instructions thoroughly on all supplements that you take.*

Neti Pot for Sinus Symptoms

❶ **Neti Pot:**
- The neti pot is a small ceramic or plastic pot with a narrow spout. It looks like a small teapot. Two manufacturers of the neti pot are the Himalayan Institute in Pennsylvania and SinuCleanse in Wisconsin.
  - **How It Helps:** The neti pot performs nasal washing (also called nasal irrigation or "jala neti"). The salt water rinses out excess mucus, washes out any irritants (dust, allergens) that might be present, and moisturizes the nasal cavity.
  - **Indications:** The neti pot is widely used as a home remedy to relieve conditions such as colds, sinus infections, and hay fever (nasal allergies).
  - **Adverse Reactions:** None. Though, not everyone likes the sensation of pouring water into their nose.
  - **YouTube Instructional Video:** There are instructional videos on how to use a neti pot both on manufacturers' Web sites and also on YouTube: www.youtube.com/watch?v=j8sDIbRAXlg.

❷ **Neti Pot Step-by-step Instructions:**
- **Step 1:** Follow the directions on the salt package to make warm salt water.
- **Step 2:** Lean forward and turn your head to one side over the sink. Keep your forehead slightly higher than your chin.
- **Step 3:** Gently insert the spout of the neti pot into the higher nostril. Put it far enough so that it forms a comfortable seal.
- **Step 4:** Raise the neti pot gradually so the salt water flows in through your higher nostril and out of the lower nostril. Breathe through your mouth.
- **Step 5:** When the neti pot is empty, blow your nose to clean out the water and mucus.
- **Step 6:** Some of the water may run into the back of your throat. Spit this out. If you swallow the salt water it will not hurt you.
- **Step 7:** Refill the neti pot and repeat on the other side. Again, blow your nose to clear the nasal passages.

❸ **How to Make Saline (Salt Water) Nasal Wash:**
- You can make your own saline nasal wash.
- Add ½ tsp of table salt to 1 cup (8 oz; 240 mL) of warm water.
- You should use sterile, distilled, or previously boiled water for nasal irrigation.

BACKGROUND

Key Points
- Colds are very common. The average adult has 3-4 colds each year.
- Colds are caused by viruses, and no medicine or "shot" will cure an uncomplicated cold.
- Colds are usually not serious. Most patients with colds do not need to be seen.
- Rarely, colds can lead to illnesses of greater seriousness like: sinusitis, bronchitis, pneumonia, and otitis media. The elderly and immunocompromised are at higher risk of developing these infectious complications.

Color of Nasal Discharge
- The nasal discharge normally changes color during different stages of a cold.
- It starts as a clear discharge and later becomes cloudy.
- Sometimes it becomes yellow or green for a few days, and this is still normal.
- Intermittent yellow or green discharge is more common with sleep, antihistamines, or low humidity. *(Reason: All of these events reduce the production of normal nasal secretions.)*
- Yellow or green nasal secretions suggest the presence of a bacterial sinusitis ONLY if they occur in combination with (1) sinus pain OR (2) the return of a fever after it has been gone for > 24 hours OR (3) nasal discharge persists > 10 days without improvement.
- Nasal secretions only become a problem when they block the nose and interfere with breathing through the nose. During a cold, if nasal breathing is noisy but the caller can't see blockage in the nose, it usually means the dried mucus is farther back. Nasal washes can remove it.
- Nasal mucus can become blood-tinged during a cold. It is just due to frequent wiping and blowing the nose.

Nasal Washes (Nasal Irrigation) for Sinus Symptoms

- **Introduction:** Saline (salt water) nasal irrigation is an effective and simple home remedy for treating cold symptoms and other conditions involving the nasal and sinus passages. Nasal irrigation consists of pouring, spraying, or squirting salt water into the nose and then letting it run back out.
- **How It Helps:** The salt water rinses out excess mucus, washes out any irritants (dust, allergens) that might be present, and moisturizes the nasal cavity.
- **Indications:** Nasal irrigation appears to be an effective treatment for chronic sinusitis. It may also help reduce sinus symptoms from acute viral upper respiratory infection (colds), irritant rhinitis (e.g., dust from the workplace), and allergic rhinitis (hay fever). Some doctors recommend it for rhinitis of pregnancy.
- **Adverse Reactions:** Nasal irrigation is safe and there are no serious adverse effects. However, not everyone likes the sensation of having water in their nose.
- **Methods:** There are several ways to perform nasal irrigation. None has been proven to be better than any other. Methods include use of a nasal spray bottle (available OTC), a rubber ear syringe, a Waterpik set on low, a 5- to 20-mL medical syringe without the needle, or a neti pot.
- **How to Make Salt Water for Nasal Irrigation:** Add ½ teaspoon of table salt to 1 cup (8 oz; 240 mL) of warm water.

Neti Pot for Sinus Symptoms

- The neti pot is a small ceramic or plastic pot with a narrow spout. It looks like a small teapot. Two manufacturers of the neti pot are the Himalayan Institute in Pennsylvania and SinuCleanse in Wisconsin.
- **How It Helps:** The neti pot performs nasal washing (also called nasal irrigation or "jala neti"). The salt water rinses out excess mucus, washes out any irritants (dust, allergens) that might be present, and moisturizes the nasal cavity.
- **Indications:** The neti pot is widely used as a home remedy to relieve conditions such as colds, sinus infections, and hay fever (nasal allergies).
- **Adverse Reactions:** None. Nasal irrigation with a neti pot is safe and there are no serious adverse effects. However, not everyone likes the sensation of having salt water poured into their nose.
- **YouTube Instructional Video:** www.youtube.com/ watch?v=j8sDlbRAXlg.

Neti Pot and Primary Amebic Meningoencephalitis

- Primary amebic meningoencephalitis (PAM) is caused by *Naegleria fowleri,* the so-called "brain-eating ameba." This is an extremely rare infection. There were 32 cases in the United States between 2001 and 2010.
- The majority of the cases of PAM have occurred in the southern United States and were linked to swimming or bathing in freshwater lakes, rivers, and ponds containing this ameba. The ameba can also be found in hot springs, geothermal water sources, and poorly maintained swimming pools.
- In 2011 there were 2 cases of PAM in Louisiana that occurred after nasal irrigation with a neti pot. These 2 cases suggest—but are not definite proof—that the nasal irrigation fluid that the individuals used was somehow contaminated with the *N fowleri* ameba.
- The Centers for Disease Control and Prevention recommends that individuals should use distilled, sterile, or previously boiled water for nasal irrigation. It's also important to rinse the irrigation device after each use and leave open to air dry.

Mineral, Vitamin, and Herbal Supplements for Colds

- **Zinc:** Some studies have reported that zinc gluconate lozenges (i.e., Cold-Eeze) may reduce the duration and severity of cold symptoms (Mossad and Prasad). Some people complain of nausea and a bad taste in their mouth when they take zinc. A zinc nasal gel (i.e., Zicam) is also available OTC. There have been a number of lawsuits claiming that Zicam causes loss of smell (anosmia); it is uncertain whether this truly happens, but for now it is reasonable for the call center nurse to not recommend this product.
- **Vitamin C:** A number of experts, including Nobel Prize–winner Linus Pauling, have promoted taking high doses of this vitamin as a treatment for the common cold. Research to date shows that vitamin C has minimal (if any) effect on the duration or degree of cold symptoms. Thus, it cannot be recommended as a treatment. Vitamin C is probably harmless in standard doses (< 2 g daily).
- **Echinacea:** There is no proven benefit of using this herbal remedy in treating or preventing the common cold. In fact, current research suggests that it does not help.

Dextromethorphan Cough Medicines for Cough

- The most common cough suppressant in OTC cough medications is dextromethorphan (DM). Usually the letters DM appear in the name. An example is Robitussin DM.
- **Research:** Dextromethorphan, in some research studies, has been shown to reduce the frequency and severity of cough in adults (≥ 18 years) without significant adverse effects. However, other studies suggest that DM is no better than placebo at reducing a cough.
- **Dextromethorphan and Adult Telephone Triage Protocols:** The care advice in these protocols continues to recommend DM containing cough syrups. The rationale for this is: DM may reduce cough to some extent in adults, adult patients may benefit from the placebo effect of DM, many patients demand a recommendation for a cough syrup, there is no OTC medicine that works better than DM, and, generally, DM has no side effects.
- **Use Cough Drop or Hard Candy Instead:** Cough drops can often be used instead of cough syrups. While some would consider them a placebo similar to cough medicines, they may actually reduce coughing by soothing an irritated throat. In addition, they have the advantage of portability. Hard candy probably works just as well as an OTC cough drop.
- **Use Honey for Nocturnal Cough:** See Honey for Cough section.
- **Dextromethorphan—a Drug of Abuse:** It is important to note that DM has become a drug of abuse. This problem is seen most commonly in the adolescent population. Overdose symptoms can range from giggling and euphoria to hallucinations or coma.

Honey for Cough

- **Recent Research Study:** A recent research study (Paul) compared honey to either DM or no treatment for the treatment of nocturnal coughing. The study group contained 105 children aged 2-18 years. Honey consistently scored the best for reducing cough frequency and cough severity. It also scored best for improving sleep. Dextromethorphan did not score significantly better than "no treatment" (showing its lack of efficacy).
- **How Might Honey Work?:** One explanation for how honey works is that sweet substances naturally cause reflex salivation and increased airway secretions. These secretions may lubricate the airway and remove the trigger (or tickle) that causes a dry, nonproductive cough.
- **Adult Dosage:** 2 teaspoons (10 mL) at bedtime.

CONFUSION (DELIRIUM)

Definition
- Diminished awareness and attention
- Confused thinking, talking "crazy," and acting strange
- Disorientation to person, place, or time
- **May Also Occur:** Hallucinations (usually visual or auditory), delusions (unrealistic thoughts), impaired judgment, decreased memory

Level of Consciousness
- **Alert:** Normal state; oriented to person, place, and time.
- **Delirious (Confused):** Awake but confused talking, thinking, behavior.
- **Lethargic:** Very sleepy but can be awakened with verbal or tactile stimuli. When awakened, not alert.
- **Stuporous:** Very difficult to awaken and only responds to painful stimuli.
- **Comatose:** Persistent loss of consciousness. Doesn't awaken to painful stimuli.

Level of consciousness can also be defined using the **AVPU** acronym:
- **A:** Awake
- **V:** Responding to verbal stimuli
- **P:** Responding to painful stimuli
- **U:** Unresponsive

TRIAGE ASSESSMENT QUESTIONS

Call EMS 911 Now
- ⬤ Difficult to awaken or acting confused (disoriented, slurred speech) and has diabetes
  R/O: hypoglycemia
- ⬤ Difficult to awaken or acting confused (disoriented, slurred speech) and new onset
  R/O: subarachnoid hemorrhage, meningitis, encephalitis, stroke
- ⬤ Weakness of the face, arm, or leg on one side of the body and new onset
  R/O: stroke
- ⬤ Numbness of the face, arm, or leg on one side of the body and new onset
  R/O: stroke
- ⬤ Loss of speech or garbled speech and new onset
  R/O: stroke

- ⬤ Difficulty breathing and bluish (or gray) lips or face
  R/O: CNS symptoms of hypoxia
- ⬤ Shock suspected (e.g., cold/pale/clammy skin, too weak to stand)
  R/O: shock
  First Aid: Lie down with the feet elevated.
- ⬤ Seeing, hearing, or feeling things that are not there (i.e., auditory, visual, or tactile hallucinations)
  R/O: psychosis, substance abuse, alcohol withdrawal, alcoholic hallucinosis
- ⬤ Followed a head injury
  R/O: concussion, cerebral contusion, epidural hematoma
- ⬤ Drug overdose suspected
- ⬤ Sounds like a life-threatening emergency to the triager

See More Appropriate Protocol
- ⬤ Alcohol use, abuse, or dependence, question or problem related to
  Go to Protocol: Alcohol Abuse and Dependence on page 12
- ⬤ Drug abuse or dependence, question or problem related to
  Go to Protocol: Substance Abuse and Dependence on page 382

Go to ED Now
- ⬤ Headache or vomiting
  R/O: meningitis, encephalitis, increased ICP, CO poisoning
- ⬤ Stiff neck (can't touch chin to chest)
  R/O: meningitis
- ⬤ Very strange or paranoid behavior
  R/O: drug-induced psychosis, schizophrenia, bipolar disorder
  Note: Factors that the nurse triager should consider in selecting the best disposition include risk of harm to self or others, how this compares to normal (baseline) behavior, and the patient's support systems (available family and friends).

Go to ED/UCC Now
(or to Office With PCP Approval)
- Fever > 100.5° F (38.1° C)
  R/O: bacterial infection
- Patient sounds very sick or weak to the triager
  Reason: severe acute illness or serious complication suspected

See Today in Office
- Brief confusion (now gone)
  Reason: course of delirium can fluctuate
- Patient wants to be seen (or caregiver requests)

See Today or Tomorrow in Office
- Long-standing confusion (e.g., dementia, stroke) and worsening
  R/O: infection, dehydration, metabolic abnormality

See Within 2 Weeks in Office
- Long-standing confusion (e.g., dementia, stroke) and NO worsening

Home Care
- Sundowning, questions about

HOME CARE ADVICE

Fever
❶ **Fever Medicines:**
- For fevers > 101° F (38.3° C), take either acetaminophen or ibuprofen.
- They are over-the-counter (OTC) drugs that help treat both fever and pain. You can buy them at the drugstore.
- The goal of fever therapy is to bring the fever down to a comfortable level. Remember that fever medicine usually lowers fever 2° F (1-1½° C).

Acetaminophen (e.g., Tylenol):
- **Regular Strength Tylenol:** Take 650 mg (two 325 mg pills) by mouth every 4-6 hours as needed. Each Regular Strength Tylenol pill has 325 mg of acetaminophen.
- **Extra Strength Tylenol:** Take 1,000 mg (two 500 mg pills) every 8 hours as needed. Each Extra Strength Tylenol pill has 500 mg of acetaminophen.
- The most you should take each day is 3,000 mg (10 Regular Strength or 6 Extra Strength pills a day).

Ibuprofen (e.g., Motrin, Advil):
- Take 400 mg (two 200 mg pills) by mouth every 6 hours.
- Another choice is to take 600 mg (three 200 mg pills) by mouth every 8 hours.
- The most you should take each day is 1,200 mg (six 200 mg pills), unless your doctor has told you to take more.

❷ **Fever Medicines—Extra Notes:**
- Use the lowest amount of medicine that makes your fever better.
- Acetaminophen is thought to be safer than ibuprofen or naproxen in people > 65 years old. Acetaminophen is in many OTC and prescription medicines. It might be in more than one medicine that you are taking. You need to be careful and not take an overdose. An acetaminophen overdose can hurt the liver.
- McNeil, the company that makes Tylenol, has different dosage instructions for Tylenol in Canada and the United States. In Canada, the maximum recommended dose per day is 4,000 mg or 12 Regular Strength (325 mg) pills. In the United States, McNeil recommends a maximum dose of 10 Regular Strength (325 mg) pills.
- CAUTION: Do not take acetaminophen if you have liver disease.
- CAUTION: Do not take ibuprofen if you have stomach problems, have kidney disease, are pregnant, or have been told by your doctor to avoid this type of anti-inflammatory drug. Do not take ibuprofen for > 7 days without consulting your doctor.
- *Before taking any medicine, read all the instructions on the package.*

❸ **Call Back If:**
- You (i.e., patient, family member) become worse.

Questions About Sundowning
❶ **Sundowning:**
- **Definition:** Sundowning, or sundown syndrome, refers to the increased confusion that is sometimes seen in the late afternoon and evening in individuals with Alzheimer disease and certain other brain conditions.
- **Symptoms:** In addition to increased confusion, there may be agitation, paranoia, hallucinations, and wandering (i.e., leaving house and getting lost).

❷ **Sundowning—General Care Advice:**
- Arrange for support from family, friends, and other caregivers.
- Ensure adequate room lighting when awake. Consider a small night-light for use during the night.
- Promote orientation by having an easily visible clock and calendar in the room.
- Provide a structured daily routine and a familiar environment (photos of family, favorite possessions).

❸ **Call Back If:**
- You have more questions.
- You (i.e., patient, family member) become worse.

FIRST AID

First Aid Advice for Hypoglycemia—Glucose

If blood glucose < 70 mg/dL (3.9 mmol/L) or unknown (pending EMS arrival) for conscious patients:
- Give sugar (10-15 g glucose) by mouth IF able to swallow.
- Each of the following is equivalent to 10 g of glucose: milk (1 cup; 240 mL); orange juice (½ cup; 120 mL); prepackaged juice box (1 box); table sugar or honey (3 teaspoons; 15 mL); glucose tablets (3 tablets); glucose paste (10-15 g).

First Aid Advice for Hypoglycemia—Glucagon

If blood glucose < 70 mg/dL (3.9 mmol/L) or unknown (pending EMS arrival):
- If family has glucagon for hypoglycemic emergencies AND the caller knows how to use it, encourage the caller to give the glucagon now.
- Inject it IM into the upper outer thigh.
- Adult dosage is 1 mg.

First Aid Advice for Narcotic Overdoes:

If narcotic overdose is known or suspected AND caller has Narcan nasal spray available, give Narcan nasal spray NOW:
- Peel back package and take out the nasal spray.
- Put the nozzle in one of the patient's nostrils.
- Press firmly down on the plunger to give the dose of Narcan.
- Turn patient on his or her side.
- Call EMS 911. Emergency care is needed even if patient improves after Narcan is given.

Each package is a single dose of Narcan. If the patient does not respond by waking up or breathing normally, give another dose. If the patient gets worse after briefly getting better, give another dose.

BACKGROUND

Delirium
- **Definition:** The term delirium is used to describe an acute alteration in level of consciousness that develops over hours to days.
- **Symptoms:** Symptoms may include disorientation, decreased attention, trouble with speech and understanding, and hallucinations. Symptoms often fluctuate.
- Most adults with delirium need to be evaluated emergently.

Causes of Delirium
- Numerous acute and chronic medical conditions
- **Medications:** Especially benzodiazepines, narcotics, anticholinergics
- Substance abuse and alcohol intoxication
- Substance withdrawal (e.g., delirium tremens from alcohol withdrawal)

Conditions That Mimic Delirium
- **Depression:** Depressive symptoms, but oriented times 3
- **Dementia:** Long-standing confusion worsening over months to years
- **Psychosis:** History of psychiatric illness, paranoid thoughts

CONSTIPATION

Definition
- **Infrequent Bowel Movements:** Patient feels like bowel movements do not occur frequently enough.
- **Difficulty Passing Bowel Movements:** Straining, hard stools, or rectal pressure.

Constipation Severity
- **Mild:** Intermittent symptoms; occasional use of dietary modifications (e.g., high fiber), stool softeners, laxatives, or enema.
- **Moderate:** Frequent or ongoing symptoms; regular use of dietary modifications (e.g., high fiber), stool softeners, laxatives, or enema.
- **Severe:** Frequent or ongoing symptoms; manual evacuation/disimpaction required.

TRIAGE ASSESSMENT QUESTIONS

See More Appropriate Protocol
- Abdomen pain is the main symptom and adult male
  Go to Protocol: Abdominal Pain (Male) on page 4
- Abdomen pain is the main symptom and adult female
  Go to Protocol: Abdominal Pain (Female) on page 1
- Rectal bleeding or blood in stool is the main symptom
  Go to Protocol: Rectal Bleeding on page 333

Go to ED/UCC Now (or to Office With PCP Approval)
- Patient sounds very sick or weak to the triager
  Reason: severe acute illness or serious complication suspected

Go to Office Now
- Constant abdominal pain lasting > 2 hours
  R/O: acute abdomen
- Vomiting bile (green color)
  R/O: intestinal obstruction
- Vomiting and abdomen looks much more swollen than usual
  R/O: intestinal obstruction

See Today in Office
- Rectal pain or fullness from fecal impaction (rectum full of stool) and NOT better after sitz bath, suppository, or enema
  R/O: fecal impaction
- Abdomen is more swollen than usual
  R/O: fecal impaction
- Last BM > 4 days ago
  R/O: fecal impaction
- Leaking stool
  R/O: encopresis due to fecal impaction
- Intermittent mild abdominal pain and fever
  R/O: diverticulitis

See Within 3 Days in Office
- Unable to have a BM without manually removing stool (using finger to pull out stool or perform disimpaction)
  Reason: SEVERE constipation; needs better treatment program
- Unable to have a BM without using a laxative, suppository, or enema
  Reason: MODERATE-SEVERE constipation; needs better treatment program
- Constipation persists > 1 week while using care advice
- Weight loss > 10 pounds (5 kg) and not dieting
  R/O: malignancy
- Pencillike, narrow stools
  R/O: malignancy
- Patient wants to be seen

See Within 2 Weeks in Office
- Uses enema or laxative (e.g., lactulose, milk of magnesia) more than once a month
- Constipation is a recurrent ongoing problem (i.e., < 3 BMs/week or straining > 25% of the time)
- Minor bleeding from rectum (e.g., blood just on toilet paper, few drops, streaks on surface of normal formed BM) occurs more than twice
  R/O: anal fissure, hemorrhoids, malignancy

Home Care

○ Mild constipation
○ Rectal pain
  R/O: hemorrhoids, anal fissure, hard stools
○ Rectal pain or fullness from fecal impaction (rectum full of stool) and has not tried a sitz bath, suppository, or enema
  R/O: fecal impaction
○ Minor bleeding from rectum (e.g., blood just on toilet paper, few drops, streaks on surface of normal formed BM), and only 1-2 times

HOME CARE ADVICE

Constipation

❶ **What You Should Know:**
  • Trouble passing a stool, hard stools, and infrequent stools are signs of constipation.
  • Healthy living habits can help treat and prevent constipation. Healthy habits include eating a diet high in fiber and regular exercise.
  • You can treat mild constipation at home.
  • *Here is some care advice that should help.*

❷ **General Constipation Instructions:**
  • Eat a high-fiber diet.
  • Drink adequate liquids.
  • Exercise regularly (even a daily 15-minute walk!).
  • Get into a rhythm—try to have a bowel movement (BM) at the same time each day.
  • Don't ignore your body's signals to have a BM.
  • Avoid enemas and stimulant laxatives.

❸ **High-Fiber Diet:**
  • A high-fiber diet will help improve your intestinal function and soften your BMs. The fiber works by holding more water in your stools.
  • Try to eat fresh fruit and vegetables at each meal (peas, prunes, citrus, apples, beans, corn).
  • Eat more grain foods (bran flakes, bran muffins, graham crackers, oatmeal, brown rice, whole wheat bread). Popcorn is a source of fiber.

❹ **Liquids:** Adequate liquid intake is important to keep your BMs soft.
  • Drink 6-8 glasses of water a day.
    (Caution: Certain medical conditions require fluid restriction.)
  • Prune juice is a natural laxative.
  • Avoid alcohol.

❺ **Get Into a Rhythm:**
  • Try to have a BM at the same time every day. The best time is about 30-60 minutes after breakfast or another meal.
    (Reason: natural increased intestinal activity)
  • Do not ignore your body's signals to have a BM.

❻ **Enemas:** Should be used rarely and only after other measures have not worked.

❼ **Narcotic Pain Medicine:**
  • Narcotic pain medicine (opioids such as Vicodin) can commonly cause constipation.
  • All persons taking narcotic pain pills, especially the elderly, should also be taking a laxative like docusate (Colace).
  • *Before taking any medicine, read all the instructions on the package.*

❽ **Call Back If:**
  • Constipation lasts > 1 week after using Home Care Advice.
  • Abdominal swelling, vomiting, or fever occur.
  • Constant or increasing abdominal pain.
  • You think you need to be seen.
  • You become worse.

Treating Constipation With Over-the-counter Medicines

❶ **Step-by-step:** A step-by-step approach to using over-the-counter (OTC) medicines for constipation is best.

❷ **Step 1—Fiber Laxatives, Every Day:**
  • You can take a fiber laxative instead of eating more fiber. An example of a fiber laxative is psyllium (Metamucil). Fiber can help soften your stools.
  • Fiber works by holding more water in your stools.
  • Be patient. Sometimes this takes a couple weeks before it starts to work.

❸ **Step 2—Use an Osmotic Laxative if Needed:**
  • You can take polyethylene glycol (PEG, MiraLAX) or milk of magnesia.
  • This type of medicine helps pull water into your intestines. This softens the stools.

❹ **Step 3—Add a Stimulant Laxative:**
  • If the constipation does not get better with the Home Care Advice in steps 1 and 2, add a stimulant laxative.
  • Use either bisacodyl (Dulcolax) or a glycerin suppository.

❺ Narcotic Pain Medicine:
- Narcotic pain medicine (opioids such as Vicodin) can commonly cause constipation.
- All persons taking narcotic pain pills, especially the elderly, should also be taking a laxative like docusate (Colace).
- *Before taking any medicine, read all the instructions on the package.*

❻ Call Back If:
- Constipation lasts > 1 week after using Home Care Advice.
- Abdominal swelling, vomiting, or fever occur.
- Constant or increasing abdominal pain.
- You think you need to be seen.
- You become worse.

Rectal Pain

❶ What You Should Know:
- The skin around the rectal area has a rich nerve supply. Pain in this area can be intense.
- Hemorrhoids (piles), anal fissures (skin cracks), and hard stools are the top causes of rectal pain.
- You can treat pain from hemorrhoids, anal fissure, or hard stool at home.
- *Here is some care advice that should help.*

❷ Warm Saline Sitz Bath—Twice Daily for Rectal Pain:
- Sit in a warm sitz bath for 20 minutes twice a day.
- A sitz bath may help relax the muscles around your rectum and make it easier to have a BM.
- Afterwards, pat area dry with unscented toilet paper.

❸ Warm Saline Sitz Bath—How to Make a Sitz Bath:
- Here is how you can make a saline sitz bath.
- Fill the tub with warm water until it is 3-4" (7-10 cm) deep.
- Add ¼ cup (80 g) of table salt or baking soda to a tub of warm water. Stir the water until it dissolves.

❹ Hydrocortisone Ointment Twice a Day for Hemorrhoid Pain:
- You can use 1% hydrocortisone ointment (Anusol HC) to decrease hemorrhoid pain and irritation.
- Hydrocortisone is available over the counter at the drugstore.

❺ Rectal Pain and Can't Pass Stool (Blocked-Up Feeling):
- **Sitz Bath:** Take a 20-minute bath in warm water. It often helps relax the anal sphincter and release the stool.
- **Glycerin Suppository:** If the sitz bath does not work, try 1 or 2 glycerin rectal suppositories.
- **Enema:** An enema should be used rarely and only after other measures have not worked.

❻ Call Your Doctor If:
- Rectal pain not better after using Home Care Advice.
- Abdominal swelling, vomiting, or fever occur.
- Constant or increasing abdominal pain.
- You think you need to be seen.
- You get worse.

Rectal Pain or Fullness From Fecal Impaction

❶ General Constipation Instructions:
- Eat a high-fiber diet.
- Drink adequate liquids.
- Exercise regularly (even a daily 15-minute walk!).
- Get into a rhythm—try to have a BM at the same time each day.
- Don't ignore your body's signals to have a BM.

❷ Warm Saline Sitz Bath—Twice Daily for Rectal Pain Due to Constipation:
- Sit in a warm sitz bath for 20 minutes twice a day.
- A sitz bath may help relax the muscles around your rectum and make it easier to have a BM.
- Afterwards, pat area dry with unscented toilet paper.

❸ Warm Saline Sitz Bath—How to Make a Sitz Bath:
- Here is how you can make a saline sitz bath.
- Fill the tub with warm water until it is 3-4" (7-10 cm) deep.
- Add ¼ cup (80 g) of table salt or baking soda to a tub of warm water. Stir the water until it dissolves.

❹ Suppository for Acute Rectal Pain: If the sitz bath doesn't work, use 1 or 2 glycerin suppositories (OTC).

❺ Fleet Enema for Acute Rectal Pain: If the sitz bath and suppository do not relieve the rectal pain, a Fleet phosphate enema may be helpful.

❻ **Fleet Enema—Step-by-step Instructions:**
- **Step 1—Body Position:** Patient should lie on left side. Keep the bottom leg (left) straight or slightly bent. The right knee should be flexed (bent upwards).
- **Step 2—Enema Bottle:** Shake well and remove the cap from the enema bottle tip.
- **Step 3—Inserting Tip of Enema Bottle:** Lubricate the tip of the enema tube with water or small amount of Vaseline. Gently insert tip of enema tube into rectum about 1-2" (3-5 cm). Gently squeeze bottle to slowly push the fluid into the rectum.
- **Step 4—Wait:** Patient should stay on side for several minutes. The patient should try to hold the enema fluid inside for at least 5 minutes.
- **Step 5—Fluid Comes Back Out:** Patient (if able) should sit on toilet. Fluid and stool should come out. Enemas usually work in 5-20 minutes but can take longer.

❼ **Caution—Fleet Enema:**
- Do not use if there is fever, abdominal pain, or rectal bleeding.
- Do not use if you have heart disease, kidney disease, or inflammatory bowel disease.
- Do not use if you have neutropenia (very low white cell count).
- Do not use if you are pregnant.

❽ **Expected Course:**
- Rectal pain should be completely relieved by these instructions.
- If the discomfort does not go away, you should be seen right away.

❾ **Call Back If:**
- Rectal pain is not relieved.
- Constant or increasing abdominal pain.
- Abdominal swelling or vomiting occur.
- You become worse.

Minor Bleeding From Hemorrhoids

❶ **Reassurance:**
- Small drops of blood can sometimes be seen on the toilet paper or stool in people with hemorrhoids or rectal irritation.
- *Here is some care advice that should help.*

❷ **General Constipation Instructions:**
- Eat a high-fiber diet.
- Drink adequate liquids.
- Exercise regularly (even a daily 15-minute walk!)
- Get into a rhythm—try to have a BM at the same time each day.
- Don't ignore your body's signals to have a BM.

❸ **Warm Saline Sitz Baths—Twice Daily for Rectal Symptoms:**
- Sit in a warm sitz bath for 20 minutes twice a day. This will decrease swelling and irritation, keep the area clean, and help with healing.
- Afterwards, pat area dry with unscented toilet paper.

❹ **Warm Saline Sitz Bath—How to Make a Sitz Bath:**
- Here is how you can make a saline sitz bath.
- Fill the tub with warm water until it is 3-4" (7-10 cm) deep.
- Add ¼ cup (80 g) of table salt or baking soda to a tub of warm water. Stir the water until it dissolves.

❺ **Hydrocortisone Ointment for Rectal Itching:**
- After sitz bath and drying your rectal area, put hydrocortisone ointment on the area 2 times a day. This will help decrease the itching.
- This is an over-the-counter (OTC) drug. You can buy it at the drugstore. It can be found in a number of OTC hemorrhoid medicines (e.g., Anusol HC, Preparation H Hydrocortisone, Anal-pram HC Cream).
- Some people like to keep the ointment in the refrigerator. It feels even better if the cream is used when it is cold.
- CAUTION: Do not use this medicine for > 1 week without talking to your doctor.
- *Before using any medicine, read all the instructions on the package.*

❻ **High-Fiber Diet:**
- A high-fiber diet will help improve your intestinal function and soften your BMs. The fiber works by holding more water in your stools.
- Try to eat fruit and vegetables at each meal (peas, prunes, citrus, apples, beans, corn).
- Eat more grain foods (bran flakes, bran muffins, graham crackers, oatmeal, brown rice, whole wheat bread).

❼ **Liquids:**
- Adequate liquid intake is important to keep your BMs soft.
- Drink 6-8 glasses of water a day.
  (Caution: Certain medical conditions require fluid restriction.)
- Prune juice is a natural laxative.
- Avoid alcohol.

❽ **Call Back If:**
- Rectal bleeding increases or occurs > 2 times.
- No BM for > 4 days.
- Constant or increasing abdominal pain.
- Fever > 100.5° F (38.1° C) occurs.
- You become worse.

BACKGROUND

Symptoms of Constipation

Some patients complain of "constipation" if they feel that their bowel movements (BMs) do not occur frequently enough. However, every person has his or her own sense of how often BMs should occur. Normal BM frequency varies from 3 times a day to 3 times a week.

Patients also complain of constipation when they have difficulty passing BMs. They may describe this in different ways, including

- Straining
- Hard or lumpy stools
- Feeling of rectal fullness or that stool cannot be passed
- Feeling of incomplete evacuation ("It won't come out.")
- Abdominal fullness or bloating
- Need to press around the anus

The passage of small, dry, rabbit-pellet–like stools is not constipation and instead reflects the desiccation mechanism and insufficient oral fluids. Additional symptoms frequently associated with constipation include abdominal bloating, cramping, malaise, and nausea.

Lifestyle Causes
- **Inadequate Fiber in Diet:** Inadequate dietary fiber reduces intestinal motility and makes BMs hard and more difficult to pass. Fiber works by helping stools to retain water. Good sources of dietary fiber are fresh fruits and vegetables, beans, and bran. Fiber can also be taken via supplements (e.g., Metamucil).
- **Insufficient Liquids:** Insufficient liquid intake cause stools to be dry and harder to pass. Adults should drink 6-8 glasses of water daily.
- **Lack of Exercise:** Inactivity reduces bowel function, whereas exercise helps stimulate the bowels and improve regularity. Patients who are bedridden have increased problems with constipation and may develop fecal impaction.
- **Postponing BMs:** Some individuals ignore their body's signals for having a BM. This can lead to chronic problems with constipation.
- **Recent Travel:** Travel can cause constipation because it interferes with your diet and normal daily cycle.

Other Causes
- **Irritable Bowel Syndrome:** Patients with this syndrome may report abdominal pain and bloating relieved with passage of BMs. This is diagnosed clinically, as there is no test that diagnoses irritable bowel syndrome.
- **Malignant Neoplasm of Colon:** Colon cancer can present initially as constipation. Suspect this in elderly patients with new onset or worsening constipation.
- **Medications:** There are a number of prescription and OTC medications that can cause or aggravate constipation. Examples include NSAIDs, antidepressants, calcium channel blockers (e.g., verapamil), and iron.
- **Medications—Narcotic (Opiate):** Narcotic pain medicine can commonly cause constipation. All persons taking narcotic pain pills, especially the elderly, should also be taking a laxative like docusate (Colace).
- **Metabolic and Endocrine Disorders:** Examples include hypercalcemia, hypokalemia, diabetes mellitus, and hypothyroidism.

- **Neurologic Disease:** Constipation can occur in patients with multiple sclerosis, Parkinson disease, and spinal cord injury.
- **Pregnancy:** Constipation is common in pregnancy, especially during the third trimester.
- **Rectal Problems:** Anal fissures and hemorrhoids cause localized pain and slight bleeding. Hard BMs cause tears in the skin (anal fissure) with passage. Chronic constipation can lead to straining at BMs, which causes enlargement of the rectal veins (hemorrhoids). The pain from these 2 disorders may cause a patient to avoid having a BM, thus aggravating the constipation further.

Caution: Constipation

Constipation is usually not a serious symptom. However, there are several red flags that can signal that additional medical evaluation is needed:

- Abdominal or rectal mass
- Blood in stool or rectal bleeding
- Iron deficiency anemia
- New onset of severe constipation and no obvious cause
- Weight loss and not dieting

COUGH

Definition
- A cough is the sound made when the cough reflex clears the lungs. It helps protect the lungs from infections.
- A coughing fit or spell is nonstop coughing that lasts > 5 minutes.
- Coughs can be dry (no mucus) or wet (with mucus).

Definition—Severe Difficulty Breathing:
- Marked respiratory effort (struggling to breathe). Can only speak in single words. Cyanosis may occur. (*Response: Activate EMS.*)

TRIAGE ASSESSMENT QUESTIONS

Call EMS 911 Now
- Bluish (or gray) lips or face
  R/O: cyanosis and need for oxygen
- SEVERE difficulty breathing (e.g., struggling for each breath, speaks in single words)
  R/O: respiratory failure, hypoxia
- Rapid onset of cough and has hives
  R/O: anaphylaxis
- Coughing started suddenly after medicine, an allergic food, or bee sting
  R/O: anaphylaxis
- Difficulty breathing after exposure to flames, smoke, or fumes
  R/O: inhalation injury
- Sounds like a life-threatening emergency to the triager

See More Appropriate Protocol
- Previous asthma attacks and this feels like asthma attack
  Go to Protocol: Asthma Attack on page 38

Go to ED Now
- Chest pain present when not coughing
  R/O: pneumonia, pneumothorax, pulmonary embolism
- Difficulty breathing
  R/O: pneumonia
- Passed out (i.e., fainted, collapsed and was not responding)
  R/O: hypoxia, cough syncope, pulmonary embolism

Go to ED/UCC Now (or to Office With PCP Approval)
- Patient sounds very sick or weak to the triager
  Reason: severe acute illness or serious complication suspected

Go to Office Now
- Coughed up > 1 tablespoon (15 mL) blood
  (Exception: blood-tinged sputum)
  Reason: significant hemoptysis
- Fever > 103° F (39.4° C)
  R/O: pneumonia
- Fever > 100.5° F (38.1° C) and > 60 years of age
  R/O: pneumonia
- Fever > 100.0° F (37.8° C) and has diabetes mellitus or a weak immune system (e.g., HIV positive, cancer chemotherapy, organ transplant, splenectomy, chronic steroids)
  R/O: pneumonia
- Fever > 100.0° F (37.8° C) and bedridden (e.g., nursing home patient, stroke, chronic illness, recovering from surgery)
  R/O: pneumonia
  Note: May need ambulance transport to ED.
- Increasing ankle swelling
  R/O: congestive heart failure
- Wheezing is present
  R/O: asthma, bronchitis

See Today in Office
- SEVERE coughing spells (e.g., whooping sound after coughing, vomiting after coughing)
  R/O: whooping cough (pertussis)
- Coughing up rusty-colored (reddish-brown) or blood-tinged sputum
  R/O: pneumonia
- Fever present > 3 days (72 hours)
  R/O: bacterial sinusitis, bronchitis, pneumonia
- Fever returns after gone > 24 hours and symptoms worse or not improved
  R/O: bacterial sinusitis, bronchitis, pneumonia
- Using nasal washes and pain medicine > 24 hours and sinus pain persists
  R/O: bacterial sinusitis

● Known COPD or other severe lung disease (i.e., bronchiectasis, cystic fibrosis, lung surgery) and worsening symptoms (i.e., increased sputum purulence or amount, increased breathing difficulty)
R/O: exacerbation
Reason: may need antibiotic therapy

See Today or Tomorrow in Office

● Continuous (nonstop) coughing interferes with work or school and no improvement using cough treatment per Home Care Advice
Reason: may need codeine or asthma medication

● Patient wants to be seen

See Within 3 Days in Office

● Cough has been present for > 3 weeks
R/O: bacterial sinusitis, bronchitis

● Allergy symptoms are also present (e.g., itchy eyes, clear nasal discharge, postnasal drip)
R/O: asthmatic cough

● Nasal discharge present > 10 days
R/O: bacterial sinusitis

● Exposure to tuberculosis (TB)

● Taking an ACE inhibitor medication (e.g., benazepril/Lotensin, captopril/Capoten, enalapril/Vasotec, lisinopril/Zestril)
R/O: ACE inhibitor as cause; see list in Background

Home Care

○ Cough with no complications
R/O: viral URI

○ Cough with cold symptoms (e.g., runny nose, postnasal drip, throat clearing)
R/O: postnasal drip syndrome (upper airway cough syndrome)

HOME CARE ADVICE

General Care Advice for Mild to Moderate Cough

❶ Reassurance:
- Coughing is the way that our lungs remove irritants and mucus. It helps protect our lungs from getting pneumonia.
- You can get a dry hacking cough after a chest cold. Sometimes this type of cough can last 1-3 weeks and be worse at night.
- You can also get a cough after being exposed to irritating substances like smoke, strong perfumes, and dust.
- *Here is some care advice that should help.*

❷ Cough Medicines:
- **OTC Cough Syrups:** The most common cough suppressant in OTC cough medications is dextromethorphan (DM). Often the letters DM appear in the name.
- **OTC Cough Drops:** Cough drops can help a lot, especially for mild coughs. They reduce coughing by soothing your irritated throat and removing that tickle sensation in the back of the throat. Cough drops also have the advantage of portability—you can carry them with you.
- **Home Remedy—Hard Candy:** Hard candy works just as well as medicine-flavored OTC cough drops. People who have diabetes should use sugar-free candy.
- **Home Remedy—Honey:** This old home remedy has been shown to help decrease coughing at night. The adult dosage is 2 teaspoons (10 mL) at bedtime. Honey should not be given to infants < 1 year of age.

❸ OTC Cough Syrup—Dextromethorphan:
- Cough syrups containing the cough suppressant DM may help decrease your cough. Cough syrups work best for coughs that keep you awake at night. They can also sometimes help in the late stages of a respiratory infection when the cough is dry and hacking. They can be used along with cough drops.
- Examples: Benylin, Robitussin DM, Vicks 44 Cough Relief.
- *Before taking any medicine, read all the instructions on the package.*

❹ Caution—Dextromethorphan:
- Do not try to completely suppress coughs that produce mucus and phlegm. Remember that coughing is helpful in bringing up mucus from the lungs and preventing pneumonia.
- **Research Notes:** Dextromethorphan, in some research studies, has been shown to reduce the frequency and severity of cough in adults (≥ 18 years) without significant adverse effects. However, other studies suggest that DM is no better than placebo at reducing a cough.
- **Drug Abuse Potential:** It should be noted that DM has become a drug of abuse. This problem is seen most often in adolescents. Overdose symptoms can range from giggling and euphoria to hallucinations and coma.

- **Contraindicated:** Do not take DM if you are taking a monoamine oxidase (MAO) inhibitor now or in the past 2 weeks. Examples of MAO inhibitors include isocarboxazid (Marplan), phenelzine (Nardil), rasagiline (Azilect), selegiline (Eldepryl, Emsam, Zelapar), and tranylcypromine (Parnate). Do not take DM if you are taking venlafaxine (Effexor).

❺ **Coughing Spasms:**
- Drink warm fluids. Inhale warm mist. *(Reason: Both relax the airway and loosen up the phlegm.)*
- Suck on cough drops or hard candy to coat the irritated throat.

❻ **Prevent Dehydration:**
- Drink adequate liquids.
- This will help soothe an irritated or dry throat and loosen up the phlegm.

❼ **Avoid Tobacco Smoke:** Smoking or being exposed to smoke makes coughs much worse.

❽ **Fever Medicines:**
- For fevers > 101° F (38.3° C) take either acetaminophen or ibuprofen.
- They are over-the-counter (OTC) drugs that help treat both fever and pain. You can buy them at the drugstore.
- The goal of fever therapy is to bring the fever down to a comfortable level. Remember that fever medicine usually lowers fever 2° F (1-1½° C).

Acetaminophen (e.g., Tylenol):
- **Regular Strength Tylenol:** Take 650 mg (two 325 mg pills) by mouth every 4-6 hours as needed. Each Regular Strength Tylenol pill has 325 mg of acetaminophen.
- **Extra Strength Tylenol:** Take 1,000 mg (two 500 mg pills) every 8 hours as needed. Each Extra Strength Tylenol pill has 500 mg of acetaminophen.
- The most you should take each day is 3,000 mg (10 Regular Strength or 6 Extra Strength pills a day).

Ibuprofen (e.g., Motrin, Advil):
- Take 400 mg (two 200 mg pills) by mouth every 6 hours.
- Another choice is to take 600 mg (three 200 mg pills) by mouth every 8 hours.
- The most you should take each day is 1,200 mg (six 200 mg pills), unless your doctor has told you to take more.

❾ **Fever Medicines—Extra Notes:**
- Use the lowest amount of medicine that makes your fever better.
- Acetaminophen is thought to be safer than ibuprofen or naproxen in people > 65 years old. Acetaminophen is in many OTC and prescription medicines. It might be in more than one medicine that you are taking. You need to be careful and not take an over- dose. An acetaminophen overdose can hurt the liver.
- McNeil, the company that makes Tylenol, has different dosage instructions for Tylenol in Canada and the United States. In Canada, the maximum recommended dose per day is 4,000 mg or 12 Regular Strength (325 mg) pills. In the United States, McNeil recommends a maximum dose of 10 Regular Strength (325 mg) pills.
- CAUTION: Do not take acetaminophen if you have liver disease.
- CAUTION: Do not take ibuprofen if you have stomach problems, have kidney disease, are pregnant, or have been told by your doctor to avoid this type of anti-inflammatory drug. Do not take ibuprofen for > 7 days without consulting your doctor.
- *Before taking any medicine, read all the instructions on the package.*

❿ **Expected Course:**
- The expected course depends on what is causing the cough.
- Viral bronchitis (chest cold) causes a cough that lasts 1-3 weeks. Sometimes you may cough up lots of phlegm (sputum, mucus). The mucus can normally be white, gray, yellow, or green.

⓫ **Call Back If:**
- Difficulty breathing.
- Cough lasts > 3 weeks.
- Fever lasts > 3 days.
- You become worse.

Cough With Cold Symptoms

❶ **Reassurance:**
- It sounds like an uncomplicated cold that we can treat at home.
- Colds are very common and may make you feel uncomfortable.
- Colds are caused by viruses, and no medicine or "shot" will cure an uncomplicated cold.
- Colds are usually not serious.
- *Here is some care advice that should help.*

❷ For a Runny Nose With Profuse Discharge: Blow the Nose
- Nasal mucus and discharge help to wash viruses and bacteria out of the nose and sinuses.
- Blowing the nose is all that is needed.
- If the skin around your nostrils gets irritated, apply a tiny amount of petroleum ointment to the nasal openings once or twice a day.

❸ Nasal Washes for a Stuffy Nose:
- **Introduction:** Saline (salt water) nasal irrigation (nasal wash) is an effective and simple home remedy for treating stuffy nose and sinus congestion. The nose can be irrigated by pouring, spraying, or squirting salt water into the nose and then letting it run back out.
- **How It Helps:** The salt water rinses out excess mucus and washes out any irritants (dust, allergens) that might be present. It also moistens the nasal cavity.
- **Methods:** There are several ways to irrigate the nose. You can use a saline nasal spray bottle (available over the counter), a rubber ear syringe, a medical syringe without the needle, or a neti pot.

❹ Nasal Washes—Step-by-step Instructions:
- **Step 1:** Lean over a sink.
- **Step 2:** Gently squirt or spray warm salt water into one of your nostrils.
- **Step 3:** Some of the water may run into the back of your throat. Spit this out. If you swallow the salt water it will not hurt you.
- **Step 4:** Blow your nose to clean out the water and mucus.
- **Step 5:** Repeat steps 1-4 for the other nostril. You can do this a couple times a day if it seems to help you.

❺ How to Make Saline (Salt Water) Nasal Wash:
- You can make your own saline nasal wash.
- Add ½ tsp of table salt to 1 cup (8 oz; 240 mL) of warm water.
- You should use sterile, distilled, or previously boiled water for nasal irrigation.

❻ Medicines for a Stuffy or Runny Nose:
- Most cold medicines that are available over the counter are not helpful.
- **Antihistamines:** Are only helpful if you also have nasal allergies.
- If you have a very runny nose and you really think you need a medicine, you can try using a nasal decongestant for a couple days.

❼ Nasal Decongestants for a Very Stuffy or Runny Nose:
- **Most people do not need to use these medicines.**
- If your nose feels blocked, you should try using nasal washes first.
- If you have a very stuffy nose, nasal decongestant medicines can shrink the swollen nasal mucosa and allow for easier breathing. If you have a very runny nose, these medicines can reduce the amount of drainage. They may be taken as pills by mouth or as a nasal spray.
- **Pseudoephedrine (Sudafed):** Available over the counter in pill form. Typical adult dosage is two 30 mg tablets every 6 hours.
- **Oxymetazoline Nasal Drops (Afrin):** Available over the counter. Clean out the nose before using. Spray each nostril once, wait 1 minute for absorption, and then spray a second time.
- **Phenylephrine Nasal Drops (Neo-Synephrine):** Available over the counter. Clean out the nose before using. Spray each nostril once, wait 1 minute for absorption, and then spray a second time.
- *Before taking any medicine, read all the instructions on the package.*

❽ Caution—Nasal Decongestants:
- Do not take these medications if you have high blood pressure, heart disease, prostate problems, or an overactive thyroid.
- Do not take these medications if you are pregnant.
- Do not take these medications if you have used an MAO inhibitor such as isocarboxazid (Marplan), phenelzine (Nardil), rasagiline (Azilect), selegiline (Eldepryl, Emsam, Zelapar), or tranylcypromine (Parnate) in the past 2 weeks. Life-threatening side effects can occur.
- Do not use these medications for > 3 days. *(Reason: rebound nasal congestion)*

❾ Pain and Fever Medicines:
- For pain or fever relief, take either acetaminophen or ibuprofen.
- They are over-the-counter (OTC) drugs that help treat both fever and pain. You can buy them at the drugstore.
- Treat fevers > 101° F (38.3° C). The goal of fever therapy is to bring the fever down to a comfortable level. Remember that fever medicine usually lowers fever 2° F (1-1½° C).

Acetaminophen (e.g., Tylenol):

- **Regular Strength Tylenol:** Take 650 mg (two 325 mg pills) by mouth every 4-6 hours as needed. Each Regular Strength Tylenol pill has 325 mg of acetaminophen.
- **Extra Strength Tylenol:** Take 1,000 mg (two 500 mg pills) every 8 hours as needed. Each Extra Strength Tylenol pill has 500 mg of acetaminophen.
- The most you should take each day is 3,000 mg (10 Regular Strength or 6 Extra Strength pills a day).

Ibuprofen (e.g., Motrin, Advil):

- Take 400 mg (two 200 mg pills) by mouth every 6 hours.
- Another choice is to take 600 mg (three 200 mg pills) by mouth every 8 hours.
- The most you should take each day is 1,200 mg (six 200 mg pills), unless your doctor has told you to take more.

❿ **Pain and Fever Medicines—Extra Notes:**

- Use the lowest amount of medicine that makes your pain or fever better.
- Acetaminophen is thought to be safer than ibuprofen or naproxen in people > 65 years old. Acetaminophen is in many OTC and prescription medicines. It might be in more than one medicine that you are taking. You need to be careful and not take an overdose. An acetaminophen overdose can hurt the liver.
- McNeil, the company that makes Tylenol, has different dosage instructions for Tylenol in Canada and the United States. In Canada, the maximum recommended dose per day is 4,000 mg or 12 Regular Strength (325 mg) pills. In the United States, McNeil recommends a maximum dose of 10 Regular Strength (325 mg) pills.
- CAUTION: Do not take acetaminophen if you have liver disease.
- CAUTION: Do not take ibuprofen if you have stomach problems, have kidney disease, are pregnant, or have been told by your doctor to avoid this type of anti-inflammatory drug. Do not take ibuprofen for > 7 days without consulting your doctor.
- *Before taking any medicine, read all the instructions on the package.*

⓫ **Contagiousness:**

- The cold virus is present in your nasal secretions.
- Cover your nose and mouth with a tissue when you sneeze or cough.
- Wash your hands frequently with soap and water.
- You can return to work or school after the fever is gone and you feel well enough to participate in normal activities.

⓬ **Expected Course:**

- Fever may last 2-3 days.
- Nasal discharge 7-14 days.
- Cough up to 2-3 weeks.

⓭ **Call Back If:**

- Difficulty breathing occurs.
- Fever lasts > 3 days.
- Nasal discharge lasts > 10 days.
- Cough lasts > 3 weeks.
- You become worse.

BACKGROUND

Key Points

- Cough is one of the most common symptoms that patients experience. It is the fifth most common reason for visits to physicians.
- A cough is the sound made when the cough reflex suddenly forces air and secretions from the lungs.
- The common cold is the single most common cause of acute cough (i.e., cough < 3 weeks in duration).
- Smokers may have a chronic cough, especially in the morning.

Why Do We Cough?

A cough has 2 important functions:

- Serves to clear the airways of infection, mucus, foreign bodies, and other irritants.
- Protects against aspiration of oral and stomach contents.

Causes of Coughing

- **Most Common Causes:** Postnasal drip syndrome from a cold, allergic rhinitis, and sinusitis
- **Other Common Causes:** Asthma, bronchitis, pneumonia, gastroesophageal reflux, and smoking
- **Less Common Causes:** Lung cancer, congestive heart failure, pulmonary embolism, tuberculosis, whooping cough, and ACE inhibitor drugs

Coughs and How They Sound

- Coughs generally are not helpful at telling us if the cause is serious. Asking about difficulty breathing or respiratory distress is the only way to determine seriousness.
- Coughs are also not helpful at determining etiology, except for the barky cough of croup in children, which is fairly distinctive. The sound of the cough in patients can vary greatly over the course of the day. A rattly cough is simply a productive cough. The chest wall usually vibrates if you feel it during a bout of coughing.

Antibiotics for Cough

- **Acute Bronchitis:** Routine antibiotic therapy provides no meaningful benefit in the treatment of acute bronchitis. There is no effect on duration of illness, severity of symptoms, or return to work.
- **Common Cold:** Colds are caused by viruses, and no medicine, "shot," or antibiotic will cure an uncomplicated cold.
- **Pneumonia:** Pneumonia is often caused by bacteria; antibiotic therapy is usually needed.
- **Whooping Cough (Pertussis):** Whooping cough is caused by bacteria (*Bordetella pertussis*). Treatment with antibiotics is indicated when whooping cough is diagnosed or strongly suspected.

Dextromethorphan Cough Medicines for Cough

- The most common cough suppressant in OTC cough medications is dextromethorphan (DM). Usually the letters DM appear in the name. An example is Robitussin DM.
- **Research:** Dextromethorphan, in some research studies, has been shown to reduce the frequency and severity of cough in adults (≥ 18 years) without significant adverse effects. However, other studies suggest that DM is no better than placebo at reducing a cough.
- **Dextromethorphan and Adult Telephone Triage Protocols:** The care advice in these protocols continues to recommend DM-containing cough syrups. The rationale for this is: DM may reduce cough to some extent in adults, adult patients may benefit from the placebo effect of DM, many patients demand a recommendation for a cough syrup, there is no OTC medicine that works better than DM, and, generally, DM has no side effects.

- **Use Cough Drop or Hard Candy Instead:** Cough drops can often be used instead of cough syrups. While some would consider them a placebo similar to cough medicines, they may actually reduce coughing by soothing an irritated throat. In addition, they have the advantage of portability. Hard candy probably works just as well as an OTC cough drop.
- **Use Honey for Nocturnal Cough:** See Honey for Cough section.
- **Dextromethorphan—a Drug of Abuse:** It is important to note that DM has become a drug of abuse. This problem is seen most commonly in the adolescent population. Overdose symptoms can range from giggling and euphoria to hallucinations or coma.

Honey for Cough

- **Recent Research Study:** A recent research study (Paul) compared honey with either DM or no treatment for the treatment of nocturnal coughing. The study group contained 105 children aged 2-18 years. Honey consistently scored the best for reducing cough frequency and cough severity. It also scored best for improving sleep. Dextromethorphan did not score significantly better than "no treatment" (showing its lack of efficacy).
- **How Might Honey Work?:** One explanation for how honey works is that sweet substances naturally cause reflex salivation and increased airway secretions. These secretions may lubricate the airway and remove the trigger (or tickle) that causes a dry, nonproductive cough.
- **Adult Dosage:** 2 teaspoons (10 mL) at bedtime.

Vicks VapoRub and Other Menthol Products for Cough

- Menthol-containing products (OTC) are sold to be added to vaporizers. Menthol fumes tend to make coughs worse. They can definitely worsen an asthma attack.
- Since they have no proven benefits, they should be avoided.

Angiotensin-Converting Enzyme (ACE) inhibitors

can cause a dry chronic cough. Generic and trade name listing:

- **Benazepril:** Lotensin
- **Captopril:** Capoten
- **Cilazapril:** Inhibace
- **Enalapril, Enalaprilat:** Vasotec
- **Fosinopril:** Monopril
- **Lisinopril:** Zestril
- **Moexipril:** Univasc
- **Perindopril:** Aceon, Coversyl
- **Quinapril:** Accupril
- **Ramipril:** Altace
- **Trandolapril:** Mavik

DENTAL PROCEDURE ANTIBIOTIC PROPHYLAXIS

Definition
- Patient is requesting antibiotic prophylaxis prior to a dental procedure.

TRIAGE ASSESSMENT QUESTIONS

Go to ED/UCC Now
(or to Office With PCP Approval)
- ● Patient sounds very sick or weak to the triager
  Reason: severe acute illness or serious complication suspected

Discuss With PCP and Callback by Nurse Today
- ◐ Has both SPECIFIED CARDIAC CONDITION and SPECIFIED DENTAL PROCEDURE, and NO standing order to call in prescription for antibiotic
  Reason: antibiotic prescription needed
  Note: See relevant definitions in Background.
- ◐ Has both SPECIFIED CARDIAC CONDITION and SPECIFIED DENTAL PROCEDURE, and already taking antibiotics for something else
  Reason: current antibiotic may or may not be effective
- ◐ Joint replacement surgery in past 2 years
  Reason: antibiotic prescription may (or may not) be needed; patient should discuss this with PCP or dentist
- ◐ Triager unable to answer question

See Within 3 Days in Office
- ◐ Patient wants to be seen

Home Care
- ○ Has both SPECIFIED CARDIAC CONDITION and SPECIFIED DENTAL PROCEDURE, and standing order to call in prescription for antibiotic
  Reason: antibiotic prescription needed
  Note: See relevant definitions in Background.
- ○ Does not have SPECIFIED CARDIAC CONDITION
  Reason: antibiotic prophylaxis is not indicated
- ○ Does not have SPECIFIED DENTAL PROCEDURE
  Reason: antibiotic prophylaxis is not indicated

HOME CARE ADVICE

Antibiotic Prophylaxis Is Indicated
❶ You Should Take Antibiotics Before the Dental Procedure:
- Given what you have told me about your heart condition and the planned dental work, it sounds like you should take antibiotics before the procedure.
- Take the antibiotic 1 hour before the start of the dental procedure.

❷ Recommended Antibiotic: Follow call center policy and the physician's practice rules. Call in prescription for one of the following antibiotics:
- Amoxicillin 2 g orally
- **Unable to Take Medications by Mouth:** Ampicillin 2 g intramuscular (IM) shot or intravenous (IV) or cefazolin 1 g IM or IV.
- **Allergic to Penicillins:** Clindamycin 600 mg orally, IM, IV, or azithromycin (Zithromax) 500 mg orally.

❸ Caution—Antibiotics:
- Ask patient about allergies.
- Intramuscular antibiotics generally should not be used in patients taking Coumadin or who have a coagulopathy.

❹ Call Back If:
- You have more questions.

Antibiotic Prophylaxis Is Not Indicated
❶ You Do NOT Need to Take Antibiotics Before This Dental Procedure: Given what you have told me about your heart condition and the planned dental work, it sounds like you do NOT need to take antibiotics before the procedure.

❷ Disclaimer:
- These are protocols for general practice. Occasionally, antibiotic prophylaxis may still be advised for an individual patient. If you have any type of heart condition, you should ask your cardiologist about this.
- The full text of the American Heart Association (AHA) guideline for prevention of infective endocarditis is available online at: http://circ.ahajournals.org/content/116/15/1736.full.pdf.

- There are some cardiac conditions that have an increased lifetime risk of endocarditis, yet the AHA has deemed that antibiotic prophylaxis is not indicated. If you develop symptoms of endocarditis, such as unexplained fever, talk with your doctor right away.

❸ Call Back If:
- You have more questions.

Additional Resources

❶ The AHA has created a wallet card that physicians can give to their patients. It is available online at: www.heart.org/idc/groups/heart-public/@wcm/@hcm/documents/downloadable/ucm_307644.pdf.

❷ The wallet card is also available in Spanish at: www.heart.org/idc/groups/heart-public/@wcm/@hcm/documents/downloadable/ucm_311663.pdf.

BACKGROUND

Key Points

- In 2007 the American Heart Association (AHA) released guidelines for antibiotic prophylaxis prior to procedures for the purpose of preventing infective endocarditis.
- There are substantive changes in the 2007 guidelines; antibiotic prophylaxis is now indicated in fewer patients than before. Antibiotic prophylaxis is indicated in patients who have *both* a SPECIFIED CARDIAC CONDITION *and* a SPECIFIED DENTAL PROCEDURE (see next sections).
- The full text of the AHA guideline for prevention of infective endocarditis is available online at: http://circ.ahajournals.org/content/116/15/1736.full.pdf.
- The AHA has created a wallet card that physicians can give to their patients. It is available online at: www.heart.org/idc/groups/heart-public/@wcm/@hcm/documents/downloadable/ucm_307644.pdf.
- The Canadian Dental Association (CDA) released a statement in November 2007 that disagreed with a part of the 2007 AHA antibiotic prophylaxis guidelines. Specifically, the CDA recommended that prophylactic antibiotics should be considered for all patient types undergoing dental procedures during the first 2 years following joint replacement.
- In 2015 the American Dental Association (ADA) stated: *"In general, for patients with prosthetic joint implants, prophylactic antibiotics are not recommended prior to dental procedures to prevent prosthetic joint infection."*

However, the ADA also recommended that this was a decision made jointly by practitioner and patient.

Specified Cardiac Conditions

Antibiotic prophylaxis prior to specified dental procedures is recommended for the following cardiac conditions (AHA 2007):
- Prosthetic cardiac valve (artificial valve)
- Previous infective endocarditis
- Congenital heart disease (CHD), specifically
  - Unrepaired cyanotic CHD, including palliative shunts and conduits
  - Completely repaired congenital heart defect with prosthetic material or device, whether placed by surgery or by catheter intervention, during the first 6 months after the procedure
  - Repaired CHD with residual defects at the site or adjacent to the site of a prosthetic patch or prosthetic device (which inhibit endothelialization)
- Or, cardiac transplantation recipients who develop cardiac valvulopathy

Note: Except for the conditions listed above, antibiotic prophylaxis is no longer recommended for any other form of CHD. Antibiotic prophylaxis is no longer recommended for mitral valve prolapse.

Specified Dental Procedures

Antibiotic prophylaxis is recommended for patients with the above specified cardiac conditions for all dental procedures that involve manipulation of gingival tissue or the periapical region of the teeth, or perforation of the oral mucosa (AHA 2007). Examples include:
- Teeth cleaning
- Dental extraction (tooth removal)
- Biopsies
- Dental implant placement and reimplantation of avulsed teeth
- Endodontic surgery (e.g., root canal)
- Periodontal procedures (e.g., surgery, scaling, root planing)
- Placement of orthodontic bands
- Suture removal

Note: The following dental procedures do not need antibiotic prophylaxis: routine anesthetic injections through noninfected tissue, taking dental radiographs, placement of removable prosthodontic or orthodontic appliances, adjustment of orthodontic appliances, placement of orthodontic brackets, shedding of primary teeth, and bleeding from trauma to the lips or oral mucosa.

DEPRESSION

Definition
- Patient/caller states that he or she has depression.
- Feelings of sadness or hopelessness.
- Decreased pleasure or interest in daily activities.

TRIAGE ASSESSMENT QUESTIONS

Call EMS 911 Now
- Patient attempted suicide
  R/O: physical injury or overdose
- Patient is threatening suicide now
  Reason: triager considers risk of harm to be moderate to severe; patient has suicidal ideation with intent
- Patient is threatening to kill a specific person
  Reason: triager considers risk of harm to be moderate to severe; patient has homicidal ideation
  Note: Triager should contact police.
- Patient is very confused (disoriented, slurred speech) and no other adult (e.g., friend or family member) available
  Reason: dispatch EMS to assess caller
  Note: Under normal circumstances, most patients are oriented times 3 and can answer questions about person, place, and day or date. Triage nurse should contact EMS.
- Difficult to awaken or acting very confused (disoriented, slurred speech) and new onset
  R/O: drug overdose, subarachnoid hemorrhage, encephalitis, stroke
- Sounds like a life-threatening emergency to the triager

See More Appropriate Protocol
- Alcohol use, abuse, or dependence, question or problem related to
  Go to Protocol: Alcohol Abuse and Dependence on page 12
- Drug abuse or dependence, question or problem related to
  Go to Protocol: Substance Abuse and Dependence on page 382

Go to ED Now
- Depression and unable to do any of normal activities (e.g., self-care, school, work; in comparison to baseline)
  Reason: triager considers functional impairment to be severe

Go to ED/UCC Now
(or to Office With PCP Approval)
- Very strange or confused behavior
  R/O: psychosis, bipolar disorder, substance abuse
  Note: Factors that the nurse triager should consider in selecting the best disposition include risk of harm to self or others, how this compares to normal (baseline) behavior, and the patient's support systems (available family and friends).
- Patient sounds very sick or weak to the triager
  Reason: severe acute illness or serious complication suspected

See Today in Office
- Fever > 101° F (38.3° C)
  R/O: bacterial infection
- Sometimes has thoughts of suicide
  Reason: triager considers risk of harm to be low; no current intent or plan

See Within 3 Days in Office
- Symptoms interfere with work or school
  R/O: major depression
- Depression is worsening (e.g., sleeping poorly, less able to do activities of daily living)
  Reason: triager considers functional impairment to be moderate
- Significant weight loss (> 10 lb or 5 kg) and not dieting
  R/O: depression, organic pathology
- Known or suspected alcohol or drug abuse
  R/O: substance abuse as cause or contributing factor for depression
- New or changed psychiatric medications > 2 weeks ago and not feeling any better
  Reason: antidepressant medications require 2-4 weeks to work
- Requesting to talk with a counselor (mental health worker, psychiatrist, etc.)
- Patient wants to be seen

See Within 2 Weeks in Office

● Started on antidepressant medications < 2 weeks ago and is not feeling any better
Reason: antidepressant medications require 2-4 weeks to work

● Feels depressed only on days just before menstrual period
R/O: PMS

● History of manic depression (bipolar disorder)

● Pregnant

Home Care

○ Mild depression

○ Recent death of a loved one
Reason: bereavement, grieving

○ Referral phone numbers for depression, questions about

HOME CARE ADVICE

General Advice for Depression

❶ Reassurance:
- People with depression do get through this—even people who feel as badly as you feel now. You can be helped.
- Encourage the caller to talk about his/her problems and feelings.
- Offer hope.

❷ Depression—Symptoms: People with depression feel sad much of the time. They often have decreased joy from or interest in daily activities. Other symptoms include:
- Anxiety
- Easily upset
- Feeling worthless or guilty
- Loss of energy
- Major weight loss or gain and not dieting
- Mental slowness
- Not able to focus
- Thoughts of death or about hurting oneself
- Trouble sleeping or sleeping too much

❸ Depression—Causes: Depression is caused by a chemical imbalance in the brain. Stresses in life can trigger a bout of depression or make it worse. Things that can trigger depression or make it worse include:
- Certain drugs
- Death of a loved one
- Divorce or other relationship problems
- Loss of a job or stress from money problems
- Major life changes, such as starting college or having a baby
- Severe or long-standing illness

❹ Depression—Tips for Healthy Living:
- There are things you can do to feel better.
- **Eat Healthy:** Eat a well-balanced diet.
- **Get More Sleep:** Most people need 7-8 hours of sleep each night. Being well rested improves your mood and your sense of well-being.
- **Talk With Friends and Family:** Share how you are feeling with someone. Make sure that your spouse, family, or friends know how you are feeling.
- **Exercise Regularly:** Take a daily walk.
- **Avoid alcohol.**

❺ Depression—Stay Active:
- Staying active can also make you feel better.
- Spend time outside of your home. Go on an outing with a family member or a friend. Go to the store. Go to a movie.
- Become involved in your community. Go to a place of worship or school. Join a club or parent-teacher association.
- Start a new hobby.
- Get outside in the fresh air. Take a walk in the nearest part or forest preserve.

❻ Call Back If:
- Sadness or depression symptoms persist > 2 weeks.
- You want to talk with a counselor.
- You feel like harming yourself.
- You become worse.

Special Situations

❶ Death of a Loved One:
- Feeling numb, sad, or even angry are common feelings and normal after the death of a loved one.
- Encourage the caller to talk about his/her troubles.
- Let the caller know that taking time to grieve is important, and it is part of the healing process.
- **Suggest:** Review a photo album or share your favorite memories with a friend or family member.
- Support of family and friends is important.

❷ Death of a Loved One—Phrases to USE or AVOID:
- **Use:** Tell me more about how you are doing; I'm sorry; what is the hardest part of your day?
- **Avoid:** I understand how you feel; he is in the Lord's hands; it is for the best.

❸ Premenstrual Syndrome:
- Some women experience depression symptoms and irritability during the couple days prior to their menstrual period. This is because of fluctuations in female hormone levels as the menstrual period approaches.
- Your doctor can help you with this.

Depression and Treatment With Counseling

❶ Treatment With Counseling:
- You doctor may suggest counseling. This is also called talk therapy.
- This type of therapy can work just as well as medicine to treat mild depression.

❷ How Does Counseling Work?
- Your counselor can provide you the support you need until you feel better. Counseling can help you gain insight into your feelings. It can also help you learn how to deal better with your problems.
- Examples of talk therapy are one-to-one counseling, family counseling, and support groups.
- Just like medicines used to treat depression, counseling may take time to work. Most people start to feel better after 6-8 weeks.
- You may need this type of therapy for just a few months. However, some people will benefit from more long-term counseling and support.
- For many people, treatment with both medicine and counseling works best.

❸ Call Back If:
- You have more questions.

Depression and Treatment With Medicines

❶ Treatment With Antidepressant Medicines:
- Some people who have depression benefit from medical treatment.
- Your doctor may prescribe drugs called antidepressants.

❷ How Do Antidepressant Drugs Work?
- Antidepressant drugs help restore the balance of chemicals in the brain.
- There are many types of drugs used to treat depression. The kind your doctor prescribes depends on a number of things. Your doctor will consider the type of symptoms you are having. Other things your doctor will consider are your age, your overall health, and other medicines you take.
- Some people start to feel a little better after taking these medicines for 1-2 weeks. However, it may take up to 4-6 weeks or longer for you to feel much better.
- Your doctor will often start you off on a lower dose of the new medicine. Your doctor may adjust your dose over time.
- If the first medicine doesn't help enough, your doctor may prescribe another type. Be patient. It may take a few months to find out which drug works best for you.
- Most often, you will need to stay on the medicine for at least 6-9 months. Some people need to take them longer or for the rest of their life. Some people may have to take more than one type.

❸ When Should You Call Your Doctor While Taking Antidepressant Drugs?
Talk to your doctor if:
- You want to stop taking your antidepressant. Never stop taking these medicines on you own. Always talk to your doctor first. Stopping them suddenly may cause serious health problems.
- You start any new medicine, including any over-the-counter or herbal medicines. There could be harmful drug interactions.
- You become pregnant or are thinking about becoming pregnant. Your doctor will help you decide which medicine is safest for you and your baby.
- You think you are having side effects from your medicine. Your doctor may suggest a change in dose or a different type of antidepressant. This often helps reduce side effects.
- Your symptoms of depression become worse.

❹ **Call Back If:**
- You have more questions.

Referral Phone Numbers for Depression and Additional Resources

❶ **Local Mental Health Program Phone Numbers:**
- If available, local mental health program:

  — — — ⁻ — — — ⁻ — — — —

- If available, local psychiatric crisis service at
  _____ hospital:

  — — — ⁻ — — — ⁻ — — — —

❷ **United States—NAMI HelpLine:**
- National Alliance on Mental Illness (NAMI).
- The NAMI HelpLine is an information and referral source for locating community mental health programs. *"Our toll-free NAMI HelpLine allows us to respond personally to hundreds of thousands of requests each year, providing free referral, information and support—a much-needed lifeline for many."*
- Toll-free phone number: 800/950-NAMI (6264), Monday through Friday, 10:00 am to 6:00 pm, Eastern time.
- E-mail: info@nami.org
- Web site: www.nami.org

❸ **United States—SAMHSA National Helpline:**
- The SAMHSA National Helpline (http://samhsa.gov/treatment) is a *"confidential, free, 24-hour-a-day, 365-day-a-year, information service, in English and Spanish, for individuals and family members facing substance abuse and mental health issues. This service provides referrals to local treatment facilities, support groups, and community-based organizations. Callers can also order free publications and other information in print on substance abuse and mental health issues."*
- The phone number is 800/662-HELP (4357).

❹ **United States—Mood Disorder Organizations:**
- Anxiety and Depression Association of America (ADAA).
- There is a "Find a Therapist" link on the home page.
- Web site: www.adaa.org.
- Telephone: 240/485-1001.

❺ **Canada—Internet Resources:**
- **New Brunswick:** Department of Health and Wellness Addiction Services. Offered by region.
- **Newfoundland and Labrador:** Newfoundland and Labrador Addictions Services. Offered by region.
- **Northwest Territories:** Nats'ejée K'éh Treatment Centre crisis line—800/661-0846.
- **Ontario:** ConnexOntario: Provides access to addiction, mental health, and problem gambling services. Available at: http://www.connexontario.ca. The phone number for the helpline is 866-531-2600.
- **Ontario—Centre for Addiction and Mental Health (CAMH):** 800/463-6273.

❻ **Canada—Mood Disorder Organizations:**
- **Ontario:** Mood Disorders Association of Ontario (MDAO)—866/363-MOOD (6663)
- Web site: www.mooddisorders.ca

❼ **Call Back If:**
- You have more questions.

BACKGROUND

Key Points

- Depression is common, with 1 in 20 Americans getting depressed each year. Women are affected twice as often as men.
- Depression is treatable.

Symptoms

People with depression feel sad much of the time. They often have decreased joy from or interest in daily activities.

Other symptoms include:

- Anxiety
- Easily upset
- Feeling worthless or guilty
- Loss of energy
- Major weight loss or gain and not dieting
- Mental slowness
- Not able to focus
- Thoughts of death or about hurting oneself
- Trouble sleeping or sleeping too much

Causes

Depression is caused by a chemical imbalance in the brain. Stresses in life can trigger a bout of depression or make it worse. Things that can trigger depression or make it worse include:

- Certain drugs
- Death of a loved one
- Divorce or other relationship problems
- Loss of a job or stress from money problems
- Major life changes, such as starting college or having a baby
- Severe or long-standing illness

Treatment

- Depression can be treated with psychiatric counseling or medications.
- Sometimes both are necessary.

Suggestions for Healthy Living

Healthy living habits can improve one's sense of well-being:

- **Eat Healthy:** Eat a well-balanced diet.
- **Get More Sleep:** Most people need 7-8 hours of sleep each night. Being well rested improves your attitude and your sense of physical well-being.
- **Communicate:** Share how you are feeling with someone in your life who is a good listener. Make certain that your spouse, family, or friends know how you are feeling.
- **Exercise Regularly:** Take a daily walk.
- **Stay Active:** Get out of the house periodically. Go on an outing with a family member or a friend. Go to the store. Go to a movie.
- **Avoid alcohol.**

Caution: Suicidal Ideation—Intent and Plan

- **Intent:** It is appropriate to directly ask patients about their intent to harm themselves or end their own life. Such questions will not provoke a suicide attempt and may instead give patients a chance to unburden themselves. Any patient who is threatening self-harm NOW needs to be seen immediately for evaluation.
- **Plan:** This refers to the extent to which the patient has prepared for a suicide attempt. Does the patient have a specific method in mind (e.g., gun, knife, overdose)? Does the patient have access to the verbalized method (e.g., hoarded pills, firearm in house)? Access to lethal methods increases the risk of suicide attempt and death. Generally, a patient with a specific plan is considered at higher suicide risk than a patient who is threatening suicide but has no plan.

DIABETES (HIGH BLOOD SUGAR)

Definition
- Patient with known diabetes mellitus
- Has a high blood sugar (hyperglycemia), defined as a blood glucose > 200 mg/dL (11 mmol/L)
- Has symptoms of high blood sugar
- Has questions about high blood sugar

Symptoms
- **Mild Hyperglycemia:** Most often patient will have no symptoms.
- **Moderate Hyperglycemia:** Polyuria, polydipsia, fatigue, blurred vision.
- **Severe Hyperglycemia:** Confusion and coma.
- **Diabetic Ketoacidosis (DKA):** Fruity odor on breath, vomiting, rapid breathing, weakness, confusion, and coma.

TRIAGE ASSESSMENT QUESTIONS

Call EMS 911 Now
- Unconscious or difficult to awaken
  R/O: DKA, severe hyperglycemia, profound hypoglycemia
- Acting confused (e.g., disoriented, slurred speech)
  R/O: DKA, severe hyperglycemia, hypoglycemia
- Very weak (can't stand)
  R/O: DKA, severe hyperglycemia, hypoglycemia
- Sounds like a life-threatening emergency to the triager

Go to ED Now
- Vomiting and signs of dehydration (e.g., very dry mouth, light-headed, etc.)
  Reason: may need IV hydration, possible DKA
- Blood glucose > 240 mg/dL (13 mmol/L) and rapid breathing
  R/O: DKA

Go to ED/UCC Now
(or to Office With PCP Approval)
- Blood glucose > 500 mg/dL (27.5 mmol/L)
- Blood glucose > 240 mg/dL (13 mmol/L) AND urine ketones moderate-large (or more than 1+)
  R/O: DKA
  Note: Most people with diabetes who use insulin do the urine ketone test.
- Blood glucose > 240 mg/dL (13 mmol/L) and blood ketones > 1.5 mmol/L
  R/O: DKA
  Note: Some patients can check their blood for ketones using a handheld device.
- Blood glucose > 240 mg/dL (13 mmol/L) AND vomiting AND unable to check for ketones (in blood or urine)
  R/O: DKA
  Note: Most people with diabetes who use insulin do the urine ketone test. Some patients can check their blood for ketones using a handheld device.
- Vomiting lasting > 4 hours
  R/O: DKA, dehydration
- Patient sounds very sick or weak to the triager
  Reason: severe acute illness or serious complication suspected

Go to Office Now
- Fever > 100.5° F (38.1° C)
  Reason: diabetics are immunocompromised, consider possibility of bacterial infection

Call Transferred to PCP Now
- Caller has URGENT medication or insulin pump question and triager unable to answer question

Discuss With PCP and Callback by Nurse Within 1 Hour
- Blood glucose > 400 mg/dL (22 mmol/L)
  Reason: significant hyperglycemia
- Blood glucose > 300 mg/dL (16.5 mmol/L) AND 2 or more times in a row
  Reason: obtain PCP input regarding medication adjustment and diet
- Urine ketones moderate-large
  Reason: obtain PCP input regarding medication adjustment and diet

See Today in Office

- New-onset diabetes suspected (e.g., frequent urination, weak, weight loss)
- Symptoms of high blood sugar (e.g., frequent urination, weak, weight loss) and not able to test blood glucose
- Patient wants to be seen

Discuss With PCP and Callback by Nurse Today

- Caller has NONURGENT medication question about medicine that PCP prescribed and triager unable to answer question

Home Care

- Blood glucose > 240 mg/dL (13 mmol/L)
  Reason: hyperglycemia
- Blood glucose 60-240 mg/dL (3.5-13 mmol/L)
- Sick-day rules for people with diabetes mellitus, questions about

HOME CARE ADVICE

Treating High Blood Sugar (Hyperglycemia)

❶ General:
- **Definition of Hyperglycemia:** Fasting blood glucose > 140 mg/dL (7.5 mmol/L) or random blood glucose > 200 mg/dL (11 mmol/L).
- **Symptoms of Mild Hyperglycemia:** Frequent urination, increased thirst, fatigue, blurred vision.
- **Symptoms of Severe Hyperglycemia:** Weakness, progressing to confusion and coma.
- **Contributing Factors:** Nonadherence to medicines, nonadherence to diet, and infection.

❷ Treatment—Liquids:
- Drink at least 1 glass (8 oz or 240 mL) of water per hour for the next 4 hours.
  (Reason: Adequate hydration will reduce hyperglycemia.)
- Generally, you should try to drink 6-8 glasses of water each day.

❸ Treatment—Insulin:
- Continue to take your insulin, as prescribed by your doctor.
- **Sliding Scale Insulin:** If your doctor has given you instructions to take extra rapid-acting (e.g., lispro, aspart) or short-acting (regular) insulin when your blood sugar is high, give yourself the insulin dose your doctor has recommended.

❹ Treatment—Diabetes Medications: Continue taking your diabetes pills.

❺ Measure and Record Your Blood Glucose:
- Measure your blood glucose before breakfast and before going to bed.
- Record the results and show them to your doctor at your next office visit.

❻ Daily Blood Glucose Goals: You and your doctor should decide on what your blood glucose goals should be. Typical goals for many people who perform daily finger-stick blood testing at home are:
- **Preprandial** (before meal): 80-130 mg/dL (4.4-7.2 mmol/L)
- **Postprandial** (1-2 hours after a meal): < 180 mg/dL (10 mmol/L)

❼ Daily Blood Glucose Goals—Gestational Diabetes in Pregnancy (Diabetes That Started in Pregnancy):
- You and your doctor should decide on what your blood glucose goals should be. Typical goals for most pregnant women who perform daily finger-stick blood testing at home are:
- **Preprandial** (before meal): < 95 mg/dL (5.3 mmol/L)
- **Postprandial:** < 140 mg/dL (7.8 mmol/L) 1 hour after eating OR < 120 mg/dL (6.7 mmol/L) 2 hours after eating

❽ Daily Blood Glucose Goals—Type 1 or 2 Diabetes in Pregnancy (Diabetes That Started Before Pregnancy):
- You and your doctor should decide on what your blood glucose goals should be. Typical goals for most pregnant women who perform daily finger-stick blood testing at home are:
- **Fasting:** <90 mg/dL (5.0 mmol/L)
- **1 Hour Postprandial** (after a meal): < 130-140 mg/dL (7.2-7.8 mmol/L)
- **2 Hour Postprandial** (after a meal): < 120 mg/dL (6.7 mmol/L)

❾ **Check for Ketones:**
- If you use insulin, you should have ketone test strips at home.
- You should check your ketones when you are sick or your blood glucose is > 240 mg/dL (13 mmol/L).
- There are 2 ways a person can test for ketones.
- **Urine Ketone Test:** Most people with diabetes use this test. Urine ketone test kits are available at your local pharmacy.
- **Blood Ketone Test:** Some people have special meters that allow them to test for blood ketones.

❿ **Expected Course:** You should call back in 3-5 days if:
- Your blood sugar continues to get > 240 mg/dL (13 mmol/L).
- Your blood sugar continues to be higher than your daily glucose goals (set by you and your doctor).
- It has been > 6 months since you had a hemoglobin A_{1c} test.

⓫ **Call Back If:**
- Blood glucose > 300 mg/dL (16.5 mmol/L) ≥ 2 times in a row.
- Urine ketones become moderate or large (or more than 1+); if you check blood ketones, blood ketone test is 1.6 or higher.
- Vomiting lasting > 4 hours or unable to drink any fluids.
- Rapid breathing occurs.
- You become worse or have more questions.

Sick-Day Rules for Patients Who Use Insulin

❶ **General:**
- **Do Not Stop Taking Your Insulin:** During illness the blood sugar often rises.
- **Check Your Blood Glucose Every 3-4 Hours:** Write down the results.
- **Check for Ketones (Urine or Blood) Every 3-4 Hours:** Ketones can be a sign of dehydration or poorly controlled diabetes.
- **Drink Liquids:** It is important to prevent dehydration. Drink small amounts frequently.
- **Avoid Hypoglycemia:** If your appetite is bad, you are not eating solid food, and your blood glucose is < 200 mg/dL (11 mmol/L), you should be drinking sugar-containing liquids. Examples are soda, clear juices, sports drinks.

❷ **Insulin—Do Not Stop Taking It:**
- If you are supposed to be using insulin, do not stop taking it.
- The reason is that during an illness you may need even more insulin than usual.

❸ **Insulin—Supplemental Insulin for Hyperglycemia:**
- **Note to Triager:** Supplemental rapid-acting (e.g., lispro, aspart) or short-acting (regular) insulin is sometimes needed in addition to usual insulin doses for treating hyperglycemia. Most patients should already have been given "sick-day rules" education by their doctor and instructions on when to use supplemental insulin. **The triage nurse must discuss all insulin dosing with the doctor before giving recommendations to the patient.** In most cases it is best if the doctor talks directly with the patient.
- **Total Daily Dose (TDD):** The TDD is calculated by adding up all insulin administered during a usual day.
- **Typical Sick-Day Insulin Supplementation— Urine Ketones Negative or Trace:** If glucose is 80-240 mg/dL (4.5-13 mmol/L), give usual dose. If glucose is 250-400 mg/dL (14-22 mmol/L), supplemental insulin dosage is 10% of TDD. If glucose is > 400 mg/dL (22 mmol/L), supplemental insulin dosage is 20% of TDD.
- **Typical Sick-Day Insulin Supplementation— Urine Ketones Moderate:** If glucose is 80-240 mg/dL (4.5-13 mmol/L), give usual dose. If glucose is 250-400 mg/dL (14-22 mmol/L), supplemental insulin dosage is 20% of TDD. If glucose is > 400 mg/dL (22 mol/L), supplemental insulin dosage is 20% of TDD.

❹ Insulin—Decreased Insulin for Hypoglycemia:
- **Note to Triager:** Decreased insulin dosing is sometimes needed in patients with a blood glucose < 80 mg/dL (4.5 mmol/L), especially if there is decreased oral intake. **The triage nurse must discuss all insulin dosing with the doctor before giving recommendations to the patient.** In most cases it is best if the doctor talks directly with the patient.
- **Typical Sick-Day Insulin Reduction—for Blood Glucose < 80 mg/dL (4.5 mmol/L) and There Is Decreased Oral Intake:** Do not give rapid-acting (e.g., lispro, aspart) or short-acting (regular) insulin. Reduce intermediate-acting insulin (e.g., NPH, Lente, 70/30) by 20%.

❺ Diet:
- **Appetite OK, Minimal Nausea:** Continue your normal diabetic meal plan. Avoid spicy or greasy foods.
- **Appetite Fair, Moderate Nausea:** Eat a bland diet. Try small amounts of food 6-8 times a day. Take ½-1 cup of food or liquids every 1-2 hours.
- **Appetite Poor, Severe Nausea, Can't Eat Solid Food:** Drink plenty of liquids. Try to drink 4-8 oz (120-240 mL) per hour. If glucose > 240 mg/dL (13 mmol/L), drink sugar-free liquids (e.g., water, broth). If glucose < 200 mg/dL (11 mmol/L), drink sugar-containing liquids (e.g., sports drinks, juice, soda).
- Advance diet as you improve.

❻ Liquids:
- Drink more fluids, at least 8-10 glasses daily (8 oz or 240 mL each glass).
- Even more liquids are needed if there is fever, vomiting, or diarrhea.

❼ Check Blood Glucose:
- When you are ill, you should measure your blood glucose every 2-4 hours.
- Write down the results.

❽ Check for Ketones:
- You should check your ketones when you are sick or your blood glucose is > 240 mg/dL (13 mmol/L).
- There are 2 ways a person can test for ketones.
- **Urine Ketone Test:** Most people with diabetes use this test. Urine ketone test kits are available at your local pharmacy.
- **Blood Ketone Test:** Some people have special meters that allow them to test for blood ketones.

❾ Call Back If:
- Blood glucose > 300 mg/dL (16.5 mmol/L) ≥ 2 times in a row.
- Urine ketones become moderate or large (or more than 1+); if you check blood ketones, blood ketone test is 1.6 or higher.
- Vomiting lasting > 4 hours or unable to drink any fluids.
- Rapid breathing occurs.
- You become worse or have more questions.

Sick-Day Rules for Patients Who Do Not Use Insulin

❶ General:
- **Do not stop taking your diabetes medications.** *(Reason: During illness the blood sugar often rises.)*
- **Check Your Blood Glucose Every 3-4 Hours:** Write down the results.
- **Check for Ketones in Your Urine:** Ketones can be a sign of dehydration or poorly controlled diabetes.
- **Drink Liquids:** It is important to prevent dehydration. Drink small amounts frequently.
- **Avoid Hypoglycemia:** If your appetite is bad, you are not eating solid food, and your blood glucose is < 200 mg/dL (11 mmol/L), you should be drinking sugar-containing liquids. Examples are soda, clear juices, sports drinks.

❷ Diet:
- **Appetite OK, Minimal Nausea:** Continue your normal diabetic meal plan. Avoid spicy or greasy foods.
- **Appetite Fair, Moderate Nausea:** Eat a bland diet. Try small amounts of food 6-8 times a day. Take ½-1 cup of food or liquids every 1-2 hours.
- **Appetite Poor, Severe Nausea, Can't Eat Solid Food:** Drink plenty of liquids. Try to drink 4-8 oz (120-240 mL) per hour. If glucose > 240 mg/dL (13 mmol/L), drink sugar-free liquids (e.g., water, broth). If glucose < 200 mg/dL (11 mmol/L), drink sugar-containing liquids (e.g., sports drinks, juice, soda).
- Advance diet as you improve.

❸ Liquids:

- Drink more fluids, at least 8-10 glasses daily (8 oz or 240 mL each glass). Even more liquids are needed if there is fever, vomiting, or diarrhea.
- If glucose > 240 mg/dL (13 mmol/L), drink sugar-free liquids (e.g., water).
- If glucose < 120 mg/dL (6.5 mmol/L), drink sugar-containing liquids (e.g., sports drinks, juice, soda).

❹ Check Blood Glucose:

- When you are ill, you should measure your blood glucose every 3-4 hours.
- Write down the results.

❺ Check for Ketones:

- You should check your ketones when you are sick or your blood glucose is > 240 mg/dL (13 mmol/L).
- There are 2 ways a person can test for ketones.
- **Urine Ketone Test:** Most people with diabetes use this test. Urine ketone test kits are available at your local pharmacy.
- **Blood Ketone Test:** Some people have special meters that allow them to test for blood ketones.

❻ Call Back If:

- Blood glucose > 300 mg/dL (16.5 mmol/L) ≥ 2 times in a row.
- Urine ketones become moderate or large (or more than 1+); if you check blood ketones, blood ketone test is 1.6 or higher.
- Vomiting lasting > 4 hours or unable to drink any fluids.
- Rapid breathing occurs.
- You become worse or have more questions.

Additional Resources

❶ American Diabetes Association:

- Telephone number: 1-800-DIABETES (800/342-2383)
- Web site: www.diabetes.org

❷ US National Diabetes Education Program (NDEP):

- "If you are living with diabetes or have a loved one with the disease, it's important to work together to manage diabetes. Use these resources to learn how to make healthy lifestyle choices to help manage diabetes, prevent complications, and improve your quality of life."
- Telephone number: 800/438-5383.
- Web site: https://www.cdc.gov/diabetes/ndep/people-with-diabetes/index.html

❸ Canadian Diabetes Association:

- Telephone number: 1-800-BANTING (226-8464)
- Web site: www.diabetes.ca

FIRST AID

First Aid Advice for Hypoglycemia—Glucose

If blood glucose < 70 mg/dL (3.9 mmol/L) or unknown for conscious patients:

- Give sugar (15-20 g glucose) by mouth IF able to swallow.
- Each of the following has the right amount of sugar: low-fat milk (1 cup; 240 mL); fruit juice or non-diet soda (½ cup; 120 mL); prepackaged juice box (1 box); table sugar or honey (3 teaspoons; 15 mL); glucose tablets (3 tablets); glucose paste (10-15 g).
- Symptoms should begin to improve within 5 minutes. Full recovery may take 10-20 minutes.

First Aid Advice for Hypoglycemia—Glucagon

If blood glucose < 70 mg/dL (3.9 mmol/L) or unknown (pending EMS arrival):

- If family has glucagon for hypoglycemic emergencies AND the caller knows how to use it, encourage the caller to give the glucagon now.
- Inject it IM into the upper outer thigh.
- Adult dosage is 1 mg.
- Glucagon can be used in unconscious patients.
- Symptoms should begin to improve within 5 minutes. Full recovery may take 10-20 minutes.

BACKGROUND

Causes of High Blood Sugar (Hyperglycemia)

- Noncompliance with taking insulin or other diabetes medicines. Forgetting to take insulin is the most common cause.
- Malfunction of an individual's insulin pump.
- Noncompliance with diabetes diet.
- Infection.
- Steroid medications (e.g., prednisone, Medrol dose pack).
- Combination of these factors.

Diabetes Mellitus

- **Definition:** Diabetes mellitus is an endocrine condition in which patients have elevated blood glucose levels (hyperglycemia). The classic symptoms of untreated or undertreated diabetes are: frequent urination (polyuria), polydipsia (excessive thirst), and involuntary weight loss.
- **The Role of Insulin:** Insulin is a hormone produced by the pancreas to help process food. Eating food makes the blood glucose rise and insulin makes the blood glucose fall.
- **Classification of Diabetes Mellitus:** There are 4 different classes of diabetes mellitus: type 1 diabetes, type 2 diabetes, gestational diabetes mellitus, and other.
- **Diagnosis:** Probably the best way to diagnose diabetes is a hemoglobin A_{1c} test with a value of $\geq 6.5\%$. There are 2 other tests that have long been used for diagnosing diabetes: a fasting plasma glucose > 126 mg/dL (7.0 mmol/L) and a 2-hour oral glucose tolerance test with a glucose > 200 mg/dL (11.1 mmol/L).

Type 1 Diabetes

- **Other Names:** Insulin-dependent diabetes mellitus, juvenile-onset diabetes.
- **Physiology:** There is no production of insulin by the body.
- **Ketosis-Prone:** Patients with this type of diabetes are ketosis-prone, which means that if they do not receive daily insulin shots their bodies break down fats and produce ketones. The ketones spill into the urine and can be measured. Patients with type 1 diabetes are susceptible to developing diabetic ketoacidosis (DKA), a life-threatening condition.

- **Onset:** It most commonly first appears in childhood or adolescence. Approximately 10% of diabetics are type 1.
- **Treatment:** Insulin therapy is always required and needs to be given subcutaneously at least once daily. Patients striving for tighter control of their blood glucose will take insulin more often than once a day. Most people with type 1 diabetes should be treated with either multiple-dose insulin injections (3–4 injections per day) or continuous subcutaneous insulin infusion therapy. It is important to learn how to match mealtime (prandial) insulin with carbohydrate intake, premeal blood glucose, and anticipated activity.

Type 2 Diabetes

- **Other Names:** Non–insulin-dependent diabetes mellitus, adult-onset diabetes.
- **Physiology:** In type 2 diabetes, there is decreased insulin production and decreased sensitivity to insulin.
- **Not Ketosis-Prone:** These patients are not prone to ketosis. DKA rarely occurs.
- **Onset:** It more commonly develops in elderly and overweight adults.
- **Treatment:** The initial and most important treatments are exercise and weight loss. When these measures fail, there are oral medications (e.g., metformin) that can be prescribed to help the body make more insulin or use the insulin more effectively. Occasionally, patients require insulin therapy.

Gestational Diabetes

- Gestational diabetes is diabetes that is found for the first time when a woman is pregnant.
- **Physiology:** In gestational diabetes, the body is not making sufficient insulin to keep pace with the weight gain and other hormonal changes of pregnancy.
- **Not Ketosis-Prone:** These patients are not prone to ketosis. DKA rarely occurs.
- **Onset:** It occurs during pregnancy.
- **Treatment:** A meal plan and regular physical activity are important.

Diabetic Ketoacidosis (DKA)

- **Definition:** Blood glucose > 250 mg/dL (12 mmol/L) with acidosis and ketosis (urine ketones moderate-large; or blood ketones > 1.5 mmol/L).
- **Symptoms of DKA:** In addition to symptoms of hyperglycemia, fruity odor on breath, vomiting, rapid/deep breathing, confusion, and coma.
- **Causes:** Noncompliance with using insulin in type 1 diabetes, infection.

Ketone Testing

- Diabetics who take insulin should test for ketones when their blood sugar is > 240 mg/dL (13 mmol/L). They should also check for ketones when they are sick or have symptoms of ketoacidosis (vomiting, fruity breath, or rapid breathing).
- Detecting ketosis early is important to help prevent life-threatening diabetes ketoacidosis.
- There are 2 ways patients can test for ketones at home.
- **Urine Ketone Tests:** Many patients test for urine ketones (urine acetoacetate) by doing a urine ketone test. Urine ketone strips are available at local pharmacies. The results indicate the amount of urine ketones as small, moderate, or large. Moderate to large amounts of ketones indicate ketosis.
- **Blood Ketone Tests:** Some blood glucose test meters now allow the patient to also test for blood ketones (blood β-hydroxybutyrate). The patient can often test for blood ketones and blood glucose at the same time. The blood ketone test does require a different strip made just for ketone tests. Blood ketone tests may detect ketones a bit sooner than urine ketone test. The blood ketone tests give the patient a number reading. A number < 0.6 mmol/L is considered normal. Numbers between 0.6 and 1.5 mmol/L mean ketosis is developing and patients should call their doctor for further instructions. Numbers > 1.6 mmol/L mean ketosis is concerning and patients should call their doctor or seek medical care now.

Five Types of Insulin for Diabetes

- **Rapid-acting** (Humalog/lispro, NovoLog/aspart): Onset 5-15 minutes; peaks 30-90 minutes; lasts 4-6 hours.
- **Short-acting** (Regular, Humulin R, Novolin R): Onset 30-60 minutes; peaks 2-3 hours; lasts 5-8 hours.
- **Intermediate-acting** (NPH, Lente, Humulin N, Humulin L, Novolin N, Novolin L): Onset 2-4 hours; peaks 4-12 hours; lasts 10-18 hours.
- **Long-acting** (Lantus/glargine, Detemir, Levemir): Onset 2-4 hours; no true peak; lasts 18-24 hours.
- **Premixed** (Humulin 70/30, Humulin 50/50, Humalog mix, NovoLog mix): 2 peaks; lasts 10-16 hours; depends on mixture.

Insulin Administration: Different Dosing Regimens

- **Sliding Insulin Scale:** Generally only used in the hospital.
- **Insulin Algorithm:** The patient checks his/her blood glucose before each meal and then adjusts insulin dosing based on BOTH the blood glucose and an estimated caloric count for the meal. This is considered "prandial" insulin because it is given with (just before) meals. Rapid-acting (Humalog/lispro or Novolog/aspart) or short-acting (regular) insulin are used for prandial insulin dosing.
- **Once-Daily Insulin:** This is not considered physiologic insulin dosing, as it only provides the "basal" insulin and does not provide the needed prandial increases. However, it may be an effective addition for some type 2 diabetic patients on oral medications, as their need for insulin is low. Intermediate-acting insulin (NPH) or long-acting insulin (Lantus/glargine) are used.
- **Twice-Daily Insulin:** Intermediate-acting insulin (NPH) or long-acting insulin (Lantus/glargine) can be used in twice-daily regimens. Twice-daily insulin dosing may be sufficient for type 2 diabetic patients because they still make sufficient insulin on their own to handle prandial (mealtime) insulin needs.
- **Flexible Insulin Regimens:** In this type of regimen, both an intermediate-acting insulin (for basal insulin needs) AND a rapid or ultrashort-acting insulin (for prandial insulin needs) are used.

Five Types of Oral Medications for Diabetes

- **Sulfonylureas:** Examples include glyburide (Micronase, DiaBeta), glipizide (Glucotrol, Glucotrol XL), and glimepiride (Amaryl).
- **Biguanides:** Examples include metformin (Glucophage, Fortamet).
- **Thiazolidinediones:** Examples include rosiglitazone (Avenida) and pioglitazone (Actos).
- **Alpha-Glucosidase Inhibitors:** Examples include acarbose (Precose) and miglitol (Glyset).
- **Meglitinides:** Examples include repaglinide (Prandin) and nateglinide (Starlix).

Goals for Diabetes Management

- **Hemoglobin A_{1c}:** Hemoglobin A_{1c} (HbA$_{1c}$) is the primary goal for diabetes management. Depending on the patient, it should be measured 2-4 times a year. The American Diabetes Association (ADA) recommends a goal of < 7.0% for nonpregnant adults.
- **Blood Glucose:** Depending on the patient, the blood glucose should be measured 1-3 times per day. The ADA recommends the following blood glucose goals:
  - **Preprandial** (before meal):
    80-130 mg/dL (4.4-7.2 mmol/L)
  - **Postprandial** (1-2 hours after a meal):
    < 180 mg/dL (10 mmol/L)

  Goals should be individualized based on age/life expectancy, duration of diabetes, comorbid conditions, hypoglycemic unawareness, history of severe hypoglycemic reactions, and other individual considerations.
  - Internet Resource: ADA "Standards of Medical Care in Diabetes" 2016; available at: http://care.diabetesjournals.org/content/39/Supplement_1

Glycosylated Hemoglobin A_{1c}

- The HbA$_{1c}$ provides a good estimate of how well a patient has managed his/her diabetes during the past 2-3 months. With good diabetes management, the HbA$_{1c}$ goes down; with poor management, it goes up. In general, the higher the HbA$_{1c}$, the greater the risk of long-term diabetic complications.
- **Goal:** The American Association of Clinical Endocrinologists and the American College of Endocrinology recommend a target glycosylated hemoglobin level (HbA$_{1c}$) of < 6.5%. The ADA recommends a goal of < 7.0% for nonpregnant adults. The Canadian Diabetes Association also recommends a goal of < 7.0%.

Long-term Complications of Diabetes Mellitus

- **Eye Disease** (e.g., retinopathy): Diabetes is a leading cause of blindness.
- **Heart Disease** (e.g., coronary heart disease, myocardial infarction).
- **Kidney Disease** (e.g., renal failure, proteinuria).
- **Nerve Disease** (e.g., peripheral and autonomic neuropathy).
- **Stroke.**

Converting Glucose Levels: mg/dL and mmol/L

- In the United States, glucose is typically measured using the units mg/dL. Nearly every country in the world (including Canada) measures glucose levels using the units mmol/L.
- To convert mmol/L of glucose to mg/dL, multiply by 18.
- To convert mg/dL of glucose to mmol/L, divide by 18 or multiply by 0.055.

DIABETES (LOW BLOOD SUGAR)

Definition

- Patient with known diabetes mellitus
- Has a low blood sugar (hypoglycemia), defined as a blood glucose < 70 mg/dL (3.9 mmol/L)
- Has symptoms of low blood sugar
- Has questions regarding low blood sugar

Symptoms

- **Mild Hypoglycemia:** Dizziness, shakiness, weakness, trembling, sweating, headache, nervousness, and hunger. Some patients with mild hypoglycemia experience no symptoms.
- **Severe Hypoglycemia:** Unable to speak, confusion, seizures, and coma.
- **Hypoglycemic Unawareness:** Some diabetics have no symptoms of hypoglycemia and can lose consciousness without ever knowing their blood glucose levels were dropping. This condition is mainly seen in adults with long-standing diabetes. These patients need more frequent checks of their blood glucose level.

TRIAGE ASSESSMENT QUESTIONS

Call EMS 911 Now

- Unconscious or difficult to awaken
  R/O: severe hypoglycemia, insulin coma
- Seizure occurs
  R/O: severe hypoglycemia
- Acting confused (e.g., disoriented, slurred speech)
  R/O: severe hypoglycemia
- Very weak (can't stand)
  R/O: symptomatic hypoglycemia
- Sounds like a life-threatening emergency to the triager

Go to ED Now

- Vomiting and signs of dehydration (e.g., no urine > 12 hours, very dry mouth, dark urine, etc.)
  Reason: may need IV hydration
- Low blood sugar symptoms persist > 15 minutes AND using low blood sugar Home Care Advice
  Reason: no improvement with Home Care Advice
- Low blood glucose (< 70 mg/dL or 3.9 mmol/L) persists > 15 minutes AND using low blood sugar Home Care Advice
  Reason: no improvement with Home Care Advice

Go to ED/UCC Now (or to Office With PCP Approval)

- Patient sounds very sick or weak to the triager
  Reason: severe acute illness or serious complication suspected

Call Transferred to PCP Now

- Diabetes medication overdose (e.g., insulin error) and triager unable to answer question
  Note: Triager should consider medication, dose, and whether patient is alone. An upgrade to EMS 911 may be indicated in some circumstances.
- Caller has URGENT medication question about medication that PCP prescribed and triager unable to answer question

Discuss With PCP and Callback by Nurse Within 1 Hour

- Low blood sugar symptoms with no other adult present AND hasn't tried Home Care Advice
  Notes: Obtain contact information. Recruit family or friend to help. Consider upgrade to EMS 911 based on social support and ability to recontact.
- Low blood glucose (< 70 mg/dL or 3.9 mmol/L) with no other adult present AND hasn't tried Home Care Advice
  Notes: Obtain contact information and callback in 15 minutes. Recruit family or friend to help. Consider upgrade to EMS 911 based on social support and ability to recontact.
- Low blood glucose (< 70 mg/dL or 3.9 mmol/L) or symptomatic, now improved with Home Care Advice, AND cause unknown
  Reason: unexplained hypoglycemia
  Note: Causes can include extra insulin, delayed meal or insufficient food, strenuous exercise.

See Today in Office

- Patient wants to be seen

Discuss With PCP and Callback by Nurse Today

- ◓ Morning (before breakfast) blood glucose < 80 mg/dL (4.5 mmol/L) and more than once in past week
  Reason: obtain PCP input regarding medication adjustment and diet
- ◓ Evening (after bedtime snack) blood glucose < 100 mg/dL (5.6 mmol/L) and more than once in past week
  Reason: obtain PCP input regarding medication adjustment and diet
- ◓ Caller has NONURGENT medication question about medication that PCP prescribed and triager unable to answer question

Home Care

- ○ Blood glucose < 70 mg/dL (3.9 mmol/L) or symptomatic AND has other adult present
  Reason: cause known, another adult is present
- ○ Low blood sugar prevention, questions about
- ○ Sick-day rules for people with diabetes mellitus, questions about

HOME CARE ADVICE

Treating Low Blood Sugar (Hypoglycemia)

❶ Reassurance:
- It sounds like an episode of low blood sugar (hypoglycemia) that we can treat at home.
- Low blood sugar can result from taking too much diabetes medication, delayed meals, strenuous exercise, or a combination of these factors.
- *Here is some care advice that should help.*

❷ Definition:
- Low blood sugar (hypoglycemia) is defined as a blood glucose < 70 mg/dL (3.9 mmol/L).
- **Symptoms of Mild Hypoglycemia:** Shakiness, weakness, not thinking clearly, headache, trembling, sweating, dizziness, palpitations, and hunger.
- **Symptoms of Severe Hypoglycemia:** Unable to speak, confusion, seizures, and coma.
- **Contributing Factors:** Too much insulin, delayed meal, insufficient food, strenuous exercise, alcohol.

❸ Low Blood Sugar—Treatment: Eat some (15 g) sugar now. Each of the following has the right amount of sugar:
- Low-fat milk (1 cup; 240 mL)
- Fruit juice or non-diet soda (½ cup; 120 mL)
- Prepackaged juice box (1 box)
- Table sugar or honey (3 teaspoons; 15 mL)
- Glucose tablets (3-4 tablets)

❹ Low Blood Sugar—Treatment: If patient is taking Precose (acarbose):
- In this case, low blood sugar must be treated with glucose tablets. Take 3-4 glucose tablets now. If glucose tablets are not available, milk may work.
- **Special Note:** Juice, candies, and table sugar are not effective because of the mechanism of action of this diabetes pill.

❺ Expected Course:
- The symptoms of hypoglycemia should resolve in 10-15 minutes. After the symptoms resolve, eat a small snack to prevent this from recurring. Examples include cheese and crackers, a glass of milk, or half a sandwich.
- If the symptoms of hypoglycemia are not better in 15 minutes, eat some more glucose (10 g).

❻ Call Back If:
- There is no improvement within 30 minutes.
- Sleepiness or confusion occur.
- You become worse.

Preventing Low Blood Sugar

❶ Prevention:
- **Meals:** Do not skip or delay meals. Try to eat meals and snacks at the same time every day.
- **Glucose:** Keep some type of sugar (e.g., glucose tablets or gels, honey, juice box) with you at all times. Do you have them available at work, at school, during exercise, and in your car?
- **Dieting:** Talk with your doctor before starting a weight-loss program.

❷ Let Your Friends and Family Know!
- If you take insulin or any other diabetic medication, you are at risk of having a hypoglycemic spell. Inform your family, close friends, and coworkers that you have diabetes and what to do if you have hypoglycemia.
- Wear a medical alert bracelet that identifies that you have diabetes.

❸ **Daily Blood Glucose Goals:** You and your doctor should decide on what your blood glucose goals should be. Typical goals for most nonpregnant adults who perform daily finger-stick blood testing at home are:
  • **Preprandial** (before meal): 80-130 mg/dL (4.4-7.2 mmol/L)
  • **Postprandial** (1-2 hours after a meal): < 180 mg/dL (10 mmol/L)
  • Hemoglobin A_{1c} level < 7%

❹ **Daily Records:**
  • Measure your blood glucose before breakfast and before going to bed.
  • Record the results and show them to your doctor at your next office visit.

❺ **Call Back If:**
  • Morning blood glucose < 80 mg/dL (4.5 mmol/L) more than once in a week.
  • Bedtime blood glucose < 100 mg/dL (5.5 mmol/L) more than once in a week.
  • You have more questions.
  • You become worse.

Sick-Day Rules
❶ **General:**
  • **Do Not Stop Taking Your Insulin:** During illness the blood sugar often rises.
  • **Check Your Blood Glucose Every 2-4 Hours:** Write down the results.
  • **Check for Ketones in Your Urine:** Ketones can be a sign of dehydration or poorly controlled diabetes.
  • **Drink Liquids:** It is important to prevent dehydration. Drink small amounts frequently.
  • **Avoid Hypoglycemia:** If your appetite is bad, you are not eating solid food, and your blood glucose is < 200 mg/dL (11 mmol/L), you should be drinking sugar-containing liquids. Examples are soda, clear juices, sports drinks.

❷ **Insulin—Do Not Stop Taking It:**
  • If you are supposed to be using insulin, do not stop taking it.
  • The reason is that during an illness, you may need even more insulin than usual.

❸ **Insulin—Supplemental Insulin for Hyperglycemia:**
  • **Note to Triager:** Supplemental rapid-acting (e.g., lispro, aspart) or short-acting (regular) insulin is sometimes needed in addition to usual insulin doses for treating hyperglycemia. Most patients should already have been given "sick-day rules" education by their doctor and instructions on when to use supplemental insulin. **The triage nurse must discuss all insulin dosing with the doctor before giving recommendations to the patient.** In most cases it is best if the doctor talks directly with the patient.
  • **Total Daily Dose (TDD):** The TDD is calculated by adding up all insulin administered during a usual day.
  • **Typical Sick-Day Insulin Supplementation—Urine Ketones Negative or Trace:** If glucose is 80-240 mg/dL (4.5-13 mmol/L), give usual dose. If glucose is 250-400 mg/dL (14-22 mmol/L), supplemental insulin dosage is 10% of TDD. If glucose is > 400 mg/dL (22 mol/L), supplemental insulin dosage is 20% of TDD.
  • **Typical Sick-Day Insulin Supplementation—Urine Ketones Moderate:** If glucose is 80-240 mg/dL (4.5-13 mmol/L), give usual dose. If glucose is 250-400 mg/dL (14-22 mmol/L), supplemental insulin dosage is 20% of TDD. If glucose is > 400 mg/dL (22 mol/L), supplemental insulin dosage is 20% of TDD.

❹ **Insulin—Decreased Insulin for Hypoglycemia:**
  • **Note to Triager:** Decreased insulin dosing is sometimes needed in patients with a blood glucose < 80 mg/dL (4.5 mmol/L), especially if there is decreased oral intake. **The triage nurse must discuss all insulin dosing with the doctor before giving recommendations to the patient.** In most cases it is best if the doctor talks directly with the patient.
  • **Typical Sick-Day Insulin Reduction—for Blood Glucose < 80 mg/dL (4.5 mmol/L) and There Is Decreased Oral Intake:** Do not give rapid-acting (e.g., lispro, aspart) or short-acting (regular) insulin. Reduce intermediate-acting insulin (e.g., NPH, Lente, 70/30) by 20%.

❺ Diet:
- **Appetite OK, Minimal Nausea:** Continue your normal diabetic meal plan. Avoid spicy or greasy foods.
- **Appetite Fair, Moderate Nausea:** Eat a bland diet. Try small amounts of food 6-8 times a day. Take ½-1 cup (120-240 mL) of food or liquids every 1-2 hours.
- **Appetite Poor, Severe Nausea, Can't Eat Solid Food:** Drink plenty of liquids. Try to drink 4-8 oz (120-240 mL) per hour. If glucose > 240 mg/dL (13 mmol/L), drink sugar-free liquids (e.g., water, broth). If glucose < 200 mg/dL (11 mmol/L), drink sugar-containing liquids (e.g., sports drinks, juice, soda).
- Advance diet as you improve.

❻ Liquids:
- Drink more fluids, at least 8-10 glasses daily (8 oz or 240 mL each glass).
- Even more liquids are needed if there is fever, vomiting, or diarrhea.

❼ Check Blood Glucose:
- When you are ill, you should measure your blood glucose every 2-4 hours.
- Write down the results.

❽ Ketone Testing:
- If you use insulin, you should have ketone test strips at home.
- You should check for ketones when you are sick or your blood glucose is > 240 mg/dL (13 mmol/L).
- There are 2 ways a person can test for ketones.
- **Urine Ketone Test:** Most people with diabetes use this test. Urine ketone test kits are available at your local pharmacy.
- **Blood Ketone Test:** Some people have special meters that allow them to test for blood ketones.

❾ Call Back If:
- Blood glucose > 300 mg/dL (16.5 mmol/L) ≥ 2 times in a row.
- Urine ketones become moderate or large.
- Vomiting lasting > 4 hours.
- Rapid breathing occurs.
- You become worse or have more questions.

Additional Resources

❶ American Diabetes Association (ADA):
- Telephone number: 1-800-DIABETES (800/342-2383)
- Web site: www.diabetes.org

❷ US National Diabetes Education Program (NDEP):
- "If you are living with diabetes or have a loved one with the disease, it's important to work together to manage diabetes. Use these resources to learn how to make healthy lifestyle choices to help manage diabetes, prevent complications, and improve your quality of life."
- Telephone number: 800/438-5383.
- Web site: https://www.cdc.gov/diabetes/ndep/people-with-diabetes/index.html.

❸ Canadian Diabetes Association:
- Telephone number: 1-800-BANTING (226-8464)
- Web site: www.diabetes.ca

FIRST AID

First Aid Advice for Hypoglycemia—Glucose

If blood glucose < 70 mg/dL (3.9 mmol/L) or unknown for conscious patients:
- Give sugar (15-20 g glucose) by mouth IF able to swallow.
- Each of the following has the right amount of sugar: low-fat milk (1 cup; 240 mL); fruit juice or non-diet soda (½ cup; 120 mL); prepackaged juice box (1 box); table sugar or honey (3 teaspoons; 15 mL); glucose tablets (3 tablets); glucose paste (10-15 g).
- Symptoms should begin to improve within 5 minutes. Full recovery may take 10-20 minutes.

First Aid Advice for Hypoglycemia—Glucagon

If blood glucose < 70 mg/dL (3.9 mmol/L) or unknown (pending EMS arrival):
- If family has glucagon for hypoglycemic emergencies AND the caller knows how to use it, encourage the caller to give the glucagon now.
- Inject it IM into the upper outer thigh.
- Adult dosage is 1 mg.
- Glucagon can be used in unconscious patients.
- Symptoms should begin to improve within 5 minutes. Full recovery may take 10-20 minutes.

BACKGROUND

Causes and Risk Factors for Low Blood Sugar (Hypoglycemia)

- **Aggressive Diabetes Control:** Intensive glycemic control reduces the long-term complications of diabetes. Unfortunately, it also increases the frequency of hypoglycemia.
- Alcohol ingestion.
- History of other recent episodes of hypoglycemia.
- Prolonged or vigorous exercise.
- Renal failure.
- Too much diabetes medication (e.g., insulin, pills) or too little food.
- Combination of these factors.

Diabetes Mellitus

- **Definition:** Diabetes mellitus is an endocrine condition in which patients have elevated blood glucose levels (hyperglycemia). The classic symptoms of untreated or undertreated diabetes are: frequent urination (polyuria), polydipsia (excessive thirst), and involuntary weight loss.
- **The Role of Insulin:** Insulin is a hormone produced by the pancreas to help process food. Eating food makes the blood glucose rise and insulin makes the blood glucose fall.
- **Classification of Diabetes Mellitus:** There are 4 different classes of diabetes mellitus: type 1 diabetes, type 2 diabetes, gestational diabetes mellitus, and other.

Type 1 Diabetes

- **Other Names:** Insulin-dependent diabetes mellitus, juvenile-onset diabetes.
- **Physiology:** There is no production of insulin by the body.
- **Ketosis-Prone:** Patients with this type of diabetes are ketosis-prone, which means that if they do not receive daily insulin shots their bodies break down fats and produce ketones. The ketones spill into the urine and can be measured. Patients with type 1 diabetes are susceptible to developing diabetic ketoacidosis (DKA), a life-threatening condition.
- **Onset:** It most commonly first appears in childhood or adolescence. Approximately 10% of diabetics are type 1.

- **Treatment:** Insulin therapy is always required and needs to be given subcutaneously at least once daily. Patients striving for tighter control of their blood glucose will take insulin more often than once a day. Recommended therapy for type 1 diabetes includes: 1) use of multiple-dose insulin injections (3–4 injections per day) and 2) matching of mealtime (prandial) insulin to carbohydrate intake, premeal blood glucose, and anticipated activity.

Type 2 Diabetes

- **Other Names:** Non–insulin-dependent diabetes mellitus, adult-onset diabetes.
- **Physiology:** In type 2 diabetes, there is decreased insulin production and decreased sensitivity to insulin.
- **Not Ketosis-Prone:** These patients are not prone to ketosis. DKA rarely occurs.
- **Onset:** It more commonly develops in elderly and overweight adults.
- **Treatment:** The initial and most important treatments are exercise and weight loss. When these measures fail, there are oral medications (e.g., metformin) that can be prescribed to help the body make more insulin or use the insulin more effectively. Occasionally, patients require insulin therapy.
- **Diagnosis:** Probably the best way to diagnose diabetes is a hemoglobin A_{1c} test with a value of $\geq 6.5\%$. There are 2 other tests that have long been used for diagnosing diabetes: a fasting plasma glucose > 126 mg/dL (7.0 mmol/L) and a 2-hour oral glucose tolerance test with a glucose > 200 mg/dL (11.1 mmol/L).

Gestational Diabetes

- Gestational diabetes is diabetes that is found for the first time when a woman is pregnant.
- **Physiology:** In gestational diabetes, the body is not making sufficient insulin to keep pace with the weight gain and other hormonal changes of pregnancy.
- **Not Ketosis-Prone:** These patients are not prone to ketosis. DKA rarely occurs.
- **Onset:** It occurs during pregnancy.
- **Treatment:** A meal plan and regular physical activity are important.

Diabetic Ketoacidosis (DKA)
- **Definition:** Blood glucose > 250 mg/dL (12 mmol/L) with acidosis and ketosis (urine ketones moderate-large; or blood ketones > 1.5 mmol/L)
- **Symptoms of DKA:** In addition to symptoms of hyperglycemia, fruity odor on breath, vomiting, rapid/deep breathing, confusion, and coma.
- **Causes:** Noncompliance with using insulin in type 1 diabetes, infection.

Ketone Testing
- Diabetics who take insulin should test for ketones when their blood sugar is > 240 mg/dL (13 mmol/L). They should also check for ketones when they are sick or have symptoms of ketoacidosis (vomiting, fruity breath, or rapid breathing).
- Detecting ketosis early is important to help prevent life-threatening diabetes ketoacidosis.
- There are now 2 ways patients can test for ketones at home.
- **Urine Ketone Tests:** Many patients test for urine ketones (urine acetoacetate) by doing a urine ketone test. Urine ketone strips are available at local pharmacies. The results indicate the amount of urine ketones as small, moderate, or large. Moderate to large amounts of ketones indicate ketosis.
- **Blood Ketone Tests:** Some blood glucose test meters now allow the patient to also test for blood ketones (blood β-hydroxybutyrate). The patient can often test for blood ketones and blood glucose at the same time. The blood ketone test does require a different strip made just for ketone tests. Blood ketone tests may detect ketones a bit sooner than urine ketone test. The blood ketone tests give the patient a number reading. A number < 0.6 mmol/L is considered normal. Numbers between 0.6 and 1.5 mmol/L mean ketosis is developing and patients should call their doctor for further instructions. Numbers > 1.6 mmol/L mean ketosis is concerning and patients should call their doctor or seek medical care now.

Five Types of Insulin for Diabetes
- **Rapid-acting** (Humalog/lispro, NovoLog/aspart): Onset 5-15 minutes; peaks 30-90 minutes; lasts 4-6 hours.
- **Short-acting** (Regular, Humulin R, Novolin R): Onset 30-60 minutes; peaks 2-3 hours; lasts 5-8 hours.
- **Intermediate-acting** (NPH, Lente, Humulin N, Humulin L, Novolin N, Novolin L): Onset 2-4 hours; peaks 4-12 hours; lasts 10-18 hours.
- **Long-acting** (Lantus/glargine, Detemir, Levemir): Onset 2-4 hours; no true peak; lasts 18-24 hours.
- **Premixed** (Humulin 70/30, Humulin 50/50, Humalog mix, NovoLog mix): 2 peaks; lasts 10-16 hours; depends on mixture.

Insulin Administration—Different Dosing Regimens
- **Sliding Insulin Scale:** Generally only used in the hospital.
- **Insulin Algorithm:** The patient checks his/her blood glucose before each meal and then adjusts insulin dosing based on BOTH the blood glucose and an estimated caloric count for the meal. This is considered "prandial" insulin because it is given with (just before) meals. Rapid-acting (Humalog/lispro or NovoLog/aspart) or short-acting (regular) are used for prandial insulin dosing.
- **Once-Daily Insulin:** This is not considered physiologic insulin dosing, as it only provides the "basal" insulin and does not provide the needed prandial increases. However, it may be an effective addition for some type 2 diabetic patients on oral medications, as their need for insulin is low. Intermediate-acting insulin (NPH) or long-acting insulin (Lantus/glargine) are used.
- **Twice-Daily Insulin:** Intermediate-acting insulin (NPH) or long-acting insulin (Lantus/glargine) can be used in twice-daily regimens. Twice-daily insulin dosing may be sufficient for type 2 diabetic patients because they still make sufficient insulin on their own to handle prandial (mealtime) insulin needs.
- **Flexible Insulin Regimens:** In this type of regimen, both an intermediate-acting insulin (for basal insulin needs) AND a rapid or ultrashort-acting insulin (for prandial insulin needs) are used.

Five Types of Oral Medications for Diabetes

- **Sulfonylureas:** Examples include glyburide (Micronase, DiaBeta), glipizide (Glucotrol, Glucotrol XL), and glimepiride (Amaryl).
- **Biguanides:** Examples include metformin (Glucophage, Fortamet).
- **Thiazolidinediones:** Examples include rosiglitazone (Avenida) and pioglitazone (Actos).
- **Alpha-Glucosidase Inhibitors:** Examples include acarbose (Precose) and miglitol (Glyset).
- **Meglitinides:** Examples include repaglinide (Prandin) and nateglinide (Starlix).

Goals for Diabetes Management

- **Hemoglobin A_{1c}:** Hemoglobin A_{1c} (HbA$_{1c}$) is the primary goal for diabetes management. Depending on the patient, it should be measured 2-4 times a year. The American Diabetes Association (ADA) recommends a goal of < 7.0% for nonpregnant adults.
- **Blood Glucose:** Depending on the patient, the blood glucose should be measured 1-3 times per day. The ADA recommends the following blood glucose goals:
  - **Preprandial** (before meal): 80-130 mg/dL (4.4-7.2 mmol/L)
  - **Postprandial** (1-2 hours after a meal): < 180 mg/dL (10 mmol/L)
  Goals should be individualized based on: age/life expectancy, duration of diabetes, comorbid conditions, hypoglycemic unawareness, history of severe hypoglycemic reactions, and other individual considerations.
  - **Internet Resource:** ADA "Standards of Medical Care in Diabetes" 2016; available at: http://care.diabetesjournals.org/content/39/Supplement_1

Glycosylated Hemoglobin A_{1c}

- The HbA$_{1c}$ provides a good estimate of how well a patient has managed his/her diabetes during the past 2-3 months. With good diabetes management, the HbA$_{1c}$ goes down; with poor management, it goes up. In general, the higher the HbA$_{1c}$, the greater the risk of long-term diabetic complications.
- **Goal:** The American Association of Clinical Endocrinologists and the American College of Endocrinology recommend a target glycosylated hemoglobin level (HbA$_{1c}$) of < 6.5%. The ADA recommends a goal of < 7.0% for nonpregnant adults. The Canadian Diabetes Association also recommends a goal of < 7.0%

Long-term Complications of Diabetes Mellitus

- **Eye Disease** (e.g., retinopathy): Diabetes is the leading cause of blindness.
- **Heart Disease** (e.g., coronary heart disease, myocardial infarction).
- **Kidney Disease** (e.g., renal failure, proteinuria).
- **Nerve Disease** (e.g., peripheral and autonomic neuropathy).
- **Stroke.**

Converting Glucose Levels: mg/dL and mmol/L

- In the United States, glucose is typically measured using the units mg/dL. Nearly every country in the world (including Canada) measures glucose levels using the units mmol/L.
- To convert mmol/L of glucose to mg/dL, multiply by 18.
- To convert mg/dL of glucose to mmol/L, divide by 18 or multiply by 0.055.

Screening for Diabetes

- **Hemoglobin A_{1c}:** < 5.7 (normal); 5.7-6.4 (impaired fasting glucose); > 6.4 (type 2 diabetes)
- **Fasting Glucose mg/dL:** < 100 (normal); 100-125 (impaired fasting glucose); > 125 (type 2 diabetes)
- **Fasting Glucose mmol/L:** < 5.6 (normal); 5.6-6.9 (impaired fasting glucose); > 6.9 (type 2 diabetes)

DIARRHEA

Definition
- Diarrhea is the sudden increase in the frequency and looseness of bowel movements (BMs; stools).

Diarrhea Severity
- **No Diarrhea.**
- **Mild:** Few loose or mushy BMs; increase of 1-3 stools over normal daily number of stools.
- **Moderate:** Increase of 4-6 stools daily over normal.
- **Severe** (or "worst possible"): Increase of ≥ 7 stools daily over normal; incontinence.

TRIAGE ASSESSMENT QUESTIONS

Call EMS 911 Now
- Shock suspected (e.g., cold/pale/clammy skin, too weak to stand)
  R/O: shock
  First Aid: Lie down with the feet elevated.
- Difficult to awaken or acting confused (e.g., disoriented, slurred speech)
- Sounds like a life-threatening emergency to the triager

See More Appropriate Protocol
- Vomiting also present and worse than the diarrhea
  Go to Protocol: Vomiting on page 433
- Blood in stool and without diarrhea
  Go to Protocol: Rectal Bleeding on page 333

Go to ED Now
- SEVERE abdominal pain (e.g., excruciating) and present > 1 hour
  R/O: appendicitis or other acute abdomen
- SEVERE abdominal pain and age > 60
  Reason: higher risk of serious cause of abdominal pain, e.g., mesenteric ischemia
- Bloody, black, or tarry BMs
  R/O: GI bleed
  (Exception: chronic unchanged black-gray BMs and is taking iron pills or Pepto-Bismol)

Go to ED/UCC Now
(or to Office With PCP Approval)
- SEVERE diarrhea (e.g., ≥ 7 times/day more than normal) and age > 60 years
  Reason: severe diarrhea, higher risk of dehydration
- Constant abdominal pain lasting > 2 hours
  R/O: acute abdomen
- Drinking very little and has signs of dehydration (e.g., no urine > 12 hours, very dry mouth, very light-headed)
  Reason: may need IV hydration
- Patient sounds very sick or weak to the triager
  Reason: severe acute illness or serious complication suspected

See Today in Office
- SEVERE diarrhea (e.g., ≥ 7 times/day more than normal) and present > 24 hours (1 day)
  Reason: high risk for dehydration
- MODERATE diarrhea (e.g., 4-6 times/day more than normal) and present > 48 hours (2 days)
  Reason: higher risk of dehydration
- MODERATE diarrhea (e.g., 4-6 times/day more than normal) and age > 70 years
  Reason: higher risk of dehydration and morbidity
- Abdominal pain
  (Exception: pain clears completely with each passage of diarrhea stool)
- Fever > 101° F (38.3° C)
  R/O: bacterial diarrhea
- Blood in the stool
  R/O: bacterial diarrhea
- Mucus or pus in stool has been present > 2 days and diarrhea is more than mild
- Weak immune system (e.g., HIV positive, cancer chemotherapy, splenectomy, organ transplant, chronic steroids)
  Reason: broader range of causes

Callback by PCP Today

● Travel to a foreign country in past month
Reason: antibiotic therapy may be indicated for traveler's diarrhea

● Recent antibiotic therapy (i.e., within last 2 months)
R/O: C difficile diarrhea, antibiotic side effect

● Tube feedings (e.g., nasogastric, gastrostomy tube, jejunostomy tube)
R/O: osmotic diarrhea

See Within 3 Days in Office

● MILD diarrhea (e.g., 1-≥ 3 stools than normal in past 24 hours) without known cause and present > 7 days

● Patient wants to be seen

See Within 2 Weeks in Office

● Diarrhea is a chronic symptom (recurrent or ongoing AND lasting > 4 weeks)

Home Care

○ SEVERE diarrhea (e.g., ≥ 7 times/day more than normal)
Reason: new or transient diarrhea without significant risk factors; may respond to homecare measures

○ MILD-MODERATE diarrhea (e.g., 1-6 times/day more than normal)
Reason: new or transient diarrhea without significant risk factors; may respond to Home Care Advice

HOME CARE ADVICE

Severe Diarrhea

❶ Reassurance:

• Sometimes the cause is an infection caused by a virus ("stomach flu") or bacteria. Diarrhea is one of the body's ways of getting rid of germs.

• Certain foods (e.g., dairy products, supplements like Ensure) can also trigger diarrhea.

• In some patients, the exact cause is never found.

• Staying well hydrated is the key for adults with diarrhea. From what you have told me, it sounds like you are not severely dehydrated at this point.

• *Here is some general care advice that should help.*

❷ Fluid Therapy During Severe Diarrhea:

• Drink more fluids, at least 8-10 cups daily. One cup equals 8 oz (240 mL).

• **Water:** Even for severe diarrhea, water is often the best liquid to drink. You should also eat some salty foods (e.g., potato chips, pretzels, saltine crackers). This is important to make sure you are getting enough salt, sugars, and fluids to meet your body's needs.

• **Sports Drinks:** You can also drink a sports drink (e.g., Gatorade, Powerade) to help treat and prevent dehydration. For it to work best, mix it half and half with water.

• Avoid caffeinated beverages.
(Reason: Caffeine is mildly dehydrating.)

• Avoid alcohol beverages (beer, wine, hard liquor).

❸ Food and Nutrition During Severe Diarrhea:

• Drinking enough liquids is more important that eating when one has severe diarrhea.

• As the diarrhea starts to get better, you can slowly return to a normal diet.

• Begin with boiled starches/cereals (e.g., potatoes, rice, noodles, wheat, oats) with a small amount of salt to taste.

• Other foods that are OK include: bananas, yogurt, crackers, soup.

❹ Contagiousness:

• Be certain to wash your hands after using the restroom.

• If your work is cooking, handling, serving, or preparing food, you should not work until the diarrhea has completely stopped.

❺ Expected Course: Viral diarrhea lasts 4-7 days. Always worse on days 1 and 2.

❻ Call Back If:

• Signs of dehydration occur (e.g., no urine > 12 hours, very dry mouth, light-headed, etc.).

• Severe diarrhea lasts > 1 day.

• Diarrhea lasts > 7 days.

• You become worse.

Mild-Moderate Diarrhea

❶ Reassurance:

- Sometimes the cause is an infection caused by a virus ("stomach flu") or bacteria. Diarrhea is one of the body's way of getting rid of germs.
- Certain foods (e.g., dairy products, supplements like Ensure) can also trigger diarrhea.
- In some patients, the exact cause is never found.
- Staying well hydrated is the key for adults with diarrhea. From what you have told me, it sounds like you are not severely dehydrated at this point.
- *Here is some general care advice that should help.*

❷ Fluid Therapy During Mild-Moderate Diarrhea:

- Drink more fluids, at least 8-10 cups daily. One cup equals 8 oz (240 mL).
- **Water:** For mild-moderate diarrhea, water is often the best liquid to drink. You should also eat some salty foods (e.g., potato chips, pretzels, saltine crackers). This is important to make sure you are getting enough salt, sugars, and fluids to meet your body's needs.
- **Sports Drinks:** You can also drink a sports drink (e.g., Gatorade, Powerade) to help treat and prevent dehydration. For it to work best, mix it half and half with water.
- Avoid caffeinated beverages. *(Reason: Caffeine is mildly dehydrating.)*
- Avoid alcohol beverages (beer, wine, hard liquor).

❸ Food and Nutrition During Mild-Moderate Diarrhea:

- You can eat when you are having diarrhea. In fact, it is healthy for your intestines.
- Begin with boiled starches/cereals (e.g., potatoes, rice, noodles, wheat, oats) with a small amount of salt to taste.
- Other foods that are OK include: bananas, yogurt, crackers, soup.
- As the diarrhea starts to get better, you can slowly return to a normal diet.

❹ Contagiousness:

- Be certain to wash your hands after using the restroom.
- If your work is cooking, handling, serving, or preparing food, you should not work until the diarrhea has completely stopped.

❺ Expected Course: Viral diarrhea lasts 4-7 days. Always worse on days 1 and 2.

❻ Call Back If:

- Signs of dehydration occur (e.g., no urine > 12 hours, very dry mouth, light-headed, etc.).
- Moderate diarrhea lasts > 2 days.
- Diarrhea lasts > 7 days.
- You become worse.

Treating Diarrhea With Over-the-counter (OTC) Medicines

❶ OTC Medicines—Loperamide (Imodium AD):

- Helps reduce diarrhea.
- **Adult Dosage:** 4 mg (2 capsules or 4 teaspoons or 20 mL) is the recommended first dose. You may take an additional 2 mg (1 capsule or 2 teaspoons or 10 mL) after each loose BM.
- **Maximum Dosage:** 16 mg (8 capsules or 16 teaspoons or 80 mL).
- Do not use for > 2 days.
- 1 capsule = 2 mg; 1 teaspoon (5 mL) = 1 mg.

❷ Caution—Loperamide (Imodium AD):

- **Do not** use if there is a fever > 100.5° F (38.1° C) or if there is blood or mucus in the stools.
- *Read and follow the package instructions carefully.*

❸ OTC Medicines—Bismuth Subsalicylate (e.g., Kaopectate, Pepto-Bismol):

- Helps reduce diarrhea, vomiting, and abdominal cramping.
- **Adult Dosage:** 2 tablets or 2 tablespoons by mouth every hour (if diarrhea continues) to a maximum of 8 doses in a 24-hour period.
- Do not use for > 2 days.

❹ Caution—Bismuth Subsalicylate (e.g., Kaopectate, Pepto-Bismol):

- May cause a temporary darkening of stool and tongue.
- Do not use if allergic to aspirin.
- Do not use in pregnancy.
- *Read and follow the package instructions carefully.*

❺ Call Back If:

- You have more questions.
- You become worse.

FIRST AID

First Aid Advice for Shock:
Lie down with the feet elevated.

BACKGROUND

Key Points
- The majority of adults with acute diarrhea (< 14 days' duration) have an infectious etiology for their diarrhea, and in most cases the infection is a virus. Other common causes of acute diarrhea are food poisoning and medications.
- Maintaining hydration is the cornerstone of treatment of adults with acute diarrhea.
- In general, an adult who is alert, feels well, and is not thirsty or dizzy is **not** dehydrated. A couple loose or runny stools do not cause dehydration. Frequent, watery stools can cause dehydration.
- Antibiotic therapy is only rarely required in the treatment of acute diarrhea. Two types of acute diarrhea that require antibiotic therapy are *C difficile* diarrhea and (sometimes) traveler's diarrhea.

Causes
- **Antibiotic Side Effect** (e.g., temporary diarrhea from Augmentin/amoxicillin clavulanic acid).
- **Bacterial Gastroenteritis** (i.e., *Campylobacter, Salmonella, Shigella*).
- **Cathartics, Excessive Use of** (e.g., magnesium citrate, milk of magnesia).
- **Food Poisoning.**
- **Giardiasis.**
- **Inflammatory Bowel Disease.**
- **Irritable Bowel Syndrome.**
- **Traveler's Diarrhea.**
- **Pseudomembranous Colitis:** An inflammation in the colon that occurs in some people from taking antibiotics. It is usually caused by an overgrowth of a specific type bacteria called *Clostridium difficile* (*C difficile*). Other names that are used to describe this illness include antibiotic-associated diarrhea and *C difficile* colitis.
- **Viral Gastroenteritis** (stomach flu).

Traveler's Diarrhea
- **Definition:** Traveler's diarrhea typically begins within 2 weeks of traveling to a foreign country. There are bacteria in the water and food that the body is not used to and a diarrheal infection is the result. Traveler's diarrhea is also called "mummy tummy," "Montezuma's revenge," and "turista."
- **Symptoms:** Passage of ≥ 3 loose stools a day; accompanying symptoms may include nausea, vomiting, abdominal cramping, fecal urgency, and fever.
- **Region and Risk:** Travelers to the following developing areas have a **high risk** (40%) of getting traveler's diarrhea: Latin America, Africa, Southern Asia. There is an **intermediate risk** (15%) with travel to Northern Mediterranean countries, the Middle East, China, and Russia. Travelers to the United States, Western Europe, Canada, and Japan have a **low risk** (2%-4%) of getting traveler's diarrhea.
- **Prevention: Diet:** Avoid uncooked foods (salad). Cooked foods (served steaming hot) are usually safe, as are dry foods (e.g., bread). Avoid ice cubes and tap water. Drink steaming beverages (e.g., coffee, tea) or carbonated drinks (e.g., bottled soft drinks, beer). Fruits that can be peeled are usually safe (e.g., oranges, bananas, apples).
- **Prevention: Bismuth Subsalicylate:** Bismuth subsalicylate (Pepto-Bismol 8 tablets daily orally) is approximately 65% effective at preventing traveler's diarrhea.
- **Prevention: Antibiotics:** Antibiotic chemoprophylaxis (prevention) during travel may be indicated in certain circumstances. Rifaximin (200 mg orally twice a day with meals) is approximately 70%-80% effective at preventing traveler's diarrhea.
- **Treatment: Antidiarrheal Agents:** Bismuth subsalicylate (Pepto-Bismol) and loperamide (Imodium AD) are both effective at reducing the diarrhea symptoms.
- **Treatment: Antibiotics:** Antibiotic therapy is sometimes recommended to treat this type of diarrhea, especially if the symptoms are more than mild. There are a number of antibiotics that are effective, including ciprofloxacin (Cipro), azithromycin (Zithromax), and rifaximin (Xifaxan 200 mg orally 3 times a day for 3 days).

Norwalk Virus

- **Definition:** The Norwalk virus is one of a number of viruses that cause stomach flu (viral gastroenteritis). It is usually acquired through contaminated food or water. In 2002 and 2003 this received significant media attention when several cruise ships had outbreaks in which hundreds of passengers were affected.
- **Symptoms:** Acute onset of diarrhea, vomiting, abdominal cramps. In adults there is usually more diarrhea than vomiting. The symptoms typically last 1-2 days.
- **Epidemiology:** The Norwalk virus is the number one cause of epidemic gastroenteritis. Outbreaks have been reported in restaurants, nursing homes, hospitals, and vacation settings like cruise ships.
- **Incubation Period:** 1-3 days.
- **Prevention:** How can one avoid exposure while on a vacation? Avoid uncooked food. Drink bottled water (avoid ice cubes). Wash your hands frequently. Do not share glassware or eating utensils.
- **Treatment:** Antibiotics are not helpful since this is a viral infection. Maintaining adequate hydration through intake of oral liquids is the most important thing. Pepto-Bismol can be used.

Dehydration—Estimation by Telephone

Mild Dehydration

1. **Urine Production:** Slightly decreased
2. **Mucous Membranes:** Normal
3. Heart rate < 100 beats/minute
4. Slightly thirsty
5. **Capillary Refill:** < 2 seconds
6. **Treatment:** Can usually treat at home

Moderate Dehydration

1. **Urine Production:** Minimal or absent.
2. **Mucous Membranes:** Dry inside of mouth.
3. Heart rate 100-130 beats/minute.
4. Thirsty, light-headed when standing.
5. **Capillary Refill:** > 2 seconds.
6. **Treatment:** Must be seen; Go to ED NOW (or PCP Triage).

Severe Dehydration

1. **Urine Production:** None > 12 hours.
2. **Mucous Membranes:** Very dry inside of mouth.
3. Heart rate > 130 beats/minute.
4. Very thirsty, very weak, and light-headed; fainting may occur.
5. **Capillary Refill:** > 2-4 seconds.
6. **Treatment:** Must be seen immediately; Go to ED Now or CALL EMS 911 NOW.

Signs of Shock

1. Confused, difficult to awaken, or unresponsive.
2. Heart rate (pulse) is rapid and weak.
3. Extremities (especially hands and feet) are bluish or gray, and cold.
4. Too weak to stand or very dizzy when tries to stand.
5. **Capillary Refill:** > 4 seconds.
6. **Treatment:** Lie down with the feet elevated; CALL EMS 911 NOW.

DIZZINESS

Definition
- Patient complains of dizziness, light-headedness, or feeling woozy.
- Patient feels like he/she might faint but has not.
- Transient blurring of vision may be associated.

Dizziness Severity
- **Mild:** Walking normally.
- **Moderate:** Interferes with normal activities (e.g., work, school).
- **Severe:** Unable to stand, requires support to walk, feels like passing out now.

TRIAGE ASSESSMENT QUESTIONS

Call EMS 911 Now
- Shock suspected (e.g., cold/pale/clammy skin, too weak to stand)
  R/O: shock
  First Aid: Lie down with the feet elevated.
- Difficult to awaken or acting confused (e.g., disoriented, slurred speech)
- Fainted, and still feels dizzy afterwards
  R/O: arrhythmia, shock
- SEVERE difficulty breathing (e.g., struggling for each breath, speaks in single words)
  R/O: respiratory failure, hypoxia
- Overdose (accidental or intentional) of medications
- New neurologic deficit that is present now:
  - Weakness of the face, arm, or leg on one side of the body
  - Numbness of the face, arm, or leg on one side of the body
  - Loss of speech or garbled speech
    R/O: stroke
- Heart beating < 50 beats per minute OR > 140 beats per minute
  Reason: symptomatic bradycardia-tachycardia
- Sounds like a life-threatening emergency to the triager

See More Appropriate Protocol
- Chest pain
  Go to Protocol: Chest Pain on page 73
- Rectal bleeding, bloody stool, or tarry-black stool
  Go to Protocol: Rectal Bleeding on page 333
- Vomiting is the main symptom
  Go to Protocol: Vomiting on page 433
- Diarrhea is the main symptom
  Go to Protocol: Diarrhea on page 123
- Headache is the main symptom
  Go to Protocol: Headache on page 207

Go to ED/UCC Now
(or to Office With PCP Approval)
- SEVERE dizziness (e.g., unable to stand, requires support to walk, feels like passing out now)
  R/O: severe labyrinthitis, CVA
- Severe headache
  R/O: migraine, aneurysm
- Extra heartbeats OR irregular heart beating (i.e., "palpitations")
  R/O: dysrhythmia
- Difficulty breathing
  R/O: hypoxia
- Drinking very little and has signs of dehydration (e.g., no urine > 12 hours, very dry mouth, very light-headed)
  Reason: IV hydration needed
- Follows bleeding (e.g., stomach, rectum, vagina)
  (Exception: became dizzy from sight of small amount of blood)
  R/O: hypovolemic shock from major blood loss
- Patient sounds very sick or weak to the triager
  Reason: severe acute illness or serious complication suspected

Go to Office Now
- Light-headedness (dizziness) present now, after 2 hours of rest and fluids
- Spinning or tilting sensation (vertigo) present now
- Fever > 103° F (39.4° C)
- Fever > 100.0° F (37.8° C) and has diabetes mellitus or a weak immune system (e.g., HIV positive, cancer chemotherapy, organ transplant, splenectomy, chronic steroids)

See Today in Office
- Vomiting occurs with dizziness
- Patient wants to be seen

Discuss With PCP and Callback by Nurse Today
- Taking a medicine that could cause dizziness (e.g., blood pressure medications, diuretics)
- Diabetes

  Note: Patient should check his/her glucose level when feeling dizzy.

See Within 2 Weeks in Office
- Dizziness not present now but is a chronic symptom (recurrent or ongoing AND lasting > 4 weeks)

Home Care
- ○ Poor fluid intake probably causing dizziness
- ○ Recent heat exposure probably causing dizziness
- ○ Sudden or prolonged standing probably causing dizziness

HOME CARE ADVICE

❶ Temporary dizziness is usually a harmless symptom. It can be caused by not drinking enough water during sports or hot weather. It can also be caused by skipping a meal, too much sun exposure, standing up suddenly, standing too long in one place, or even a viral illness.

❷ Some Causes of Temporary Dizziness:
- **Poor Fluid Intake:** Not drinking enough fluids and being a little dehydrated is a common cause of temporary dizziness. This is always worse during hot weather.
- **Standing Up Suddenly:** Standing up suddenly (especially getting out of bed) and prolonged standing in one place are common causes of temporary dizziness. Not drinking enough fluids always makes it worse. Certain medications can cause or increase this type of dizziness (e.g., blood pressure medications).
- **Heat Exposure:** Hot weather, hot tubs, and too much sun exposure are common causes of temporary dizziness. Not drinking enough fluids always makes it worse.

❸ Drink Fluids: Drink several glasses of fruit juice, other clear fluids, or water. This will improve hydration and blood glucose. If you have a fever or have had heat exposure, make sure the fluids are cold.

❹ Cool Off: If the weather is hot, apply a cold compress to the forehead or take a cool shower or bath.

❺ Rest for 1-2 Hours: Lie down with the feet elevated for 1 hour. This will improve blood flow and increase blood flow to the brain.

❻ Stand Up Slowly:
- In the mornings, sit up for a few minutes before you stand up. That will help your blood flow make the adjustment.
- If you have to stand up for long periods, contract and relax your leg muscles to help pump the blood back to the heart.
- Sit down or lie down if you feel dizzy.

❼ Call Back If:
- Still feel dizzy after 2 hours of rest and fluids.
- Passes out (faints).
- You become worse.

FIRST AID

First Aid Advice for Shock:
Lie down with the feet elevated.

First Aid Advice for Anaphylaxis—Epinephrine:
- If the patient has an epinephrine autoinjector, **give it now.** Do not delay.
- Use the autoinjector on the upper outer thigh. You may give it through clothing if necessary.
- Give epinephrine first, then call 911.
- Epinephrine is available in autoinjectors under trade names: EpiPen, EpiPen Jr, and Auvi-Q (Allerject in Canada). Auvi-Q has an audio chip and talks patients and caregivers through injection process.
- You may give a second (repeat) dose of epinephrine 10-15 minutes later, IF the person with anaphylaxis does not respond to the first dose AND ambulance arrival takes > 10 minutes.

First Aid Advice for Anaphylaxis—Benadryl:
- Give antihistamine by mouth **NOW** if able to swallow.
- Use Benadryl (diphenhydramine; adult dose: 50 mg) or any other available antihistamine medicine.

BACKGROUND

Key Points

- There are 2 main types of dizziness: light-headedness and vertigo.
- **Light-headedness:** This type of dizziness results from decreased blood flow to the brain. Equivalent terms that patients may use include feeling faint, spacey, weak, giddy, or woozy. Light-headedness is often aggravated by standing up and relieved by lying down.
- **Vertigo:** Patients with vertigo have the sensation that they are or their environment is spinning. They may complain that the floor seems to be tilting. As a result, patients with vertigo often report difficulty with walking and standing because they feel like they are going to fall down. Vertigo typically has a neurologic etiology, resulting from some condition affecting the ear or the brain. Vertigo is usually aggravated by changes in head position.

Causes of Light-headedness

- Anyone can develop temporary dizziness or light-headedness from standing up suddenly, standing too long in one place, skipping a meal, dehydration, too much sun or hot tub exposure, or overexertion.
- Acute blood loss (e.g., gastrointestinal bleeding, vaginal bleeding).
- Cardiac disorders with decreased cardiac output (e.g., arrhythmias, valvular heart disease, cardiomyopathies).
- Fever.
- Heat exhaustion.
- Medication side effect.
- Metabolic disorder (e.g., hypoglycemia).
- Orthostatic hypotension (e.g., antihypertensive medications).
- Panic disorder and hyperventilation.
- **Viral Syndrome:** Patients with viral illnesses (e.g., colds, flu) often report some dizziness along with all the other symptoms that they are experiencing.
- **Volume Depletion and Dehydration:** From vomiting, diarrhea, sweating.

EAR, SWIMMER'S (OTITIS EXTERNA)

Definition
- An infection or irritation of the skin that lines the ear canal.
- Typically, the patient has been swimming recently or uses Q-tips frequently.
- *Use this guideline only if the patient has symptoms that match swimmer's ear.*

Symptoms
- Ear canal may feel itchy, plugged, or full.
- Ear becomes painful as the swimmer's ear becomes worse.
- Ear pain occurs or increases whenever the earlobe is moved up and down or with pushing on the tragus. This finding of movement causing pain is always present.
- Sometimes there is a discharge from the ear; it may be clear, white, or yellow.
- There are no cold symptoms (e.g., runny nose, cough). The symptoms just involve the ear.

TRIAGE ASSESSMENT QUESTIONS

See More Appropriate Protocol
- Symptoms do not match swimmer's ear
  Go to Protocol: Earache on page 139

Go to ED/UCC Now
(or to Office With PCP Approval)
- Pink or red swelling behind the ear
  R/O: mastoiditis
- Stiff neck (can't touch chin to chest)
  R/O: meningitis, cervical lymphadenitis
- Patient sounds very sick or weak to the triager
  Reason: severe acute illness or serious complication suspected

Go to Office Now
- Diabetes mellitus or a weak immune system (e.g., HIV positive, cancer chemotherapy, transplant patient)
  Reason: higher risk for malignant otitis externa, should be examined
- Outer ear (earlobe) is red and/or swollen
  R/O: cellulitis
- Fever > 100.5° F (38.1° C)
  Reason: fever is uncommon in otitis externa

See Today in Office
- Severe earache pain
- Yellow or green discharge from ear canal
  R/O: otitis externa or otitis media with perforation
- Decreased hearing (or another adult says that the ear canal is completely blocked with discharge)
  Reason: debris/discharge will need to be removed manually
- Swollen lymph node near ear
  R/O: lymphadenitis
- Patient wants to be seen

See Today or Tomorrow in Office
- Diagnosis is uncertain
  Reason: see physician for confirmation of diagnosis
- Ear symptoms persist after 3 days of home treatment

Home Care
- Swimmer's ear with no complications
- Preventing swimmer's ear, questions about

HOME CARE ADVICE

Treatment of Mild Swimmer's Ear

❶ **White Vinegar Rinses:** Vinegar (acetic acid) restores the normal acid pH of the ear canal. This helps swimmer's ear to get better. Rinse the ear canals twice daily with ½-strength white vinegar (dilute it with equal parts water). Here are some instructions on how to do this:
- Lie down with the affected ear upward. Fill the ear canal.
- After 5 minutes, remove the fluid by tilting the head to one side and gently pulling on the ear.
- Continue doing this twice daily until the ear canal returns to normal.
- CAUTION: Do not do if you have ear tubes or hole in eardrum.

❷ **Pain Medicines:**
- For pain relief, you can take either acetaminophen, ibuprofen, or naproxen.
- They are over-the-counter (OTC) pain drugs. You can buy them at the drugstore.

Acetaminophen (e.g., Tylenol):
- **Regular Strength Tylenol:** Take 650 mg (two 325 mg pills) by mouth every 4-6 hours as needed. Each Regular Strength Tylenol pill has 325 mg of acetaminophen.
- **Extra Strength Tylenol:** Take 1,000 mg (two 500 mg pills) every 8 hours as needed. Each Extra Strength Tylenol pill has 500 mg of acetaminophen.
- The most you should take each day is 3,000 mg (10 Regular Strength or 6 Extra Strength pills a day).

Ibuprofen (e.g., Motrin, Advil):
- Take 400 mg (two 200 mg pills) by mouth every 6 hours.
- Another choice is to take 600 mg (three 200 mg pills) by mouth every 8 hours.
- The most you should take each day is 1,200 mg (six 200 mg pills), unless your doctor has told you to take more.

Naproxen (e.g., Aleve):
- Take 220 mg (one 220 mg pill) by mouth every 8 hours as needed. You may take 440 mg (two 220 mg pills) for your first dose.
- The most you should take each day is 660 mg (three 220 mg pills a day), unless your doctor has told you to take more.

❸ **Pain Medicines—Extra Notes:**
- Use the lowest amount of medicine that makes your pain better.
- Acetaminophen is thought to be safer than ibuprofen or naproxen in people > 65 years old. Acetaminophen is in many OTC and prescription medicines. It might be in more than one medicine that you are taking. You need to be careful and not take an overdose. An acetaminophen overdose can hurt the liver.
- McNeil, the company that makes Tylenol, has different dosage instructions for Tylenol in Canada and the United States. In Canada, the maximum recommended dose per day is 4,000 mg or 12 Regular Strength (325 mg) pills. In the United States, McNeil recommends a maximum dose of 10 Regular Strength (325 mg) pills.
- CAUTION: Do not take acetaminophen if you have liver disease.
- CAUTION: Do not take ibuprofen or naproxen if you have stomach problems, have kidney disease, are pregnant, or have been told by your doctor to avoid this type of anti-inflammatory drug. Do not take ibuprofen or naproxen for > 7 days without consulting your doctor.
- *Before taking any medicine, read all the instructions on the package.*

❹ **Local Heat:** If pain is moderate-severe, apply a heating pad (set on low) or hot water bottle (wrapped in a towel) to outer ear for 20 minutes. *(Caution: Avoid burns.)* This will also increase drainage.

❺ **Avoid Earplugs:** If pus or cloudy fluid is draining from the ear canal, wipe the pus away as it appears. Avoid plugging with cotton. *(Reason: Retained pus causes irritation or infection of the ear canal.)*

❻ **Avoid Swimming:** Try to avoid swimming until symptoms are gone.

❼ **Contagiousness:** Swimmer's ear is not contagious.

❽ **Expected Course:** With treatment, symptoms should improve in 3 days and resolve within 7 days.

❾ **Call Back If:**
- Ear symptoms last > 7 days with treatment.
- You become worse.

Prevention of Swimmer's Ear

❶ **Prevention—Keep Ear Canals Dry:**
- Try to keep your ear canals dry.
- After showers, hair washing, and swimming, help the water run out by tilting the head to one side. You can also use a hair dryer set on the lowest setting to dry out your ears.

❷ **Prevention—Avoid Cotton Swabs:**
- Avoid cotton swabs (i.e., Q-tips, cotton tip applicator).
- These remove the protective earwax of the ear canal.

❸ **Prevention—Rinse Ear Canal With Vinegar After Swimming:**
- After swimming, place several drops of ½-strength white vinegar (dilute it with equal parts water) in your ear canals.
- After 5 minutes, remove the fluid by tilting the head to one side and gently pulling on the ear.
- **Reason:** Vinegar (acetic acid) restores the normal acid pH of the ear canal.
- **Indication:** You may want to try this if you tend to get swimmer's ear frequently.
- CAUTION: Do not use if you have ear tubes or hole in eardrum.

BACKGROUND

Key Points

- Otitis externa is an infection of the skin that lines the ear canal. It is also referred to as swimmer's ear.
- **Cause:** When water repeatedly gets trapped in the ear canal (usually from swimming), the lining becomes wet and swollen. This makes the skin of the ear canal susceptible to superficial infection (swimmer's ear). Ear canals were meant to be dry.
- **Earwax (Cerumen):** Cerumen is produced by the ear canal as a natural waterproofing agent. Thus, frequent use of cotton ear swabs depletes the wax barrier and increases the likelihood of developing otitis externa. On the other hand, excessive amounts of earwax can inhibit water drainage from the ear, leading to chronic wetness, ear canal skin maceration, and then on to otitis externa.
- **Wrong Diagnosis:** The triager should question the diagnosis of swimmer's ear if there is no pain on movement of the ear. The triager should also question the diagnosis if the patient has cold symptoms. In such cases, otitis media (middle ear infection) is the more likely explanation.

Treatment

- **Antibiotic Ear Drops:** Otitis externa is usually treated with antibiotic ear drops. Examples include Cortisporin Otic, Floxin Otic, and Cipro HC Otic.
- **Oral Antibiotics:** Occasionally, more severe cases are treated with oral antibiotics.
- **Acetic Acid Solution:** Milder cases of otitis externa can be treated with an acetic acid solution. Household white vinegar contains acetic acid; instructions for use are to rinse the ear canals twice daily with ½-strength white vinegar (dilute it with equal parts water). Acetic acid is also available by prescription (e.g., Acetic Acid Otic, Vosol).
- Pain medications.

EAR PIERCING

Definition
- Area around pierced earring is red, tender, or swollen.
- Earlobes can also become torn or lacerated.

TRIAGE ASSESSMENT QUESTIONS

Go to ED/UCC Now
(or to Office With PCP Approval)
- ● Earring tore completely through the earlobe
  Reason: may need sutures
- ● Skin is split open or gaping
  (or length > ¼" or 6 mm)
  Reason: may need sutures
- ● Bleeding at the piercing site has not stopped after 10 minutes of direct pressure
- ● Part of jewelry (clasp) is stuck inside the earlobe
  Reason: removal of foreign body
- ● Patient sounds very sick or weak to the triager
  Reason: severe acute illness or serious complication suspected

Go to Office Now
- ● Ear pain and entire lower ear is red or swollen
  R/O: cellulitis of earlobe
- ● Ear pain and entire upper ear is red or swollen
  R/O: auricular chondritis of helix
- ● Ear pain and fever
  R/O: cellulitis, chondritis

See Today or Tomorrow in Office
- ◐ Swollen lymph node (in front of or behind earlobe)
  R/O: lymphadenitis
- ◐ Symptoms of minor pierced ear infection (e.g., localized redness just at earring site, slight discharge), and not improving 3 days following Home Care Advice (e.g., cleaning, antibiotic ointment)
  R/O: minor local infection, inadequate cleaning of area, contact dermatitis
- ◐ Small tear in earlobe from earring injury and no tetanus booster > 10 years
  Reason: may need a tetanus booster shot (vaccine)
- ◐ Patient wants to be seen

See Within 2 Weeks in Office
- ◐ Large thick scar has developed at the earring site over the last couple months
  R/O: keloid

Home Care
- ○ Symptoms of minor pierced ear infection (e.g., localized redness just at earring site, slight discharge)
- ○ Small tear in earlobe from earring injury
- ○ Aftercare instructions for new ear piercings, questions about

HOME CARE ADVICE

Caring of Minor Infection at a Ear-Piercing Site
❶ **Reassurance:**
- This sounds like a minor infection that you can treat at home.
- The most important thing to do is to keep the piercing site clean. It's also important to apply an antibiotic ointment; it should get better. I can give you instructions on how to do both of these.

❷ **General Care Advice for New Piercings (< 6 Weeks Old):**
- Leave the earring in at all times. If you take it out, the hole can close, sometimes even within a few minutes.
- Posts should be made out of surgical steel, 14-18 karat gold, or some other metal (e.g., titanium) that does not cause skin allergy. However, some piercing salons recommend that gold posts be avoided immediately after a piercing, because even higher quality gold can contain trace amounts of nickel.
- Make certain that phones are clean.
- Be careful when brushing your hair.
- Change and use a clean pillowcase every 2 days.
- **Avoid** playing with the earring/jewelry.
- **Avoid** smoking during the healing period.
  (Reason: It prolongs healing.)
- **Avoid** wearing heavy/large/dangling earrings.
- **Avoid** hanging any accessories from piercing until it is completely healed.

❸ General Care Advice for Established Piercings (≥ 6 Weeks):
- Make certain that phones are clean.
- Be careful when brushing your hair.
- Change and use a clean pillowcase every 2 days.
- **Avoid** playing with the earring/jewelry.
- **Avoid** smoking during the healing period. *(Reason: It prolongs healing.)*
- **Avoid** wearing heavy/large/dangling earrings.
- **Avoid** hanging any accessories from piercing until it is completely healed.

❹ Treatment—Cleaning Instructions:
- **Step 1:** Wash your hands with soap and water.
- **Step 2:** Soak the area in warm saline (salt water) solution 3 times per day for 5-10 minutes. For ear piercings it is easiest to place a saline-soaked cotton ball directly on the piercing site.
- **Step 3:** Wash the piercing site 3 times a day. Use a cotton swab (e.g., Q-tip) dipped in an ear care antiseptic solution (usually contains benzalkonium chloride). If you do not have ear care antiseptic, you can use just a tiny amount of liquid antibacterial soap (e.g., Dial); be certain to rinse it off completely.
- **Step 4:** Gently pat area dry using clean gauze or a disposable tissue.

❺ Treatment—Antibiotic Ointment:
- Apply a small amount of antibiotic ointment to piercing site 3 times per day.
- Use bacitracin ointment (OTC in United States) or Polysporin ointment (OTC in Canada) or one that you already have.
- Rotate (turn) the earring several times to prevent the skin from sticking to the post.

❻ Expected Course:
- With proper care, most minor piercing site infections should clear up in a couple days.
- You should see a doctor if it does not improve within 3 days or if it gets worse.

❼ Saline Solution—How to Make It:
- Place ½ teaspoon of non-iodized (iodine-free) salt into a cup (8 oz or 240 mL) of warm water. You can use sea salt to make the saline (salt) solution.
- Stir the water until the salt dissolves.

❽ Call Back If:
- Not improved after 3 days.
- Pain increases.
- Spreading redness occurs.
- You become worse.

Very Small Tear in Earlobe

❶ General Care Advice for Ear Piercings:
- Make certain that phones are clean.
- Be careful when brushing your hair.
- Change and use a clean pillowcase every 2 days.
- **Avoid** playing with the earring/jewelry.
- **Avoid** smoking during the healing period. *(Reason: It prolongs healing.)*
- **Avoid** wearing heavy/large/dangling earrings.
- **Avoid** hanging any accessories from piercing until it is completely healed.

❷ Bleeding:
- Using gauze or clean cloth, apply direct pressure to the area from both sides.
- Call back if the bleeding does not stop after 10 minutes.

❸ Tetanus Vaccine: If your last tetanus shot was given > 10 years ago, you need a booster.

❹ Call Back If:
- Ear looks infected.
- You become worse.

Aftercare Instructions for a New Ear Piercing

❶ General Care Advice for New Piercings (< 6 Weeks Old):
- Leave the earring in at all times. If you take it out, the hole can close, sometimes even within a few minutes.
- Posts should be made out of surgical steel, 14-18 karat gold, or some other metal (e.g., titanium) that does not cause skin allergy. However, some piercing salons recommend that gold posts be avoided immediately after a piercing, because even higher quality gold can contain trace amounts of nickel.
- Make certain that phones are clean.
- Be careful when brushing your hair.
- Change and use a clean pillow case every 2 days.
- **Avoid** playing with the earring/jewelry.
- **Avoid** smoking during the healing period. *(Reason: It prolongs healing.)*
- **Avoid** wearing heavy/large/dangling earrings.
- **Avoid** hanging any accessories from piercing until it is completely healed.

❷ **Treatment—Cleaning Instructions:**
- **Step 1:** Wash your hands with soap and water.
- **Step 2:** Soak the area in warm saline (salt water) solution 3 times per day for 5-10 minutes. For ear piercings it is easiest to place a saline-soaked cotton ball directly on the piercing site.
- **Step 3:** Wash the piercing site 3 times a day. Use a cotton swab (e.g., Q-tip) dipped in an ear care antiseptic solution (usually contains benzalkonium chloride). If you do not have ear care antiseptic, you can use just a tiny amount of liquid antibacterial soap (e.g., Dial); be certain to rinse it off completely.
- **Step 4:** Gently pat area dry using clean gauze or a disposable tissue.

❸ **Saline Solution—How to Make It:**
- Place ½ teaspoon of non-iodized (iodine-free) salt into a cup (8 oz or 240 mL) of warm water. You can use sea salt to make the saline (salt) solution.
- Stir the water until the salt dissolves.

❹ **Expected Course:**
- **First 1-3 Days:** There might be some mild bruising, mild swelling, and mild tenderness. Rarely, there might be very slight bleeding (a couple spots of blood at piercing site).
- **During Healing Period:** You may note some itching at the site. You also may note whitish-yellow fluid (not pus) that coats the jewelry and forms a crust when it dries.
- **After Healing Period:** Sometimes jewelry will not move freely within the piercing tract; this is OK, and you should not try to force the jewelry to move. If you forget to clean the piercing for a couple days, you may note normal but slightly smelly secretions. This should be prevented; thus, it is important to remember to clean the piercing as part of your normal daily good hygiene.

❺ **Healing Period—How Long Does It Take?**
- A piercing heals from the outside in, so it can look healed on the outside and still be fragile on the inside.
- Reputable piercing studios provide aftercare instructions, and these aftercare instructions should be followed for the duration of the healing time.
- Healing times vary from person to person. The values below are averages.
- **Earlobe** (soft lower part of ear): 6-8 weeks.
- **Ear Cartilage:** 6-9 months.

❻ **Call Back If:**
- You have more questions.

BACKGROUND

Key Points
- Piercing guns should not be used. Two problems with piercing guns are tissue injury and exposure to body fluids from repeated prior use. The Association of Professional Piercers recommends against using piercing guns.
- Individuals should have their ears pierced by someone who is experienced and uses sterile technique.
- Reputable piercing studios provide aftercare instructions, and these instructions should be followed for the entire duration of the healing time.

Healing Times for Ear Piercings
Healing times vary from person to person. The values below are averages.
- **Earlobe** (soft lower part of ear): 6-8 weeks
- **Ear Helix** (folded rim of skin and cartilage of the upper outer ear): 6-9 months

Complications of Ear Piercing—Common
Minor complications occur in about 30% of people who have their ears pierced. These complications most commonly happen in the first few days or weeks after piercing.
- **Contact Dermatitis:** Contact dermatitis is fairly common and most often is the result of an allergic reaction to nickel (contained in some piercing jewelry). Piercing jewelry should be made of hypoallergenic metal. Examples of metals that cause the least amount of allergy are stainless steel, titanium, platinum, palladium, and niobium. Titanium has the least risk of allergic reaction. Even gold posts should be avoided immediately after a piercing because even higher quality gold can contain trace amounts of nickel.
- **Embedded Clasp:** The backing (clasp, ball) gets stuck (embedded) under the skin. The most common cause is that the earring post is too short (the thickness of earlobes varies) or the clasp is squeezed on too tightly. A visit to the doctor is often necessary to extract the embedded clasp.
- **Local Infection:** A minor local infection at the piercing site may occur in 10%-30% of individuals, even when the piercing is performed in a sterile manner by professionals. Symptoms of a local infection include yellow discharge, crusting, and mild irritation.

- **Traumatic Injury:** Tears of skin can occur because of a pulling injury on jewelry. The most common site is the earlobe, and a common scenario is the earring getting hooked on an article of clothing during dressing or undressing.

Complications of Ear Piercing—Uncommon
- **Auricular Chondritis:** This is a serious infection of the ear cartilage that occurs in a piercing through the cartilage of the helix. The helix is the folded rim of skin and cartilage of the upper outer ear. This infection can begin weeks after an ear piercing and it usually requires IV antibiotics.
- **Blood-borne Infections—Hepatitis B and C:** Blood-borne infections can be transmitted by sharing earrings with other people or through use of unsanitary piercing needles. Professional piercing studios follow strict sanitation guidelines and utilize sterile single-use piercing needles.
- **Cellulitis:** Rarely, a local infection at a piercing site can spread into the surrounding skin and cause cellulitis; symptoms are spreading redness and increasing pain at the site. In such cases, oral antibiotic therapy is needed.
- **Blood-borne Infections—HIV**
- **Keloid:** A keloid is the medical term for excessive scar formation at a wound or surgical site. It develops over months. It occurs because some individuals are simply prone to developing excessive scar formation and not because of how the piercing was performed.

Causes of Pierced Ear Infections
- The most common causes of infection are piercing the ears with unsterile equipment, inserting unsterile posts, or frequently touching the earlobes with dirty hands.
- Another frequent cause is earrings that are too tight either because the post is too short (the thickness of earlobes varies) or the clasp is closed too tightly. Tight earrings don't allow air to enter the channel through the earlobe. Also, the pressure from tight earrings reduces blood flow to the earlobe and makes it more vulnerable to infection. Often, this can be prevented by leaving the clasp at the notch on the post.

- Some inexpensive earrings have rough areas on the posts that scratch the channel and can result in infection. Heavy earrings can cause breaks in the skin lining the channel. Inserting the post at the wrong angle also can scratch the channel, so a mirror should be used until insertion becomes second nature. Posts containing nickel can also cause an itchy, allergic reaction.

Aftercare Instructions for Newly Pierced Ears—General
- Maintain good personal hygiene.
- Leave the jewelry in at all times. *(Reason: The hole can close, sometimes even within a few minutes.)*
- Posts should be made out of surgical steel, 14-18 karat gold, or some other metal (e.g., titanium) that does not cause skin allergy. Some piercing salons recommend that gold posts be avoided immediately after a piercing, because even higher quality gold can contain trace amounts of nickel.
- Make certain that phones are clean.
- Be careful when brushing hair.
- **Avoid** playing with the jewelry.
- **Avoid** smoking during the healing period. *(Reason: It prolongs healing.)*
- **Avoid** wearing heavy/large/dangling earrings.
- **Avoid** hanging any accessories from piercing until it is completely healed.

Aftercare Instructions for Newly Pierced Ears—Cleaning
- **Wash hands** with soap and water.
- **Soak** the area in warm saline (salt water) solution 3 times per day for 5-10 minutes. For ear piercings it is easiest to place a saline-soaked cotton ball directly on the piercing site.
- **Wash** the piercing site 3 times a day. Use a cotton swab (Q-tip) dipped in an ear care antiseptic solution (usually contains benzalkonium chloride). If ear antiseptic solution is not available, a tiny amount of liquid antibacterial soap (e.g., Dial) can be used instead; be certain to rinse it off completely.
- Gently pat area **dry** using clean gauze or a disposable tissue.

Saline Solution—How to Make It

- Place ½ teaspoon (3 g) of non-iodized (iodine-free) salt into a cup (8 oz or 240 mL) of warm water. You can use sea salt to make the saline (salt) solution.
- Stir the water until the salt dissolves.

Contact Dermatitis From Nickel

- **Definition:** > 10% of adults have an allergy to nickel-containing metals. Nickel is often present in less expensive jewelry. Even gold posts should be avoided immediately after a piercing because even higher quality gold can contain trace amounts of nickel.
- **Symptoms:** People with nickel allergy can get an itchy rash where the metal touches their skin: finger (rings), earlobes (earrings), neck (neck chains), mid-abdomen (metal fasteners on jeans or belt buckle), wrist (bracelets and wristwatches), and face (eyeglass frames).
- **Diagnosis:** See doctor if diagnosis is uncertain.
- **Treatment:** Avoid further contact with nickel. Apply a small amount of hydrocortisone cream 3 times a day for 7 days to the red, itchy area.
- **Expected Course:** Once the person stops wearing the nickel-containing jewelry, the redness and itching should go away in 7-14 days.
- **Prevention:** Avoid nickel-containing jewelry. Piercing jewelry should be made of hypoallergenic metal. Examples of metals that cause the least amount of allergy are titanium, platinum, palladium, niobium, and nickel-free stainless steel. Significant amounts of nickel are present in white gold, yellow gold (≤ 12 karat), regular stainless steel, and "costume" jewelry.

EARACHE

Definition
- Pain or discomfort in or around ear
- Not due to a traumatic injury

Pain Severity Scale
- **Mild (1-3):** Doesn't interfere with normal activities.
- **Moderate (4-7):** Interferes with normal activities or awakens from sleep.
- **Severe (8-10):** Excruciating pain, unable to do any normal activities.

TRIAGE ASSESSMENT QUESTIONS

Call EMS 911 Now
- ● Sounds like a life-threatening emergency to the triager

See More Appropriate Protocol
- ● Moving the earlobe or touching the ear clearly increases the pain
  Go to Protocol: Ear, Swimmer's (Otitis Externa) on page 131

Go to ED/UCC Now (or to Office With PCP Approval)
- ● Pink or red swelling behind the ear
  R/O: mastoiditis
- ● Stiff neck (can't touch chin to chest)
  R/O: meningitis
- ● Patient sounds very sick or weak to the triager
  Reason: severe acute illness or serious complication suspected

Go to Office Now
- ● SEVERE earache pain
- ● Fever > 103° F (39.4° C)
- ● Pointed object was inserted into the ear canal (e.g., a pencil, stick, or wire)
  R/O: TM perforation

See Today in Office
- ● White, yellow, or green discharge
  R/O: otitis externa or otitis media with perforation
- ● Diabetes mellitus or a weak immune system (e.g., HIV positive, cancer chemotherapy, transplant patient)
  Reason: higher risk for malignant otitis externa, should be examined
- ● Bloody discharge or unexplained bleeding from ear canal
  R/O: otitis media with perforation, otitis externa
- ● New blurred vision or vision changes
  R/O: temporal arteritis

See Today or Tomorrow in Office
- ● All other earaches
  (Exceptions: earache lasting < 1 hour, earache from air travel)
  R/O: otitis media or otitis externa
- ● Patient wants to be seen

Home Care
- ○ Mild earache and ear congestion (fullness) occurring during air travel
  R/O: barotitis media
- ○ Earache < 60 minutes' duration that is now completely gone

HOME CARE ADVICE

Earache
❶ **Pain Medicines:**
- For pain relief, you can take either acetaminophen, ibuprofen, or naproxen.
- They are over-the-counter (OTC) pain drugs. You can buy them at the drugstore.

Acetaminophen (e.g., Tylenol):
- **Regular Strength Tylenol:** Take 650 mg (two 325 mg pills) by mouth every 4-6 hours as needed. Each Regular Strength Tylenol pill has 325 mg of acetaminophen.
- **Extra Strength Tylenol:** Take 1,000 mg (two 500 mg pills) every 8 hours as needed. Each Extra Strength Tylenol pill has 500 mg of acetaminophen.
- The most you should take each day is 3,000 mg (10 Regular Strength or 6 Extra Strength pills a day).

Ibuprofen (e.g., Motrin, Advil):
- Take 400 mg (two 200 mg pills) by mouth every 6 hours.
- Another choice is to take 600 mg (three 200 mg pills) by mouth every 8 hours.
- The most you should take each day is 1,200 mg (six 200 mg pills), unless your doctor has told you to take more.

Naproxen (e.g., Aleve):

- Take 220 mg (one 220 mg pill) by mouth every 8 hours as needed. You may take 440 mg (two 220 mg pills) for your first dose.
- The most you should take each day is 660 mg (three 220 mg pills a day), unless your doctor has told you to take more.

❷ **Pain Medicines—Extra Notes:**

- Use the lowest amount of medicine that makes your pain better.
- Acetaminophen is thought to be safer than ibuprofen or naproxen in people < 65 years old. Acetaminophen is in many OTC and prescription medicines. It might be in more than one medicine that you are taking. You need to be careful and not take an overdose. An acetaminophen overdose can hurt the liver.
- McNeil, the company that makes Tylenol, has different dosage instructions for Tylenol in Canada and the United States. In Canada, the maximum recommended dose per day is 4,000 mg or 12 Regular Strength (325 mg) pills. In the United States, McNeil recommends a maximum dose of 10 Regular Strength (325 mg) pills.
- CAUTION: Do not take acetaminophen if you have liver disease.
- CAUTION: Do not take ibuprofen or naproxen if you have stomach problems, have kidney disease, are pregnant, or have been told by your doctor to avoid this type of anti-inflammatory drug. Do not take ibuprofen or naproxen for > 7 days without consulting your doctor.
- *Before taking any medicine, read all the instructions on the package.*

❸ **Apply Cold to the Area for Pain:** Apply a cold pack or a cold, wet washcloth to the outer ear for 20 minutes to reduce pain while the pain medicine takes effect.
(Note: Some individuals prefer local heat instead of cold for 20 minutes.)

❹ **Avoid Earplugs:** If pus or cloudy fluid is draining from the ear canal, wipe the pus away as it appears. Avoid plugging with cotton.
(Reason: Retained pus causes irritation or infection of the ear canal.)

❺ **Contagiousness:** Ear infections are not contagious.

❻ **Call Back If:**

- Earache lasts > 1 hour.
- High fever, severe headache, or stiff neck occurs.
- You become worse.

Earache During Air Travel

❶ **Reassurance:**

- Ear pain and stuffiness can occur during air travel. Nearly everybody experiences ear pressure symptoms during air travel.
- **Barotitis Media:** Changes in altitude while flying cause a difference between air pressure and the pressure behind your eardrum. The medical term for this is barotitis media.
- **Eustachian Tube:** Your eustachian tube is a small tube connecting your nose and middle ear. It allows tiny amounts of air to move in and out of the middle ear. This helps reduce any pressure buildup.
- There are things that you can do to decrease ear congestion symptoms during air travel.
- *Here is some care advice that should help.*

❷ **Treatment for Symptoms on Takeoff (for Positive Ear Pressure):**

- Chew gum.
- Yawn.
- Swallow.
- Swallow while pinching your nostrils.

❸ **Treatment for Symptoms on Landing (Valsalva Maneuver for Negative Ear Pressure):**

- Take a small breath, pinch off your nose, and then attempt to gently force air through the pinched-off nostrils.
- You should feel a slight clicking or popping in your ears as air moves into the middle ear.

❹ **Prevention—Decongestant Nasal Spray:**

- Nasal decongestant drops help shrink swollen nasal passages and open up the eustachian tubes. These drops can be very helpful during a flight if you have a cold or a flare of your nasal allergies.
- **Oxymetazoline Nasal Drops (e.g., Afrin):** Available OTC. One hour before takeoff, spray each nostril twice. Wait 1 minute and then spray each nostril once more. For flights > 4 hours, spray each nostril once more 30 minutes before the plane lands.

- **Phenylephrine Nasal Drops (e.g., Neo-Synephrine):** Available OTC. One hour before takeoff, spray each nostril twice. Wait 1 minute and then spray each nostril once more. For flights > 4 hours, spray each nostril once more 30 minutes before the plane lands.
- *Before taking any medicine, read all the instructions on the package.*

❺ **Caution—Nasal Decongestants:**
- Do not take these medications if you have high blood pressure, heart disease, prostate problems, or an overactive thyroid.
- Do not take these medications if you are pregnant.
- Do not take these medications if you have used a monoamine oxidase (MAO) inhibitor such as isocarboxazid (Marplan), phenelzine (Nardil), rasagiline (Azilect), selegiline (Eldepryl, Emsam), or tranylcypromine (Parnate) in the past 2 weeks. Life-threatening side effects can occur.
- Do not use these medications for > 3 days. *(Reason: rebound nasal congestion)*

❻ **Call Back If:**
- Ear congestion, pressure, or pain lasts > 48 hours.
- Fever or severe ear pain occurs.
- You become worse.

BACKGROUND

Causes
- Ear pain can be primary or referred. Primary ear pain originates from the ear itself. Examples include otitis media and otitis externa.
- **Otitis Media:** An infection of the middle portion of the ear behind the tympanic membrane. It is very common in children but less common in adults.
- **Otitis Externa:** Also called swimmer's ear; it is an infection of the external ear canal. Swimmers and people who use Q-tips frequently are more likely to get it. Otitis externa is more common than otitis media in adults.
- **Referred Ear Pain:** Referred ear pain means that the pain originates from a disease process outside of the ear. Because of the manner in which the nerves run in the head, the pain may be perceived as being in the ear. Examples of referred ear pain include dental abscess, temporomandibular disorder, and tonsillitis.

ELBOW INJURY

Definition
- Injuries to a bone, muscle, joint, or ligament of the elbow.
- Associated skin and soft tissue injuries are also included.

TRIAGE ASSESSMENT QUESTIONS

Call EMS 911 Now
- Major bleeding (actively dripping or spurting) that can't be stopped
  First Aid: Apply direct pressure to the entire wound with a clean cloth.
- Amputation or bone sticking through the skin
- Serious injury with multiple fractures
- Bullet, stabbed by knife, or other serious penetrating wound
  First Aid: If penetrating object is still in place, don't remove it.
- Sounds like a life-threatening emergency to the triager

See More Appropriate Protocol
- Wound looks infected
  Go to Protocol: Wound Infection on page 443
- Shoulder injury
  Go to Protocol: Shoulder Injury on page 348
- Hand or wrist injury
  Go to Protocol: Hand and Wrist Injury on page 189

Go to ED Now
- Looks like a broken bone or dislocated joint (crooked or deformed)

Go to ED/UCC Now
(or to Office With PCP Approval)
- Can't bend injured elbow at all
  R/O: fracture
- Skin is split open or gaping (length > ½" or 12 mm)
  Reason: may need laceration repair (e.g., sutures)
- Bleeding won't stop after 10 minutes of direct pressure (using correct technique)

- Dirt in the wound and not removed after 15 minutes of scrubbing
  Reason: needs irrigation or debridement
- Numbness (loss of sensation) of finger(s), present now
  R/O: nerve injury
- Sounds like a serious injury to the triager

See Today in Office
- SEVERE pain (e.g., excruciating)
- Can't move injured elbow normally (i.e., bend or straighten completely)
  R/O: minor fracture
- Large swelling or bruise and size > palm of person's hand
  R/O: fracture, large contusion
- Patient wants to be seen

See Today or Tomorrow in Office
- Wound and no tetanus booster in > 5 years (or > 10 years for clean cuts)
  Reason: may need a tetanus booster shot (vaccine)
- High-risk adult (e.g., age > 60, osteoporosis, chronic steroid use)
  Reason: greater risk of fracture in patients with osteoporosis
- Suspicious history for the injury
  R/O: domestic violence or elder abuse

See Within 3 Days in Office
- Injury and pain has not improved after 3 days
- Injury is still painful or swollen after 2 weeks

Home Care
- Minor elbow injury
  R/O: bruise, strain, or sprain

HOME CARE ADVICE

Treatment of a Minor Bruise, Sprain, or Strain

❶ Reassurance—Direct Blow (Contusion, Bruise):
- A direct blow to your elbow can cause a contusion. Contusion is the medical term for bruise.
- Symptoms are mild pain, swelling, and/or bruising.
- *Here is some care advice that should help.*

❷ Reassurance—Bending or Twisting Injury (Strain, Sprain):
- Strain and sprain are the medical terms used to describe overstretching of the muscles and ligaments of the elbow. A twisting or bending injury can cause a strain or sprain.
- The main symptom is pain that is worse with movement. Swelling can occur.
- *Here is some care advice that should help.*

❸ Apply a Cold Pack:
- Apply a cold pack or an ice bag (wrapped in a moist towel) to the area for 20 minutes. Repeat in 1 hour, then every 4 hours while awake.
- Continue this for the first 48 hours after an injury.
- This will help decrease pain and swelling.

❹ Apply Heat to the Area:
- Beginning 48 hours after an injury, apply a warm washcloth or heating pad for 10 minutes 3 times a day.
- This will help increase blood flow and improve healing.

❺ Wrap With an Elastic Bandage:
- Wrap the injured part with a snug, elastic bandage for 48 hours.
- The pressure from the bandage can make it feel better and help prevent swelling.
- If your start to get numbness or tingling in your hand or fingers, the bandage may be too tight. Loosen the bandage wrap.

❻ Elevate the Arm:
- Lie down and put your arm on a pillow. This puts (elevates) the elbow above the heart.
- Do this for 15-20 minutes, 2-3 times a day, for the first 2 days.
- This can also help decrease swelling, bruising, and pain.

❼ Rest Versus Movement:
- Movement is generally more healing in the long term than rest.
- Continue normal activities as much as your pain permits.
- Avoid heavy lifting and active sports for 1-2 weeks or until the pain and swelling are gone.
- Complete rest should only be used for the first day or two after an injury. If it really hurts to use that arm at all, you will need to see the doctor.

❽ Expected Course:
- Pain, swelling, and bruising usually start to get better 2-3 days after an injury.
- Swelling most often is gone after 1 week.
- Bruises fade away slowly over 1-2 weeks.
- It may take 2 weeks for pain and tenderness of the injured area to go away.

❾ Call Back If:
- Pain becomes severe.
- Pain does not improve after 3 days.
- Pain or swelling lasts > 2 weeks.
- You become worse.

Treatment of a Small Cut or Scrape

❶ Reassurance—Superficial Laceration (Cut or Scratch) or Abrasion (Scrape):
- This sounds like a small cut or scrape that we can treat at home.
- *Here is some care advice that should help.*

❷ Bleeding: Apply direct pressure for 10 minutes with a sterile gauze to stop any bleeding.

❸ Cleaning the Wound:
- Wash the wound with soap and water for 5 minutes.
- For any dirt, scrub gently with a washcloth.
- For any bleeding, apply direct pressure with a sterile gauze or clean cloth for 10 minutes.

❹ Antibiotic Ointment:
- Apply an antibiotic ointment (e.g., OTC bacitracin), covered by a Band-Aid or dressing. Change daily or if it becomes wet.
- Option: A Telfa dressing won't stick to the wound when it is removed.
- Option: Another option is to use a liquid skin bandage that only needs to be applied once. Don't use antibiotic ointment if you use a liquid skin bandage.

❺ **Liquid Skin Bandage:**
- You can use a liquid skin bandage instead of antibiotic ointment and a dressing or a Band-Aid.
- **Benefits:** Liquid skin bandage has several benefits when compared with a regular bandage (e.g., a dressing or a Band-Aid). You only need to put a liquid bandage on once to minor cuts and scrapes. It helps stop minor bleeding. It seals the wound and may promote faster healing and lower infection rates. However, it also costs more.
- **How to Use It:** First clean and dry the wound. You put on the liquid as spray or with a swab. It dries in < 1 minute and usually lasts a week. You can get it wet.
- **Examples:** Liquid skin bandage is available over the counter. Examples are Band-Aid Liquid Bandage, New Skin, Curad Spray Bandage, and 3M No Sting Liquid Bandage Spray.

❻ **Call Back If:**
- Looks infected (pus, redness, increasing tenderness).
- Doesn't heal within 10 days.
- You become worse.

Over-the-counter Pain Medicines

❶ **Pain Medicines:**
- For pain relief, you can take either acetaminophen, ibuprofen, or naproxen.
- They are over-the-counter (OTC) pain drugs. You can buy them at the drugstore.

Acetaminophen (e.g., Tylenol):
- **Regular Strength Tylenol:** Take 650 mg (two 325 mg pills) by mouth every 4-6 hours as needed. Each Regular Strength Tylenol pill has 325 mg of acetaminophen.
- **Extra Strength Tylenol:** Take 1,000 mg (two 500 mg pills) every 8 hours as needed. Each Extra Strength Tylenol pill has 500 mg of acetaminophen.
- The most you should take each day is 3,000 mg (10 Regular Strength or 6 Extra Strength pills a day).

Ibuprofen (e.g., Motrin, Advil):
- Take 400 mg (two 200 mg pills) by mouth every 6 hours.
- Another choice is to take 600 mg (three 200 mg pills) by mouth every 8 hours.
- The most you should take each day is 1,200 mg (six 200 mg pills), unless your doctor has told you to take more.

Naproxen (e.g., Aleve):
- Take 220 mg (one 220 mg pill) by mouth every 8 hours as needed. You may take 440 mg (two 220 mg pills) for your first dose.
- The most you should take each day is 660 mg (three 220 mg pills a day), unless your doctor has told you to take more.

❷ **Pain Medicines—Extra Notes:**
- Use the lowest amount of medicine that makes your pain better.
- Acetaminophen is thought to be safer than ibuprofen or naproxen in people > 65 years old. Acetaminophen is in many OTC and prescription medicines. It might be in more than one medicine that you are taking. You need to be careful and not take an overdose. An acetaminophen overdose can hurt the liver.
- McNeil, the company that makes Tylenol, has different dosage instructions for Tylenol in Canada and the United States. In Canada, the maximum recommended dose per day is 4,000 mg or 12 Regular Strength (325 mg) pills. In the United States, McNeil recommends a maximum dose of 10 Regular Strength (325 mg) pills.
- CAUTION: Do not take acetaminophen if you have liver disease.
- CAUTION: Do not take ibuprofen or naproxen if you have stomach problems, have kidney disease, are pregnant, or have been told by your doctor to avoid this type of anti-inflammatory drug. Do not take ibuprofen or naproxen for > 7 days without consulting your doctor.
- *Before taking any medicine, read all the instructions on the package.*

❸ **Call Back If:**
- You have more questions.
- You become worse.

Bruised "Funny Bone"

❶ Reassurance:
- It sounds like a "bruised funny bone" that we can treat at home.
- A blow to the back of the elbow can cause numbness, tingling, and burning in the hand. The involved fingers are usually the middle, ring, and pinky (little).
- Your "funny bone" is actually a nerve (ulnar) which wraps around the back part of your elbow.

❷ Expected Course:
- Symptoms from "bruising your funny bone" usually last only a few minutes.
- If the symptoms last > 30 minutes, you should see your doctor.
- If this happens often, you should see your doctor.

❸ Call Back If:
- You become worse.

FIRST AID

First Aid Advice for Bleeding:
Apply direct pressure to the entire wound with a clean cloth.

First Aid Advice for Penetrating Object:
If penetrating object is still in place, don't remove it. *Reason: Removal could increase bleeding.*

First Aid Advice for Shock:
Lie down with the feet elevated.

First Aid Advice for Suspected Fracture or Dislocation of the Elbow:
- Use a sling to support the arm. Make the sling with a triangular piece of cloth.
- Or, at the very least, the patient can support the injured arm with the other hand or a pillow.

BACKGROUND

Types of Elbow Injuries
- Bone bruise from a direct blow (e.g., elbow)
- Dislocations (bone out of joint)
- Fractures (broken bones)
- Muscle overuse injuries from sports or exercise (e.g., tennis elbow)
- Muscle bruise from a direct blow
- **Sprains:** Stretches and tears of ligaments
- **Strains:** Stretches and tears of muscles (e.g., pulled muscle)
- Traumatic olecranon bursitis

Bruised "Funny Bone"
- A direct blow to the near side of the posterior elbow can cause numbness, tingling, and burning in the hand. The involved fingers are usually the middle, ring, and pinky (little).
- The "funny bone" is actually a nerve (ulnar) which wraps around the posterior part of your elbow.
- Symptoms from bruising your funny bone usually last only a few minutes. If the symptoms last > 30 minutes or if this problem seems to happen too frequently, the patient will need to see the doctor for evaluation.

What Cuts Need to be Sutured?
Any cut that is split open or gaping probably needs sutures. Cuts > ½" (1 cm) usually need sutures. Any open wound that may need sutures should be evaluated by a physician regardless of the time that has passed since the initial injury.

When Does an Adult Need a Tetanus Booster (Tetanus Shot)?
- **Clean Cuts and Scrapes—Tetanus Booster Needed Every 10 Years:** Patients with clean minor wounds AND who have previously had ≥ 3 tetanus shots (full series) need a booster every 10 years. Examples of minor wounds include a superficial abrasion or a shallow cut from a clean knife blade. Obtain booster within 72 hours.
- **Dirty Wounds—Tetanus Booster Needed Every 5 Years:** Patients with dirty wounds need a booster if it has been > 5 years since the last booster. Examples of dirty wounds include those contaminated with soil, feces, and/or saliva and more serious wounds from deep punctures, crushing, and burns. Obtain booster within 72 hours.

ELBOW PAIN

Definition
- Pain in the elbow.
- Not due to a traumatic injury.
- Minor muscle strain and overuse are covered in this protocol.

Pain Severity Scale
- **Mild (1-3):** Doesn't interfere with normal activities.
- **Moderate (4-7):** Interferes with normal activities (e.g., work or school) or awakens from sleep.
- **Severe (8-10):** Excruciating pain, unable to do any normal activities, unable to hold a cup of water.

TRIAGE ASSESSMENT QUESTIONS

Call EMS 911 Now
- Shock suspected (e.g., cold/pale/clammy skin, too weak to stand)
  R/O: shock
  First Aid: Lie down with the feet elevated.
- Similar pain previously and it was from "heart attack"
  R/O: cardiac ischemia, myocardial infarction
- Similar pain previously and it was from "angina," and not relieved by nitroglycerin
  R/O: cardiac ischemia
- Sounds like a life-threatening emergency to the triager

See More Appropriate Protocol
- Chest pain
  Go to Protocol: Chest Pain on page 73
- Followed an elbow injury
  Go to Protocol: Elbow Injury on page 142
- Wound looks infected
  Go to Protocol: Wound Infection on page 443

Go to ED Now
- Difficulty breathing or unusual sweating (e.g., sweating without exertion)
  R/O: cardiac ischemia
- Age > 40 and associated chest or jaw pain, and pain lasting > 5 minutes
  R/O: cardiac ischemia

Go to ED/UCC Now
(or to Office With PCP Approval)
- Red area or streak and fever
  R/O: cellulitis, lymphangitis
  Note: It may be difficult to determine the rash color in people with darker-colored skin.
- Swollen joint and fever
  R/O: septic arthritis, infected bursitis
- Entire arm is swollen
  R/O: DVT of upper extremity
- Patient sounds very sick or weak to the triager
  Reason: severe acute illness or serious complication suspected

Go to Office Now
- SEVERE pain (e.g., excruciating, unable to do any normal activities)
- Weakness (i.e., loss of strength) in hand or fingers
  (Exception: not truly weak; hand feels weak because of pain)
  R/O: herniated cervical disk

See Today in Office
- Swollen joint
  R/O: arthritis
- Fluid-filled sac located directly over point of elbow
  R/O: olecranon bursitis, infected bursitis
  Note: The "point" refers to the posterior elbow and the skin area directly over the olecranon process.
- Looks like a boil, infected sore, deep ulcer, or other infected rash (spreading redness, pus)
  R/O: impetigo, abscess, cellulitis
- Painful rash with multiple small blisters grouped together (i.e., dermatomal distribution or "band" or "stripe")
  R/O: herpes zoster (shingles)
- Numbness (i.e., loss of sensation) in hand or fingers
  R/O: cervical radiculopathy, herniated cervical disk, carpal tunnel syndrome
- Can't move joint normally (bend and straighten completely)
  R/O: arthritis, unobserved injury

See Within 3 Days in Office

- MODERATE pain (e.g., interferes with normal activities) and present > 3 days
  R/O: arthritis, tendonitis, carpal tunnel syndrome
- Patient wants to be seen

See Within 2 Weeks in Office

- MILD pain (e.g., does not interfere with normal activities) and present > 7 days
- Elbow pain is a chronic symptom (recurrent or ongoing AND lasting > 4 weeks)

Home Care

- ○ Elbow pain
- ○ Caused by bumping elbow and had brief (now gone) burning pain shooting (radiating) into hand and fingers
  R/O: "bruised funny bone"
- ○ Caused by overuse from recent vigorous activity (e.g., golf, tennis, throwing a baseball)
  R/O: muscle strain, overuse, tendinitis

HOME CARE ADVICE

Elbow Pain

❶ **Reassurance—Elbow Pain:**
- Usually elbow pain is not serious. You have told me that there is no redness, numbness, or swelling.
- Causes of elbow pain can include a strained muscle, a forgotten minor injury, and tendinitis.
- *Here is some care advice that should help.*

❷ **Pain Medicines:**
- For pain relief, you can take either acetaminophen, ibuprofen, or naproxen.
- They are over-the-counter (OTC) pain drugs. You can buy them at the drugstore.

Acetaminophen (e.g., Tylenol):
- **Regular Strength Tylenol:** Take 650 mg (two 325 mg pills) by mouth every 4-6 hours as needed. Each Regular Strength Tylenol pill has 325 mg of acetaminophen.
- **Extra Strength Tylenol:** Take 1,000 mg (two 500 mg pills) every 8 hours as needed. Each Extra Strength Tylenol pill has 500 mg of acetaminophen.
- The most you should take each day is 3,000 mg (10 Regular Strength or 6 Extra Strength pills a day).

Ibuprofen (e.g., Motrin, Advil):
- Take 400 mg (two 200 mg pills) by mouth every 6 hours.
- Another choice is to take 600 mg (three 200 mg pills) by mouth every 8 hours.
- The most you should take each day is 1,200 mg (six 200 mg pills), unless your doctor has told you to take more.

Naproxen (e.g., Aleve):
- Take 220 mg (one 220 mg pill) by mouth every 8 hours as needed. You may take 440 mg (two 220 mg pills) for your first dose.
- The most you should take each day is 660 mg (three 220 mg pills a day), unless your doctor has told you to take more.

❸ **Pain Medicines—Extra Notes:**
- Use the lowest amount of medicine that makes your pain better.
- Acetaminophen is thought to be safer than ibuprofen or naproxen in people > 65 years old. Acetaminophen is in many OTC and prescription medicines. It might be in more than one medicine that you are taking. You need to be careful and not take an overdose. An acetaminophen overdose can hurt the liver.
- McNeil, the company that makes Tylenol, has different dosage instructions for Tylenol in Canada and the United States. In Canada, the maximum recommended dose per day is 4,000 mg or 12 Regular Strength (325 mg) pills. In the United States, McNeil recommends a maximum dose of 10 Regular Strength (325 mg) pills.
- CAUTION: Do not take acetaminophen if you have liver disease.
- CAUTION: Do not take ibuprofen or naproxen if you have stomach problems, have kidney disease, are pregnant, or have been told by your doctor to avoid this type of anti-inflammatory drug. Do not take ibuprofen or naproxen for > 7 days without consulting your doctor.
- *Before taking any medicine, read all the instructions on the package.*

❹ **Expected Course:** If this does not get better during the next week or if it recurs, you should make an appointment with your doctor.

❺ Call Back If:
- Moderate pain (e.g., interferes with normal activities) lasts > 3 days.
- Mild pain lasts > 7 days.
- Swollen joint or fever occurs.
- You become worse.

Overuse of Elbow

❶ Reassurance—Overuse:
- **Definition:** Activities associated with repetitive forceful use of the elbow can cause soreness, muscle strain, and tendinitis. Such activities can include tennis, throwing of a baseball, golf, and certain types of repetitive forceful motions (e.g., washing the car, scrubbing the floor).
- **Symptoms:** Soreness and tenderness of the elbow. Pain increases with certain movements.

❷ Apply Cold to the Area:
- Apply a cold pack or an ice bag (wrapped in a moist towel) to the area for 20 minutes. Repeat in 1 hour, then every 4 hours while awake.
- Continue this for the first 48 hours after an injury. *(Reason: Reduce the swelling and pain.)*

❸ Apply Heat to the Area:
- Beginning 48 hours after an injury, apply a warm washcloth or heating pad for 10 minutes 3 times a day.
- This will help increase blood flow and improve healing.

❹ Pain Medicines:
- For pain relief, you can take either acetaminophen, ibuprofen, or naproxen.
- They are over-the-counter (OTC) pain drugs. You can buy them at the drugstore.

Acetaminophen (e.g., Tylenol):
- **Regular Strength Tylenol:** Take 650 mg (two 325 mg pills) by mouth every 4-6 hours as needed. Each Regular Strength Tylenol pill has 325 mg of acetaminophen.
- **Extra Strength Tylenol:** Take 1,000 mg (two 500 mg pills) every 8 hours as needed. Each Extra Strength Tylenol pill has 500 mg of acetaminophen.
- The most you should take each day is 3,000 mg (10 Regular Strength or 6 Extra Strength pills a day).

Ibuprofen (e.g., Motrin, Advil):
- Take 400 mg (two 200 mg pills) by mouth every 6 hours.
- Another choice is to take 600 mg (three 200 mg pills) by mouth every 8 hours.
- The most you should take each day is 1,200 mg (six 200 mg pills), unless your doctor has told you to take more.

Naproxen (e.g., Aleve):
- Take 220 mg (one 220 mg pill) by mouth every 8 hours as needed. You may take 440 mg (two 220 mg pills) for your first dose.
- The most you should take each day is 660 mg (three 220 mg pills a day), unless your doctor has told you to take more.

❺ Pain Medicines—Extra Notes:
- Use the lowest amount of medicine that makes your pain better.
- Acetaminophen is thought to be safer than ibuprofen or naproxen in people > 65 years old. Acetaminophen is in many OTC and prescription medicines. It might be in more than one medicine that you are taking. You need to be careful and not take an overdose. An acetaminophen overdose can hurt the liver.
- McNeil, the company that makes Tylenol, has different dosage instructions for Tylenol in Canada and the United States. In Canada, the maximum recommended dose per day is 4,000 mg or 12 Regular Strength (325 mg) pills. In the United States, McNeil recommends a maximum dose of 10 Regular Strength (325 mg) pills.
- CAUTION: Do not take acetaminophen if you have liver disease.
- CAUTION: Do not take ibuprofen or naproxen if you have stomach problems, have kidney disease, are pregnant, or have been told by your doctor to avoid this type of anti-inflammatory drug. Do not take ibuprofen or naproxen for > 7 days without consulting your doctor.
- *Before taking any medicine, read all the instructions on the package.*

❻ Rest: You should try to avoid any exercise or activity that caused this pain for the next 3 days.

❼ Expected Course:
- For minor injuries, pain should improve over a 2- to 3-day period and disappear within 7 days.
- If this does not get better during the next week or if it recurs, you should make an appointment with your doctor.

❽ Call Back If:
- Moderate pain (e.g., interferes with normal activities) lasts > 3 days.
- Mild pain lasts > 7 days.
- Swollen joint or fever occurs.
- You become worse.

Bruised "Funny Bone"

❶ Reassurance:
- It sounds like a "bruised funny bone" that we can treat at home.
- A blow to the back of the elbow can cause numbness, tingling, and burning in the hand. The involved fingers are usually the middle, ring, and pinky (little).
- Your "funny bone" is actually a nerve (ulnar) which wraps around the back part of your elbow.

❷ Expected Course:
- Symptoms from "bruising your funny bone" usually last only a few minutes.
- If the symptoms last > 30 minutes, you should call your doctor.
- If this happens often, you should see your doctor.

❸ Call Back If: You become worse.

FIRST AID

First Aid Advice for Shock:
Lie down with the feet elevated.

BACKGROUND

Key Points
- Elbow pain is a common symptom and there are a number of causes.
- Elbow pain is almost always not serious, and it generally originates from the muscles or tendons of the elbow region, as a result of overuse or injury.

Causes of Elbow Pain
- Arthritis
- Cancer (rare; in a patient with known cancer metastasis)
- Cardiac ischemia (rare)
- Cellulitis
- Fracture, dislocation, contusion
- Lateral epicondylitis (tennis elbow)
- Medial epicondylitis (golfer's elbow)
- Olecranon bursitis
- Muscle strain

Serious Signs and Symptoms
- Severe pain.
- Red area with streak.
  R/O: cellulitis with lymphangitis; common
- Joint swelling with fever.
  R/O: septic arthritis; rare
- Entire arm is swollen.
  R/O: deep vein thrombosis of upper extremity; rare

Caution: Cardiac Ischemia
- Rarely, patients may present with elbow pain as the sole symptom of a myocardial infarction. Usually there will be other associated symptoms of cardiac ischemia: chest pain, shortness of breath, nausea, and/or diaphoresis.
- Cardiac ischemia should be suspected in any patients with risk factors for cardiac disease. These include: hypertension, smoking, diabetes, hyperlipidemia, a strong family history of heart disease, and age > 50.

EYE, CHEMICAL IN

Definition
- Chemical gets into the eye from fingers, contaminated object, spray, or splash.

TRIAGE ASSESSMENT QUESTIONS

Go to ED Now
- Acid or alkali was the chemical
  (Exception: mild agents such as household bleach or ammonia—instead call Poison Center)
  First Aid: Irrigate eye immediately before going to the ED.
  Note: Acid and alkali defined in Background.
- Shortness of breath
  Reason: possible bronchospasm or pulmonary involvement

Go to ED/UCC Now
(or to Office With PCP Approval)
- Sounds like a serious injury to the triager

Call Poison Center Now
- Possibly harmful substance in the eye
  (Exception: mace, pepper spray, soap, sunscreen lotion, or other obviously harmless substance)
  First Aid: Irrigate eye immediately before calling Poison Center.

Go to Office Now
- Cloudy spot or sore on the cornea (clear central part of eye)
  First Aid: Irrigate eye immediately after exposure to harmful substance.
- Blurred vision that persists > 1 hour after irrigation
  R/O: corneal damage
- Eye pain that persists > 1 hour after irrigation
  R/O: corneal damage
- Continued tearing or blinking that persists > 1 hour after irrigation
  R/O: corneal damage

See Today in Office
- Redness persists > 24 hours
  First Aid: Irrigate eye immediately afterwards.
- R/O: conjunctivitis
- Patient wants to be seen

Home Care
- Mace or "pepper spray" was sprayed into face/eyes
  First Aid: Irrigate eye immediately.
- Eye irritation from harmless chemical
  First Aid: Irrigate eye immediately.
  Note: See Harmless Chemicals list.

HOME CARE ADVICE

❶ **Irrigate the eye immediately.**
❷ **Eye Irrigation Method #1—Immersion:**
  - Immerse the entire face into a sink or basin filled with lukewarm tap water.
  - With the face under water, open and close the eyelids. You may need to use your fingers. Look from side to side.

❸ **Eye Irrigation Method #2—Flushing:**
  - Slowly pour lukewarm water into the eye from a pitcher or glass.
  - Or place your head under a gently running faucet or shower.
  - Hold the eyelid open during this process.

❹ **Duration of Irrigation for Harmless Substances:**
  - For harmless substances (e.g., household soap, sunscreen, hair spray), irrigation only needs to be carried out for 2-3 minutes.
  - For stronger chemicals that cause more irritation and stinging (e.g., ammonia, vinegar, alcohol, household bleach), flush the eye for 5-10 minutes.

❺ **Vasoconstrictor Eye Drops:** Red eyes from irritants usually feel much better after the irritant has been washed out. If they remain uncomfortable and blood-shot, use some long-acting vasoconstrictor eyedrops (e.g., Visine). Use 1-2 drops. May repeat once in 8-12 hours.

❻ **Contacts:** Patients with contact lenses need to switch to glasses temporarily.
  (Reason: to prevent damage to the cornea)

❼ **Expected Course:** The pain and discomfort usually pass 1 hour after irrigation.

❽ **Call Back If:**
  - Pain or blurred vision lasts > 1 hour after irrigation.
  - Redness lasts > 24 hours.
  - You become worse.

FIRST AID

First Aid Advice for Chemical in the Eye:

- Immediate and thorough irrigation of the eye with tap water should be done as quickly as possible. *(Reason: to prevent damage to the cornea)*
- If one eye is not burned, cover it (if possible) while irrigating the other.

Duration of Irrigation:

- For **harmless substances** (e.g., sunscreen or hair spray), irrigation only needs to be carried out for 2-3 minutes.
- For **stronger chemicals** that cause more irritation and stinging (e.g., ammonia, vinegar, alcohol, household bleach), flush the eye for 5-10 minutes.
- For **acids,** irrigate the eye continuously for 10 minutes.
- For **alkalis,** irrigate the eye continuously for 20 minutes.
- For any **chemical particles** that can't be flushed away, wipe them away with a moistened cotton swab.

Special Notes:

- Never irrigate with antidotes such as vinegar. *(Reason: The chemical reaction can cause more damage.)*
- Tell the patient to call back immediately if he/she is unable to carry out the irrigation. *(Reason: needs a topical anesthetic in the ED)*

BACKGROUND

Causes

- **Harmless Chemicals:** These include soap, hair spray, and sunscreen. They cause no symptoms or transient irritation.
- **Harmless Chemicals That Cause More Stinging:** Examples are alcohol or hydrocarbons. They cause temporary stinging and superficial irritation (pink sclera) but no lasting damage.
- **Harmful Chemicals:** Acids (e.g., toilet bowl cleaners) and alkalis (e.g., oven cleaners) splashed into the eye can cause severe eye pain and permanently damage the cornea. Alkali burns cause more damage than acid burns.

- **Mace and Pepper Spray:** Mace and pepper spray are used in personal protection devices. Eye exposure results in marked eye pain and tearing. Usually these symptoms subside in 30 minutes and there is no lasting damage.

Harmless Chemicals

- The following liquid products are harmless to the eye: bubble bath, cosmetics, deodorant, foods (e.g., lemon juice), glow stick liquid, hair conditioner, hair spray, hand lotion, laundry detergent (liquid), medications, shampoo, shaving cream, soap, sunscreen, and toothpaste.
- The following substances are also harmless but will cause transient irritation: hydrogen peroxide, ethyl alcohol (ethanol), automobile gasoline, and vinegar. Brief irrigation of the eye is indicated.

Harmful Chemicals

- *Eye contact with acids or alkalis can cause severe damage to the eye.* Both need immediate irrigation followed by immediate referral to an ED.
- **Acids:** Acids include hydrochloric acid, nitric acid, sulfuric acid, phosphoric acid, oxalic acid, or any other product labeled as an acid. Products that are called drain cleaners, toilet bowl cleaners, metal cleaners, or battery fluid can be assumed to contain acid until proven otherwise.
- **Alkalis:** Alkalis include lime, lye, potassium hydroxide, sodium hydroxide, calcium hydroxide, and industrial-strength ammonia. Any product that is called a drain cleaner, oven cleaner, bathroom cleaner, or industrial cleaner should be assumed to contain alkali until proven otherwise.
- Two weak alkalis that usually don't cause any harm are household bleach and household ammonia. For these exposures, instruct the caller to call the Poison Center after irrigation to determine if the particular product is harmful.

First Aid Advice for All Patients With Chemical in the Eye

- Immediate and thorough irrigation of the eye with tap water should be done as quickly as possible. *(Reason: to prevent damage to the cornea)*
- If one eye is not burned, cover it (if possible) while irrigating the other.
- **Duration:** For harmless substances (e.g., sunscreen or hair spray), irrigation only needs to be carried out for 2 minutes. For stronger chemicals that cause more irritation and stinging (e.g., ammonia, vinegar, alcohol, household bleach), flush the eye for 5 minutes. For acids, irrigate the eye continuously for 10 minutes. For alkalis, irrigate the eye continuously for 20 minutes.
- For any chemical particles that can't be flushed away, wipe them away with a moistened cotton swab.
- Never irrigate with antidotes such as vinegar. *(Reason: The chemical reaction can cause more damage.)*
- Tell the patient to call back immediately if he/she is unable to carry out the irrigation. *(Reason: needs a topical anesthetic in the ED)*

Eye Irrigation Method #1: Flushing

- Have the patient lie down and slowly pour lukewarm water into the eye from a pitcher or glass. Alternatively, the patient can hold his/her eye under a faucet or shower.
- Hold the eyelid open during this process if the patient can't keep it open.

Eye Irrigation Method #2: Immersion

- Immerse the entire face into a sink or basin filled with tap water.
- With the face under water, open and close the eyelids. You may need to use your fingers. Look from side to side.

Call Poison Center

- *Tell the caller to call the Poison Center immediately after irrigation is completed.* One exception to this would be a definitely harmless chemical. Another exception to this would be a definitely harmful chemical like an acid or alkali (since for these the victim should go immediately to the ED after irrigation).
- **United States:** Give them the national toll-free number: **1-800-222-1222.**
- **Canada:** Call local poison control center.
- **If a Poison Center Is Unavailable:** Triager, call back the patient in 10-20 minutes after the irrigation time is up. Ask the remaining triage questions.

EYE, FOREIGN BODY

Definition

- A foreign body (FB) or object becomes lodged in the eye.
- The main symptoms are irritation, pain, tearing, and blinking.
- Also includes calls about a contact stuck in the eye.

TRIAGE ASSESSMENT QUESTIONS

See More Appropriate Protocol

- ● Doesn't sound like FB in the eye
  Go to Protocol: Eye, Red Without Pus on page 158
- ● FB is a chemical
  Go to Protocol: Eye, Chemical In on page 150

Go to ED/UCC Now
(or to Office With PCP Approval)

- ● FB stuck on eyeball
  R/O: embedded FB
- ● FB hit eye at high speed (e.g., small metallic chip from hammering, lawn mower, BB gun, explosion)
  R/O: intraocular FB
- ● Cloudy spot on the cornea (clear part of the eye)
  R/O: retained FB, tiny abrasion
- ● Sounds like a serious injury to the triager

Go to Office Now

- ● Severe eye pain
- ● Sharp FB (even if FB was removed)
  R/O: corneal abrasion, other eye damage
- ● Eye has been washed out > 30 minutes ago and still feels like FB is still present
  Reason: FB can cause corneal abrasion
- ● Eye has been washed out > 30 minutes ago and pain persists
  Reason: FB can cause corneal abrasion
- ● Eye has been washed out > 30 minutes ago and tearing or blinking persists
  Reason: FB can cause corneal abrasion
- ● Eye has been washed out > 30 minutes ago and blurred vision persists
  Reason: FB can cause corneal abrasion

See Today in Office

- ◐ Yellow or green pus occurs
  R/O: retained FB
- ◐ Contact lens stuck in eye and unable to remove using Home Care Advice
- ◐ Patient wants to be seen

Home Care

- ○ Minor FB in the eye (e.g., eyelash, dirt, sand)
  Reason: probably can be removed at home
- ○ FB was successfully removed, and now no symptoms
- ○ Contact lens stuck in eye

HOME CARE ADVICE

Removing a Foreign Body From the Eye

❶ Treatment for Numerous Particles (e.g., Dirt or Sand):
  - Clean around the eye with a wet washcloth first.
  - Try to open and close the eye repeatedly while submerging that side of the face in a pan of water.

❷ Treatment for a Particle in a Corner of the Eye:
  Try to get it out with a moistened cotton swab or the corner of a moistened cloth.

❸ Treatment for a Particle Under the Lower Lid:
  - Pull the lower lid out by pulling down on the skin over the cheekbone.
  - Touch the particle with a moistened cotton swab.
  - If that does not work, try pouring water on the speck while pulling the lower lid out.

❹ Treatment for a Particle Under the Upper Lid:
  - If particle cannot be seen, it is probably under the upper lid, the most common hiding place.
  - Try to open and close the eye several times while it is submerged in a pan or bowl of water. Or turn your head to the side and flush the eye using the faucet.
  - If this fails, pull the upper lid out and draw it over the lower lid. This maneuver, and tears, will sometimes dislodge the particle. By doing this the lower eyelashes may sweep the particle out from under the upper eyelid.

❺ Expected Course: The discomfort, redness, and excessive tearing usually pass 1-2 hours after the foreign body is removed.

❻ **Contacts:** Patients with contact lenses need to switch to glasses temporarily.
(Reason: to prevent damage to the cornea)

❼ **Call Back If:**
- This approach does not remove all the foreign material from the eye (i.e., the sensation of "grittiness" or pain does not go away).
- Vision does not return to normal after the eye has been irrigated.
- Foreign object has been removed, but tearing and blinking do not stop.
- You become worse.

Removing a Contact Lens

❶ **Reassurance:**
- It sounds like something you should be able to remove at home.
- It may reassure you to know, if you did not know this already, that a contact lens cannot go behind the eyeball. A contact lens can sometimes get hidden under your upper or lower eyelid.
- I am going to give you some instructions.
- Your first step will be to wash your hands with soap and water.

❷ **Moisten the Contact Lens:**
- Place several drops of saline into the eye.
- You may need to repeat this in 5 minutes.
(Reason: hydrates soft contacts; helps lubricate and float soft and hard contacts)

❸ **Removing a Soft Contact Lens:**
- Look upward.
- Pull down your lower eyelid with your middle finger.
- Touch contact lens with your index finger and slide the lens downward to the lower white part of your eye.
- Gently pinch the contact lens between your thumb and index finger and remove it from your eye.

❹ **Removing a Hard Contact Lens—
Blink Method:**
- Pull outward on the skin at the corner of the eye (right index finger for right eye; left index finger for left eye).
- Cup your other hand under the eye to catch the contact lens.
- Blink several times.

❺ **Removing a Hard Contact Lens—
Plunger Method:**
- Use a contact lens "plunger" to remove the contact lens.
- If you do not have one, you can get one at a local pharmacy. This is a small, flexible plastic tool that has a suction cup on it.

❻ **Call Back If:**
- Unable to remove the contact lens.
- Pain or foreign body sensation lasts > 2 hours after removing the contact lens.
- You become worse.

FIRST AID

First Aid Advice for Glass Fragments on the Eyelids:
- **Method 1:** Bend forward and close the eyes. Have someone blow on the closed eyelids to get the flakes of glass off the skin.
- **Method 2:** Another technique is to touch the flakes of glass with a piece of tape.
- To get off any remaining glass, splash water on the eyelids and face. Cover the eyes with a wet washcloth. Do not rub your eyes.

BACKGROUND

Key Points
- Foreign bodies of the eye need to be removed, as they can damage the eye.
- If there is any persisting blurred vision or pain, evaluation is needed.

Causes
- The most common objects that get in the eye are an eyelash or a piece of dried mucus ("sleep").
- Particulate matter such as sand, dirt, sawdust, or other grit also can be blown into the eyes.
- Tree and plant pollen can blow into the eye.
- Rubbing the eye can lead to the foreign object scratching the cornea (clear part) and causing a secondary corneal abrasion.

EYE, PUS OR DISCHARGE

Definition
- Yellow or green discharge (pus) in one or both eyes.
- Dried pus on the eyelids and eyelashes. The eye-lashes are especially likely to be matted together following sleep.
- The white portions of the eye (sclera) may be pink or red (not required).
- The eyelids are usually puffy due to irritation from the infection.
- Includes calls about adults receiving antibiotic eye drops who are not improving or may be allergic to the eye drops.

TRIAGE ASSESSMENT QUESTIONS

See More Appropriate Protocol
- Eye exposure to chemical or fumes
  Go to Protocol: Eye, Chemical In on page 150
- Redness of white of eye (sclera), but no pus or only a small amount of brief pus
  Go to Protocol: Eye, Red Without Pus on page 158

Go to ED/UCC Now
(or to Office With PCP Approval)
- SEVERE pain (e.g., excruciating)
  R/O: corneal ulcer
- Patient sounds very sick or weak to the triager
  Reason: severe acute illness or serious complication suspected

Go to Office Now
- MODERATE eye pain (e.g., interferes with normal activities)
  R/O: corneal ulcer, herpes, hyperacute bacterial conjunctivitis
- Blurred vision
- Cloudy spot or sore seen on the cornea (clear part of the eye)
  R/O: corneal ulcer, herpes
- Eyelids are very swollen (shut or almost)
  R/O: periorbital cellulitis or preseptal cellulitis
- Eyelid (outer) is very red and painful (or tender to touch)
- Fever > 103° F (39.4° C)

See Today in Office
- Discharge from penis
  R/O: sexually transmitted infection (STI), chlamydia conjunctivitis
- New or abnormal vaginal discharge
  R/O: STI, chlamydia conjunctivitis
- Using antibiotic eye drops > 3 days but pus persists
  R/O: resistant bacteria
- Lots of yellow or green nasal discharge
  R/O: concurrent sinusitis
- Weak immune system (e.g., HIV positive, cancer chemotherapy, splenectomy, organ transplant, chronic steroids)
- Patient wants to be seen

See Today or Tomorrow in Office
- Fever present > 3 days (72 hours)
- Bleeding on white of the eye
  Reason: probably hemorrhagic conjunctivitis from adenovirus or enterovirus, but patient needs reassurance

Callback by PCP Today
- Eye with yellow/green discharge or eyelashes stick together, but NO standing order to call in antibiotic eye drops
  Reason: probably mild viral or bacterial eye infection
  CANADA: Continue with triage; antibiotic eye drops are available OTC.
- Using antibiotic eye drops and now eyes have become very itchy (especially after eye drops are put in)
  R/O: eye allergy to antibiotic
- Using antibiotic eye drops > 72 hours (3 days) and pus in eye persists
  Reason: possibly resistant bacteria
- Taking oral antibiotic > 48 hours (2 days) and pus in eye persists
  Reason: possibly resistant bacteria

Home Care

○ Eye with yellow/green discharge or eyelashes stick together, and PCP standing order to call in antibiotic eye drops
Reason: probable mild bacterial or viral conjunctivitis without complications
CANADA: Antibiotic eye drops are available OTC and a PCP prescription not required. See Home Care Advice for more detail.

○ Very small amount of discharge and only in corner of eye
Reason: probable viral conjunctivitis without complications

HOME CARE ADVICE

General Care Advice for Pinkeye

❶ **Reassurance:**
• A small amount of pus or mucus in the inner corner of the eye is often due to a cold or virus. Sometimes it's just a reaction to an irritant in the eye.
• You can get pinkeye from someone who has had it recently.
• Pinkeye will not harm your eyesight.
• Viral conjunctivitis (pinkeye) does not need antibiotic treatment. It gets better by itself. Usually it's gone in 2 or 3 days.
• *Here is some care advice that should help.*

❷ **Eyelid Cleansing:**
• Gently wash eyelids and lashes with warm water and wet cotton balls (or cotton gauze). Remove all the dried and liquid pus.
• Do this as often as needed.

❸ **Contact Lenses:**
• Switch to glasses for a short time. This will help stop damage to your eye.
• Clean your contacts before wearing them again.
• Throw away used contacts if they are meant to be thrown away.

❹ **Contagiousness:**
• Pinkeye is contagious. It is very easy to spread to other people. You can spread it by shaking hands.
• Try not to touch your eyes. Wash your hands often. Do not share towels.
• You may return to work or school. Avoid physical contact (e.g., shaking hands) until the symptoms have resolved.

❺ **Call Back If:**
• Pus increases in amount.
• Pus in corner of eye lasts > 3 days.
• Eyelid becomes red or swollen.
• You become worse.

Antibiotic Eye Drops for Mild Bacterial Conjunctivitis

❶ **Reassurance:**
• People often get pinkeye (conjunctivitis) when they have a cold.
• You can also get pinkeye from someone who has had it recently.
• Pinkeye will not harm your eyesight.
• Antibiotic eye drops work well to treat pinkeye.
• *Here is some care advice that should help.*

❷ **Prescription Option for Antibiotic Eye Drops Per Protocol—United States:**
• If PCP approves calling in prescription, do so per protocol.
• **Prescription:** Polytrim (polymyxin-trimethoprim) eye drops, 5 mL bottle ($12).
• **Dosing:** 1-2 drops 4 times daily for 5-7 days. *(Note: Drop covers the adult eye.)*
• **Additional Instructions:** Continue using eye drops until you have awakened 2 mornings without pus in the eyes.
• *Before taking any medicine, read all the instructions on the package.*

❸ **OTC Antibiotic Eye Drops—Canada:**
• Polysporin eye drops are available over the counter. Use 2 drops 4-6 times daily.
• Continue using the eye drops until you have awakened 2 mornings without pus in the eyes.
• *Before using any medicine, read all the instructions on the package.*

❹ **Expected Course:** With treatment, the yellow discharge should clear up in 3 days. The red eyes may persist for several more days.

❺ **Call Back If:**
• Pus lasts > 3 days (72 hours) on treatment.
• Blurred vision develops.
• More than just mild discomfort.
• You become worse.

BACKGROUND

Causes of Eye Discharge

Red eyes without a discharge are presumed to not be bacterial. A small amount of pus (or mucus) that's only present in the corner of the eye is usually viral or due to an irritant. Even matting (sticking together) of the eyelids after a night's sleep and that doesn't recur during the day is viral, unless it progresses.

Eye discharge that recurs throughout the day is 80% bacterial (Weiss 1993). *Note:* Some viruses can cause purulent conjunctivitis (e.g., adenovirus).

The 4 main causes of red eye with discharge are:
• **Bacterial Conjunctivitis** (thick white-yellow discharge; eyelashes sticky or eyes feel "glued" shut in morning)
• **Viral Conjunctivitis** (thin, clear-white discharge)
• **Allergic Conjunctivitis** (itching, clear-white discharge)
• **Chemical conjunctivitis** from exposure to chemicals, fumes (eye irritation, tearing)

Bacterial Conjunctivitis

Purulent discharge from the eye with redness is suggestive of a bacterial conjunctivitis. Bacterial conjunctivitis requires treatment with antibiotic eye drops. It can be a common complication of a cold and starts off as a viral conjunctivitis.

The symptoms can occur in one or both eyes. Other symptoms include:
• Mild discomfort or mild burning of the eye(s).
• Dried pus on the eyelids and eyelashes; eyelids are stuck together on awakening; eye discharge tends to recur throughout the day.
• Eyelids may be puffy due to irritation from the infection.
• Tearing.

Antibiotic Drops (or Ointment) for Bacterial Conjunctivitis

• **Polytrim** (polymyxin B and trimethoprim) eye drops (generic) is the current prescription of choice recommended in this protocol. It was selected because of its efficacy, safety, availability, and cost-effectiveness. The dosage is 1-2 drops 4 times daily for 5-7 days.
• **Other Options:** Erythromycin ophthalmic ointment, azithromycin drops.
• Fluoroquinolone eye drops are not recommended because they cost much more than Polytrim eye drops. However, fluoroquinolone eye drops are the antibiotic eye drop of choice for contact lens wearers with purulent discharge, because of the higher risk of *Pseudomonas*.

Caution: Eye Pain or Blurred Vision

Patients with eye pain that is more than mild or any blurred vision need to be seen within 4 hours. Significant eye pain and blurred vision do not generally occur in patients with regular conjunctivitis.

EYE, RED WITHOUT PUS

Definition
- Redness or pinkness of the sclera and inner eyelids.
- May have increased tearing (watery eye).
- Not due to a traumatic injury.
- **Excluded:** Yellow or green pus in the eyes; see Eye, Pus or Discharge protocol on page 155.

TRIAGE ASSESSMENT QUESTIONS

See More Appropriate Protocol
- ● Chemical got in the eye
  Go to Protocol: Eye, Chemical In on page 150
- ● Piece of something got in the eye
  Go to Protocol: Eye, Foreign Body on page 153
- ● Followed an eye injury
  Go to Protocol: Eye Injury on page 161
- ● Yellow or green pus in the eyes
  Go to Protocol: Eye, Pus or Discharge on page 155

Go to ED/UCC Now
(or to Office With PCP Approval)
- ● Severe eye pain
  R/O: acute angle-closure glaucoma
- ● Patient sounds very sick or weak to the triager
  Reason: severe acute illness or serious complication suspected

Go to Office Now
- ● Blurred vision
- ● Cloudy spot or sore seen on the cornea (clear part of the eye)
  R/O: corneal ulcer, herpes
- ● Eyelids are very swollen (shut or almost)
  R/O: periorbital cellulitis or preseptal cellulitis
- ● Eyelid (outer) is very red
  R/O: periorbital cellulitis or preseptal cellulitis
- ● Vomiting
  R/O: acute angle-closure glaucoma, migraine headache
- ● Foreign body sensation ("feels like something is in there")
  R/O: corneal abrasion, foreign body
- ● Recent eye surgery and has increasing eye pain
  R/O: endophthalmitis
- ● Eye pain/discomfort that is more than mild
  R/O: corneal ulcer, herpes, iritis

See Today in Office
- ◐ Patient wants to be seen
- ◐ Eye pain present > 24 hours
  R/O: forgotten corneal abrasion, occult foreign body, iritis, herpes simplex
- ◐ Bleeding on white of the eye and is taking Coumadin or known bleeding disorder (e.g., thrombocytopenia)
  Reason: need for testing of INR, prothrombin time
  Notes: Besides Coumadin, other strong blood thinners include Arixtra (fondaparinux), Eliquis (apixaban), Pradaxa (dabigatran), and Xarelto (rivaroxaban).
- ◐ Only 1 eye is red, and persists > 48 hours
  R/O: tiny foreign body

See Today or Tomorrow in Office
- ◐ Red eyes present > 7 days
- ◐ Bleeding on white of the eye
  R/O: subconjunctival hemorrhage, conjunctivitis

Home Care
- ○ Red eye caused by sunscreen, smoke, smog, chlorine, food, soap, or other mild irritant
  Reason: probable minor chemical conjunctivitis
- ○ Red eye caused by contact lens
  Reason: probable contact lens overuse
- ○ Red eye and no complications
  R/O: viral conjunctivitis (pinkeye)

HOME CARE ADVICE

❶ **Red Eye Caused by Mild Irritant** (e.g., sunscreen, smoke, smog, chlorine, food, soap, or other mild irritant):

- **Reassurance:** Most eye irritants cause transient redness of the eyes.
- **Face Cleansing:** Wash the face, then the eyelids, with a mild soap and water. This will remove any irritants. Also try to avoid the irritant.
- **Eye Irrigation:** Irrigate the eye with warm water for 2-3 minutes.
- **Vasoconstrictor Eye Drops:** If your eyes remain uncomfortable after irrigation and are still bloodshot, use some long-acting over-the-counter vasoconstrictor eye drops (e.g., Visine). Use 1-2 drops. May repeat once in 8-12 hours.
- **Remove Contacts:** Remove your contact lenses; you need to switch to glasses temporarily. *(Reason: to prevent damage to the cornea)*
- **Expected Course:** After removal of the irritant, the eyes usually return to normal color in 1-2 hours.

❷ **Red Eye Caused by Contacts:**

- **Reassurance:** It is reassuring that you have no blurred vision and that there is minimal to no discomfort. Sometimes people who wear contacts can develop eye irritation, especially if they wear their contacts too long.
- **Remove Contacts:** Remove your contact lenses; you need to switch to glasses temporarily. *(Reason: to prevent damage to the cornea)*
- **No Rubbing:** Do not rub your eyes. *(Reason: can cause a corneal abrasion or worsen an existing abrasion)*
- **Expected Course:** The pain and irritation should go away over the next 12-24 hours. If it does not, you will need an examination. *(Reason: possible corneal abrasion or ulcer)*

❸ **Red Eye Caused by Pinkeye:**

- **Reassurance:** It is reassuring that you have no blurred vision and that there is minimal to no discomfort. One cause of minor eye redness is pinkeye (viral conjunctivitis). People with pinkeye may often note mild eye irritation and a watery discharge. Often it affects both eyes. It can occur with a cold. It generally is not serious.
- **Remove Contacts:** Remove your contact lenses; you need to switch to glasses temporarily. *(Reason: to prevent damage to the cornea)*
- **No Rubbing:** Do not rub your eyes. *(Reason: can cause a corneal abrasion or worsen an existing abrasion)*
- **Contagiousness:** Pinkeye is extremely contagious. Try not to touch your eyes. Wash your hands frequently. Do not share towels.
- **Expected Course:** Pinkeye with a cold usually lasts about 7 days.

❹ **Call Back If:**

- Blurred vision or increasing pain.
- No improvement.
- You become worse.

BACKGROUND

Key Points

- The presence of either severe pain or blurring of the vision in a patient with a red eye requires urgent evaluation.
- Common causes of a red eye include blepharitis, conjunctivitis, allergy, and subconjunctival hemorrhage.

Causes

- Abrasion of cornea
- Acute angle-closure glaucoma
- Blepharitis
- Conjunctivitis, allergic
- Conjunctivitis, chemical/irritants (e.g., sunscreen, soap, chlorinated pool water, smoke, smog)
- Conjunctivitis, viral
- Corneal foreign body
- Corneal ulcer
- Episcleritis and scleritis
- Glaucoma
- Keratitis (inflammation of the cornea)
- Subconjunctival hemorrhage
- Trauma
- Uveitis (iritis, iridocyclitis)

Blepharitis

- **Definition:** Blockage of the oil glands along the eyelid margins results in inflammation. Crusting and flaking skin are present at the base of the eyelashes.
- **Pain:** Minimal to absent. May describe chronic irritation of eyelids and eyes.
- **Vision Loss:** None.
- **Treatment:** Gentle daily scrubbing of the eyelid margins with a dilute baby shampoo solution and frequent application of warm compresses.

Viral Conjunctivitis

- **Definition:** Viral infection of the conjunctiva of the eye. The whites of the eyes become diffusely red or pink because of blood vessel dilatation in the conjunctiva. A watery discharge is common. Mild eyelid swelling may occur. Usually both eyes are affected.
- **Layperson Term:** Pinkeye.
- **Pain:** Minimal to absent. May describe mild irritation or itching.
- **Vision Loss:** None.
- **Treatment:** Viral conjunctivitis resolves on its own. Some physicians will prescribe antibiotic drops to prevent bacterial superinfection. Viral conjunctivitis is contagious; the patient should not share towels, should wash hands frequently, and should avoid close contact with others for 2 weeks.

Subconjunctival Hemorrhage

- **Definition:** Localized area of bleeding into the white area (sclera) of the eye. The fragile blood vessels in this area can rupture as a result of minor and sometimes forgotten trauma or from forceful coughing or vomiting. It can also occur spontaneously. It is nearly always unilateral.
- **Pain:** None.
- **Vision Loss:** None.
- **Treatment:** No specific treatment is required. Area of hemorrhage should gradually clear in 2-3 weeks.

EYE INJURY

Definition
- Injuries to the eye, eyelid, and area around the eye

TRIAGE ASSESSMENT QUESTIONS

Call EMS 911 Now
- Knocked out (unconscious) > 1 minute
  R/O: concussion
- Sounds like a life-threatening emergency to the triager

See More Appropriate Protocol
- Wound looks infected
  Go to Protocol: Wound Infection on page 443
- Foreign body in the eye
  Go to Protocol: Eye, Foreign Body on page 153
- Head injury is main concern
  Go to Protocol: Head Injury on page 201

Go to ED Now
- Vision is blurred or lost in either eye
  R/O: acute hyphema
- Double vision or unable to look upward
  R/O: blowout fracture
- Bloody or cloudy fluid behind the cornea (clear part)
  R/O: acute hyphema

Go to ED/UCC Now
(or to Office With PCP Approval)
- Object hit the eye at high speed (e.g., from a lawn mower)
  R/O: penetrating injury or foreign body
- Sharp object hit the eye (e.g., metallic chip)
- Any cut on the eyelid or eyeball
  R/O: eyeball perforation
- Skin is split open or gaping (length > ¼" or 6 mm)
  Reason: may need laceration repair (e.g., sutures)
  R/O: deeper injury
- Bleeding won't stop after 10 minutes of direct pressure (using correct technique)
- Two black eyes (both sides)
  R/O: "raccoon eyes" from basilar skull fracture
- Sounds like a serious injury to the triager

Go to Office Now
- SEVERE pain (e.g., excruciating)
  R/O: penetrating injury or foreign body
- Constant tearing or blinking
- Patient keeps the eye covered or refuses to open it
  R/O: corneal abrasion

See Today in Office
- Large swelling or bruise (> 2" or 5 cm)
  R/O: fracture, large contusion
- Eyelids swollen shut
- Scratch on white of the eye (sclera)
- Patient wants to be seen

See Today or Tomorrow in Office
- Wound and no tetanus booster in > 5 years (or > 10 years for clean cuts)
  Reason: may need a tetanus booster shot (vaccine)
- Suspicious history for the injury
  R/O: domestic violence or elder abuse

See Within 3 Days in Office
- Injury and pain has not improved after 3 days
- Pain or swelling persisting > 7 days

Home Care
- Minor eye injury
  R/O: superficial cut or abrasion, bruise
- Minor flame-shaped bruise on sclera (white part of eyeball)
  R/O: small subconjunctival hemorrhage

HOME CARE ADVICE

❶ Treatment of Superficial Cuts and Scrapes (Abrasions) to Eyelid or Area Around Eye:
- Apply direct pressure with a sterile gauze or clean cloth for 10 minutes to stop any bleeding.
- Wash the wound with soap and water for 5 minutes (protect the eye with a clean cloth).
- Apply an antibiotic ointment. Cover large scrapes with a Band-Aid or dressing. Change daily.

❷ Treatment of Swelling or Bruise With Intact Skin:
- Apply an ice pack to the area for 20 minutes each hour for 4 consecutive hours.
- 48 hours after the injury, use local heat for 10 minutes 3 times each day to help reabsorb the blood.

❸ Treatment of Subconjunctival Hemorrhage (flame-shaped bruise of the white area of eyeball): No specific treatment is required. It usually goes away in 2-3 weeks.

❹ Pain Medicines:
- For pain relief, you can take either acetaminophen, ibuprofen, or naproxen.
- They are over-the-counter (OTC) pain drugs. You can buy them at the drugstore.

Acetaminophen (e.g., Tylenol):
- **Regular Strength Tylenol:** Take 650 mg (two 325 mg pills) by mouth every 4-6 hours as needed. Each Regular Strength Tylenol pill has 325 mg of acetaminophen.
- **Extra Strength Tylenol:** Take 1,000 mg (two 500 mg pills) every 8 hours as needed. Each Extra Strength Tylenol pill has 500 mg of acetaminophen.
- The most you should take each day is 3,000 mg (10 Regular Strength or 6 Extra Strength pills a day).

Ibuprofen (e.g., Motrin, Advil):
- Take 400 mg (two 200 mg pills) by mouth every 6 hours.
- Another choice is to take 600 mg (three 200 mg pills) by mouth every 8 hours.
- The most you should take each day is 1,200 mg (six 200 mg pills), unless your doctor has told you to take more.

Naproxen (e.g., Aleve):
- Take 220 mg (one 220 mg pill) by mouth every 8 hours as needed. You may take 440 mg (two 220 mg pills) for your first dose.
- The most you should take each day is 660 mg (three 220 mg pills a day), unless your doctor has told you to take more.

❺ Pain Medicines—Extra Notes:
- Use the lowest amount of medicine that makes your pain better.
- Acetaminophen is thought to be safer than ibuprofen or naproxen in people > 65 years old. Acetaminophen is in many OTC and prescription medicines. It might be in more than one medicine that you are taking. You need to be careful and not take an overdose. An acetaminophen overdose can hurt the liver.
- McNeil, the company that makes Tylenol, has different dosage instructions for Tylenol in Canada and the United States. In Canada, the maximum recommended dose per day is 4,000 mg or 12 Regular Strength (325 mg) pills. In the United States, McNeil recommends a maximum dose of 10 Regular Strength (325 mg) pills.
- CAUTION: Do not take acetaminophen if you have liver disease.
- CAUTION: Do not take ibuprofen or naproxen if you have stomach problems, have kidney disease, are pregnant, or have been told by your doctor to avoid this type of anti-inflammatory drug. Do not take ibuprofen or naproxen for > 7 days without consulting your doctor.
- *Before taking any medicine, read all the instructions on the package.*

❻ Call Back If:
- Pain becomes severe.
- Pain does not improve after 3 days.
- Changes in vision.
- You become worse.

FIRST AID

First Aid Advice for Bleeding:

- Apply direct pressure to the entire wound with a clean cloth.
- Try to avoid pressure on the eyeball.

First Aid Advice for Penetrating Object:

If penetrating object is still in place, don't remove it. *Reason: Removal could cause bleeding or more damage.*

First Aid Advice for Shock:

Lie down with the feet elevated.

BACKGROUND

Vision and Trauma to the Eye

- The main concern in all eye injuries is whether the vision is damaged.
- It is important to test vision in both eyes. If there has been no damage to the vision, then most likely there is no serious injury to the eyeball. Test vision at home by covering each eye in turn and looking at a near object and then at a distant object. Is the vision blurred in comparison with normal?

Common Injuries to the Eye and Orbital Area

- **Black Eye:** Bruising and purple discoloration of the eyelids and upper cheek is referred to as a black eye. Usually it is the result of a direct blow to this area (e.g., a punch). It gets worse for the first couple days. It usually goes away in 2-3 weeks.
- **Corneal Abrasion (Scratch):** A corneal abrasion is one of the most common eye injuries. The typical mechanism is an accidental scratch from a fingernail, a piece of paper, or the branch of a tree. It can be quite painful. Generally, a minor corneal abrasion will heal in 1-2 days; it is treated with antibiotic eye drops and (sometimes) patching.
- **Eye Laceration, Puncture Wound:** Penetrating eye injuries are always very serious. They may be caused by a sharp object (laceration) or from a small object traveling at high speed (puncture wound with intraocular foreign body).

- **Eyelid Laceration, Puncture Wound:** Always consider the possibility that the wound went through the eyelid into the eye.
- **Hyphema:** Blood is visible inside the front portion of eye (anterior chamber) just behind the cornea. This finding is serious and can occur with either blunt or penetrating eye trauma.
- **Orbital Fracture (Blow-out Fracture):** The bony walls of the socket in which the eye sits are somewhat thin and can be fractured with blunt trauma. The appearance is similar to a black eye. The pain and swelling are usually worse, and sometimes the patient may complain of double vision.
- **Subconjunctival Hemorrhage:** This is the medical term for a flame-shaped bruise of the white area of the eyeball. It sometimes happens after a direct blow to the eye. It looks as though a red patch was "painted" onto the eye. It usually goes away in 2-3 weeks.

Unilateral Dilated Pupil (Anisocoria)

- Anisocoria is the medical term for unequal pupil sizes.
- **Normal Variant:** Most commonly unequal pupils are a normal variant. Approximately 10% of the population has anisocoria. This is almost always the reason in alert individuals without other serious neurologic symptoms. One simple way to check to see if someone always has anisocoria is to look at a driver's license photo or other photo that shows the pupils.
- **Local Eye Trauma (Traumatic Mydriasis):** Blunt trauma to one eye can cause unilateral dilation of the pupil (traumatic mydriasis). Associated symptoms will include eye pain, eye redness, blurred vision, and photophobia.
- **As a Sign of Brain Stem Herniation:** A unilaterally dilated pupil in the setting of head trauma always raises the concern about brain hemorrhage, swelling, and herniation. A dilated pupil from brain herniation is always accompanied by altered mental status, severe headache, and other neurologic symptoms. Thus, if a patient is comatose AND has a unilateral widely dilated pupil, brain stem herniation should be suspected.

What Cuts Need to Be Sutured?

- Any cut that is split open or gaping probably needs sutures (or skin glue).
- Cuts on the face > ¼" (6 mm) usually need sutures.
- Any open wound that may need sutures should be evaluated by a physician regardless of the time that has passed since the initial injury.

When Does an Adult Need a Tetanus Booster (Tetanus Shot)?

- **Clean Cuts and Scrapes—Tetanus Booster Needed Every 10 Years:** Patients with clean minor wounds AND who have previously had ≥ 3 tetanus shots (full series) need a booster every 10 years. Examples of minor wounds include a superficial abrasion or a shallow cut from a clean knife blade. Obtain booster within 72 hours.
- **Dirty Wounds—Tetanus Booster Needed Every 5 Years:** Patients with dirty wounds need a booster if it has been > 5 years since the last booster. Examples of dirty wounds include those contaminated with soil, feces, and/or saliva and more serious wounds from deep punctures, crushing, and burns. Obtain booster within 72 hours.

Caution: Associated Head and Neck Trauma

- Head trauma should be considered in all patients with a facial injury. Signs of significant head injury include loss of consciousness, amnesia, unsteady walking, confusion, and slurred speech.
- Neck trauma should also be considered in all patients with a facial injury. Concerning findings include numbness, weakness, and neck pain.
- After using the Eye Injury protocol, if the triager or caller has remaining concerns about head or neck trauma, the patient also should be triaged using the Head Injury and/or Neck Injury protocols on pages 201 and 290, respectively.

FAINTING

Definition

- Fainting is a brief (transient) loss of consciousness (passing out) with falling down.
- Spontaneous recovery with return to full awareness usually occurs in < 1 minute.
- Also called passing out or syncope.
- **Note:** Remaining unconscious (coma) is an emergency.

TRIAGE ASSESSMENT QUESTIONS

Call EMS 911 Now

- Still unconscious
  R/O: coma, postictal after unwitnessed seizure
- Still feels dizzy or light-headed
  R/O: hypovolemia, arrhythmia
- Difficult to awaken or acting confused (e.g., disoriented, slurred speech)
  R/O: shock, CVA, hypoglycemia, postictal
- Difficulty breathing
  R/O: hypoxia and need for oxygen
- Bluish (or gray) lips or face
  R/O: cyanosis and need for oxygen
- Shock suspected (e.g., cold/pale/clammy skin, too weak to stand)
  R/O: shock
  First Aid: Lie down with the feet elevated.
- Bleeding (e.g., vomiting blood, rectal bleeding or tarry stools, severe vaginal bleeding)
- Chest pain
  R/O: cardiac ischemia, myocardial infarction, pulmonary embolism
- Extra heartbeats or heart is beating fast (i.e., palpitations)
  R/O: dysrhythmia
- Heart beating < 50 beats per minute OR > 140 beats per minute
- Fainted suddenly after medicine, allergic food, or bee sting
  R/O: anaphylaxis
- Sounds like a life-threatening emergency to the triager

See More Appropriate Protocol

- Has diabetes (diabetes mellitus) and fainting from low blood sugar (i.e., < 70 mg/dL or 3.9 mmol/L)
  Go to Protocol: Diabetes (Low Blood Sugar) on page 116
- Seizure suspected (e.g., muscle jerking or shaking followed by confusion)
  Go to Protocol: Seizure on page 340
- Heat exhaustion suspected
  Go to Protocol: Heat Exposure (Heat Exhaustion and Heatstroke) on page 214

Go to ED Now

- Fainted > 15 minutes ago and still looks pale (pale skin, pallor)
  R/O: anemia, GI bleeding
- Fainted > 15 minutes ago and still feels weak or dizzy
  R/O: hypovolemia, dehydration
- History of heart problems or congestive heart failure
  Reason: greater risk of arrhythmia as cause of syncope
- Occurred during exercise
  R/O: cardiac arrhythmia, structural heart disease
- Any head or face injury
  Reason: suggests sudden loss of consciousness from dysrhythmia (short duration of warning)

Go to ED/UCC Now (or to Office With PCP Approval)

- Age > 50 years
  Reason: higher risk for cardiac disease and other serious causes of syncope
- Drinking very little and has signs of dehydration (e.g., no urine > 12 hours, very dry mouth)
- Fainted 2 times in one day
- Patient sounds very sick or weak to the triager
  Reason: severe acute illness or serious complication suspected

See Today in Office

- All other patients, and now alert and feels fine
  (Exception: simple faint due to stress, pain, prolonged standing, or suddenly standing)
- Patient wants to be seen

See Within 2 Weeks in Office

- Simple fainting is a chronic symptom (has occurred multiple times)

Home Care

- ○ Sudden standing caused simple fainting, and now alert and feels fine
  R/O: simple faint
- ○ Prolonged standing caused simple fainting, and now alert and feels fine
  R/O: simple faint
- ○ Fear, stress, or pain caused simple fainting, and now alert and feels fine
  R/O: simple faint (vasovagal syncope)

HOME CARE ADVICE

General Care Advice

❶ **Treatment:**
- Lie down with the feet elevated for 10 minutes.
  (Reason: Simple fainting is due to temporarily decreased blood flow to the brain.)
- Drink some fruit juice, especially if you have missed a meal or have not eaten in > 6 hours.

❷ **Expected Course:** Most adults with a simple faint are back to normal after lying down for 10 minutes.

❸ **Warning Symptoms for Fainting:**
- Fainting usually has early warning symptoms (e.g., dizziness, blurred vision, nausea, feeling cold or warm).
- If you feel these warning symptoms, immediately lie down to prevent falling down. You only have 5 seconds to act.
  (Reason: almost impossible to faint when lying down)
- Lying down (even on the floor) is less embarrassing than fainting, no matter where you are.
- Sitting down (with head between knees) is certainly better than staying standing up but is less effective than lying down.

❹ **Pregnancy Test, When in Doubt:**
- If there is a chance that you might be pregnant, use a urine pregnancy test.
- You can buy a pregnancy test at the drugstore.
- It works best if you test your first urine in the morning.
- *Follow the instructions included in the package.*
- Call back if you are pregnant.

❺ **Call Back If:**
- You pass out again on the same day.
- You are pregnant.
- You become worse.

Simple Faint From Standing Up Suddenly

❶ **Reassurance:**
- Standing up suddenly after lying down can cause temporary dizziness in anyone. If you don't sit back down when this happens, fainting can sometimes occur.
- It is caused by temporary blood pooling in the legs and not enough blood getting to the brain.
- It is usually not serious, and it is preventable.

❷ **Prevention:**
- Most fainting can be prevented.
- When getting out of bed, sit on the edge for a few minutes before standing. If you feel dizzy, sit or lie down.
- **Water and Salt Are Key:** If you have this tendency, drink extra fluids every day. Also, add some mildly salty foods (saltine crackers, soup) to your diet.

Simple Faint From Prolonged Standing

❶ **Reassurance:**
- Standing for too long in one position is a common cause of fainting.
- It is caused by temporary blood pooling in the legs and not enough blood getting to the brain.
- It is usually not serious, and it is preventable.

❷ **Prevention:**
- If prolonged standing is required, repeatedly contract and relax the leg muscles. This will pump the blood back to the heart.
- Try to avoid standing in one place for too long with your knees locked.
- **Water and Salt Are Key:** If you have this tendency, drink extra fluids every day. Also, add some mildly salty foods (saltine crackers, soup) to your diet.

Simple Faint From Fear/Stress/Pain

❶ Reassurance:
- Some people faint if they experience a painful, frightening, or emotional event. Examples include getting a shot, having a bloody wound, or seeing someone else bleed.
- For some people this is a normal reaction to stress and shouldn't cause any lasting effects.
- It is caused by temporary blood pooling in the legs and not enough blood getting to the brain.
- It is usually not serious, and it is preventable.

❷ Prevention:
- Preventing fainting from stressful events is not always possible. However, here are some important tips that may help.
- If you know you are at risk for fainting under certain circumstances (e.g., a shot in the doctor's office), lie down in advance.
- Try thinking about something else. Visualize yourself on the beach or with a friend.
- You can also learn relaxation exercises (relaxing every muscle in the body).

FIRST AID

First Aid Advice for Fainting:
Lie down with the feet elevated.

First Aid Advice for Shock:
Lie down with the feet elevated.

BACKGROUND

Key Points
- Fainting (syncope) is a transient loss of consciousness due to a reduction in cerebral blood flow. Thus, anything that temporarily reduces blood flow to the brain can cause a person to faint. If sitting, the person loses postural tone and slumps over; if standing, the person falls to the ground.
- There are serious and nonserious causes of syncope.

Findings Suggestive of Serious Cause for Syncope
- Age > 50
- Known cardiac disease
- Presence of head or face injury
- Persisting decreased level of alertness after syncopal event
- Occurs during exercise
- Has other symptoms: cardiorespiratory, neurologic, GI, or genitourinary

Causes of Syncope That Require Emergent Evaluation
- Abdominal aortic aneurysm
- Arrhythmias and cardiac conduction disorders resulting in bradycardia and tachycardia
- Cerebrovascular accident/transient ischemic attack
- Ectopic pregnancy
- Gastrointestinal (GI) bleeding
- Myocardial infarction
- Pulmonary embolism
- Seizure (may be mistaken for syncope)
- Subarachnoid hemorrhage

Findings Suggestive of Nonserious Cause for Syncope
- Age < 50
- No injury from fainting
- Now feels normal and is fully alert
- No other symptoms—cardiorespiratory, neurologic, GI, or genitourinary

Simple Faints

- **Introduction:** Simple faints can occur in healthy individuals due to stress, pain, prolonged standing, or suddenly standing up. It is the most common reason for syncope; perhaps 80% of all fainting occurs in this manner. It is also called vasovagal or vasomotor syncope.
- **Physiology:** When an individual is exposed to some sort of stimulus (e.g., pain, stress, prolonged standing), a reflex controlled by the vasomotor center in the brain stem is triggered. It tells the blood vessels in the legs to dilate, causing pooling of blood in the legs; there is less blood flow to the brain; and as a result, fainting occurs.
- **Warning Signs** (pre-syncope): There are a number of warning signs that occur immediately before a simple faint. These include pallor, dizziness (light-headedness), feeling cold or warm, blurred vision, nausea or vague stomach discomfort, sweating, and feeling cold. These warning symptoms last for 5-10 seconds before passing out occurs. Fainting can sometimes be prevented by sitting down or, even better, lying down.
- **Symptoms:** A brief period of warning symptoms (e.g., dizziness, nausea), followed by unconsciousness, with return to full awareness usually in < 1 minute; afterward, feeling normal.
- **Expected Course:** There is often a feeling of tiredness or mild malaise (e.g., being "washed out") for a period after a vasovagal fainting episode.
- **Predisposing Factors:** Mild dehydration, fasting, hot weather, sleep deprivation, recent illness, pregnancy, change in altitude, reaction to vaccination.

Simple Faints—Causes

- **Prolonged Standing in One Position Prior to Fainting** (called orthostatic syncope): This is a common cause of simple faints. It commonly occurs at church, graduations, weddings, school assemblies, parades, etc. It is more common if one keeps one's knees "locked"—due to pooling of blood in the legs. Anyone who stands long enough in one position will eventually faint.
- **Standing Up Suddenly** (*especially after lying down*) prior to fainting (called orthostatic syncope): Usually this just causes transient dizziness. It is more common in the morning after overnight fasting and relative dehydration.
- **Sudden Fearful or Disgusting Event (Emotional Pain) Prior to Fainting** (called vasovagal syncope): Examples are any kind of blood-and-guts scenario, such as seeing someone vomit, bleed, or pass a stool. Seeing a badly injured person or pet can precipitate syncope. It can also occur prior to an injection or public performance (e.g., a speech or musical recital).
- **Sudden Physical Pain Prior to Fainting** (called vasovagal syncope): Examples are receiving an injection (e.g., postimmunization syncope), having a sliver or sutures removed, or blood draw for laboratory tests. The stress of the experience probably has more to do with the syncope than the pain itself.

FEVER

Definition
- Fever is the only symptom.

Measurements:
- Oral temperature > 100.0° F (37.8° C).
- Ear (tympanic) temperature > 100.4° F (38.0° C).
- Rectal temperature > 100.4° F (38.0° C).
- Forehead temperature strips are unreliable.

Note: If another acute symptom is present, see that protocol (e.g., symptoms of cough, runny nose, sore throat, earache, abdominal pain, diarrhea, vomiting).

TRIAGE ASSESSMENT QUESTIONS

Call EMS 911 Now
- Difficult to awaken or acting confused (e.g., disoriented, slurred speech)
  R/O: sepsis, shock
- Pale cold skin and very weak (can't stand)
- Difficulty breathing and bluish (or gray) lips or face
  R/O: cyanosis and need for oxygen
- New onset rash with purple (or blood-colored) spots or dots
  R/O: meningococcemia
- Sounds like a life-threatening emergency to the triager

See More Appropriate Protocol
- Fever onset within 24 hours of receiving vaccine
  Go to Protocol: Immunization Reactions on page 230

Go to ED Now
- Headache and stiff neck (can't touch chin to chest)
  R/O: meningitis
- Difficulty breathing
  R/O: pneumonia
- IV drug abuse
  R/O: endocarditis

Go to ED/UCC Now
(or to Office With PCP Approval)
- Fever > 103° F (39.4° C)
  R/O: bacterial infection
- Fever > 100.5° F (38.1° C) and > 60 years of age
  R/O: bacterial infection
- Fever > 100.0° F (37.8° C) and diabetes mellitus or a weak immune system (e.g., HIV positive, chemotherapy, splenectomy)
  R/O: bacterial infection
- Fever > 100.0° F (37.8° C) and bedridden (e.g., nursing home patient, stroke, chronic illness, recovering from surgery)
  Reason: higher risk of bacterial infection
  Note: May need ambulance transport to ED.
- Fever > 100.0° F (37.8° C) and indwelling urinary catheter (e.g., Foley, coudé)
  R/O: bacterial infection
- Fever > 100.5° F (38.1° C) and has port (Port-A-Cath), central line, or PICC line
  R/O: catheter-related bacteremia
- Drinking very little and has signs of dehydration (e.g., no urine > 12 hours, very dry mouth, very light-headed)
  Reason: may need IV hydration
- Patient sounds very sick or weak to the triager
  Reason: severe acute illness or serious complication suspected

Go to Office Now
- Fever > 100.5° F (38.1° C) and surgery in the past month
  R/O: UTI or other bacterial infection
- Transplant patient (e.g., liver, heart, lung, kidney)
  R/O: bacterial infection
- Widespread rash and cause unknown

See Today in Office
- Patient wants to be seen

See Today or Tomorrow in Office

- Fever present > 3 days (72 hours)
  Reason: unexplained fever
- Intermittent fever > 100.5° F (38.1° C) persists > 3 weeks
- Fever > 100.0° F (37.8° C) and foreign travel to a developing country in the past month
  R/O: malaria, typhoid fever, dengue, leptospirosis, rickettsia, et al

Home Care

- Fever with no signs of serious infection or localizing symptoms

HOME CARE ADVICE

❶ **Reassurance:** The presence of a fever usually means that you have an infection. Most fevers are good and help the body fight infection. The goal of fever therapy is to bring the fever down to a comfortable level. Use the following definitions to help put the level of fever into proper perspective:
  - **100° F-102° F (37.8° C-38.9° C):** Low-grade fevers and may help body fight infection.
  - **102° F-104° F (38.9° C-40° C):** Moderate-grade fevers; cause discomfort.
  - **> 104° F (> 40° C):** High fevers; cause discomfort, weakness, headache, lethargy.
  - **> 107° F (> 41.7° C):** The fever itself can be harmful.

❷ **For All Fevers:**
  - Drink cold fluids to prevent dehydration. *(Reason: Good hydration replaces sweat and improves heat loss via skin.)* Adults should drink 6-8 glasses of water daily.
  - Dress in one layer of lightweight clothing and sleep with one light blanket.
  - For fevers 100° F-101° F (37.8° C-38.3° C) this is the only treatment and fever medicine is not needed.

❸ **Fever Medicines:**
  - For fevers > 101° F (38.3° C) take either acetaminophen or ibuprofen.
  - They are over-the-counter (OTC) drugs that help treat both fever and pain. You can buy them at the drugstore.
  - The goal of fever therapy is to bring the fever down to a comfortable level. Remember that fever medicine usually lowers fever 2° F (1-1½° C).

❹ **Acetaminophen (e.g., Tylenol):**
  - **Regular Strength Tylenol:** Take 650 mg (two 325 mg pills) by mouth every 4-6 hours as needed. Each Regular Strength Tylenol pill has 325 mg of acetaminophen.
  - **Extra Strength Tylenol:** Take 1,000 mg (two 500 mg pills) every 8 hours as needed. Each Extra Strength Tylenol pill has 500 mg of acetaminophen.
  - The most you should take each day is 3,000 mg (10 Regular Strength or 6 Extra Strength pills a day).

❺ **Ibuprofen (e.g., Motrin, Advil):**
  - Take 400 mg (two 200 mg pills) by mouth every 6 hours.
  - Another choice is to take 600 mg (three 200 mg pills) by mouth every 8 hours.
  - The most you should take each day is 1,200 mg (six 200 mg pills), unless your doctor has told you to take more.

❻ **Fever Medicines—Extra Notes:**
  - Use the lowest amount of medicine that makes your fever better.
  - Acetaminophen is thought to be safer than ibuprofen or naproxen in people > 65 years old. Acetaminophen is in many OTC and prescription medicines. It might be in more than one medicine that you are taking. You need to be careful and not take an overdose. An acetaminophen overdose can hurt the liver.
  - McNeil, the company that makes Tylenol, has different dosage instructions for Tylenol in Canada and the United States. In Canada, the maximum recommended dose per day is 4,000 mg or 12 Regular Strength (325 mg) pills. In the United States, McNeil recommends a maximum dose of 10 Regular Strength (325 mg) pills.
  - CAUTION: Do not take acetaminophen if you have liver disease.
  - CAUTION: Do not take ibuprofen if you have stomach problems, have kidney disease, are pregnant, or have been told by your doctor to avoid this type of anti-inflammatory drug. Do not take ibuprofen for > 7 days without consulting your doctor.
  - *Before taking any medicine, read all the instructions on the package.*

❼ **Lukewarm Shower for Reducing Fever:** Take the fever medicine first. Take a lukewarm shower or bath for 10 minutes. Lukewarm water should be warm enough that it does not make you shiver but cold enough that it helps cool you off and reduce your temperature. Do not sponge yourself with rubbing alcohol.

❽ **Expected Course:** Most fevers from a viral illness, such as a cold, fluctuate between 99.5° F and 103° F (37.5° C-39.5° C) and last for 2 or 3 days.

❾ **Contagiousness:** You can return to work or school after the fever is gone.

❿ **Call Back If:**
  • Fever lasts > 3 days (72 hours).
  • You become worse.

FIRST AID

First Aid Advice for Shock:

Lie down with the feet elevated.

BACKGROUND

Key Points

• In most clinical situations, fever does no major harm and may actually benefit the host defense mechanism. But nonetheless, fever is an abnormal finding that can signal a serious illness, especially in the old, frail, or immunocompromised adult. The absence of fever in a significant or overwhelming infection forebodes poorly.

• Adults tend to run lower fevers than children. Fever may be further blunted or even absent in elderly patients.

• Rectal temperatures are generally about 1° F (0.6° C) above oral temperatures.

Commonly Associated Symptoms

• The fever itself can cause significant muscle aches, nausea, light-headedness, weakness, and headache.

• **Chills:** Chills can sometimes precede fever. A fever occurs because the "thermostat" in the hypothalamus gets set to a higher temperature. The hypothalamus then causes the body temperature to rise in 2 ways. First, vasoconstriction of the peripheral blood vessels occurs, and blood is shunted centrally. The patient notices a cold sensation in the hands and feet ("I feel really cold") and will often seek blankets or extra warmth. Second, shivering occurs from muscular contractions ("I am shivering; I have the chills").

• **Sweats:** These occur when the hypothalamic "thermostat" gets reset downwards. Body temperature falls from vasodilation and sweating ("I feel hot and sweaty").

Broad Categories: Causes of Fever

• Infections
• Neoplasms
• Collagen vascular disorders
• Drugs

Normal Body Temperature

• Most physicians, nurses, laypersons, and medical references state the "normal" temperature is 98.6° F (37° C). Sometimes people forget to qualify this result by including the site at which the temperature was taken (oral, tympanic, rectal).

• However, a study (Mackowiak) showed that the correct average-daily oral temperature is 98.2° F (36.8° C) in healthy adults.

• The average temperature of healthy elderly patients is the same as younger adults. Though, there are some data to suggest that the average temperature in chronically ill elderly patients is lower than that of other healthy adults. Interpretation of a temperature reading in a chronically ill elderly adult must be done with some caution. Given that lower baseline temperatures are expected in this group of patients, it would be easy to miss a fever if the conventional fever standards were applied to chronically ill elderly patients.

Normal Variations of Body Temperature

• There is a normal daily awake-sleep cycle variation in temperature, with the low occurring at 6:00 am and the high occurring at 6:00 pm. The low and high temperatures vary by 0.9° F (0.6° C).

• In women, temperature increases about 0.9° F (0.6° C) at the time of ovulation.

• Temperature can go up in response to exercise and as a result of climatic factors.

Recording the Temperature During the Triage Phone Call

• Record the temperature that the patient gives you and the site at which it was taken. For example, *"Patient reports a temperature this morning of 101.2° F (oral)."*

FINGER INJURY

Definition
- Injuries to finger(s).
- Finger injuries include cuts, abrasions, jammed finger, smashed finger, fingernail injury, subungual hematoma, dislocations, and fractures.

TRIAGE ASSESSMENT QUESTIONS

Call EMS 911 Now
- ● Major bleeding (actively dripping or spurting) that can't be stopped
  First Aid: Apply direct pressure to the entire wound with a clean cloth.
- ● Sounds like a life-threatening emergency to the triager

See More Appropriate Protocol
- ● Wound looks infected
  Go to Protocol: Wound Infection on page 443
- ● Caused by animal bite
  Go to Protocol: Animal Bite on page 22

Go to ED Now
- ● Amputation
  First Aid: Apply direct pressure to the entire wound with a clean cloth.
- ● High-pressure injection injury (e.g., from paint gun, usually work related)
  Reason: deep tissue damage may exceed superficial injury

Go to ED/UCC Now
(or to Office With PCP Approval)
- ● Looks like a broken bone or dislocated joint (e.g., crooked or deformed)
  R/O: dislocation or angulated fracture
- ● Skin is split open or gaping (length > ½" or 12 mm)
  Reason: may need laceration repair (e.g., sutures)
- ● Cut or scrape is very deep (e.g., can see bone or tendons)
  R/O: tendon injury
- ● Bleeding won't stop after 10 minutes of direct pressure (using correct technique)
  R/O: need for sutures

- ● Dirt in the wound and not removed after 15 minutes of scrubbing
  Reason: needs irrigation or debridement
- ● Cut with numbness (loss of sensation) of finger
  R/O: digital nerve laceration
- ● Fingernail is partially torn from a crush injury
  (Exception: torn nail from catching it on something)
- ● Sounds like a serious injury to the triager

Go to Office Now
- ● Looks infected (e.g., spreading redness, pus, red streak)
  R/O: cellulitis, lymphangitis
- ● Fingernail is completely torn off
- ● Base of fingernail has popped out from under skinfold (cuticle)
  Reason: needs to be reinserted under the skin

See Today in Office
- ● SEVERE pain (e.g., excruciating)
  R/O: fracture
- ● MODERATE-SEVERE pain and blood present under the nail (usually > 50% of nail bed)
  R/O: severe subungual hematoma needing drainage
- ● Finger joint can't be opened (straightened) or closed (bent) completely
  R/O: fracture, tendon injury
- ● Patient wants to be seen

See Today or Tomorrow in Office
- ● Injury interferes with work or school
- ● Wound and no tetanus booster in > 5 years (or > 10 years for clean cuts)
  Reason: may need a tetanus booster shot (vaccine)
- ● Suspicious history for the injury
  R/O: domestic violence or elder abuse

See Within 3 Days in Office
- ● Injury and pain has not improved after 3 days
- ● Injury is still painful or swollen after 2 weeks

Home Care
- ○ Minor finger injury
  R/O: minor bruise or sprain, scrapes, small subungual hematoma

HOME CARE ADVICE

Treatment of a Minor Bruise of the Fingernail or Finger

❶ **Reassurance—Bruised Fingernail (Subungual Hematoma):**
- A direct blow to your fingertip can cause bruising under the fingernail. There is bleeding underneath the nail. The medical term for this is subungual hematoma.
- Symptoms are bruising under the fingernail and mild-moderate pain. Usually, the larger the bruise under the nail, the greater the pain.
- *Here is some care advice that should help.*

❷ **Reassurance—Bruised Finger (Contusion, Bruise):**
- A direct blow to your finger can cause a contusion. Contusion is the medical term for bruise.
- Symptoms are mild pain, swelling, and/or bruising.
- *Here is some care advice that should help.*

❸ **Apply a Cold Pack:**
- Apply a cold pack or an ice bag (wrapped in a moist towel) to the area for 20 minutes. Repeat in 1 hour, then every 4 hours while awake.
- Continue this for the first 48 hours after an injury.
- This will help decrease pain and swelling.

❹ **Keep the Hand Elevated:**
- When you are up walking around, try not to let the hand hang down. If you do you will notice that the finger hurts and throbs more.
- When you are sitting down reading or watching TV, place your arm up on a pillow. This puts (elevates) the hand above the heart.
- This can also help decrease swelling and pain.

❺ **Rest Versus Movement:**
- Movement is generally more healing in the long term than rest.
- Continue normal activities as much as your pain permits.
- If it really hurts to use the finger at all, you will need to see the doctor.

❻ **Expected Course:**
- Pain, swelling, and bruising usually start to get better 2-3 days after an injury.
- It may take 2 weeks for pain and tenderness of the injured area to go away.
- A fingernail bruise can take 6-12 weeks to go away. That is the amount of time needed for a nail to grow back completely. Sometimes the fingernail falls off.

❼ **Call Back If:**
- Pain becomes severe.
- Pain does not improve after 3 days.
- Pain or swelling lasts > 2 weeks.
- You become worse.

Treatment of a Minor Sprain (Jammed Finger)

❶ **Reassurance—Sprained Finger (Jammed, Overstretched):**
- Sprain is the medical terms used to describe overstretching of the ligaments of the finger. This can happen when the finger is twisted or bent in the wrong way. It can happen when the finger is "jammed," for example, when the end of a softball hits a finger.
- The main symptom is pain that is worse with movement. Swelling can occur. There is usually no bruising; if bruising is present it can be a sign that there is a small fracture.
- *Here is some care advice that should help.*

❷ **Apply a Cold Pack:**
- Apply a cold pack or an ice bag (wrapped in a moist towel) to the area for 20 minutes. Repeat in 1 hour, then every 4 hours while awake.
- Continue this for the first 48 hours after an injury.
- This will help decrease pain and swelling.

❸ **Apply Heat to the Area:**
- Beginning 48 hours after an injury, apply a warm washcloth or heating pad for 10 minutes 3 times a day.
- This will help increase blood flow and improve healing.

❹ **Buddy-Tape Splinting:**
- Protect your injured finger by "buddy-taping" it to the next finger.
- Use 2 pieces of tape. Place one around the base of both fingers. Place the other around the ends of both fingers.

❺ Rest Versus Movement:
- Movement is generally more healing in the long term than rest.
- Continue normal activities as much as your pain permits.
- If it really hurts to use the finger at all, you will need to see the doctor.

❻ Expected Course:
- Pain and swelling usually start to get better 2-3 days after an injury.
- Swelling most often is gone after 1 week.
- It may take 2 weeks for the pain and stiffness of the finger to go away.

❼ Call Back If:
- Pain becomes severe.
- Pain does not improve after 3 days.
- Pain or swelling lasts > 2 weeks.
- You become worse.

Treatment of a Small Cut or Scrape

❶ Reassurance—Superficial Laceration (Cut or Scratch) or Abrasion (Scrape):
- This sounds like a small cut or scrape that we can treat at home.
- *Here is some care advice that should help.*

❷ Bleeding: Apply direct pressure for 10 minutes with a sterile gauze to stop any bleeding.

❸ Cleaning the Wound:
- Wash the wound with soap and water for 5 minutes.
- For any dirt, scrub gently with a washcloth.
- For any bleeding, apply direct pressure with a sterile gauze or clean cloth for 10 minutes.

❹ Antibiotic Ointment:
- Apply an antibiotic ointment (e.g., OTC bacitracin), covered by a Band-Aid or dressing. Change daily or if it becomes wet.
- Option: A Telfa dressing won't stick to the wound when it is removed.
- Option: Another option is to use a liquid skin bandage that only needs to be applied once. Don't use antibiotic ointment if you use a liquid skin bandage.

❺ Liquid Skin Bandage:
- You can use a liquid skin bandage instead of antibiotic ointment and a dressing or a Band-Aid.
- **Benefits:** Liquid skin bandage has several benefits when compared with a regular bandage (e.g., a dressing or a Band-Aid). You only need to put a liquid bandage on once to minor cuts and scrapes. It helps stop minor bleeding. It seals the wound and may promote faster healing and lower infection rates. However, it also costs more.
- **How to Use It:** First clean and dry the wound. You put on the liquid as spray or with a swab. It dries in < 1 minute and usually lasts a week. You can get it wet.
- **Examples:** Liquid skin bandage is available over the counter. Examples are Band-Aid Liquid Bandage, New Skin, Curad Spray Bandage, and 3M No Sting Liquid Bandage Spray.

❻ Call Back If:
- Looks infected (pus, redness, increasing tenderness).
- Doesn't heal within 10 days.
- You become worse.

Treatment of a Torn Fingernail

❶ Reassurance—Torn Fingernail (From Catching It on Something):
- Symptoms are mild pain and a torn or cracked nail.
- *Here is some care advice that should help.*

❷ Trimming the Nail:
- For a cracked nail without rough edges, leave it alone.
- For a large flap of nail that is almost torn through, use a sterile scissors to cut it off along the line of the tear. This will keep the nail from catching on clothes or other things and tearing further.
- Apply an antibiotic ointment and cover with a Band-Aid. Change daily.

❸ Expected Course:
- After about 7 days, the nail bed should be covered by new skin and no longer hurt.
- It takes about 6-12 weeks for a fingernail to grow back completely.

❹ Call Back If:
- Looks infected (pus, redness, increasing tenderness).
- You become worse.

Over-the-counter Pain Medicines

❶ **Pain Medicines:**
- For pain relief, you can take either acetaminophen, ibuprofen, or naproxen.
- They are over-the-counter (OTC) pain drugs. You can buy them at the drugstore.

Acetaminophen (e.g., Tylenol):
- **Regular Strength Tylenol:** Take 650 mg (two 325 mg pills) by mouth every 4-6 hours as needed. Each Regular Strength Tylenol pill has 325 mg of acetaminophen.
- **Extra Strength Tylenol:** Take 1,000 mg (two 500 mg pills) every 8 hours as needed. Each Extra Strength Tylenol pill has 500 mg of acetaminophen.
- The most you should take each day is 3,000 mg (10 Regular Strength or 6 Extra Strength pills a day).

Ibuprofen (e.g., Motrin, Advil):
- Take 400 mg (two 200 mg pills) by mouth every 6 hours.
- Another choice is to take 600 mg (three 200 mg pills) by mouth every 8 hours.
- The most you should take each day is 1,200 mg (six 200 mg pills), unless your doctor has told you to take more.

Naproxen (e.g., Aleve):
- Take 220 mg (one 220 mg pill) by mouth every 8 hours as needed. You may take 440 mg (two 220 mg pills) for your first dose.
- The most you should take each day is 660 mg (three 220 mg pills a day), unless your doctor has told you to take more.

❷ **Pain Medicines—Extra Notes:**
- Use the lowest amount of medicine that makes your pain better.
- Acetaminophen is thought to be safer than ibuprofen or naproxen in people > 65 years old. Acetaminophen is in many OTC and prescription medicines. It might be in more than one medicine that you are taking. You need to be careful and not take an overdose. An acetaminophen overdose can hurt the liver.

- McNeil, the company that makes Tylenol, has different dosage instructions for Tylenol in Canada and the United States. In Canada, the maximum recommended dose per day is 4,000 mg or 12 Regular Strength (325 mg) pills. In the United States, McNeil recommends a maximum dose of 10 Regular Strength (325 mg) pills.
- CAUTION: Do not take acetaminophen if you have liver disease.
- CAUTION: Do not take ibuprofen or naproxen if you have stomach problems, have kidney disease, are pregnant, or have been told by your doctor to avoid this type of anti-inflammatory drug. Do not take ibuprofen or naproxen for > 7 days without consulting your doctor.
- *Before taking any medicine, read all the instructions on the package.*

❸ **Call Back If:**
- You have more questions.
- You become worse.

FIRST AID

First Aid Advice for Bleeding:
Apply direct pressure to the entire wound with a clean cloth.

First Aid Advice for Penetrating Object:
If penetrating object is still in place, don't remove it. *Reason: Removal could increase bleeding.*

First Aid Advice for Shock:
Lie down with the feet elevated.

First Aid Advice for a Sprain of the Finger:
- Remove any rings or jewelry from the injured finger.
- Tape the injured finger to the finger next to it (this is called a buddy splint).
- Apply a cold pack or an ice bag (wrapped in a moist towel) to the area for 20 minutes.

First Aid Advice for Suspected Fracture or Dislocation of the Finger:
- Remove any rings or jewelry from the injured finger.
- Tape the injured finger to the finger next to it (this is called a buddy splint).
- Apply a cold pack or an ice bag (wrapped in a moist towel) to the area for 20 minutes.

First Aid Advice for Transport of an Amputated Finger:
- Briefly rinse amputated part with water (to remove any dirt).
- Place amputated part in plastic bag (to protect and keep clean).
- Place plastic bag containing part in a cup of ice water (to keep cool and preserve tissue).

BACKGROUND

Type of Finger Injuries

❶ **Cuts, Abrasions (Skinned Knuckles), and Bruises:** The most common injuries.

❷ **Jammed Finger:**
- **Description:** The end of a straightened finger or thumb receives a blow (usually from a ball). The energy is absorbed by the ligaments (sprain) and the finger joints.
- For jammed fingers, always check carefully that the injured person can fully straighten (extend) the end of the finger. If the person cannot straighten the finger, the diagnosis may be a mallet finger.

❸ **Mallet Finger:**
- **Description:** The injured person will report that he or she is not able to straighten the end of the finger (DIP joint) completely.
- **Mechanism:** The most common mechanism is being "jammed" by a ball (e.g., playing softball without a glove).
- **Pathology:** This occurs because of either a tear of the extensor tendon at the DIP joint or an avulsion fracture where the extensor tendon attaches to the distal phalanx.

❹ **Crushed or Smashed Fingertip** (e.g., slammed door, machine accident):
- **Minor Injuries:** The most common injuries are bruising, a blood blister, or a small cut.
- **Moderate Injuries:** Lacerations of skin or nail bed that require suturing. Fractures of the fingertip (distal phalanx) can occur and are painful but usually not serious. There is a slight risk for osteomyelitis if there is an open wound overlying the fractured bone.
- **Major Injuries:** Severe crush injuries, amputation, or near-amputation.

❺ **Fingernail Injury:**
- Most fingernail injuries are not in and of themselves serious.
- **Nail Bed Laceration:** With significant crush injuries (e.g., slammed door, machine accident) a minor injury of the nail may be covering up a major laceration of the nail bed. If the nail bed is lacerated, suturing may be required to prevent a future deformed fingernail. Sometimes the surgeon or ED doctor will use the old nail during the repair; this is the reason the patient should bring the nail.

❻ **Finger Amputation:** Patients with this type of injury need to go to the ED. In some cases, reimplantation is possible. In most cases, a repair-revision of the remaining portion of the finger is the best surgical treatment.

❼ **Subungual Hematoma** (bruised fingernail):
- **Definition:** Bleeding under the nail.
- **Mechanism:** Usually caused by a crush injury from a door or a heavy object falling on the finger while it is on a firm surface.
- **Treatment of a Small Subungual Hematoma:** Small subungual hematomas have blood under < 50% of the nail. Pain is mild-moderate. Treatment consists of pain medications, application of cold packs, and time. After a couple days the pain will feel better. The bruising disappears over 2-4 weeks.
- **Treatment of a Large Subungual Hematoma:** Large subungual hematomas have blood under > 50% of the nail. Pain can be moderate-severe and throbbing. The doctor may need to drill (or burn) a tiny hole in the nail to reduce the pressure and to relieve pain. Additional treatment consists of pain medications and application of cold packs. Many of these patients will lose the nail sometime in the next couple weeks.

❽ Fractures or Dislocations:
- **Fractures:** Fractures of the finger can occur and are painful but usually not serious. If there is no deformity, most can be treated with a simple finger splint. There is a slight risk for osteomyelitis if there is an open wound overlying the fractured bone.
- **Dislocation:** The injured person will report pain and visible deformity of one of the finger joints. Treatment consists of reducing the dislocation and splinting.

What Cuts Need to Be Sutured?

- Any cut that is split open or gaping probably needs sutures (or staples or skin glue).
- Cuts > ½" (1 cm) usually need sutures.
- Any open wound that may need sutures should be evaluated by a physician regardless of the time that has passed since the initial injury.

When Does an Adult Need a Tetanus Booster (Tetanus Shot)?

- **Clean Cuts and Scrapes—Tetanus Booster Needed Every 10 Years:** Patients with clean minor wounds AND who have previously had ≥ 3 tetanus shots (full series) need a booster every 10 years. Examples of minor wounds include a superficial abrasion or a shallow cut from a clean knife blade. Obtain booster within 72 hours.
- **Dirty Wounds—Tetanus Booster Needed Every 5 Years:** Patients with dirty wounds need a booster if it has been > 5 years since the last booster. Examples of dirty wounds include those contaminated with soil, feces, and/or saliva and more serious wounds from deep punctures, crushing, and burns. Obtain booster within 72 hours.

FINGER PAIN

Definition
- Pain in the finger
- Not due to a traumatic injury

TRIAGE ASSESSMENT QUESTIONS

See More Appropriate Protocol
- ● Followed an injury
  Go to Protocol: Finger Injury on page 172
- ● Wound looks infected
  Go to Protocol: Wound Infection on page 443
- ● Caused by an animal bite
  Go to Protocol: Animal Bite on page 22
- ● Caused by frostbite
  Go to Protocol: Frostbite on page 186
- ● Hand or wrist pain is the main symptom
  Go to Protocol: Hand and Wrist Pain on page 193

Go to ED/UCC Now (or to Office With PCP Approval)
- ● Looks infected (spreading redness, red streak, pus) and severe pain with movement
  R/O: infectious tenosynovitis
- ● Patient sounds very sick or weak to the triager
  Reason: severe acute illness or serious complication suspected

Go to Office Now
- ● SEVERE pain (e.g., excruciating, unable use hand at all)
  R/O: gouty arthritis, felon, tenosynovitis

See Today in Office
- ● Looks infected (e.g., spreading redness, pus, red streak)
  R/O: early cellulitis, impetigo, gouty arthritis
- ● Yellow pus under skin around fingernail (cuticle) or pus under fingernail
  Reason: possible paronychia, incision and drainage may be needed
- ● Painful blisters on fingertip
  R/O: herpetic whitlow
- ● Numbness (i.e., loss of sensation) in hand or fingers of new onset
  R/O: neuropathy, cervical radiculopathy, herniated cervical disk, carpal tunnel syndrome

See Within 3 Days in Office
- ● MODERATE pain (e.g., interferes with normal activities) and present > 3 days
  R/O: arthritis, tendonitis, carpal tunnel syndrome
- ● Swollen joint and no fever or redness
  R/O: arthritis
- ● Redness and painful skin around fingernail (cuticle, nail fold)
  R/O: early paronychia
- ● Neck pain and pain shoots into fingers
  R/O: cervical radiculopathy, herniated disk
- ● Numbness or tingling is a chronic symptom (recurrent or ongoing AND present > 4 weeks)
  Reason: chronic problem
  R/O: peripheral neuropathy, carpal tunnel syndrome
- ● Patient wants to be seen

See Within 2 Weeks in Office
- ● MILD pain (e.g., does not interfere with normal activities) and present > 7 days
- ● Finger pain is a chronic symptom (recurrent or ongoing AND present > 4 weeks)
  R/O: arthritis, tendonitis, carpal tunnel syndrome
- ● Morning stiffness of fingers is a chronic symptom (recurrent or ongoing AND present > 4 weeks)
  R/O: degenerative arthritis
- ● Finger locking (gets stuck in one position) is a chronic symptom (recurrent or ongoing AND present > 4 weeks)
  R/O: trigger finger
- ● Caused or worsened by exposure to cold (eg, finger hurts and changes color when taking something out of freezer)
  R/O: Raynaud disease
- ● Caused or worsened by using computer keyboard and/or mouse
  R/O: carpal tunnel syndrome

Home Care
- ○ Finger pain
- ○ Caused by overuse from recent vigorous activity (e.g., repetitive motions, scrubbing, waxing)
  R/O: overuse injury, strain
- ○ Caused by bumping elbow and now has burning pain (or tingling) in hand and fingers
  R/O: bruised ulnar nerve ("funny bone")

HOME CARE ADVICE

Finger Pain—General Care Advice

❶ Reassurance:
- The symptoms you describe do not sound serious.
- You have told me that there is no joint swelling or fever. You told me that there are no signs of infection, like redness or pus. You also told me that there has been no recent major injury.
- *Here is some care advice that should help.*

❷ Pain Medicines:
- For pain relief, you can take either acetaminophen, ibuprofen, or naproxen.
- They are over-the-counter (OTC) pain drugs. You can buy them at the drugstore.

Acetaminophen (e.g., Tylenol):
- **Regular Strength Tylenol:** Take 650 mg (two 325 mg pills) by mouth every 4-6 hours as needed. Each Regular Strength Tylenol pill has 325 mg of acetaminophen.
- **Extra Strength Tylenol:** Take 1,000 mg (two 500 mg pills) every 8 hours as needed. Each Extra Strength Tylenol pill has 500 mg of acetaminophen.
- The most you should take each day is 3,000 mg (10 Regular Strength or 6 Extra Strength pills a day).

Ibuprofen (e.g., Motrin, Advil):
- Take 400 mg (two 200 mg pills) by mouth every 6 hours.
- Another choice is to take 600 mg (three 200 mg pills) by mouth every 8 hours.
- The most you should take each day is 1,200 mg (six 200 mg pills), unless your doctor has told you to take more.

Naproxen (e.g., Aleve):
- Take 220 mg (one 220 mg pill) by mouth every 8 hours as needed. You may take 440 mg (two 220 mg pills) for your first dose.
- The most you should take each day is 660 mg (three 220 mg pills a day), unless your doctor has told you to take more.

❸ Pain Medicines—Extra Notes:
- Use the lowest amount of medicine that makes your pain better.
- Acetaminophen is thought to be safer than ibuprofen or naproxen in people > 65 years old. Acetaminophen is in many OTC and prescription medicines. It might be in more than one medicine that you are taking. You need to be careful and not take an overdose. An acetaminophen overdose can hurt the liver.
- McNeil, the company that makes Tylenol, has different dosage instructions for Tylenol in Canada and the United States. In Canada, the maximum recommended dose per day is 4,000 mg or 12 Regular Strength (325 mg) pills. In the United States, McNeil recommends a maximum dose of 10 Regular Strength (325 mg) pills.
- CAUTION: Do not take acetaminophen if you have liver disease.
- CAUTION: Do not take ibuprofen or naproxen if you have stomach problems, have kidney disease, are pregnant, or have been told by your doctor to avoid this type of anti-inflammatory drug. Do not take ibuprofen or naproxen for > 7 days without consulting your doctor.
- *Before taking any medicine, read all the instructions on the package.*

❹ Expected Course:
- Most of the time mild finger pain will get better over 2-3 days and goes away within a week.
- If you do not get better during the next week, you will need an appointment to see the doctor.

❺ Call Back If:
- Fever occurs.
- Redness or swelling appears.
- Pain lasts > 7 days.
- You become worse.

Overuse Injury

❶ Reassurance—Overuse:

- It sounds like an overuse injury. We can treat that at home.
- Finger pain from joint irritation can occur following vigorous and repetitive activity using the hand (e.g., washing the car, scrubbing the floor).
- *Here is some care advice that should help.*

❷ Apply Cold to the Area:

- Apply a cold pack or an ice bag (wrapped in a moist towel) to the area for 20 minutes. Repeat in 1 hour, then every 4 hours while awake.
- Continue this for the first 48 hours after an injury. *(Reason: to reduce the swelling and pain)*

❸ Apply Heat to the Area:

- Beginning 48 hours after an injury, apply a warm washcloth or heating pad for 10 minutes 3 times a day.
- This will help increase blood flow and improve healing.

❹ Pain Medicines:

- For pain relief, you can take either acetaminophen, ibuprofen, or naproxen.
- They are over-the-counter (OTC) pain drugs. You can buy them at the drugstore.

Acetaminophen (e.g., Tylenol):
- **Regular Strength Tylenol:** Take 650 mg (two 325 mg pills) by mouth every 4-6 hours as needed. Each Regular Strength Tylenol pill has 325 mg of acetaminophen.
- **Extra Strength Tylenol:** Take 1,000 mg (two 500 mg pills) every 8 hours as needed. Each Extra Strength Tylenol pill has 500 mg of acetaminophen.
- The most you should take each day is 3,000 mg (10 Regular Strength or 6 Extra Strength pills a day).

Ibuprofen (e.g., Motrin, Advil):
- Take 400 mg (two 200 mg pills) by mouth every 6 hours.
- Another choice is to take 600 mg (three 200 mg pills) by mouth every 8 hours.
- The most you should take each day is 1,200 mg (six 200 mg pills), unless your doctor has told you to take more.

Naproxen (e.g., Aleve):
- Take 220 mg (one 220 mg pill) by mouth every 8 hours as needed. You may take 440 mg (two 220 mg pills) for your first dose.
- The most you should take each day is 660 mg (three 220 mg pills a day), unless your doctor has told you to take more.

❺ Pain Medicines—Extra Notes:

- Use the lowest amount of medicine that makes your pain better.
- Acetaminophen is thought to be safer than ibuprofen or naproxen in people > 65 years old. Acetaminophen is in many OTC and prescription medicines. It might be in more than one medicine that you are taking. You need to be careful and not take an overdose. An acetaminophen overdose can hurt the liver.
- McNeil, the company that makes Tylenol, has different dosage instructions for Tylenol in Canada and the United States. In Canada, the maximum recommended dose per day is 4,000 mg or 12 Regular Strength (325 mg) pills. In the United States, McNeil recommends a maximum dose of 10 Regular Strength (325 mg) pills.
- CAUTION: Do not take acetaminophen if you have liver disease.
- CAUTION: Do not take ibuprofen or naproxen if you have stomach problems, have kidney disease, are pregnant, or have been told by your doctor to avoid this type of anti-inflammatory drug. Do not take ibuprofen or naproxen for > 7 days without consulting your doctor.
- *Before taking any medicine, read all the instructions on the package.*

❻ Rest: You should try to avoid any exercise or activity that caused this pain for the next 3 days.

❼ Expected Course: For minor injuries, pain should get better over a 2- to 3-day period and go away within 1 week.

❽ Call Back If:

- Swelling or severe pain occurs.
- Pain lasts > 7 days.
- You become worse.

Bruised "Funny Bone"

❶ **Reassurance:**

- It sounds like a "bruised funny bone" that we can treat at home.
- A blow to the back of the elbow can cause numbness, tingling, and burning in the hand. The involved fingers are usually the middle, ring, and pinky (little).
- Your "funny bone" is actually a nerve (ulnar) which wraps around the back part of your elbow.

❷ **Expected Course:**

- Symptoms from "bruising your funny bone" usually last only a few minutes.
- If the symptoms last > 30 minutes, you should see your doctor.
- If this happens often, you should see your doctor.

❸ **Call Back If:**

- You become worse.

BACKGROUND

Common Causes

- Arthritis (e.g., degenerative, gouty, infectious, inflammatory, traumatic).
- **Carpal Tunnel Syndrome:** Caused by compression of the median nerve at the wrist. Numbness is typically noted in the thumb, index, and ring fingers. However, sometimes it can feel like the whole hand is numb. It is seen more commonly in people with diabetes, pregnancy, rheumatoid arthritis, and individuals whose jobs require repetitive wrist movements.
- Cellulitis.
- Overuse injury (tendonitis).
- Paronychia (infection of nail fold).
- Raynaud phenomenon (RP).
- Trauma (e.g., contusion, dislocation, fracture, sprain, strain).

Raynaud Phenomenon

- **General:** Normally when the body is exposed to cold, the blood vessels narrow. This helps decrease heat loss from the body. In patients who have RP, the blood vessels in the fingers or toes narrow in an exaggerated manner. The affected finger or toe first becomes pale (a "white attack") and then blue or purple in color (a "blue attack"). Often it starts with just one finger or toe but then can spread to others.
- **Causes:** Cold exposure, sometimes emotional stress.
- **Symptoms:** Color changes (pallor), "pins and needles" feeling, aching discomfort, clumsiness.
- **Prevention:** Patients with RP should avoid sudden exposure to the cold. Dressing warmly is important, as is wearing good mittens or gloves. Do not smoke; nicotine causes blood vessels to narrow.
- **Treatment:** Rewarming of the hands (or feet) can help end an attack of RP. Patients can place their fingers under their armpits. Even better, place the hands in warm water.

Caution: Some Signs of a Possibly Serious Problem

- Severe pain
- Red area with streak
  R/O: cellulitis with lymphangitis; common
- Joint swelling with fever
  R/O: septic arthritis; rare

FOOT PAIN

Definition
- Pain in the foot
- Not due to a traumatic injury

Pain Severity Scale
- **Mild (1-3):** Doesn't interfere with normal activities.
- **Moderate (4-7):** Interferes with normal activities (e.g., work or school), awakens from sleep, or limping.
- **Severe (8-10):** Excruciating pain, unable to do any normal activities, unable to walk.

TRIAGE ASSESSMENT QUESTIONS

See More Appropriate Protocol
- ● Followed an ankle or foot injury
  Go to Protocol: Ankle and Foot Injury on page 27
- ● Ankle pain is the main symptom
  Go to Protocol: Ankle Pain on page 31

Go to ED Now
- ● Entire foot is cool or blue in comparison to other foot
  R/O: iliofemoral arterial occlusion (ischemic foot)
- ● Purple or black skin on foot or toe
  R/O: iliofemoral arterial occlusion (ischemic foot or arterial emboli)

Go to ED/UCC Now
(or to Office With PCP Approval)
- ● Red area or streak and fever
  R/O: cellulitis, lymphangitis
  Note: It may be difficult to determine the rash color in people with darker-colored skin.
- ● Swollen foot and fever
  R/O: cellulitis
- ● Patient sounds very sick or weak to the triager
  Reason: severe acute illness or serious complication suspected

See Today in Office
- ● SEVERE pain (e.g., excruciating, unable to do any normal activities)
  R/O: forgotten trauma, ischemic foot, acute gouty arthritis
- ● Looks like a boil, infected sore, deep ulcer, or other infected rash (spreading redness, pus)
  R/O: abscess, cellulitis, ulcer
- ● Swollen foot
  (Exceptions: localized bump from bunions, calluses, insect bite, sting)
  R/O: forgotten trauma, cellulitis
- ● Numbness in one foot (i.e., loss of sensation)
  R/O: nerve root compression, herniated disk

See Within 3 Days in Office
- ● MODERATE pain (e.g., interferes with normal activities, limping) and present > 3 days
  R/O: sciatica, arthritis, stress fracture
- ● Numbness or tingling in feet and new or increased
  R/O: diabetic neuropathy
- ● Pain in the big toe joint
  R/O: acute gouty arthritis of first MTP joint
- ● Patient wants to be seen

See Within 2 Weeks in Office
- ● MILD pain (e.g., does not interfere with normal activities) and present > 7 days
  R/O: arthritis, Achilles tendonitis, plantar heel pain, bunions
- ● Foot pain is a chronic symptom (recurrent or ongoing AND lasting > 4 weeks)
  R/O: arthritis, Achilles tendonitis, plantar heel pain, callus
- ● Caused by known bunions, plantar wart, or flatfeet

Home Care
- ○ Foot pain
- ○ Caused by overuse from recent vigorous activity (e.g., aerobics, jogging/running, physical work, prolonged walking, sports)
  R/O: overuse injury
- ○ Caused by brief (now gone) muscle cramps in the foot
  R/O: muscle cramps, nocturnal cramps

HOME CARE ADVICE

Foot Pain and Overuse

❶ **Reassurance—Foot Pain:** The symptoms you describe do not sound serious. You have told me that there is no redness, swelling, or fever. You have also told me that there has been no recent major injury.

❷ **Reassurance—Overuse:**
- It sounds like an overuse injury.
- Foot pain and soreness are very common following vigorous activity. Such activities include sports like tennis and basketball, jogging, and certain types of work (lots of walking).

❸ **Aggravating Factors:** There are a number of things that can cause or aggravate foot pain:
- **Aging:** Foot pain is more common in the elderly. During the aging process, the feet widen and flatten, and the skin becomes drier.
- **Pregnancy:** Foot pain is more common in pregnant women. During pregnancy hormones cause the ligaments to relax, and the extra weight causes increased stress on the feet.
- **Obesity:** Foot pain is also more common in overweight individuals. Being overweight puts excess stress on the bones and soft tissues of the feet.
- **Overuse:** People that are in professions that require prolonged standing and walking commonly report foot pain.
- **Shoes:** Poorly fitting or overly tight shoes are the underlying cause of many painful foot conditions. High heels are bad for feet.

❹ **Pain Medicines:**
- For pain relief, you can take either acetaminophen, ibuprofen, or naproxen.
- They are over-the-counter (OTC) pain drugs. You can buy them at the drugstore.

Acetaminophen (e.g., Tylenol):
- **Regular Strength Tylenol:** Take 650 mg (two 325 mg pills) by mouth every 4-6 hours as needed. Each Regular Strength Tylenol pill has 325 mg of acetaminophen.
- **Extra Strength Tylenol:** Take 1,000 mg (two 500 mg pills) every 8 hours as needed. Each Extra Strength Tylenol pill has 500 mg of acetaminophen.
- The most you should take each day is 3,000 mg (10 Regular Strength or 6 Extra Strength pills a day).

Ibuprofen (e.g., Motrin, Advil):
- Take 400 mg (two 200 mg pills) by mouth every 6 hours.
- Another choice is to take 600 mg (three 200 mg pills) by mouth every 8 hours.
- The most you should take each day is 1,200 mg (six 200 mg pills), unless your doctor has told you to take more.

Naproxen (e.g., Aleve):
- Take 220 mg (one 220 mg pill) by mouth every 8 hours as needed. You may take 440 mg (two 220 mg pills) for your first dose.
- The most you should take each day is 660 mg (three 220 mg pills a day), unless your doctor has told you to take more.

❺ **Pain Medicines—Extra Notes:**
- Use the lowest amount of medicine that makes your pain better.
- Acetaminophen is thought to be safer than ibuprofen or naproxen in people > 65 years old. Acetaminophen is in many OTC and prescription medicines. It might be in more than one medicine that you are taking. You need to be careful and not take an overdose. An acetaminophen overdose can hurt the liver.
- McNeil, the company that makes Tylenol, has different dosage instructions for Tylenol in Canada and the United States. In Canada, the maximum recommended dose per day is 4,000 mg or 12 Regular Strength (325 mg) pills. In the United States, McNeil recommends a maximum dose of 10 Regular Strength (325 mg) pills.
- CAUTION: Do not take acetaminophen if you have liver disease.
- CAUTION: Do not take ibuprofen or naproxen if you have stomach problems, have kidney disease, are pregnant, or have been told by your doctor to avoid this type of anti-inflammatory drug. Do not take ibuprofen or naproxen for > 7 days without consulting your doctor.
- *Before taking any medicine, read all the instructions on the package.*

❻ **Call Back If:**
- Swelling, redness, or fever occur.
- Severe pain not relieved by pain medication.
- Pain lasts > 7 days.
- You become worse.

Muscle Cramps

❶ Reassurance—Muscle Cramps:
- Muscle cramps can occur in the feet.
- During attacks, break the muscle spasm by stretching the muscle in the direction opposite to how it is being pulled by the cramp or spasm. For example, for a foot cramp, pull the foot and toes backward as far as they will go.

❷ Expected Course:
- Muscle cramps usually last 5-30 minutes. Once the muscle cramp stops, the muscle quickly returns to normal. The pain should go away completely.
- If you have frequent muscle cramps, you may need to see your doctor. Sometimes the doctor can give medications to reduce the muscle cramps.

❸ Call Back If:
- Fever or redness occurs.
- Foot is cool or blue in comparison to other side.
- You become worse.

General Foot Care

❶ Keep Your Feet Healthy:
- Examine your feet on a regular basis. Check for sores, redness, and calluses.
- Avoid going barefoot in warm, damp places like locker rooms.
- Change your socks or hose daily or whenever they get damp.
- If you are overweight, work on losing weight.

❷ Keep Your Feet Clean:
- Wash your feet daily using a mild soap (e.g., Dove) and lukewarm water. Rinse off all soap.
- Dry your feet thoroughly, especially between the toes.
- Put a small amount of lotion (unscented with lanolin) on your feet after bathing; this will help seal moisture in the skin. Do not put lotion between your toes.

❸ Wear Shoes That Fit:
- Shoes should have a wide toe box, so that your toes do not feel cramped.
- The shoe's toe cap should be 0.25-0.5" (6-12 mm, or approximately one finger width) longer than the longest toe in the foot.
- Buy new shoes later in the day. *(Reason: Feet swell during the day and become larger.)*
- Avoid high heels. Heels should not be taller than 2" (5 cm).

❹ Wear the Right Shoe for the Right Activity:
- Wear running shoes for running.
- Wear the correct type of protective shoes for your workplace.

❺ Call Back If:
- You have more questions.

BACKGROUND

General Causes of Foot Pain
- Foot pain is common.
- **Aging:** Foot pain is more common in the elderly. During the aging process, the feet widen and flatten, and the skin becomes drier.
- **Pregnancy:** Foot pain is more common in pregnant women. During pregnancy hormones cause the ligaments to relax, and the extra weight causes increased stress on the feet.
- **Obesity:** Foot pain is also more common in overweight individuals. Being overweight puts excess stress on the bones and soft tissues of the feet.
- **Overuse:** People who are in professions that require prolonged standing and walking commonly report foot pain.
- **Shoes:** Poorly fitting or overly tight shoes are the underlying cause of many painful foot conditions. High heels are bad for feet.

Some Common Conditions Causing Heel Pain

- **Achilles Tendinitis:** This is an inflammation of the Achilles tendon where it attaches to the back of the heel bone. It can be caused by inadequate warming up and overuse.
- **Haglund Deformity (Pump Bump):** This is a bursitis that develops on the posterior aspect of the heel. It is caused by the pressure of the rim of the shoe rubbing up against the heel.
- **Heel Spurs:** These are bony growths on the underside of the heel bone where the plantar tendons attach. The pain is located on the front portion of the underside of the heel.
- **Plantar Fasciitis:** This is an inflammation of the band of connective tissue (fascia) that runs along the sole (plantar aspect) of the foot. This band of fascia runs from the heel to the ball of the foot.

Some Common Conditions Causing Arch and Ball of Foot Pain

- **Flatfeet:** Flatfeet (no arch) can be inherited or can develop in adulthood. When it develops in adulthood it is also called posterior tibial tendon dysfunction.
- **Bunion (Hallux Valgus):** An enlargement of the foot joint (first MTP) at the base of the big toe. The big toe angles inward and the joint protrudes outward. A bunion can be caused by poorly fitting shoes, can be inherited, or can sometimes develop without any known cause. It can be painful. Surgery by a podiatrist is sometimes needed.

- **Bunionette (Tailor's Bunion):** An enlargement of the foot joint (fifth MTP) at the base of the little toe. The little toe angles inward and the joint protrudes outward.
- **Calluses:** Areas of thickened skin on the bottom (sole) of the foot. They can be painful or painless. Poor fitting and overly tight shoes are the most common cause of this condition. The constant rubbing is what causes the skin to thicken.
- **Morton Neuroma:** This is a pinched nerve. The most common location is on the sole of the foot between the third and fourth metatarsals. It can be caused by wearing shoes that are too tight, which then squeeze the bones together.
- **Muscle Cramps:** Brief pains (1-15 minutes) may be due to muscle spasms. Foot or calf muscles are especially prone to cramps that awaken from sleep. The pain should resolve completely after an episode of muscle spasm. Muscle cramps can occur more commonly in pregnancy.
- **Plantar Fasciitis:** This is an inflammation of the band of connective tissue (fascia) that runs along the sole (plantar aspect) of the foot. This band of fascia runs from the heel to the ball of the foot.
- **Plantar Warts:** A plantar wart looks a lot like a callus on the sole of the foot. The difference is that it is caused by a viral infection. The skin is thickened and slightly raised and may contain tiny black specks. The black specks are thrombosed capillaries.
- **Stress Fracture:** This is a hairline partial fracture of the foot. Strenuous activities like jogging, high-impact aerobics, and hiking can cause this overuse injury.

FROSTBITE

Definition
- Frostbite is a cold injury to the skin.
- *Use this protocol only if the patient has symptoms that match Frostbite.*

Symptoms
- Numbness, tingling, and pain of frostbitten part.
- Frostbitten hand and fingers may feel stiff or clumsy.
- Significant pain occurs during rewarming.
- True frostbite causes white, hard, completely numb skin. It can cause serious skin damage and always requires medical attention after rewarming.
- Common sites for frostbite are the toes, fingers, nose, ears, and penis.

Frostbite Severity
- **Frostnip:** There is temporary numbness and tingling that goes away after rewarming. This is actually not true frostbite because there is no injury to the skin.
- **First Degree (Mild):** White and waxy (hard) while frozen; erythema and swelling persist after rewarming.
- **Second Degree:** Same as first degree, plus blisters with clear fluid that appear in 6-24 hours.
- **Third Degree (Severe):** Hemorrhagic blisters progressing to skin necrosis.
- **Fourth Degree:** Skin necrosis (tissue death), gangrene.

TRIAGE ASSESSMENT QUESTIONS

Call EMS 911 Now
- ● Unconscious
  R/O: moderate-severe hypothermia
  First Aid: Wrap adult in warm blankets.
- ● Slurred speech
  R/O: mild-moderate hypothermia
  First Aid: Wrap adult in warm blankets.
- ● Confused thinking
  R/O: mild-moderate hypothermia
  First Aid: Wrap adult in warm blankets.
- ● Stumbling or falling
  R/O: mild-moderate hypothermia
  First Aid: Wrap adult in warm blankets.

Go to ED Now
- ● Body temperature < 95° F (35° C) rectally or < 94° F (34.4° C) orally
  R/O: mild hypothermia
  First Aid: Wrap adult in warm blankets.
- ● Severe shivering that persists > 10 minutes after rewarming and drying
  R/O: mild hypothermia
  First Aid: Wrap adult in warm blankets.

Go to ED/UCC Now
(or to Office With PCP Approval)
- ● Patient sounds very sick or weak to the triager
  Reason: severe acute illness or serious complication suspected

Go to Office Now
- ● After hour of rewarming and skin color and sensation don't return to normal
  R/O: severe frostbite
- ● Looks infected (e.g., spreading redness, red streak, pus)
  R/O: cellulitis, lymphangitis
- ● Unusually severe cold exposure and any other symptoms

See Today in Office
- ◐ White, hard, completely numb skin (before rewarming)
  R/O: severe frostbite (especially of the fingers or toes)
- ◐ Frostbitten part develops blisters
  R/O: second-degree frostbite
- ◐ Patient wants to be seen

See Today or Tomorrow in Office
- ◐ No tetanus booster in > 5 years
  Reason: mild frostbite or frostnip, may need a tetanus booster shot (vaccine)
- ◐ No prior tetanus shot
  Reason: mild frostbite or frostnip, needs to get full tetanus vaccination (a series of 3 shots)

Home Care
- ○ Mild frostbite symptoms
  R/O: frostnip, mild frostbite

HOME CARE ADVICE

❶ **Frostbite Treatment—Rewarming:** Rewarm the area rapidly with wet heat:
- Move into a warm room.
- **For Frostbite of an Extremity** (e.g., fingers, toes): Place the frostbitten part in very warm water. A bathtub or sink is often the quickest approach. The water should be very warm (104° F-108° F, or 40° C-42° C) but not hot enough to burn. Immersion in this warm water should continue until a pink flush signals the return of blood flow to the frostbitten part (usually 30 minutes). At this point, the numbness should disappear.
- **For Frostbite of the Face** (e.g., ears, nose): Apply warm, wet washcloths to frostbitten area of the face. Continue doing this until a pink flush signals the return of blood flow to the frostbitten area (usually 30 minutes).
- With more severe frostbite, the last 10 minutes of rewarming is usually quite painful.
- If not using a tub, keep the rest of your body warm by covering yourself with plenty of blankets.

❷ **Frostbite Treatment—Common Mistakes:**
- A common error is to apply snow to the frostbitten area or to massage it. Both can cause damage to thawing tissues.
- Do not rewarm with dry heat, such as a heat lamp or electric heater, because frostbitten skin cannot sense burning.
- Do not rewarm if there is a high likelihood of refreezing in the next couple hours. Freezing-warming-freezing causes more damage than freezing-warming.

❸ **Drink Warm Liquids:** Drink warm liquids (e.g., hot chocolate).

❹ **Pain Medicines:**
- For pain relief, you can take either acetaminophen, ibuprofen, or naproxen.
- They are over-the-counter (OTC) pain drugs. You can buy them at the drugstore.

Acetaminophen (e.g., Tylenol):
- **Regular Strength Tylenol:** Take 650 mg (two 325 mg pills) by mouth every 4-6 hours as needed. Each Regular Strength Tylenol pill has 325 mg of acetaminophen.
- **Extra Strength Tylenol:** Take 1,000 mg (two 500 mg pills) every 8 hours as needed. Each Extra Strength Tylenol pill has 500 mg of acetaminophen.
- The most you should take each day is 3,000 mg (10 Regular Strength or 6 Extra Strength pills a day).

Ibuprofen (e.g., Motrin, Advil):
- Take 400 mg (two 200 mg pills) by mouth every 6 hours.
- Another choice is to take 600 mg (three 200 mg pills) by mouth every 8 hours.
- The most you should take each day is 1,200 mg (six 200 mg pills), unless your doctor has told you to take more.

Naproxen (e.g., Aleve):
- Take 220 mg (one 220 mg pill) by mouth every 8 hours as needed. You may take 440 mg (two 220 mg pills) for your first dose.
- The most you should take each day is 660 mg (three 220 mg pills a day), unless your doctor has told you to take more.

❺ **Pain Medicines—Extra Notes:**
- Use the lowest amount of medicine that makes your pain better.
- Acetaminophen is thought to be safer than ibuprofen or naproxen in people > 65 years old. Acetaminophen is in many OTC and prescription medicines. It might be in more than one medicine that you are taking. You need to be careful and not take an overdose. An acetaminophen overdose can hurt the liver.
- McNeil, the company that makes Tylenol, has different dosage instructions for Tylenol in Canada and the United States. In Canada, the maximum recommended dose per day is 4,000 mg or 12 Regular Strength (325 mg) pills. In the United States, McNeil recommends a maximum dose of 10 Regular Strength (325 mg) pills.
- CAUTION: Do not take acetaminophen if you have liver disease.
- CAUTION: Do not take ibuprofen or naproxen if you have stomach problems, have kidney disease, are pregnant, or have been told by your doctor to avoid this type of anti-inflammatory drug. Do not take ibuprofen or naproxen for > 7 days without consulting your doctor.
- *Before taking any medicine, read all the instructions on the package.*

❻ **Aloe Vera Ointment:** Apply aloe vera ointment to the area of frostbite twice daily for 5 days.

❼ **Tetanus Booster for Frostbite:** If your last tetanus shot was given > 5 years ago, you need a booster.

❽ **Call Back If:**
- Color and sensation do not return to normal after 1 hour of rewarming.
- Frostbitten part develops blisters.
- You become worse.

FIRST AID

First Aid Advice for Hypothermia:
- Remove wet clothing.
- Wrap in warm blankets (or clothing, sleeping bag, even newspaper).
- Move into a warm space (e.g., home, building, car, tent).

First Aid Advice for Frostbite:
Rewarm the frostbitten area rapidly with wet heat.
- Move into a warm room.
- **For Frostbite of an Extremity** (e.g., fingers, toes): Place the frostbitten part in very warm water. A bathtub or sink is often the quickest approach. The water should be very warm (104° F-108° F, or 40° C-42° C) but not hot enough to burn. Immersion in this warm water should continue until a pink flush signals the return of circulation to the frostbitten part (usually 30 minutes).
- **For Frostbite of the Face** (e.g., ears, nose): Apply warm, wet washcloths to frostbitten area of the face. Continue doing this until a pink flush signals the return of circulation to the frostbitten area (usually 30 minutes).

Note: Do not rewarm a frostbitten area if there is a chance of refreezing.

BACKGROUND

Key Points
- Frostbite and hypothermia are 2 distinct and independent medical problems.
- **Frostbite** results from a cold injury to the skin. The body's core temperature can be normal. In frostbite, the nerves, blood vessels, and skin cells of a part of the body are temporarily frozen. The ears, nose, penis, fingers, and toes are most commonly affected.

- In contrast, **hypothermia** signifies a marked decrease in the body's core temperature, and frostbite may not be present. Hypothermia is defined as a body temperature < 95° F (35° C) rectally and can be fatal without intervention.

Factors Contributing to Frostbite
- **Alcohol, Mental Illness:** Impairs judgment and reduces normal self-protective actions.
- **Medical Conditions:** A number of medical conditions predispose to frostbite. Patients with diabetes, congestive heart failure, peripheral vascular condition, Raynaud disease, and previous frostbite are all at greater risk.
- **Type of Contact:** The frostbite is much worse if the skin and clothing are also wet at the time of cold exposure. Touching bare hands to cold metal and volatile products (like gasoline) stored outside during freezing weather can cause immediate frostbite.
- **Duration of Contact:** The longer the cold exposure, the greater both the heat loss and the likelihood of frostbite. The wind velocity on a cold day (windchill index) also determines how quickly frostbite occurs.

Frostbite Prevention—General
- Change wet gloves or socks immediately.
- Set limits on the time spent outdoors when the windchill temperature falls < 0° F (–17.8° C).
- Know the earliest warnings of frostbite. Pain, tingling, and numbness are signals from your body that you are not dressed adequately for the weather and that you need to go indoors.

Frostbite Prevention—Clothing
- **Clothing:** Dress in layers for cold weather. The first layer should be long underwear, preferably made of polypropylene or polyester (wicks moisture away from skin). The middle layer(s) should be fleece or wool. The outer layer serves as a windbreaker and also needs to be waterproof. The layers should be loose, not tight.
- **Hand Protection:** Mittens are warmer than gloves. You may wish to wear a thin glove under the mitten.
- **Footwear:** Avoid tight shoes that might interfere with circulation. Wear 1-2 pairs of socks made from wool or a wool blend. You may also wish to wear a thin liner sock made from polyester or polypropylene (wicks away moisture) under the wool socks.
- **Headwear:** Wear a hat because, during cold weather, > 50% of heat loss can occur from the head. Keep your ears covered.

HAND AND WRIST INJURY

Definition

- Injuries to a bone, muscle, joint, or ligament in the hand.
- Associated skin and soft tissue injuries are also included.

TRIAGE ASSESSMENT QUESTIONS

Call EMS 911 Now

- Major bleeding (actively dripping or spurting) that can't be stopped
  First Aid: Apply direct pressure to the entire wound with a clean cloth.
- Amputation or bone sticking through the skin
  First Aid: Apply direct pressure to the entire wound with a clean cloth.
- Sounds like a life-threatening emergency to the triager

See More Appropriate Protocol

- Finger injury is main concern
  Go to Protocol: Finger Injury on page 172
- Caused by an animal bite
  Go to Protocol: Animal Bite on page 22
- Wound looks infected
  Go to Protocol: Wound Infection on page 443

Go to ED Now

- Bullet, stabbed by knife, or other serious penetrating wound
  First Aid: If penetrating object is still in place, don't remove it.
- High-pressure injection injury (e.g., from paint gun, usually work related)
  Reason: deep tissue damage may exceed superficial injury

Go to ED/UCC Now
(or to Office With PCP Approval)

- Looks like a broken bone or dislocated joint (crooked or deformed)
  R/O: fracture, dislocation
- Skin is split open or gaping (length > ½" or 12 mm)
  Reason: may need laceration repair (e.g., sutures)

- Bleeding won't stop after 10 minutes of direct pressure (using correct technique)
- Dirt in the wound and not removed after 15 minutes of scrubbing
  Reason: needs irrigation or debridement
- Numbness (loss of sensation) of finger(s)
  R/O: nerve injury
- Sounds like a serious injury to the triager

Go to Office Now

- Looks infected (e.g., spreading redness, pus, red streak)
  R/O: cellulitis, lymphangitis

See Today in Office

- SEVERE pain (e.g., excruciating)
  R/O: fracture, severe sprain
- Large swelling or bruise and size > palm of person's hand
  R/O: fracture, large contusion
- Patient wants to be seen

See Today or Tomorrow in Office

- Injury interferes with work or school
- High-risk adult (e.g., age > 60, osteoporosis, chronic steroid use)
  Reason: greater risk of fracture in patients with osteoporosis
- Wound and no tetanus booster in > 5 years (or > 10 years for clean cuts)
  Reason: may need a tetanus booster shot (vaccine)
- Suspicious history for the injury
  R/O: domestic violence or elder abuse

See Within 3 Days in Office

- Injury and pain has not improved after 3 days
- Injury is still painful or swollen after 2 weeks

Home Care

- Minor wrist or hand injury
  R/O: bruise, strain, or sprain

HOME CARE ADVICE

Treatment of a Minor Bruise, Sprain, or Strain

❶ **Reassurance—Direct Blow (Contusion, Bruise):**
- A direct blow to your hand or wrist can cause a contusion. Contusion is the medical term for bruise.
- Symptoms are mild pain, swelling, and/or bruising.
- *Here is some care advice that should help.*

❷ **Reassurance—Bending or Twisting Injury (Strain, Sprain):**
- Strain and sprain are the medical terms used to describe overstretching of the muscles and ligaments of the hand or wrist. A twisting or bending injury can cause a strain or sprain.
- The main symptom is pain that is worse with movement. Swelling can occur.
- *Here is some care advice that should help.*

❸ **Apply a Cold Pack:**
- Apply a cold pack or an ice bag (wrapped in a moist towel) to the area for 20 minutes. Repeat in 1 hour, then every 4 hours while awake.
- Continue this for the first 48 hours after an injury.
- This will help decrease pain and swelling.

❹ **Apply Heat to the Area:**
- Beginning 48 hours after an injury, apply a warm washcloth or heating pad for 10 minutes 3 times a day.
- This will help increase blood flow and improve healing.

❺ **Wrap With an Elastic Bandage:**
- Wrap the injured part with a snug elastic bandage for 48 hours.
- The pressure from the bandage can make it feel better and help prevent swelling.
- If your start to get numbness or tingling of your hand or fingers, the bandage may be too tight. Loosen the bandage wrap.

❻ **Elevate the Arm:**
- Lay down and put your arm on a pillow. This puts (elevates) the hand and wrist above the heart.
- Do this for 15-20 minutes, 2-3 times a day, for the first 2 days.
- This can also help decrease swelling, bruising, and pain.

❼ **Rest Versus Movement:**
- Movement is generally more healing in the long term than rest.
- Continue normal activities as much as your pain permits.
- Avoid heavy lifting and active sports for 1-2 weeks or until the pain and swelling are gone.
- Complete rest should only be used for the first day or two after an injury. If it really hurts to use the hand at all, you will need to see the doctor.

❽ **Expected Course:**
- Pain, swelling, and bruising usually start to get better 2-3 days after an injury.
- Swelling most often is gone after 1 week.
- Bruises fade away slowly over 1-2 weeks.
- It may take 2 weeks for pain and tenderness of the injured area to go away.

❾ **Call Back If:**
- Pain becomes severe.
- Pain does not improve after 3 days.
- Pain or swelling lasts > 2 weeks.
- You become worse.

Treatment of a Small Cut or Scrape

❶ **Reassurance—Superficial Laceration (Cut or Scratch) or Abrasion (Scrape):**
- This sounds like a small cut or scrape that we can treat at home.
- *Here is some care advice that should help.*

❷ **Bleeding:** Apply direct pressure for 10 minutes with a sterile gauze to stop any bleeding.

❸ **Cleaning the Wound:**
- Wash the wound with soap and water for 5 minutes.
- For any dirt, scrub gently with a washcloth.
- For any bleeding, apply direct pressure with a sterile gauze or clean cloth for 10 minutes.

❹ **Antibiotic Ointment:**
- Apply an antibiotic ointment (e.g., OTC bacitracin), covered by a Band-Aid or dressing. Change daily or if it becomes wet.
- Option: A Telfa dressing won't stick to the wound when it is removed.
- Option: Another option is to use a liquid skin bandage that only needs to be applied once. Don't use antibiotic ointment if you use a liquid skin bandage.

❺ **Liquid Skin Bandage:**
- You can use a liquid skin bandage instead of antibiotic ointment and a dressing or a Band-Aid.
- **Benefits:** Liquid skin bandage has several benefits when compared with a regular bandage (e.g., a dressing or a Band-Aid). You only need to put a liquid bandage on once to minor cuts and scrapes. It helps stop minor bleeding. It seals the wound and may promote faster healing and lower infection rates. However, it also costs more.
- **How to Use It:** First clean and dry the wound. You put on the liquid as spray or with a swab. It dries in < 1 minute and usually lasts a week. You can get it wet.
- **Examples:** Liquid skin bandage is available over-the-counter. Examples are Band-Aid Liquid Bandage, New Skin, Curad Spray Bandage, and 3M No Sting Liquid Bandage Spray.

❻ **Call Back If:**
- Looks infected (pus, redness, increasing tenderness).
- Doesn't heal within 10 days.
- You become worse.

Over-the-counter Pain Medicines

❶ **Pain Medicines:**
- For pain relief, you can take either acetaminophen, ibuprofen, or naproxen.
- They are over-the-counter (OTC) pain drugs. You can buy them at the drugstore.

Acetaminophen (e.g., Tylenol):
- **Regular Strength Tylenol:** Take 650 mg (two 325 mg pills) by mouth every 4-6 hours as needed. Each Regular Strength Tylenol pill has 325 mg of acetaminophen.
- **Extra Strength Tylenol:** Take 1,000 mg (two 500 mg pills) every 8 hours as needed. Each Extra Strength Tylenol pill has 500 mg of acetaminophen.
- The most you should take each day is 3,000 mg (10 Regular Strength or 6 Extra Strength pills a day).

Ibuprofen (e.g., Motrin, Advil):
- Take 400 mg (two 200 mg pills) by mouth every 6 hours.
- Another choice is to take 600 mg (three 200 mg pills) by mouth every 8 hours.
- The most you should take each day is 1,200 mg (six 200 mg pills), unless your doctor has told you to take more.

Naproxen (e.g., Aleve):
- Take 220 mg (one 220 mg pill) by mouth every 8 hours as needed. You may take 440 mg (two 220 mg pills) for your first dose.
- The most you should take each day is 660 mg (three 220 mg pills a day), unless your doctor has told you to take more.

❷ **Pain Medicines—Extra Notes:**
- Use the lowest amount of medicine that makes your pain better.
- Acetaminophen is thought to be safer than ibuprofen or naproxen in people > 65 years old. Acetaminophen is in many OTC and prescription medicines. It might be in more than one medicine that you are taking. You need to be careful and not take an overdose. An acetaminophen overdose can hurt the liver.
- McNeil, the company that makes Tylenol, has different dosage instructions for Tylenol in Canada and the United States. In Canada, the maximum recommended dose per day is 4,000 mg or 12 Regular Strength (325 mg) pills. In the United States, McNeil recommends a maximum dose of 10 Regular Strength (325 mg) pills.
- CAUTION: Do not take acetaminophen if you have liver disease.
- CAUTION: Do not take ibuprofen or naproxen if you have stomach problems, have kidney disease, are pregnant, or have been told by your doctor to avoid this type of anti-inflammatory drug. Do not take ibuprofen or naproxen for > 7 days without consulting your doctor.
- *Before taking any medicine, read all the instructions on the package.*

❸ **Call Back If:**
- You have more questions.
- You become worse.

FIRST AID

First Aid Advice for Bleeding:
Apply direct pressure to the entire wound with a clean cloth.

First Aid Advice for Severe Bleeding:
- Place 2 or 3 sterile dressings (or a clean towel or washcloth) over the wound immediately.
- Apply direct pressure to the wound, using your entire hand.
- If bleeding continues, apply pressure more forcefully or move the pressure to a slightly different spot.
- Act quickly because ongoing blood loss can cause shock.
- Do not use a tourniquet.

First Aid Advice for Penetrating Object:
If penetrating object is still in place, don't remove it. *Reason: Removal could increase bleeding.*

First Aid Advice for Shock:
Lie down with the feet elevated.

First Aid Advice for a Sprain or Twisting Injury of Hand or Wrist:
- Apply a cold pack or an ice bag (wrapped in a moist towel) to the area for 20 minutes.
- Wrap area with an elastic bandage.

First Aid Advice for Suspected Fracture or Dislocation of Hand or Wrist:
- Immobilize the hand and wrist by placing them on a rigid splint (e.g., small board, magazine folded in half, folded-up newspaper).
- Tie several cloth strips around hand/wrist to keep the splint in place.
- Place injured arm in a sling. If no sling is available, victim can support the injured arm with the other non-injured hand.
- **Option—Soft Splint:** Immobilize the hand and wrist by wrapping them with a soft splint (e.g., pillow, rolled-up blanket, towel). Use tape to keep this splint in place.

Transport of an Amputated Body Part:
- Briefly rinse amputated part with water (to remove any dirt).
- Place amputated part in plastic bag (to protect and keep clean).
- Place plastic bag containing part in a container of ice (to keep cool and preserve tissue).

BACKGROUND

Types of Hand Injuries
- Fractures (broken bones)
- Dislocations (bone out of joint)
- **Sprains:** Stretches and tears of ligaments
- **Strains:** Stretches and tears of muscles (e.g., pulled muscle)
- Muscle overuse injuries from sports or exercise (e.g., strain, bursitis, tendonitis)
- Muscle bruise from a direct blow (e.g., contusion)

What Cuts Need to Be Sutured?
- Any cut that is split open or gaping probably needs sutures (or staples or skin glue).
- Cuts > ½" (1 cm) usually need sutures.
- Any open wound that may need sutures should be evaluated by a physician regardless of the time that has passed since the initial injury.

When Does an Adult Need a Tetanus Booster (Tetanus Shot)?
- **Clean Cuts and Scrapes—Tetanus Booster Needed Every 10 Years:** Patients with clean minor wounds AND who have previously had ≥ 3 tetanus shots (full series) need a booster every 10 years. Examples of minor wounds include a superficial abrasion or a shallow cut from a clean knife blade. Obtain booster within 72 hours.
- **Dirty Wounds—Tetanus Booster Needed Every 5 Years:** Patients with dirty wounds need a booster if it has been more than 5 years since the last booster. Examples of dirty wounds include those contaminated with soil, feces, and/or saliva and more serious wounds from deep punctures, crushing, and burns. Obtain booster within 72 hours.

HAND AND WRIST PAIN

Definition
- Pain in the hand or wrist.
- Not due to a traumatic injury.
- Minor muscle strain and overuse are covered in this protocol.

Pain Severity Scale
- **Mild (1-3):** Doesn't interfere with normal activities.
- **Moderate (4-7):** Interferes with normal activities (e.g., work or school) or awakens from sleep.
- **Severe (8-10):** Excruciating pain, unable to use hand at all.

TRIAGE ASSESSMENT QUESTIONS

Call EMS 911 Now
- Similar pain previously and it was from "heart attack"
  R/O: cardiac ischemia, myocardial infarction
- Similar pain previously from "angina" and not relieved by nitroglycerin
  R/O: cardiac ischemia
- Sounds like a life-threatening emergency to the triager

See More Appropriate Protocol
- Followed a hand or wrist injury
  Go to Protocol: Hand and Wrist Injury on page 189
- Chest pain
  Go to Protocol: Chest Pain on page 73
- Caused by an animal bite
  Go to Protocol: Animal Bite on page 22
- Wound looks infected
  Go to Protocol: Wound Infection on page 443

Go to ED/UCC Now (or to Office With PCP Approval)
- Fever and red area (or area very tender to touch)
  R/O: cellulitis, lymphangitis
- Fever and swollen joint
  R/O: septic arthritis, cellulitis
- Patient sounds very sick or weak to the triager
  Reason: severe acute illness or serious complication suspected

Go to Office Now
- SEVERE pain (e.g., excruciating, unable to use hand at all)
  R/O: unwitnessed trauma, inflammatory arthritis
- Red area or streak and large (> 2" or 5 cm)
  R/O: cellulitis, erysipelas, lymphangitis
  Note: It may be difficult to determine the rash color in people with darker-colored skin.

See Today in Office
- Weakness (i.e., loss of strength) of new onset in hand or fingers
  R/O: herniated cervical disk
  (Exception: not truly weak, hand feels weak because of pain)
  Note: This question describes a patient with both hand pain and weakness. In contrast, a stroke patient will have sudden onset of painless weakness.
- Numbness (i.e., loss of sensation) of new onset in hand or fingers
  R/O: neuropathy, cervical radiculopathy, herniated cervical disk, carpal tunnel syndrome
  Exception: slight tingling; numbness present > 2 weeks
  Note: This question describes a patient with both hand pain and numbness. In contrast, a stroke patient will have sudden onset of painless numbness/weakness.
- Looks like a boil, infected sore, deep ulcer, or other infected rash (spreading redness, pus)
  R/O: impetigo, abscess, cellulitis
- Localized rash is very painful (no fever)
  R/O: early cellulitis, bee sting, inflammatory arthritis

See Within 3 Days in Office
- MODERATE pain (e.g., interferes with normal activities) and present > 3 days
  R/O: arthritis, tendonitis, carpal tunnel syndrome
- Weakness or numbness in hand or fingers and present > 2 weeks
  R/O: tendonitis, carpal tunnel syndrome, cervical radiculopathy
  Reason: chronic symptoms
- Pain is worsened or caused by bending the neck
  R/O: cervical radiculopathy, herniated cervical disk

● Pain is worsened by using computer keyboard and/or mouse
R/O: carpal tunnel syndrome
● Swollen joint of new onset
R/O: inflammatory arthritis
● Patient wants to be seen

See Within 2 Weeks in Office

● MILD pain (e.g., does not interfere with normal activities) and present > 7 days
● Morning stiffness of hand(s) is a chronic symptom (recurrent or ongoing AND lasting > 4 weeks)
R/O: degenerative or inflammatory arthritis
● Hand or wrist pain is a chronic symptom (recurrent or ongoing AND lasting > 4 weeks)
R/O: arthritis, tendonitis, carpal tunnel syndrome

Home Care

○ Caused by bumping elbow and had brief (now gone) burning pain shooting (radiating) into hand and fingers
R/O: "bruised funny bone"
○ Caused by overuse injury from recent vigorous activity (e.g., sports, repetitive motions, heavy lifting)
R/O: muscle strain, overuse, tendinitis
○ Hand or wrist pain

HOME CARE ADVICE

Muscle Strain and Overuse

❶ **Reassurance:**
  • Muscle strain and irritation are very common following vigorous activity (e.g., throwing a ball, playing tennis), repetitive forceful motions (e.g., washing the car, scrubbing the floor), or heavy lifting.
  • *Here is some care advice that should help.*

❷ **Apply Cold to the Area for First 48 Hours:**
  • Apply a cold pack or an ice bag (wrapped in a moist towel) to the area for 20 minutes. Repeat in 1 hour, then every 4 hours while awake.
  • Continue this for the first 48 hours after an injury.
  (Reason: to reduce the swelling and pain)

❸ **Apply Heat to the Area:**
  • Beginning 48 hours after an injury, apply a warm washcloth or heating pad for 10 minutes 3 times a day.
  • This will help increase blood flow and improve healing.

❹ **Rest:** You should try to avoid any exercise or activity that caused this pain for the next 3 days.

❺ **Pain Medicines:**
  • For pain relief, you can take either acetaminophen, ibuprofen, or naproxen.
  • They are over-the-counter (OTC) pain drugs. You can buy them at the drugstore.

Acetaminophen (e.g., Tylenol):
  • **Regular Strength Tylenol:** Take 650 mg (two 325 mg pills) by mouth every 4-6 hours as needed. Each Regular Strength Tylenol pill has 325 mg of acetaminophen.
  • **Extra Strength Tylenol:** Take 1,000 mg (two 500 mg pills) every 8 hours as needed. Each Extra Strength Tylenol pill has 500 mg of acetaminophen.
  • The most you should take each day is 3,000 mg (10 Regular Strength or 6 Extra Strength pills a day).

Ibuprofen (e.g., Motrin, Advil):
  • Take 400 mg (two 200 mg pills) by mouth every 6 hours.
  • Another choice is to take 600 mg (three 200 mg pills) by mouth every 8 hours.
  • The most you should take each day is 1,200 mg (six 200 mg pills), unless your doctor has told you to take more.

Naproxen (e.g., Aleve):
  • Take 220 mg (one 220 mg pill) by mouth every 8 hours as needed. You may take 440 mg (two 220 mg pills) for your first dose.
  • The most you should take each day is 660 mg (three 220 mg pills a day), unless your doctor has told you to take more.

❻ Pain Medicines—Extra Notes:
- Use the lowest amount of medicine that makes your pain better.
- Acetaminophen is thought to be safer than ibuprofen or naproxen in people > 65 years old. Acetaminophen is in many OTC and prescription medicines. It might be in more than one medicine that you are taking. You need to be careful and not take an overdose. An acetaminophen overdose can hurt the liver.
- McNeil, the company that makes Tylenol, has different dosage instructions for Tylenol in Canada and the United States. In Canada, the maximum recommended dose per day is 4,000 mg or 12 Regular Strength (325 mg) pills. In the United States, McNeil recommends a maximum dose of 10 Regular Strength (325 mg) pills.
- CAUTION: Do not take acetaminophen if you have liver disease.
- CAUTION: Do not take ibuprofen or naproxen if you have stomach problems, have kidney disease, are pregnant, or have been told by your doctor to avoid this type of anti-inflammatory drug. Do not take ibuprofen or naproxen for > 7 days without consulting your doctor.
- *Before taking any medicine, read all the instructions on the package.*

❼ Expected Course: For minor injuries, pain should improve over a 2- to 3-day period and disappear within 7 days.

❽ Call Back If:
- Moderate pain (e.g., interferes with normal activities) lasts > 3 days.
- Mild pain lasts > 7 days.
- Arm swelling occurs.
- Signs of infection occur (e.g., spreading redness, warmth, fever).
- You become worse.

Bruised "Funny Bone"

❶ Reassurance:
- It sounds like a "bruised funny bone" that we can treat at home.
- A blow to the back of the elbow can cause numbness, tingling, and burning in the hand. The involved fingers are usually the middle, ring, and pinky (little).
- Your "funny bone" is actually a nerve (ulnar) which wraps around the back part of your elbow.

❷ Expected Course: Symptoms from bruising your funny bone usually last only a few minutes. If the symptoms last > 30 minutes or if this problem seems to happen to you frequently, you should see your doctor for evaluation.

❸ Call Back If: You become worse.

Hand and Wrist Pain—General Care Advice

❶ Reassurance: Hand and wrist pain can be caused by strained muscles, tendonitis, and mild arthritis.

❷ Pain Medicines:
- For pain relief, you can take either acetaminophen, ibuprofen, or naproxen.
- They are over-the-counter (OTC) pain drugs. You can buy them at the drugstore.

Acetaminophen (e.g., Tylenol):
- **Regular Strength Tylenol:** Take 650 mg (two 325 mg pills) by mouth every 4-6 hours as needed. Each Regular Strength Tylenol pill has 325 mg of acetaminophen.
- **Extra Strength Tylenol:** Take 1,000 mg (two 500 mg pills) every 8 hours as needed. Each Extra Strength Tylenol pill has 500 mg of acetaminophen.
- The most you should take each day is 3,000 mg (10 Regular Strength or 6 Extra Strength pills a day).

Ibuprofen (e.g., Motrin, Advil):
- Take 400 mg (two 200 mg pills) by mouth every 6 hours.
- Another choice is to take 600 mg (three 200 mg pills) by mouth every 8 hours.
- The most you should take each day is 1,200 mg (six 200 mg pills), unless your doctor has told you to take more.

Naproxen (e.g., Aleve):

- Take 220 mg (one 220 mg pill) by mouth every 8 hours as needed. You may take 440 mg (two 220 mg pills) for your first dose.
- The most you should take each day is 660 mg (three 220 mg pills a day), unless your doctor has told you to take more.

❸ **Pain Medicines—Extra Notes:**

- Use the lowest amount of medicine that makes your pain better.
- Acetaminophen is thought to be safer than ibuprofen or naproxen in people > 65 years old. Acetaminophen is in many OTC and prescription medicines. It might be in more than one medicine that you are taking. You need to be careful and not take an overdose. An acetaminophen overdose can hurt the liver.
- McNeil, the company that makes Tylenol, has different dosage instructions for Tylenol in Canada and the United States. In Canada, the maximum recommended dose per day is 4,000 mg or 12 Regular Strength (325 mg) pills. In the United States, McNeil recommends a maximum dose of 10 Regular Strength (325 mg) pills.
- CAUTION: Do not take acetaminophen if you have liver disease.
- CAUTION: Do not take ibuprofen or naproxen if you have stomach problems, have kidney disease, are pregnant, or have been told by your doctor to avoid this type of anti-inflammatory drug. Do not take ibuprofen or naproxen for > 7 days without consulting your doctor.
- *Before taking any medicine, read all the instructions on the package.*

❹ **Call Back If:**

- Moderate pain (e.g., interferes with normal activities) lasts > 3 days.
- Mild pain lasts > 7 days.
- Signs of infection occur (e.g., spreading redness, warmth, fever).
- You become worse.

BACKGROUND

Causes

- **Arthritis** (e.g., degenerative, gouty, infectious, inflammatory, traumatic).
- **Carpal Tunnel Syndrome:** Caused by compression of the median nerve at the wrist. Numbness is typically noted in the thumb, index, and ring fingers but may be poorly localized. It is seen more commonly in people with diabetes, pregnancy, rheumatoid arthritis, and individuals whose jobs require repetitive wrist movements.
- **Cellulitis.**
- **Overuse Injury** (tendonitis).
- **Trauma** (e.g., contusion, dislocation, fracture, sprain, strain).

Serious Signs and Symptoms

- Severe pain
- Red area with streak
  R/O: cellulitis with lymphangitis; common
- Joint swelling with fever
  R/O: septic arthritis; rare
- Entire arm is swollen
  R/O: deep vein thrombosis of upper extremity; rare

Caution: Cardiac Ischemia

- Rarely, patients may present with arm pain as the sole symptom of a myocardial infarction. Usually there will be other associated symptoms of cardiac ischemia: chest pain, shortness of breath, nausea, and/or diaphoresis.
- Cardiac ischemia should be suspected in any patients with risk factors for cardiac disease. These include: hypertension, smoking, diabetes, hyperlipidemia, a strong family history of heart disease, male gender, and age > 60.

HAY FEVER (NASAL ALLERGIES)

Definition
- An allergic reaction of the nose and sinuses to an inhaled substance (eg, pollen, mold, dust).
- An itchy nose and clear discharge are common.
- *Use this protocol only if the patient has symptoms that match Hay Fever.*

Symptoms
- Runny nose (clear nasal discharge)
- Stuffy nose (nasal congestion)
- Sneezing and sniffing
- Itching of nose, eyes, and roof of mouth
- Watery eyes
- Ear fullness (ear congestion)
- No fever

TRIAGE ASSESSMENT QUESTIONS

See More Appropriate Protocol
- ● Wheezing (high-pitched whistling sound) and previous asthma attacks or use of asthma medicines
  Go to Protocol: Asthma Attack on page 38
- ● Doesn't match the SYMPTOMS for nasal allergy
  Go to Protocol: Common Cold on page 79

Go to ED/UCC Now
(or to Office With PCP Approval)
- ● Patient sounds very sick or weak to the triager
  Reason: severe acute illness or serious complication suspected

See Today in Office
- ● Lots of coughing
  R/O: associated asthma
- ● Lots of yellow or green discharge from nose, present > 3 days
  R/O: bacterial sinusitis

See Today or Tomorrow in Office
- ● Nasal discharge present > 10 days
  R/O: bacterial sinusitis
- ● MODERATE-SEVERE nasal allergy symptoms (i.e., interfere with sleep, school, or work) and taking antihistamines > 2 days
  R/O: poor control
- ● Patient wants to be seen

See Within 2 Weeks in Office
- ● Nasal allergies occur only certain times of year and diagnosis of hay fever has never been confirmed by a physician
  R/O: seasonal allergic rhinitis (hay fever)
- ● Nasal allergies occur year-round
  R/O: perennial allergic rhinitis; multiple allergies to pollens, house dust, pets, foods
- ● Snores most nights of month
  R/O: chronic nasal congestion, sleep apnea

Home Care
- ○ Nasal allergies occur only certain times of year
  R/O: seasonal allergic rhinitis (hay fever)

HOME CARE ADVICE

General Care Advice for Hay Fever
❶ **Wash Off Pollen Daily:** Remove pollen from the body with hair washing and a shower, especially before bedtime.

❷ **Avoiding Pollen:**
- Stay indoors on windy days.
- Keep windows closed in home, at least in bedroom; use air conditioner (AC).
- Use a high-efficiency house air filter (HEPA or electrostatic).
- Keep windows closed in car, turn AC on recirculate.
- Avoid playing with outdoor dog.

❸ **Nasal Washes for a Stuffy Nose:**
- **Introduction:** Saline (salt water) nasal irrigation (nasal wash) is an effective and simple home remedy for treating stuffy nose and sinus congestion. The nose can be irrigated by pouring, spraying, or squirting salt water into the nose and then letting it run back out.
- **How It Helps:** The salt water rinses out excess mucus and washes out any irritants (dust, allergens) that might be present. It also moistens the nasal cavity.
- **Methods:** There are several ways to irrigate the nose. You can use a saline nasal spray bottle (available over the counter [OTC]), a rubber ear syringe, a medical syringe without the needle, or a neti pot.

❹ Nasal Washes—Step-by-step Instructions:
- **Step 1:** Lean over a sink.
- **Step 2:** Gently squirt or spray warm salt water into one of your nostrils.
- **Step 3:** Some of the water may run into the back of your throat. Spit this out. If you swallow the salt water, it will not hurt you.
- **Step 4:** Blow your nose to clean out the water and mucus.
- **Step 5:** Repeat steps 1 through 4 for the other nostril. You can do this a couple times a day if it seems to help you.

❺ How to Make Saline (Salt Water) Nasal Wash:
- You can make your own saline nasal wash.
- Add ½ tsp of table salt to 1 cup (8 oz; 240 mL) of warm water.
- You should use sterile, distilled, or previously boiled water for nasal irrigation.

❻ Antihistamine Medicines for Hay Fever:
- Antihistamine medicines help reduce sneezing, itching, and runny nose. They are the drug of choice for treating symptoms of hay fever
- **Benadryl** (diphenhydramine) and Chlor-Trimeton (chlorpheniramine; Chlor-Tripolon) are available OTC. Both of these antihistamine medicines work well. They can cause sleepiness.
- **Loratadine** is a newer (second-generation) antihistamine that is now available OTC. The dosage of loratadine (e.g., OTC Claritin, Alavert) is 10 mg once a day. Alavert is not available in Canada.
- **Cetirizine** is another newer (second-generation) antihistamine and is now available OTC. The dosage of cetirizine (e.g., OTC Zyrtec, Reactine) is 10 mg once a day.
- *Before taking any medicine, read all the instructions on the package.*

❼ Caution—Antihistamines:
- Examples include diphenhydramine (Benadryl) and chlorpheniramine (Chlor-Trimeton, Chlor-Tripolon).
- May cause sleepiness. Do not drink alcohol, drive, or operate dangerous machinery while taking antihistamines.
- Do not take these medicines if you have prostate problems.

❽ Nasal Decongestants for a Very Stuffy or Runny Nose:
- **Most people do not need to use these medicines.**
- If your nose feels blocked, you should try using nasal washes first.
- If you have a very stuffy nose, nasal decongestant medicines can shrink the swollen nasal mucosa and allow for easier breathing. If you have a very runny nose, these medicines can reduce the amount of drainage. They may be taken as pills by mouth or as a nasal spray.
- **Pseudoephedrine (Sudafed):** Available OTC in pill form. Typical adult dosage is two 30 mg tablets every 6 hours.
- **Oxymetazoline Nasal Drops (Afrin):** Available OTC. Clean out the nose before using. Spray each nostril once, wait 1 minute for absorption, and then spray a second time.
- **Phenylephrine Nasal Drops (Neo-Synephrine):** Available OTC. Clean out the nose before using. Spray each nostril once, wait 1 minute for absorption, and then spray a second time.
- *Before taking any medicine, read all the instructions on the package.*

❾ Caution—Nasal Decongestants:
- Do not take these medications if you have high blood pressure, heart disease, prostate problems, or an overactive thyroid.
- Do not take these medications if you are pregnant.
- Do not take these medications if you have used a monoamine oxidase (MAO) inhibitor such as isocarboxazid (Marplan), phenelzine (Nardil), rasagiline (Azilect), selegiline (Eldepryl, Emsam), or tranylcypromine (Parnate) in the past 2 weeks. Life-threatening side effects can occur.
- Do not use these medications for > 3 days. *(Reason: rebound nasal congestion)*

❿ For Eye Allergies: For eye symptoms, wash pollen off the face and eyelids. Then apply cold wet compresses. Oral antihistamines will usually bring all eye symptoms under control.

⓫ Call Back If:
- Symptoms are not controlled in 2 days with continuous antihistamines.
- You become worse.

Neti Pot for Sinus Symptoms

❶ Neti Pot:

- The neti pot is a small ceramic or plastic pot with a narrow spout. It looks like a small teapot. Two manufacturers of the neti pot are the Himalayan Institute in Pennsylvania and SinuCleanse in Wisconsin.
- **How It Helps:** The neti pot performs nasal washing (also called nasal irrigation or "jala neti"). The salt water rinses out excess mucus and washes out any irritants (dust, allergens) that might be present. It also moisturizes the nasal cavity.
- **Indications:** The neti pot is widely used as a home remedy to relieve conditions such as colds, sinus infections, and hay fever (nasal allergies).
- **Adverse Reactions:** None. However, some people do not like how it feels to pour water into their nose.
- **YouTube Instructional Video:** There are instructional videos on how to use a neti pot on manufacturers' Web sites and also on YouTube: www.youtube.com/watch?v=j8sDIbRAXIg.

❷ Neti Pot Step-by-step Instructions:

- **Step 1:** Follow the directions on the salt package to make warm salt water.
- **Step 2:** Lean forward and turn your head to one side over the sink. Keep your forehead slightly higher than your chin.
- **Step 3:** Gently insert the spout of the neti pot into the higher nostril. Put it far enough so that it forms a comfortable seal.
- **Step 4:** Raise the neti pot gradually so the salt water flows in through your higher nostril and out of the lower nostril. Breathe through your mouth.
- **Step 5:** When the neti pot is empty, blow your nose to clean out the water and mucus.
- **Step 6:** Some of the water may run into the back of your throat. Spit this out. If you swallow the salt water, it will not hurt you.
- **Step 7:** Refill the neti pot and repeat on the other side. Again, blow your nose to clear the nasal passages.

❸ How to Make Saline (Salt Water) Nasal Wash:

- You can make your own saline nasal wash.
- Add ½ tsp of table salt to 1 cup (8 oz; 240 mL) of warm water.
- You should use sterile, distilled, or previously boiled water for nasal irrigation.

❹ Call Back If:

- You have other questions or concerns.
- You become worse.

BACKGROUND

Key Points

- Many patients correctly self-diagnose this condition. Confirmation of this diagnosis by a physician is helpful and becomes essential if symptoms are more than mild.
- 10%-20% of the population has allergic rhinitis.
- Many patients with allergic rhinitis also have symptoms of allergic conjunctivitis (watery itchy eyes).

Two Types of Allergic Rhinitis

- **Seasonal Allergic Rhinitis:** Also known as hay fever. Hay fever is the nonmedical term people use to describe seasonal allergic rhinitis due to pollens. Patients who suffer from hay fever note that their symptoms are worse during certain seasons of the year. Such individuals usually have an allergy to pollen, grasses, or trees. Depending on the specific allergy, the symptoms may be worse in the spring, summer, or fall. A few unfortunate individuals may experience allergic symptoms in all 3 seasons. Hay fever is not specifically an allergy to hay, nor do sufferers have a fever.
- **Perennial Allergic Rhinitis:** Patients with this type of allergic rhinitis may report nasal symptoms all year long. Alternatively they may complain of sporadic symptoms throughout the year, not confined to any particular season. Such individuals often have an allergy to dust mites, mold, mildew, feathers, or animal dander.

Nasal Washes (Nasal Irrigation) for Sinus Symptoms

- **Introduction:** Saline (salt water) nasal irrigation is an effective and simple home remedy for treating cold symptoms and other conditions involving the nasal and sinus passages. Nasal irrigation consists of pouring, spraying, or squirting salt water into the nose and then letting it run back out.
- **How It Helps:** The salt water rinses out excess mucus, washes out any irritants (dust, allergens) that might be present, and moisturizes the nasal cavity.

- **Indications:** Nasal irrigation appears to be an effective treatment for chronic sinusitis. It may also help reduce sinus symptoms from acute viral upper respiratory infection (colds), irritant rhinitis (e.g., dust from the workplace), and allergic rhinitis (hay fever). Some doctors recommend it for rhinitis of pregnancy.
- **Adverse Reactions:** Nasal irrigation is safe, and there are no serious adverse effects. However, not everyone likes the sensation of having water in their nose.
- **Methods:** There are several ways to perform nasal irrigation. None has been proven to be better than any other. Methods include use of a nasal spray bottle (available OTC), a rubber ear syringe, a Waterpik set on "low," a 5- to 20-mL medical syringe without the needle, or a neti pot.
- **How to Make Salt Water for Nasal Irrigation:** Add ½ teaspoon of table salt to 1 cup (8 oz; 240 mL) of warm water.

Neti Pot for Sinus Symptoms

- The neti pot is a small ceramic or plastic pot with a narrow spout. It looks like a small teapot. Two manufacturers of the neti pot are the Himalayan Institute in Pennsylvania and SinuCleanse in Wisconsin.
- **How It Helps:** The neti pot performs nasal washing (also called nasal irrigation or "jala neti"). The salt water rinses out excess mucus, washes out any irritants (dust, allergens) that might be present, and moisturizes the nasal cavity.
- **Indications:** The neti pot is widely used as a home remedy to relieve conditions such as colds, sinus infections, and hay fever (nasal allergies).
- **Adverse Reactions:** None. Nasal irrigation with a neti pot is safe, and there are no serious adverse effects. However, not everyone likes the sensation of having salt water poured into their nose.
- **YouTube Instructional Video:** www.youtube.com/watch?v=j8sDIbRAXlg.

Neti Pot and Primary Amebic Meningoencephalitis (PAM)

- Primary amebic meningoencephalitis (PAM) is caused by *Naegleria fowleri,* the so-called "brain-eating ameba." This is an extremely rare infection. There were 32 cases in the United States between 2001 and 2010.
- The majority of the cases of PAM have occurred in the southern United States and were linked to swimming or bathing in fresh water lakes, rivers, and ponds containing this ameba. The ameba can also be found in hot springs, geothermal water sources, and poorly maintained swimming pools.
- In 2011 there were 2 cases of PAM in Louisiana that occurred after nasal irrigation with a neti pot. These 2 cases suggest—but are not definite proof—that the nasal irrigation fluid that the individuals used was somehow contaminated with the *N fowleri* ameba.
- The Centers for Disease Control and Prevention recommends that individuals should use distilled, sterile, or previously boiled water for nasal irrigation. It's also important to rinse the irrigation device after each use and leave open to air dry.

Caution: There are other illnesses that present with similar nasal symptoms:

- **Viral Rhinitis:** Also known as the common cold. Runny or stuffy nose is the main symptom. The nasal discharge may be clear, cloudy, yellow, or green. The patient usually has other symptoms of a cold: fever, muscle aches, sore throat, and headache.
- **Bacterial and Viral Sinusitis:** Yellow or green nasal secretions suggest the possibility of sinusitis if they occur in combination with 1) sinus pain OR 2) the return of a fever after it has been gone for > 24 hours OR 3) secretions persist > 10 days without improvement.
- **Rhinitis Medicamentosa:** Prolonged continuous use (> 5 days) of decongestant nose drops can lead to "rebound" congestion in which the nose becomes even more stuffy.
- **Occupational Exposure:** Airborne irritants in the workplace can cause nasal problems.

HEAD INJURY

Definition
- Injuries to the head, including scalp, skull, and brain trauma
- **Acute Neurologic Symptoms:** Difficult to awaken OR confused thinking and talking OR slurred speech OR weakness of arms OR unsteady walking

TRIAGE ASSESSMENT QUESTIONS

Call EMS 911 Now
- ACUTE NEUROLOGIC SYMPTOM and symptom present now
  R/O: cerebral contusion, subdural or epidural hematoma
- Knocked out (unconscious) > 1 minute
  R/O: concussion, intracranial bleeding
- Seizure (convulsion) occurred
  (Exception: prior history of seizures and now alert and without acute neurologic symptoms)
  Note: Consider using Seizure protocol on page 340 after triage with Head Injury protocol.
- Neck pain after dangerous injury (e.g., MVA, diving, trampoline, contact sports, fall > 10 feet or 3 m)
  (Exception: neck pain began > 1 hour after injury)
  First Aid: Protect the neck from movement.
- Major bleeding (actively dripping or spurting) that can't be stopped
  First Aid: Apply direct pressure to the entire wound with a clean cloth.
- Penetrating head injury (e.g., knife, gunshot wound, metal object)
  First Aid: Don't remove penetrating object.
- Sounds like a life-threatening emergency to the triager

Go to ED Now
- Can't remember what happened (amnesia)
  Reason: probable concussion, needs neurological examination
- Vomiting once or more
  R/O: concussion
- Watery or blood-tinged fluid dripping from the nose or ears
  R/O: basilar skull fracture

Go to ED/UCC Now
(or to Office With PCP Approval)
- ACUTE NEUROLOGIC SYMPTOM and now fine
- Knocked out (unconscious) < 1 minute and now fine
- Severe headache
- Dangerous injury (e.g., MVA, diving, trampoline, contact sports, fall > 10 feet or 3 m) or severe blow from hard object (e.g., golf club, baseball bat)
  Reason: increased risk of injury
- Large swelling or bruise and size > palm of person's hand
  R/O: fracture, hematoma
- Skin is split open or gaping (length > ½" or 12 mm)
  Reason: may need laceration repair (e.g., sutures)
- Bleeding won't stop after 10 minutes of direct pressure (using correct technique)
- One or two "black eyes" (bruising, purple color of eyelids)
  Reason: periorbital ecchymoses (raccoon eyes in the setting of head injury is suspicious for the possibility of a basilar skull fracture)
- Taking Coumadin (warfarin) or other strong blood thinner, or known bleeding disorder (e.g., thrombocytopenia)
  Reason: higher risk of serious bleeding; may need testing of INR, prothrombin time, or platelet count
  Notes: Besides Coumadin, other strong blood thinners include Arixtra (fondaparinux), Eliquis (apixaban), Pradaxa (dabigatran), and Xarelto (rivaroxaban). Plavix (clopidogrel; antiplatelet drug) also increases risk in head injury.
- Sounds like a serious injury to the triager

See Today in Office
- Patient is confused or is an unreliable provider of information (e.g., dementia, profound intellectual disability, alcohol intoxication)
- Patient wants to be seen

See Today or Tomorrow in Office

- Wound and no tetanus booster in > 5 years (or > 10 years for clean cuts)
  Reason: may need a tetanus booster shot (vaccine)
- After 3 days and headache persists
  R/O: fracture, concussion
- Suspicious history for the injury
  R/O: domestic violence or elder abuse

Home Care

- Minor head injury
  R/O: bruise, superficial cut or abrasion

HOME CARE ADVICE

Treatment of a Minor Bruise, Sprain, or Strain

❶ Reassurance—Direct Blow (Contusion, Bruise):
- This sounds like a scalp injury rather than a brain injury or concussion. Treatment at home should be safe. A direct blow to your scalp can cause a contusion. Contusion is the medical term for bruise.
- Symptoms are mild pain, swelling, and/or bruising. Sometimes there can also be mild dizziness and nausea.
- *Here is some care advice that should help.*

❷ Apply a Cold Pack:
- Apply a cold pack or an ice bag (wrapped in a moist towel) to the area for 20 minutes. Repeat in 1 hour, then every 4 hours while awake.
- Continue this for the first 48 hours after an injury.
- This will help decrease pain and swelling.

❸ Apply Heat to the Area:
- Beginning 48 hours after an injury, apply a warm washcloth or heating pad for 10 minutes 3 times a day.
- This will help increase blood flow and improve healing.

❹ Observation After Head Injury:
- Watch a person with a head injury very closely during the first 2 hours following the injury.
- Wake the head-injured person every 4 hours for the first 24 hours. Check to see if he/she can walk and talk.

❺ Expected Course:
- Most head trauma only causes an injury to the scalp. Pain, swelling, and bruising usually start to get better 2-3 days after an injury.
- Swelling most often is gone after 1 week.
- Bruises fade away slowly over 1-2 weeks.
- It may take 2 weeks for pain and tenderness of the injured area to go away.

❻ Diet: Clear fluids to drink at first, in case of vomiting. May resume a regular diet after 2 hours.

❼ Call Back If:
- Severe headache.
- Extremity weakness or numbness occurs.
- Slurred speech or blurred vision occurs.
- Vomiting occurs.
- You become worse.

Treatment of a Small Cut or Scrape

❶ Reassurance—Superficial Laceration (Cut or Scratch) or Abrasion (Scrape):
- This sounds like a small cut or scrape that we can treat at home.
- *Here is some care advice that should help.*

❷ Bleeding: Apply direct pressure for 10 minutes with a sterile gauze to stop any bleeding.

❸ Cleaning the Wound:
- Wash the wound with soap and water for 5 minutes.
- For any dirt, scrub gently with a washcloth.
- For any bleeding, apply direct pressure with a sterile gauze or clean cloth for 10 minutes.

❹ Antibiotic Ointment: Apply an antibiotic ointment (e.g., OTC bacitracin) to the wound twice a day.

❺ Call Back If:
- Looks infected (pus, redness, increasing tenderness).
- Doesn't heal within 10 days.
- You become worse.

Over-the-counter Pain Medicines

❶ Pain Medicines:
- For pain relief, you can take either acetaminophen, ibuprofen, or naproxen.
- They are over-the-counter (OTC) pain drugs. You can buy them at the drugstore.

Acetaminophen (e.g., Tylenol):
- **Regular Strength Tylenol:** Take 650 mg (two 325 mg pills) by mouth every 4-6 hours as needed. Each Regular Strength Tylenol pill has 325 mg of acetaminophen.
- **Extra Strength Tylenol:** Take 1,000 mg (two 500 mg pills) every 8 hours as needed. Each Extra Strength Tylenol pill has 500 mg of acetaminophen.
- The most you should take each day is 3,000 mg (10 Regular Strength or 6 Extra Strength pills a day).

Ibuprofen (e.g., Motrin, Advil):
- Take 400 mg (two 200 mg pills) by mouth every 6 hours.
- Another choice is to take 600 mg (three 200 mg pills) by mouth every 8 hours.
- The most you should take each day is 1,200 mg (six 200 mg pills), unless your doctor has told you to take more.

Naproxen (e.g., Aleve):
- Take 220 mg (one 220 mg pill) by mouth every 8 hours as needed. You may take 440 mg (two 220 mg pills) for your first dose.
- The most you should take each day is 660 mg (three 220 mg pills a day), unless your doctor has told you to take more.

❷ Pain Medicines—Extra Notes:
- Use the lowest amount of medicine that makes your pain better.
- Acetaminophen is thought to be safer than ibuprofen or naproxen in people > 65 years old. Acetaminophen is in many OTC and prescription medicines. It might be in more than one medicine that you are taking. You need to be careful and not take an overdose. An acetaminophen overdose can hurt the liver.
- McNeil, the company that makes Tylenol, has different dosage instructions for Tylenol in Canada and the United States. In Canada, the maximum recommended dose per day is 4,000 mg or 12 Regular Strength (325 mg) pills. In the United States, McNeil recommends a maximum dose of 10 Regular Strength (325 mg) pills.
- CAUTION: Do not take acetaminophen if you have liver disease.
- CAUTION: Do not take ibuprofen or naproxen if you have stomach problems, have kidney disease, are pregnant, or have been told by your doctor to avoid this type of anti-inflammatory drug. Do not take ibuprofen or naproxen for > 7 days without consulting your doctor.
- *Before taking any medicine, read all the instructions on the package.*

❸ Call Back If:
- You have more questions.
- You become worse.

FIRST AID

First Aid Advice for Bleeding:
Apply direct pressure to the entire wound with a clean cloth.

First Aid Advice for Penetrating Object:
If penetrating object is still in place, don't remove it. *Reason: Removal could increase bleeding.*

First Aid Advice for Shock:
Lie down with the feet elevated.

First Aid Advice for Suspected Spinal Cord Injury:
Do not move until a spine board is applied.

First Aid Advice for Bruise:
Apply a cold pack or an ice bag (wrapped in a moist towel) to the area for 20 minutes.

BACKGROUND

Types of Head Injury

- **Skin Trauma:** Cut, scrape, bruise, or scalp hematoma (goose egg).
- **Skull Trauma:** Fracture.
- **Brain Trauma:** Concussion and other brain injuries can be recognized by the presence of loss of consciousness, amnesia, or other **acute neurological symptoms.**

Acute Neurologic Symptoms—Requiring an EMS 911 Disposition

The following acute neurologic symptoms after a head injury should receive an EMS 911 disposition:

❶ Difficult to awaken

❷ Confused or slow thinking and talking

❸ Slurred speech

❹ Weakness of arms or legs

❺ Unsteady walking

Raccoon Eyes (Bilateral Black Eyes) Following Head Trauma

The cause of bilateral black eyes often can be determined by the timing of their onset.

- **Forehead hematomas** cause most of them. The black eyes appear 2-3 days after the initial minor forehead injury. Mechanism is the seepage of blood downward through the tissue planes with the help of gravity.
- **Basilar skull fracture** is occasionally the cause. A fracture of the frontal part of the base of skull can cause blood to seep anteriorly into the orbits. The black eyes usually appear within 24 hours of the initial injury but can occur later. Often there is no forehead bruise. Basilar skull fractures usually only follow major head trauma. Acute neurologic findings (e.g., altered mental status) are usually present.

Unilateral Dilated Pupil (Anisocoria)

- Anisocoria is the medical term for unequal pupil sizes.
- **Normal Variant:** Most commonly unequal pupils are a normal variant. Approximately 10% of the population has anisocoria. This is almost always the reason in alert individuals without other serious neurologic symptoms. One way to check to see if someone always has anisocoria is to look at a good-resolution (image size/detail) photo that shows the pupils; a driver's license photo is handy, but the resolution is often too poor to be of use.

- **Local Eye Trauma (Traumatic Mydriasis):** Blunt trauma to one eye can cause unilateral dilation of the pupil (traumatic mydriasis). Associated symptoms will include eye pain, eye redness, blurred vision, and photophobia.
- **As a Sign of Brain Stem Herniation:** A unilaterally dilated pupil in the setting of head trauma always raises the concern about brain hemorrhage (intracranial hematoma, swelling, and herniation). A dilated pupil from brain herniation is always accompanied by altered mental status, severe headache, and other neurologic symptoms. Thus, if a patient is comatose AND has a unilateral widely dilated pupil, brain stem herniation should be suspected.

Concussion

- **Definition:** A temporary impairment in neurologic function following a traumatic injury to the brain. A concussion is a functional disturbance in brain activity, and not a structural injury. Loss of consciousness is not required.
- **Symptoms:** Headache, nausea, and feeling irritable and sleepy are common, especially during the first couple days after a concussion. Other symptoms of a concussion include amnesia (can't remember what happened), dizziness, difficulty concentrating or "foggy" feeling, poor memory, feeling tired, feeling dazed or not your normal self, and decreased coordination.
- **Diagnosis:** The diagnosis is made by a doctor based on the clinical examination of the injured person. The computed tomography (CT) scan of a patient with a concussion (and no other brain injuries) is normal. Often a head CT scan does not need to be performed.
- **Expected Course:** The majority (80%-90%) of concussions resolve in 7-10 days.
- **Prognosis:** Most people who sustain a concussion recover completely and there are no signs of permanent damage. Sometimes a person can have concussion symptoms that last for weeks or months afterwards.
- **Cognitive Rest:** See next page.
- **Return to Sports:** See next page.
- All individuals with concussions need a neurologic examination by a health care professional.

Cognitive Rest After a Concussion
- Brain rest (cognitive rest) can help a person get better after a concussion.
- Too much mental activity can put extra strain on the brain. Intense mental activity increases neurometabolic processes in the brain.
- It is best to avoid or decrease activities such as: working on a computer, tablet, phone, or any screen; listening to loud music; reading; texting; and playing video or computer games.

Sports-Related Concussion and Sideline Evaluation (*Clin J Sport Med.* 2009;19[3]:185–200)
- *"The player should be medically evaluated onsite using standard emergency management principles, and particular attention should be given to excluding a cervical spine injury."*
- *"The appropriate disposition of the player must be determined by the treating health care provider in a timely manner. If no health care provider is available, the player should be safely removed from practice or play and urgent referral to a physician arranged."*
- *"Once the first aid issues are addressed, then an assessment of the concussive injury should be made using the SCAT2 or other similar tool."*
- *"The player should not be left alone following the injury, and serial monitoring for deterioration is essential over the initial few hours following injury."*
- *"A player with diagnosed concussion should not be allowed to return to play on the day of injury."*

Sports-Related Concussion and When to Return to Play
Return to play following a concussion should be individualized. The athlete should be free of concussion symptoms at rest and during exertion before returning to full participation. Return to play should follow a stepwise process as outlined in the following stages.

The stepwise process through these stages may take days to weeks. It depends on the person. Typically, each step should take 24 hours; a patient-athlete would typically take 1 week to proceed through the 6 stages, assuming that he/she has no post-concussion symptoms. If concussion symptoms recur at any stage, the patient should drop back to the previous level for another 24 hours.

- **Stage 1:** No activity
- **Stage 2:** Light aerobic activity (walking, swimming, stationary cycling)
- **Stage 3:** Sports-specific exercise
- **Stage 4:** Noncontact training drills
- **Stage 5:** Full-contact practice
- **Stage 6:** Return to play

Multiple concussions require longer periods of recovery before returning to sports. The reason we sideline athletes who have a concussion is to prevent the "second impact injury." This is a second concussion that occurs before the first one has healed, usually within 1 or 2 weeks after the first one. It can sometimes cause a more serious brain injury.

Sources:
- McCrory P, Meeuwisse W, Johnston K, et al. Consensus statement on concussion in sport. 3rd International Conference on Concussion in Sport held in Zurich, November 2008. *Clin J Sport Med.* 2009;19(3):185–200
- Harmon KG, Drezner JA, Gammons M, et al. American Medical Society for Sports Medicine position statement: concussion in sport. *Br J Sports Med.* 2013;47(1):15–26
- Rocky Mountain Youth Sports Medicine Group. *REAP the Benefits of Good Concussion Management.* Centennial, CO: Rocky Mountain Youth Sports Medicine Institute; 2011. http://concussiontreatment.com/images/REAP_Program.pdf. Accessed April 18, 2018
- Centers for Disease Control and Prevention (CDC). Heads Up. Managing return to activities. https://www.cdc.gov/headsup/providers/return_to_activities.html. Published February 8, 2016. Accessed April 18, 2018

Airbag Deployment
- Airbags inflate within 50 ms of impact and at a speed of 100 mph.
- The gas produced to inflate the airbag is harmless. The CDC reports no poisoning from airbag deployment (2009).
- In adults, airbag injuries are mainly minor abrasions or bruises. The areas most commonly affected are the face, arms, and hands; the skin may look red or abraded from being "slapped" by the airbag as it deployed.

What Cuts Need to Be Sutured?

- Any cut that is split open or gaping probably needs sutures (or staples or skin glue).
- Cuts > ½" (1 cm) usually need sutures.
- Any open wound that may need sutures should be evaluated by a physician regardless of the time that has passed since the initial injury.

When Does an Adult Need a Tetanus Booster (Tetanus Shot)?

- **Clean Cuts and Scrapes—Tetanus Booster Needed Every 10 Years:** Patients with clean minor wounds AND who have previously had ≥ 3 tetanus shots (full series) need a booster every 10 years. Examples of minor wounds include a superficial abrasion or a shallow cut from a clean knife blade. Obtain booster within 72 hours.
- **Dirty Wounds—Tetanus Booster Needed Every 5 Years:** Patients with dirty wounds need a booster if it has been > 5 years since the last booster. Examples of dirty wounds include those contaminated with soil, feces, and/or saliva and more serious wounds from deep punctures, crushing, and burns. Obtain booster within 72 hours.

Caution: Associated Neck Trauma

- Neck trauma should also be considered in all patients with a head injury. Concerning findings include numbness, weakness, and neck pain.
- After using the Head Injury protocol, if the triager or caller has remaining concerns about neck trauma, the patient also should be triaged using the Neck Injury protocol on page 290.

HEADACHE

Definition
- Pain or discomfort of the head.
- The face and ears are excluded.
- Not due to a traumatic injury.

Pain Severity Scale
- **Mild (1-3):** Doesn't interfere with normal activities.
- **Moderate (4-7):** Interferes with normal activities or awakens from sleep.
- **Severe (8-10):** Excruciating pain, unable to do any normal activities.

TRIAGE ASSESSMENT QUESTIONS

Call EMS 911 Now
- Difficult to awaken or acting confused (e.g., disoriented, slurred speech)
  R/O: subarachnoid hemorrhage, meningitis
- Weakness of the face, arm, or leg on one side of the body and new onset
  R/O: stroke
- Numbness of the face, arm, or leg on one side of the body and new onset
  R/O: stroke
- Loss of speech or garbled speech and new onset
  R/O: stroke
- Passed out (i.e., fainted, collapsed and was not responding)
- Sounds like a life-threatening emergency to the triager

See More Appropriate Protocol
- Followed a head injury within last 3 days
  Go to Protocol: Head Injury on page 201
- Sinus pain of forehead and yellow or green nasal discharge
  Go to Protocol: Sinus Pain and Congestion on page 352

Go to ED Now
- Unable to walk without falling
  R/O: cerebellar stroke
- Stiff neck (can't touch chin to chest)
  R/O: meningitis
- Possibility of carbon monoxide exposure
  R/O: CO poisoning

Go to ED/UCC Now (or to Office With PCP Approval)
- SEVERE headache, states "worst headache" of life
  R/O: migraine, CNS bleed
- SEVERE headache, sudden onset (i.e., reaching maximum intensity within 30 seconds)
  R/O: migraine, CNS bleed
- Severe pain in one eye
  R/O: angle-closure glaucoma
- Loss of vision or double vision
  R/O: stroke, temporal arteritis, sphenoid sinusitis, cerebral aneurysm, brain tumor, migraine (Exception: same as prior migraines)
- Patient sounds very sick or weak to the triager
  Reason: severe acute illness or serious complication suspected

Go to L&D Now (or PCP Triage)
- Pregnant > 20 weeks with new hand or face swelling
- Pregnant > 20 weeks with new blurred vision or vision changes

Go to Office Now
- Fever > 103° F (39.4° C)
  R/O: bacterial infection
- Fever > 100.0° F (37.8° C) and has diabetes mellitus or a weak immune system (e.g., HIV positive, cancer chemotherapy, organ transplant, splenectomy, chronic steroids)
  R/O: meningitis, encephalitis

Callback by PCP Within 1 Hour
- SEVERE headache (e.g., excruciating) and has had severe headaches before
  R/O: migraine
- SEVERE headache and not relieved by pain medications
  R/O: new-onset migraine, CNS bleed, brain tumor
- SEVERE headache and vomiting
  R/O: migraine, increased ICP
- SEVERE headache and fever

See Today in Office

- New headache and weak immune system (e.g., HIV positive, cancer chemotherapy, chronic steroid treatment)
  Reason: greater risk of organic pathology
- Fever present > 3 days (72 hours)
  R/O: sinusitis
- Patient wants to be seen

See Today or Tomorrow in Office

- Unexplained headache that is present > 24 hours
  R/O: sinusitis or other treatable cause
- New headache and age > 50
  Reason: greater risk of organic pathology

See Within 3 Days in Office

- Headache started during sex
  R/O: sexual headache (pre-orgasmic, orgasmic, tension headache CA)

See Within 2 Weeks in Office

- Headache is a chronic symptom (recurrent or ongoing AND lasting > 4 weeks)
  R/O: tension headache, migraine headache

Home Care

- MILD-MODERATE headache
  R/O: tension headache
- Similar to previously diagnosed migraine headaches
  R/O: migraine headache
- Similar to previously diagnosed muscle-tension headaches

HOME CARE ADVICE

❶ **Reassurance—Migraine Headache:**
- You have told me that this headache is similar to previous migraine headaches that you have had. If the pattern or severity of your headache changes, you will need to see your physician.
- Migraine headaches are also called vascular headaches. A migraine can be anywhere from mild to severely painful. Sufferers often describe it as throbbing or pulsing. It is often just on one side. Associated symptoms include nausea and vomiting. Some individuals will have visual or other neurological warning symptoms (aura) that a migraine is coming.

- This sounds like a painful headache that you are having, but there are pain medications you can take and other instructions I can give you to reduce the pain.
- *Here is some care advice that should help.*

❷ **Reassurance—Muscle Tension Headache:**
- You have told me that this headache is similar to your previously diagnosed muscle tension headaches.
- The majority of headaches are caused by muscle tension.
- The discomfort is usually diffuse and may be described as a "tight band" around the head. It may radiate down into the neck and shoulders. The discomfort can be aggravated by emotional stress.
- This sounds like a painful headache that you are having, but there are pain medications you can take and other instructions I can give you to reduce the pain.
- *Here is some care advice that should help.*

❸ **Pain Medicines:**
- For pain relief, you can take either acetaminophen, ibuprofen, or naproxen.
- They are over-the-counter (OTC) pain drugs. You can buy them at the drugstore.

Acetaminophen (e.g., Tylenol):
- **Regular Strength Tylenol:** Take 650 mg (two 325 mg pills) by mouth every 4-6 hours as needed. Each Regular Strength Tylenol pill has 325 mg of acetaminophen.
- **Extra Strength Tylenol:** Take 1,000 mg (two 500 mg pills) every 8 hours as needed. Each Extra Strength Tylenol pill has 500 mg of acetaminophen.
- The most you should take each day is 3,000 mg (10 Regular Strength or 6 Extra Strength pills a day).

Ibuprofen (e.g., Motrin, Advil):
- Take 400 mg (two 200 mg pills) by mouth every 6 hours.
- Another choice is to take 600 mg (three 200 mg pills) by mouth every 8 hours.
- The most you should take each day is 1,200 mg (six 200 mg pills), unless your doctor has told you to take more.

Naproxen (e.g., Aleve):
- Take 220 mg (one 220 mg pill) by mouth every 8 hours as needed. You may take 440 mg (two 220 mg pills) for your first dose.
- The most you should take each day is 660 mg (three 220 mg pills a day), unless your doctor has told you to take more.

❹ **Pain Medicines—Extra Notes:**
- Use the lowest amount of medicine that makes your pain better.
- Acetaminophen is thought to be safer than ibuprofen or naproxen in people > 65 years old. Acetaminophen is in many OTC and prescription medicines. It might be in more than one medicine that you are taking. You need to be careful and not take an overdose. An acetaminophen overdose can hurt the liver.
- McNeil, the company that makes Tylenol, has different dosage instructions for Tylenol in Canada and the United States. In Canada, the maximum recommended dose per day is 4,000 mg or 12 Regular Strength (325 mg) pills. In the United States, McNeil recommends a maximum dose of 10 Regular Strength (325 mg) pills.
- CAUTION: Do not take acetaminophen if you have liver disease.
- CAUTION: Do not take ibuprofen or naproxen if you have stomach problems, have kidney disease, are pregnant, or have been told by your doctor to avoid this type of anti-inflammatory drug. Do not take ibuprofen or naproxen for > 7 days without consulting your doctor.
- *Before taking any medicine, read all the instructions on the package.*

❺ **Migraine Medication:** If your doctor has prescribed specific medication for your migraine, take it as directed as soon as the migraine starts.

❻ **Rest:** Lie down in a dark, quiet place and try to relax. Close your eyes and imagine your entire body relaxing.

❼ **Apply Cold to the Area:** Apply a cold, wet washcloth or cold pack to the forehead for 20 minutes.

❽ **Stretching:** Stretch and massage any tight neck muscles.

❾ **Call Back If:**
- Headache lasts > 24 hours.
- You become worse.

BACKGROUND

Common Causes
- During the course of a year, the majority of adults suffer headaches.
- **Migraine Headaches:** Also referred to as vascular headaches. The headache is moderate-severe in intensity, described as throbbing or pulsing in nature, and usually unilateral. Associated symptoms include nausea and vomiting. Some individuals will have visual or other neurological warning symptoms (aura) that a migraine is coming.
- **Muscle Tension Headaches:** The majority of headaches are caused by muscle tension. The discomfort is usually diffuse and may be described as a "tight band" around the head. It may radiate down into the neck and shoulders. The discomfort can be aggravated by emotional stress.
- **Sinusitis:** Headaches occur with sinusitis. The headache is usually located in the forehead area and the individual has associated sinus symptoms (nasal discharge, congestion, postnasal drip).
- **Viral Illness:** A mild-moderate headache frequently accompanies many febrile illnesses (cold, flu, pharyngitis). Sometimes the headache is related to fever. A moderate headache that persists after the fever has resolved is a red flag that something more serious may be causing the headache.

Less Common Causes
- **Acute Glaucoma:** The affected individual will have eye pain.
- **Brain Tumor:** Approximately 60%-70% of patients with a brain tumor will complain of headaches. The headache is typically described as dull, slowly but steadily worsening over weeks, worse in the morning, and frontal in location.
- **Caffeine Withdrawal:** This occurs in individuals who drink large amounts of caffeine (e.g., coffee, tea, colas) and suddenly stop. Some caffeine drinkers will note a headache on arising that goes away after their first cup of coffee.
- **Carbon Monoxide Exposure:** Frequently there will be a group (e.g., the entire family) of people with the same symptoms.

- **Subarachnoid Hemorrhage:** Subarachnoid hemorrhage needs to be considered in any severe, sudden-onset headache. A typical presentation is the "worst headache ever" (79%). Other supporting symptoms of subarachnoid hemorrhage include neck pain or stiffness (33%), vomiting (28%), and loss of consciousness (64%). Subarachnoid hemorrhage is a life-threatening problem.
- **Temporal Arteritis:** The other term for this is giant cell arteritis. Typically, this presents as a unilateral headache in an individual > 55 years old. There may be tenderness of the scalp over the area of the temporal artery. Fifty percent of patients report painful chewing from jaw claudication. Other symptoms can include muscle aches, fever, and malaise. Permanent visual loss can occur in 20% of patients with temporal arteritis; any change in vision requires emergent evaluation, as immediate steroid therapy is indicated.
- **Lumbar Puncture Headache:** This is a complication of lumbar puncture. Typically occurs 12-24 hours after the procedure and the headache is aggravated by sitting up or standing.
- **Meningitis, Encephalitis:** Accompanying symptoms may include fever, confusion, stiff neck.
- **Preeclampsia:** Should be considered in any patient who is > 20 weeks' pregnant and any postpartum patient in the first 4 weeks after delivery. Clinical presentation typically consists of persistent headache, visual symptoms (spots or flashing lights), epigastric pain, hand and face swelling, sudden weight gain (e.g., > 3 lb or 1.4 kg in 1 week), proteinuria, and blood pressure > 140/90.
- **Pseudotumor Cerebri:** This is also known as benign intracranial hypertension.

HEART RATE AND HEARTBEAT QUESTIONS

Definition
- **Fast Heart Rate:** > 100 beats/minute.
- **Slow Heart Rate:** < 60 beats/minute.
- Skipped or extra heartbeats (irregular heartbeat).
- Palpitations are an increased sensation (or awareness) of an unduly rapid, forceful, or irregular heartbeat.
- **Stimulants:** Caffeine, cocaine, tobacco.

TRIAGE ASSESSMENT QUESTIONS

Call EMS 911 Now
- Passed out (i.e., fainted, collapsed and was not responding)
  R/O: arrhythmia
- Shock suspected (e.g., cold/pale/clammy skin, too weak to stand)
  R/O: arrhythmia, shock
- Difficult to awaken or acting confused (e.g., disoriented, slurred speech)
  R/O: arrhythmia, shock
- Visible sweat on face or sweat dripping down face
  R/O: hypoglycemia, arrhythmia, or serious pathology
- Unable to walk, or can only walk with assistance (e.g., requires support)
  R/O: arrhythmia, shock
- Received SHOCK from implantable cardiac defibrillator and has persisting symptoms (i.e., palpitations, light-headedness)
  R/O: recurrent ventricular tachyarrhythmia, defibrillator system failure
- Sounds like a life-threatening emergency to the triager

See More Appropriate Protocol
- Chest pain
  Go to Protocol: Chest Pain on page 73

Go to ED Now
- Difficulty breathing
  R/O: arrhythmia
- Dizziness, light-headedness, or weakness
- Heart beating very rapidly (e.g., > 140/minute) and present now
  (Exception: during exercise)
  R/O: SVT, tachyarrhythmia
- Heart beating very slowly (e.g., < 50/minute)
  (Exception: athlete)
- *R/O: bradycardia*

Go to ED/UCC Now
(or to Office With PCP Approval)
- New or worsened shortness of breath with activity (dyspnea on exertion)
  R/O: new onset atrial fibrillation
- Patient sounds very sick or weak to the triager
  Reason: severe acute illness or serious complication suspected

Call Transferred to PCP Now
- Wearing a Holter monitor or "cardiac event monitor"
  Reason: notify PCP
- Received SHOCK from implantable cardiac defibrillator (and now feels well)
  Reason: notify PCP

See Today in Office
- Heart beating very rapidly (e.g., > 140/minute) and not present now
  (Exception: during exercise)
  R/O: SVT, tachyarrhythmia
- Skipped or extra beat(s) and increases with exercise or exertion
- Skipped or extra beat(s) and occurs ≥ 4 times per minute
  R/O: PVCs, PACs
- History of heart disease (i.e., heart attack, bypass surgery, angina, angioplasty)
  Reason: higher risk of serious cardiac dysrhythmias

- Age > 60 years
  Reason: higher risk of serious cardiac dysrhythmias
- Taking water pill (i.e., diuretic) or heart medication (e.g., digoxin)
  R/O: hypokalemia, digoxin toxicity
- Patient wants to be seen

See Within 3 Days in Office

- History of hyperthyroidism or taking thyroid medication
  Reason: may be causing symptoms
- Known or suspected substance abuse (e.g., cocaine, alcohol abuse)
  Reason: needs counseling
- Palpitations and no improvement after following Home Care Advice

See Within 2 Weeks in Office

- Problems with anxiety or stress
- Palpitations are a chronic symptom (recurrent or ongoing AND present > 4 weeks)

Home Care

- ○ Palpitations
- ○ Skipped or extra beat(s) and occurs < 4 times/minute

HOME CARE ADVICE

❶ Reassurance:
- Everybody has palpitations at some point in their lives. Sometimes it is simply a heightened awareness of the heart's normal beating.
- Occasional extra heartbeats are experienced by most everyone. Lack of sleep, stress, and caffeinated beverages can make palpitations worse.
- Patients with anxiety or stress may describe a "rapid heartbeat" or "pounding" in their chest from their heart beating.

❷ Health Basics:
- **Sleep:** Try to get a sufficient amount of sleep. Lack of sleep can aggravate palpitations. Most people need 7-8 hours of sleep each night.
- **Exercise:** Regular exercise will improve your overall health and mood and is a simple method to reduce stress.
- **Diet:** Eat a balanced healthy diet.
- **Liquid Intake:** Drink adequate liquids, 6-8 glasses of water daily.

❸ Avoid Caffeine:
- Avoid caffeine-containing beverages. *(Reason: Caffeine is a stimulant and can aggravate palpitations.)*
- Examples of caffeine-containing beverages include coffee, tea, colas, Mountain Dew, Red Bull, and some energy drinks.

❹ Avoid Diet Pills: Do not use diet pills. *(Reason: They act as stimulants.)*

❺ Limit Alcohol: Limit your alcohol consumption to no more than 2 drinks a day. Ideally, eliminate alcohol entirely for the next 2 weeks.

❻ Limit Smoking: Stop or reduce your smoking.

❼ Expected Course: If your symptoms do not improve over the next couple days, you should make an appointment to see your doctor.

❽ Call Back If:
- Chest pain, light-headedness, or difficulty breathing occurs.
- Heart beating > 140 beats/minute.
- > 3 extra or skipped beats/minute.
- You become worse.

BACKGROUND

Key Points

- **Normal Heart Rate:** The normal heart rate is regular and between 60 and 100 beats per minute. The heart rate increases with exercise, emotional stress, and fever. Athletes may have a resting pulse of < 60.
- **Palpitations:** Everybody experiences palpitations at some point in their lives. In most circumstances it is simply a heightened awareness of the heart's normal beating.
- **Rapid Heart Rate:** Patients with anxiety or stress may describe a "rapid heartbeat" or "pounding" in their chest from their heart beating. If they are able to measure their own heart rate, they will relate that the heart is beating regularly at < 130 beats/minute. Patients with a heart rate > 130 (excluding during exercise) require evaluation.
- **Extra Heartbeats:** Occasional extra heartbeats are also experienced by almost everyone. Patients may state that their heart "jumps," "skips a beat," or "flip-flops." Lack of sleep, stress, and caffeinated beverages can aggravate this condition. If the patient states that this is occurring ≥ 4 times per minute on an ongoing basis, he/she requires physician evaluation.

- **Automatic Implantable Cardioverter Defibrillator (AICD):** This internal device analyzes the cardiac rhythm and automatically delivers a shock to the heart when needed. The patient can feel the shock. A patient with an AICD typically has a past history of either ventricular fibrillation, symptomatic ventricular tachycardia, or unexplained syncope.

Causes

- **Anxiety:** Stress, panic disorder, hyperventilation.
- **Endocrine:** Hyperthyroidism, hypoglycemia.
- **Exercise:** Exercise and physical work are the most common cause of temporary tachycardia.
- **Cardiac Disease:** Underlying cardiac disease predisposes an individual to cardiac dysrhythmias: angina, myocardial infarction, congestive heart failure, valvular heart disease.
- **Cardiac Dysrhythmias:** PACs, PVCs, SVT, VT, atrial fibrillation, etc.
- **Dehydration:** The heart rate speeds up with volume depletion.
- **Medication:** Thyroid hormone, digoxin (Lanoxin), diet pills.
- **Stimulants:** Caffeine, cocaine, tobacco.

HEAT EXPOSURE (HEAT EXHAUSTION AND HEATSTROKE)

Definition
- Symptoms following exposure to high environmental temperatures or vigorous physical activity during hot weather

TRIAGE ASSESSMENT QUESTIONS

Call EMS 911 Now
- Fever > 103° F (39.4° C)
  R/O: heatstroke
- Unconscious or difficult to awaken
  R/O: heatstroke
- Acting confused (e.g., disoriented, slurred speech)
  R/O: heatstroke
- Seizure has occurred
  R/O: heatstroke
- Very weak (can't stand)
  R/O: heatstroke, severe heat exhaustion
- Has fainted (passed out)
  R/O: heat syncope
- Sounds like a life-threatening emergency to the triager

See More Appropriate Protocol
- Swelling of both ankles (i.e., pedal edema) and worsened by hot weather
  Go to Protocol: Leg Swelling and Edema on page 279

Go to ED Now
- Unable to walk or can only walk with assistance (e.g., requires support)
  R/O: heat exhaustion
  First Aid for Heat Exhaustion
- Fever > 103° F (39.4° C)

Go to ED/UCC Now
(or to Office With PCP Approval)
- Vomiting interferes with drinking fluids
  R/O: need for IV fluids
- Dizziness, fever, or muscle cramps persist after 2 hours of oral fluids and rest
  R/O: need for IV fluids
- Patient sounds very sick or weak to the triager
  Reason: severe acute illness or serious complication suspected

Go to Office Now
- Fever > 100.5° F (38.1° C) and > 60 years of age
  R/O: heat exhaustion or bacterial illness
- Fever > 100.0° F (37.8° C) and has diabetes mellitus or a weak immune system (e.g., HIV positive, cancer chemotherapy, organ transplant, splenectomy, chronic steroids)
  R/O: heat exhaustion or bacterial illness
- Fever > 100.0° F (37.8° C) and bedridden (e.g., nursing home patient, stroke, chronic illness, recovering from surgery)
  R/O: heat exhaustion or bacterial illness
  Note: May need ambulance transport to ED.

See Today in Office
- Patient wants to be seen

Home Care
- Normal muscle cramps or sore muscles from heat exposure
  R/O: heat cramps
- Normal brief (1-2 hours) fever (< 103° F or 39.4° C) from heat exposure
  R/O: mild heat exhaustion
- Normal hot, flushed (pink) skin from heat exposure
  R/O: mild heat exhaustion
- Normal mild dehydration suspected (e.g., dizziness, weakness, nausea) from heat exposure
  R/O: mild heat exhaustion, dehydration

HOME CARE ADVICE

❶ Mild Heat Exposure Symptoms:
- **Heat Cramps:** Heat cramps are a common reaction to excessive heat exposure. They are not usually serious but can be a warning sign of impending heat exhaustion. Heat cramps mean that your body needs more liquids and salt.
- **Temperature Elevation:** The body can normally become overheated from sun exposure and/or exercise. The temperature should come down to normal after lost fluids are replaced and you have been able to rest for 1 or 2 hours.
- **Facial Flushing:** Your skin can become very pink or flushed when you become overheated. The skin color should return to normal in 1 or 2 hours.
- **Dizziness:** Dizziness is usually due to mild dehydration from all the sweating that occurs with heat exposure. It should disappear in 1-2 hours after the lost fluids are replaced.

❷ Move to a Cool, Shady Area:
- Move to a cool, shady area. If possible, move into an air-conditioned place.
- Remove excess clothing or equipment (e.g., sports gear, protective work uniforms).
- Rest until feeling better.

❸ Drink Liquids to Rehydrate:
- **What?** Drink a sports rehydration drink (e.g., Gatorade or Powerade), which contains sugar and salt. Or, drink water and eat some salty foods (e.g., potato chips or pretzels).
- **How Much?** Approximately 1 cup (240 mL) every 15 minutes for the next 1-2 hours. Your urine (pee) color can help you tell if you have drunk enough liquids. Dark-yellow urine suggests dehydration. Clear or light-yellow urine suggests that you have drunk enough liquids.

❹ Avoid:
- Don't take salt tablets.
  (Reason: They may cause vomiting.)
- Don't drink carbonated beverages.
  (Reason: Bubbles fill up stomach.)
- Don't drink alcohol or caffeinated beverages.
  (Reason: They are dehydrating.)

❺ Cool Bath for Elevated Temperature:
- After you drink some water, take a cool bath or shower for 5 minutes.
  (Reason: brings down the temperature more quickly)
- **Fever Medications:** Fever medications like acetaminophen (Tylenol) are of no value in reducing a body temperature elevated from heat exposure.

❻ Call Back If:
- Fever rises > 103° F (39.4° C).
- Dizziness, fever, or muscle cramps last > 2 hours.
- Vomiting interferes with taking fluids.
- You become worse.

FIRST AID

First Aid Advice for Heatstroke (Sunstroke):
- **Call EMS 911 immediately.**
- Move the victim to a cool, shady area. If possible, move into an air-conditioned place.
- Lay the victim down on his/her back. Elevate the feet.
- Remove excess clothing or equipment (e.g., sports gear, protective work uniforms).
- Sponge the entire body surface continuously with cool water. Fan the victim to increase evaporation.
- If the victim is awake, give as much cold water or sports drink (e.g., Gatorade, Powerade) as he/she can drink. An awake adult or teen should drink 2-3 cups (480-720 mL) of liquids right away to replace what was lost.
- Fever medicines are of no value for the fever seen with heatstroke.

First Aid for Heat Exhaustion:
- Move the victim to a cool, shady area. If possible, move into an air-conditioned place.
- The victim should lie down. Elevate the feet.
- Undress victim (except for underwear) so the body surface can give off heat.
- Sponge the entire body surface continuously with cool water. Fan the victim to increase evaporation.
- Give as much cold water or sports drink (e.g., Gatorade, Powerade) as the victim can tolerate. An adult or teen with heat exhaustion should drink 2-3 cups (480-720 mL) of liquids right away to replace what was lost. Then the adult or teen should drink approximately 1 cup (240 mL) every 15 minutes for the next 1-2 hours.

BACKGROUND

Cause

- Heat-related illness is caused by exposure to high temperatures. High humidity increases the risk. The primary way the body cools itself off is through sweating and evaporation of the sweat. On days with high humidity, evaporation does not occur as rapidly and the body has trouble releasing heat.
- The body's temperature rises when internal heat production and external heat exposure exceed the capacity of the body to dispel heat.

Types of Heat Injuries: There are 5 main reactions to hot environmental temperatures:

❶ **Heatstroke or Sunstroke:** Symptoms include hot, flushed skin; high fever > 105° F (40.5° C) rectally; the absence of sweating (in 50%); confusion or unconsciousness; and shock. Exertional heatstroke occurs with exertion/exercise and the onset is usually rapid. Classic heatstroke typically occurs during heat waves and the onset is usually gradual. A rectal temperature is more accurate than an oral temperature in these disorders. Heatstroke is a life-threatening emergency with a 10%-70% mortality rate if not treated promptly. EMS 911 transport is required.

❷ **Heat Exhaustion:** Symptoms may include profuse sweating, headache, nausea, vomiting, dizziness, and weakness. The body temperature can range from normal to 104° F (40° C). The onset is usually gradual. Patients with heat exhaustion are dehydrated and depleted of electrolytes (sodium, potassium). Treatment consists of rest, fluid, and electrolyte replacement.

❸ **Heat Syncope:** This is an orthostatic syncope that develops from standing up too suddenly or from prolonged standing.

❹ **Heat Cramps:** Severe muscle cramps in the limbs (especially calf or thigh muscles) and abdomen are present. No fever. Heat tetany (manifested by carpopedal spasm) may occur. Heat cramps are caused by decreased electrolytes and fluids in the muscle tissues. Treatment consists of rest, fluid, and electrolyte replacement.

❺ **Heat Edema:** Many individuals experience heat edema during the first few days of hot weather or after traveling to a warmer climate. There may be mild swelling of the feet and ankles and some puffiness of the fingers. Typically, the body adjusts to the higher temperatures (acclimatizes) in a couple of days and the swelling resolves.

Risk Factors for Heat-Related Illness

The very young, the very old, and obese individuals are at greater risk of heat-related illness.

- **Dehydration:** Sweating is the primary way that the body cools itself during hot weather. An adult athlete can lose 1-2 L (4-8 cups) of sweat per hour. The evaporation of this sweat is the main way in which the body dissipates extra heat. Dehydration inhibits sweating and, thus, predisposes toward heat injury.
- **Drugs of Abuse:** Amphetamines, cocaine, and PCP are all stimulants and increase internal heat production.
- **Elderly:** The elderly are at greater risk because they have a decreased ability to sweat. They also often have underlying cardiac and other medical conditions that further reduce their ability to compensate.
- **Environmental Factors:** Examples include lack of air-conditioning and wearing heavy clothing or sports gear.
- **Exertion:** Exercising or other vigorous activity/labor during hot weather causes heat production to exceed heat loss.
- **Fever:** Febrile illnesses increase heat production and raise the likelihood of heat injury.
- **Lack of Heat Acclimatization:** Adults who are vacationing in a hot climate and who have not acclimatized are at increased risk of heat injury. The first heat wave of the summer can cause similar problems. It takes 8-10 days to acclimate to high temperatures. After physiological acclimatization has occurred, sweating begins at lower body temperature and the sweat rate doubles.
- **Lack of Fitness:** A higher level of fitness increases the body's capability of sweating and handling heat generated by exertion.
- **Medications:** Certain classes of medications reduce the body's ability to sweat. These include antihistamines, phenothiazines, and tricyclic antidepressants.
- **Obesity:** Individuals with a higher percentage of body fat have a decreased ability to disperse heat.

Preventing Heat-Related Illness

- **Drink More:** When working or exercising in a hot environment, a person needs to drink large amounts of cool liquids. This means 1 cup every 15 minutes. Water is the ideal solution for replacing lost sweat. Very little salt is lost. Special glucose-electrolyte solutions (sports drinks) offer no advantage over water unless exercising for > 1 hour.
- **Take Water Breaks:** It is important to take 5-minute water breaks in the shade every 25 minutes. It is important to drink water even when not thirsty. Thirst is often delayed until a person is almost dehydrated. A healthy person can't drink too much water during hot weather.
- **No Salt Tablets:** Avoid salt tablets because they slow down stomach emptying and delay the absorption of fluids.
- **Dress Cool:** Wear a single layer of lightweight clothing. Change it if it becomes wet with perspiration.
- **Stay Cool:** During heat waves, spend as much time as possible in cool environments (e.g., with air-conditioning) or use an electric fan. Slow down. It takes at least a week to acclimate to a hot environment.
- **Exercise Smart:** Athletic coaches recommend that exercise sessions be shortened and less vigorous if the temperature exceeds 82° F (28° C), especially if the humidity is high.
- **Limit Hot Tub Time:** When using a hot tub, limit exposure to 15 minutes and have a "buddy" system in case a heat reaction suddenly occurs. Hot tubs and saunas should be avoided by people with a fever or following vigorous exercise when the body needs to release heat.

Heat Index Chart

A heat index chart is available on the National Oceanic and Atmospheric Administration National Weather Service Web site at www.nws.noaa.gov/os/heat/heat_index.shtml. It helps estimate the risk of heat-related illness on any given day using the temperature and relative humidity.

HIGH BLOOD PRESSURE

Definition
- Systolic blood pressure > 130 or
- Diastolic blood pressure > 80 or
- Taking medications for high blood pressure

If adult is having symptoms (e.g., headache, chest pain, difficulty breathing), go to that protocol first and use this protocol afterward.

TRIAGE ASSESSMENT QUESTIONS

Call EMS 911 Now
- Sounds like a life-threatening emergency to the triager

Go to L&D Now (or to Office With PCP Approval)
- Pregnant > 20 weeks and new hand or face swelling
  R/O: preeclampsia
- Pregnant > 20 weeks and BP > 140/90
  R/O: preeclampsia

Go to ED/UCC Now (or to Office With PCP Approval)
- Systolic BP ≥ 160 OR diastolic ≥ 100, and any cardiac or neurologic symptoms (e.g., chest pain, difficulty breathing, unsteady gait, blurred vision)
  R/O: hypertensive emergency
- Patient sounds very sick or weak to the triager
  Reason: severe acute illness or serious complication suspected

Discuss With PCP and Callback by Nurse Within 1 Hour
- Systolic BP ≥ 180 OR diastolic ≥ 110, and missed most recent dose of blood pressure medication
  Reason: needs to take medicine and recheck blood pressure

See Today in Office
- Systolic BP ≥ 180 OR diastolic ≥ 110
  Reason: asymptomatic hypertension, stage 2; may need medication adjustment or initiation
- Patient wants to be seen
  Reason: for BP check

Discuss With PCP and Callback by Nurse Today
- Ran out of BP medications
  Reason: refill
- Taking BP medications and feels is having side effects (e.g., impotence, cough, dizziness)
  Reason: may need dose adjustment or new medication

See Within 3 Days in Office
- Systolic BP ≥ 160 OR diastolic ≥ 100
  Reason: asymptomatic hypertension, stage 2; needs medication adjustment or initiation
- Systolic BP ≥ 130 OR diastolic ≥ 80, and pregnant
  Reason: high BP and pregnant; needs medical evaluation

See Within 2 Weeks in Office
- Systolic BP ≥ 130 OR diastolic ≥ 80, and is taking BP medications
  Reason: may need medication adjustment or new medicine; treatment goal usually is < 130/80 for most people; goal may be higher in elderly and based on other factors
- Systolic BP ≥ 130 OR diastolic ≥ 80, and is not taking BP medications
  R/O: hypertension
  Reason: may need medication initiation and counseling regarding lifestyle modifications
- Systolic BP ≥ 130 OR diastolic ≥ 80, and history of heart problems, kidney disease, or diabetes
  Reason: high BP and higher-risk patient; may need medication adjustment or initiation

Home Care
- Systolic BP < 130 with diastolic < 80, and taking BP medications
  Reason: hypertension; treatment goal usually is < 130/80 for most people; goal may be higher in elderly and based on other factors
- Systolic BP between 120 and 129 with diastolic < 80
  Reason: elevated BP (prehypertension, lifestyle modification recommended)
- Systolic BP < 120 with diastolic < 80
  Reason: normal blood pressure
- Healthy diet, questions about

HOME CARE ADVICE

General Care Advice for High Blood Pressure (BP)

❶ Introduction:
- Untreated high BP may cause damage to the heart, brain, kidneys, and eyes.
- Treatment of high BP can reduce the risk of stroke, heart attack, and heart failure.
- The goal of BP treatment for most patients with hypertension is to keep the BP < 140/90.

❷ BP 120-129/80:
- This is considered "elevated BP" or prehypertension.
- Sometimes, changes in your lifestyle can reduce your BP without medications.
- If your BP stays elevated during the next month, you should go in to see the doctor and get your BP checked.

❸ BP < 120/80:
- This is considered normal BP.

❹ Lifestyle Modifications—The following things can help you reduce your BP:
- **Eat Healthy:** Eat a diet rich in fresh fruits and vegetables, dietary fiber, nonanimal protein (e.g., soy), and low-fat dairy products. Avoid foods with a high content of saturated fat or cholesterol.
- **Decrease Sodium Intake:** Aim to eat < 2.4 g (100 mmol) of sodium each day. Unfortunately, 75% of the salt in the average person's diet is in preprocessed foods.
- **Limit Alcohol:** Limit alcohol to 0-2 standard drinks each day. Men should have < 14 dinks per week. Women should have < 9 drinks per week. A drink is 1.5 oz hard liquor (one shot or jigger; 45 mL), 5 oz wine (small glass; 150 mL), 12 oz beer (one can; 360 mL).
- **Exercise, Be More Physically Active:** Do at least 30 minutes of aerobic exercise (e.g., brisk walking) most days of the week. Other examples of aerobic activities include cycling, jogging, and swimming.
- **Reduce Weight and Waistline:** It is important to maintain a normal body weight. The goal should be a body mass index (BMI) < 25 for men and women, a waist circumference < 40" (102 cm) in men, and a waist circumference < 35" (88 cm) in women.

- **Reduce Stress:** Find activities that help reduce your stress. Examples might include meditation, yoga, or even a restful walk in a park.
- **If You Smoke…You Should Stop!**

❺ Call Back If:
- Headache, blurred vision, difficulty talking, or difficulty walking occurs.
- Chest pain or difficulty breathing occurs.
- You want to go in to the office for a BP check.
- You become worse.

Missed Dose of BP Medication

❶ What to Do When You Miss a Dose of Your BP Medication:
- Generally, you should take a missed dose as soon as you remember.
- If it is > 8 hours until your next dose, take the missed dose of medication now.
- If it is < 8 hours until your next dose, skip the missed dose and take the medicine at the next regularly scheduled time.
- Do NOT take 2 doses of a BP medication at the same time because you missed a dose.

❷ Call Back If:
- Headache, blurred vision, difficulty talking, or difficulty walking occurs.
- Chest pain or difficulty breathing occurs.
- You want to come in to the office for a BP check.
- You become worse.

Questions About Eating a Healthy Diet

❶ What Is a Healthy Diet?
- Eat a variety of vegetables and fruits. Aim for 5 servings per day.
- Eat a variety of grains. Aim for 6 servings per day.
- Eat fish at least twice each week. Fatty fish such as salmon and tuna are best.

❷ Choose:
- Choose reduced-fat dairy, skinless poultry, and lean meats. These are healthier than red meat.
- Choose fats with no more than 2 g of saturated fat per tablespoon. Examples include liquid and tub margarine, canola, corn, safflower, and olive oil.

❸ **Limit:**
- Limit your sugar intake. Avoid high-calorie, low-nutrition foods like soft drinks and candy.
- Limit foods high in saturated fat, trans fat, and cholesterol.
- Limit alcoholic beverages to no more than 1 drink per day for women and no more than 2 drinks for men.

❹ **Call Back If:**
- You have more questions.

Questions About Eating a Low-Salt Diet

❶ **How Much Sodium (Salt) Should You Eat Each Day?**
- Aim to eat < 2.4 g of sodium each day.
- Remember that 1 teaspoon of salt has 2,300 mg (2.3 g) of sodium.
- Unfortunately, 75% of the salt in the average person's diet is in preprocessed foods.

❷ **How to Reduce Your Sodium (Salt) Intake—DO:**
- Buy and eat more fresh foods, especially fruit and vegetables.
- Read the label on processed foods you buy. Choose processed foods with low-salt labels or brands with the lowest percentage of sodium on the food label.
- Use other spices to make food taste better.
- Eat less food at restaurants and fast-food outlets. Ask for less salt to be added in your food.

❸ **How to Reduce Your Sodium (Salt) Intake— DO NOT:**
- Do not buy or eat heavily salted foods. Examples include pickled foods, salted crackers or chips, and processed meats.
- Do not add salt while cooking or at the table.

❹ **Call Back If:**
- You have more questions.

❺ **Internet Resource—National High Blood Pressure Education Program**
- My Blood Pressure Wallet Card. Available at: https://www.nhlbi.nih.gov/files/docs/public/heart/hbpwallet.pdf
- Your Guide to Lowering Blood Pressure. Available at: https://www.nhlbi.nih.gov/files/docs/public/heart/hbp_low.pdf

BACKGROUND

Key Points
- **Definition of Hypertension:** An adult has hypertension (high blood pressure [BP]) if the BP readings consistently show a BP > 130/80; that is, a systolic BP > 130 OR a diastolic BP > 80.
- Untreated hypertension may cause damage to the heart, brain, kidneys, and eyes.
- There are age-related increases in BP, such that > 50% of adults > 60 years of age have hypertension.
- Automatic home BP measurement devices can sometimes be unreliable. Have patient check BP in both arms. If there is another adult in the home, consider checking his/her BP to see if the device is functioning correctly.
- Research casts some doubt on the common belief that hypertension causes headaches. However, it is important to emphasize that a patient who has a severe headache, which he/she describes as being the "worst headache," or is having sudden onset (thunderclap) headache, deserves an emergency evaluation.

BP Classification in Adults*
- **Normal:** < 120/80 (i.e., systolic < 120 mm Hg and diastolic < 80 mm Hg)
- **Elevated:** 120-129/80
- **Hypertension—Stage 1:** 130-139/80-89
- **Hypertension—Stage 2:** ≥ 140/90

*Source: Whelton PK, Carey RM, Aronow WS, et al. 2017 ACC/AHA/AAPA/ABC/ACPM/AGS/APhA/ASH/ASPC/NMA/PCNA guideline for the prevention, detection, evaluation, and management of high blood pressure in adults: a report of the American College of Cardiology/American Heart Association Task Force on Clinical Practice Guidelines. *Hypertension.* 2017

Causes of High BP
- Chronic kidney disease
- Coarctation of the aorta
- Cushing syndrome and other glucocorticoid excess states (including chronic steroid therapy)
- Drug withdrawal (e.g., narcotic withdrawal)
- Drugs—over the counter (e.g., NSAIDs)
- Drugs—prescription (e.g., steroids)
- Drugs—street (e.g., anabolic steroids, cocaine, phencyclidine)
- Obstructive uropathy
- Pheochromocytoma
- Primary aldosteronism and other mineralocorticoid excess states
- Renovascular hypertension
- Sleep apnea
- Thyroid or parathyroid disease

Treatment

The doctor or other health care professional will work with the patient to develop a treatment plan.

A **healthy lifestyle** can help decrease high BP. Here are some healthy living teaching points to share with patients.

- **Eat Healthy:** Eat a diet rich in fresh fruits and vegetables, dietary fiber, nonanimal protein (e.g., soy), and low-fat dairy products. Avoid foods with a high content of saturated fat or cholesterol.
- **Decrease Sodium Intake:** Aim to eat < 2.4 g (100 mmol) of sodium each day. Unfortunately, 75% of the salt in the average person's diet is in preprocessed foods.
- **Limit Alcohol:** Limit alcohol to 0-2 standard drinks each day. Men should have < 14 dinks per week. Women should have < 9 drinks per week. A drink is 1.5 oz hard liquor (one shot or jigger; 45 mL), 5 oz wine (small glass; 150 mL), 12 oz beer (one can; 360 mL).
- **Exercise, Be More Physically Active:** Do at least 30 minutes of aerobic exercise (e.g., brisk walking) most days of the week. Other examples of aerobic activities include cycling, jogging, and swimming.
- **Reduce Weight and Waistline:** It is important to maintain a normal body weight. The goal should be a body mass index (BMI) < 25 for men and women, a waist circumference < 40" (102 cm) in men, and a waist circumference < 35" (88 cm) in women.
- **Reduce Stress:** Find activities that help reduce your stress. Examples might include meditation, yoga, or even a restful walk in a park.
- **If You Smoke…Stop!**

The doctor may prescribe a **BP medicine.** This will depend on how high the BP is and whether healthy lifestyle changes help. There are many different types of BP medicines.

Benefits of Antihypertensive Medicines

- Reduce incidence of stroke by 35%-40%.
- Reduce incidence of myocardial infarction by 20%-25%.
- Reduce incidence of congestive heart failure by > 50%.

Internet Resources

- My Blood Pressure Wallet Card. Available at: https://www.nhlbi.nih.gov/files/docs/public/heart/hbpwallet.pdf
- Your Guide to Lowering Blood Pressure. Available at: https://www.nhlbi.nih.gov/files/docs/public/heart/hbp_low.pdf
- Hypertension Canada, 2013 recommendations: http://guidelines.hypertension.ca

Frequently Asked Questions

How do I know if I have hypertension?
Hypertension and high BP mean the same thing. An adult has hypertension if most of his/her BP readings are > 130/80. This means that the systolic BP is > 130 or the diastolic BP is > 80.

What do the words systolic *and* diastolic *mean?*
The BP reading is written as 2 numbers. The 2 numbers are the systolic pressure and the diastolic pressure. If a person has a BP of 130/65, 130 is the systolic BP and 65 is the diastolic BP. Systolic pressure is the BP when the heart beats. Diastolic pressure is the BP when the heart is resting between beats.

My doctor has given me BP medicine. What should my BP be? What is the target BP?
The treatment goal usually is < 130/80 for most people. The goal may be higher in elderly patients and based on other factors.

HIP INJURY

Definition
- Injuries to a bone, muscle, joint, or ligament of the hip.
- Associated skin and soft tissue injuries are also included.

TRIAGE ASSESSMENT QUESTIONS

Call EMS 911 Now
- Major bleeding (actively dripping or spurting) that can't be stopped
  First Aid: Apply direct pressure to the entire wound with a clean cloth.
- Bullet, stabbed by knife, or other serious penetrating wound
  First Aid: If penetrating object is still in place, don't remove it.
- Looks like a dislocated joint (crooked or deformed)
  R/O: fracture
- Can't stand (bear weight) or walk
- Sounds like a life-threatening emergency to the triager

See More Appropriate Protocol
- Wound looks infected
  Go to Protocol: Wound Infection on page 443
- Puncture wound of hip area
  Go to Protocol: Puncture Wound on page 319

Go to ED/UCC Now
(or to Office With PCP Approval)
- SEVERE pain (e.g., excruciating)
- Skin is split open or gaping (length > ½" or 12 mm)
  Reason: may need laceration repair (e.g., sutures)
- Bleeding won't stop after 10 minutes of direct pressure (using correct technique)
- Dirt in the wound and not removed after 15 minutes of scrubbing
  Reason: needs irrigation or debridement
- Sounds like a serious injury to the triager

Go to Office Now
- Looks infected (e.g., spreading redness, pus, red streak)
  R/O: cellulitis, lymphangitis

See Today in Office
- Patient wants to be seen

See Today or Tomorrow in Office
- Injury interferes with work or school
- Large swelling or bruise and size > palm of person's hand
  R/O: fracture, large contusion
- High-risk adult (e.g., age > 60, osteoporosis, chronic steroid use)
  Reason: greater risk of fracture in patients with osteoporosis
- Suspicious history for the injury
  R/O: domestic violence or elder abuse
- Wound and no tetanus booster in > 5 years (or > 10 years for clean cuts)
  Reason: may need a tetanus booster shot (vaccine)

See Within 3 Days in Office
- Injury and pain has not improved after 3 days
- Injury is still painful or swollen after 2 weeks

Home Care
- Minor hip injury
  R/O: minor bruise, strain, or sprain

HOME CARE ADVICE

Treatment of a Minor Bruise, Sprain, or Strain

❶ Reassurance—Direct Blow (Contusion, Bruise):
- A direct blow to your hip can cause a contusion. Contusion is the medical term for bruise.
- Symptoms are mild pain, swelling, and/or bruising.
- *Here is some care advice that should help.*

❷ Reassurance—Bending or Twisting Injury (Strain, Sprain):
- Strain and sprain are the medical terms used to describe overstretching of the muscles and ligaments of the hip. A twisting or bending injury can cause a strain or sprain.
- The main symptom is pain that is worse with movement.
- *Here is some care advice that should help.*

❸ Apply a Cold Pack:
- Apply a cold pack or an ice bag (wrapped in a moist towel) to the area for 20 minutes. Repeat in 1 hour, then every 4 hours while awake.
- Continue this for the first 48 hours after an injury.
- This will help decrease pain and swelling.

❹ Apply Heat to the Area:
- Beginning 48 hours after an injury, apply a warm washcloth or heating pad for 10 minutes 3 times a day.
- This will help increase blood flow and improve healing.

❺ Rest Versus Movement:
- Movement is generally more healing in the long term than rest.
- Continue normal activities as much as your pain permits.
- Avoid running and active sports for 1-2 weeks or until the pain and swelling are gone.
- Complete rest should only be used for the first day or two after an injury. If it really hurts too much to walk, you will need to see the doctor.

❻ Expected Course:
- Pain, swelling, and bruising usually start to get better 2-3 days after an injury.
- Swelling most often is gone after 1 week.
- Bruises fade away slowly over 1-2 weeks.
- It may take 2 weeks for pain and tenderness of the injured area to go away.

❼ Call Back If:
- Pain becomes severe.
- Pain does not improve after 3 days.
- Pain or swelling lasts > 2 weeks.
- You become worse.

Treatment of a Small Cut or Scrape

❶ Reassurance—Superficial Laceration (Cut or Scratch) or Abrasion (Scrape):
- This sounds like a small cut or scrape that we can treat at home.
- *Here is some care advice that should help.*

❷ Bleeding: Apply direct pressure for 10 minutes with a sterile gauze to stop any bleeding.

❸ Cleaning the Wound:
- Wash the wound with soap and water for 5 minutes.
- For any dirt, scrub gently with a washcloth.
- For any bleeding, apply direct pressure with a sterile gauze or clean cloth for 10 minutes.

❹ Antibiotic Ointment:
- Apply an antibiotic ointment (e.g., OTC bacitracin), covered by a Band-Aid or dressing. Change daily or if it becomes wet.
- Option: A Telfa dressing won't stick to the wound when it is removed.
- Option: Another option is to use a liquid skin bandage that only needs to be applied once. Don't use antibiotic ointment if you use a liquid skin bandage.

❺ Liquid Skin Bandage:
- You can use a liquid skin bandage instead of antibiotic ointment and a dressing or a Band-Aid.
- **Benefits:** Liquid skin bandage has several benefits when compared with a regular bandage (e.g., a dressing or a Band-Aid). You only need to put a liquid bandage on once to minor cuts and scrapes. It helps stop minor bleeding. It seals the wound and may promote faster healing and lower infection rates. However, it also costs more.
- **How to Use It:** First clean and dry the wound. You put on the liquid as spray or with a swab. It dries in < 1 minute and usually lasts a week. You can get it wet.
- **Examples:** Liquid skin bandage is available over the counter. Examples are Band-Aid Liquid Bandage, New Skin, Curad Spray Bandage, and 3M No Sting Liquid Bandage Spray.

❻ Call Back If:
- Looks infected (pus, redness, increasing tenderness).
- Doesn't heal within 10 days.
- You become worse.

Over-the-counter Pain Medicines
❶ Pain Medicines:
- For pain relief, you can take either acetaminophen, ibuprofen, or naproxen.
- They are over-the-counter (OTC) pain drugs. You can buy them at the drugstore.

Acetaminophen (e.g., Tylenol):
- **Regular Strength Tylenol:** Take 650 mg (two 325 mg pills) by mouth every 4-6 hours as needed. Each Regular Strength Tylenol pill has 325 mg of acetaminophen.
- **Extra Strength Tylenol:** Take 1,000 mg (two 500 mg pills) every 8 hours as needed. Each Extra Strength Tylenol pill has 500 mg of acetaminophen.
- The most you should take each day is 3,000 mg (10 Regular Strength or 6 Extra Strength pills a day).

Ibuprofen (e.g., Motrin, Advil):
- Take 400 mg (two 200 mg pills) by mouth every 6 hours.
- Another choice is to take 600 mg (three 200 mg pills) by mouth every 8 hours.
- The most you should take each day is 1,200 mg (six 200 mg pills), unless your doctor has told you to take more.

Naproxen (e.g., Aleve):
- Take 220 mg (one 220 mg pill) by mouth every 8 hours as needed. You may take 440 mg (two 220 mg pills) for your first dose.
- The most you should take each day is 660 mg (three 220 mg pills a day), unless your doctor has told you to take more.

❷ Pain Medicines—Extra Notes:
- Use the lowest amount of medicine that makes your pain better.
- Acetaminophen is thought to be safer than ibuprofen or naproxen in people > 65 years old. Acetaminophen is in many OTC and prescription medicines. It might be in more than one medicine that you are taking. You need to be careful and not take an overdose. An acetaminophen overdose can hurt the liver.
- McNeil, the company that makes Tylenol, has different dosage instructions for Tylenol in Canada and the United States. In Canada, the maximum recommended dose per day is 4,000 mg or 12 Regular Strength (325 mg) pills. In the United States, McNeil recommends a maximum dose of 10 Regular Strength (325 mg) pills.
- CAUTION: Do not take acetaminophen if you have liver disease.
- CAUTION: Do not take ibuprofen or naproxen if you have stomach problems, have kidney disease, are pregnant, or have been told by your doctor to avoid this type of anti-inflammatory drug. Do not take ibuprofen or naproxen for > 7 days without consulting your doctor.
- *Before taking any medicine, read all the instructions on the package.*

❸ Call Back If:
- You have more questions.
- You become worse.

FIRST AID

First Aid Advice for Bleeding:
Apply direct pressure to the entire wound with a clean cloth.

First Aid Advice for Penetrating Object:
If penetrating object is still in place, don't remove it. *Reason: Removal could increase bleeding.*

First Aid Advice for Shock:
Lie down with the feet elevated.

BACKGROUND

Types of Hip Injuries

- Fractures (broken bones).
- Dislocations (bone out of joint).
- **Sprains:** Stretches and tears of ligaments.
- **Strains:** Stretches and tears of muscles (e.g., pulled muscle).
- **Contusion:** A direct blow or crushing injury results in bruising of the skin, muscle, and underlying bone.
- Cuts, abrasions.

What Cuts Need to Be Sutured?

- Any cut that is split open or gaping probably needs sutures (or staples or skin glue).
- Cuts > ½" (1 cm) usually need sutures.
- Any open wound that may need sutures should be evaluated by a physician regardless of the time that has passed since the initial injury.

When Does an Adult Need a Tetanus Booster (Tetanus Shot)?

- **Clean Cuts and Scrapes—Tetanus Booster Needed Every 10 Years:** Patients with clean minor wounds AND who have previously had ≥ 3 tetanus shots (full series) need a booster every 10 years. Examples of minor wounds include a superficial abrasion or a shallow cut from a clean knife blade. Obtain booster within 72 hours.
- **Dirty Wounds—Tetanus Booster Needed Every 5 Years:** Patients with dirty wounds need a booster if it has been > 5 years since the last booster. Examples of dirty wounds include those contaminated with soil, feces, and/or saliva and more serious wounds from deep punctures, crushing, and burns. Obtain booster within 72 hours.

HIVES

Definition
- A very itchy rash made up of flat raised/swollen spots or patches of skin.
- *Use this protocol only if the patient has symptoms that match hives.*

Symptoms
- Itchy, swollen patches or bumps that appear suddenly.
- Patches change shape and location frequently; any one patch generally only lasts for a few hours, then fades away.
- Sizes of patches vary from ½" (6 mm) to several inches across.
- In whites and individuals with lighter skin tones, hives appear pink or red in color, with a central area of paleness (welts).

Itching Severity
- **Mild:** Doesn't interfere with normal activities.
- **Moderate-Severe:** Interferes with work, school, sleep, or other activities.

TRIAGE ASSESSMENT QUESTIONS

Call EMS 911 Now
- Difficulty breathing or wheezing now
  R/O: anaphylaxis
- Rapid onset of swollen tongue
  R/O: anaphylaxis
- Rapid onset of hoarseness or cough
  R/O: anaphylaxis
- Very weak (can't stand)
  R/O: anaphylaxis
- Difficult to awaken or acting confused (e.g., disoriented, slurred speech)
  R/O: anaphylaxis
- Life-threatening reaction (anaphylaxis) in the past to similar substance (e.g., food, insect bite/sting, chemical, etc.) and < 2 hours since exposure
  Reason: high likelihood of recurrent severe reaction
- Sounds like a life-threatening emergency to the triager

See More Appropriate Protocol
- Bee, wasp, or yellow jacket sting within last 24 hours
  Go to Protocol: Bee Sting on page 52
- Taking a new medicine now or within last 3 days *(Exception: antihistamine, decongestant, or other OTC cough/cold medicines)*
  Go to Protocol: Rash, Widespread on Drugs (Drug Reaction) on page 332
- Doesn't match the SYMPTOMS of hives
  Go to Protocol: Rash or Redness, Localized on page 326

Go to ED Now
- Swollen tongue
  R/O: angioedema
- Widespread hives and onset < 2 hours of exposure to high-risk allergen (e.g., peanuts, tree nuts, fish, or shellfish)

Go to ED/UCC Now (or to Office With PCP Approval)
- Patient sounds very sick or weak to the triager
  Reason: severe acute illness or serious complication suspected

See Today in Office
- MODERATE-SEVERE hives persist (i.e., hives interfere with normal activities or work) and taking antihistamine (e.g., Benadryl, Claritin) > 24 hours
- Hives have become worse and taking oral steroids (e.g., prednisone) > 24 hours
- Abdominal pain
  R/O: gastrointestinal angioedema
- Joint swelling
  R/O: serum sickness reaction
- Fever
  R/O: treatable infection as cause of hives
- Patient wants to be seen

See Today or Tomorrow in Office
- Hives persist > 1 week

See Within 3 Days in Office

- Widespread hives and onset > 2 hours of exposure to high-risk allergen (e.g., peanuts, tree nuts, fish, or shellfish)
- Hives from food reaction and diagnosis never confirmed by a physician
- Hives has occurred ≥ 3 times in the last year and the cause is not known
  Reason: needs diagnosis confirmed, possible further workup

Home Care

- ○ Hives from food reaction
- ○ Localized hives
- ○ Widespread hives

HOME CARE ADVICE

Hives From Food Reaction

❶ **Food-Related Hives:**
- Foods can cause transient hives, especially around the mouth.
- Some are mild food allergies; others can occur in anyone (e.g., with strawberries).
- Hives from foods usually disappear within 6 hours.

❷ **Antihistamine (e.g., Benadryl) for Hives From Food:**
- One or two dosages of an antihistamine will accelerate the clearing of this type of hives.
- Benadryl (diphenhydramine) is an antihistamine. The adult dose is 25-50 mg. If the hives are still present after 6 hours, repeat the Benadryl.
- If Benadryl is not available, use any hay fever or cold medicine that contains an antihistamine. Examples of other antihistamines are chlorpheniramine (Chlor-Trimeton, Chlor-Tripolon) and loratadine (Claritin, Alavert). Loratadine is a newer (second-generation) antihistamine and it causes less sedation than diphenhydramine.
- CAUTION: This type of medication may cause sleepiness. Do not drink alcohol, drive, or operate dangerous machinery while taking antihistamines. Do not take these medications if you have prostate problems.
- *Before taking any medicine, read all the instructions on the package.*

❸ **Prevention:** In the future, avoid any food you think caused the hives.

❹ **Call Back If:**
- Severe hives or severe itching persists > 24 hours despite taking an antihistamine (e.g., Benadryl).
- You become worse.

Localized Hives

❶ **Localized Hives:**
- For localized hives, wash the allergic substance off the skin with soap and water.
- If itchy, massage the area with a cold washcloth or ice.
- Localized hives usually disappear in a few hours and don't need treatment with an oral antihistamine (e.g., Benadryl).

❷ **Hydrocortisone Cream for Itching:**
- You can use hydrocortisone for very itchy spots.
- Put 1% hydrocortisone cream on the itchy area(s) 3 times a day. Use it for a couple days, until it feels better. This will help decrease the itching.
- This is an over-the-counter (OTC) drug. You can buy it at the drugstore.
- Some people like to keep the cream in the refrigerator. It feels even better if the cream is used when it is cold.
- CAUTION: Do not use hydrocortisone cream for > 1 week without talking to your doctor.
- *Read the instructions and warnings on the package insert for all medicines you take.*

❸ **Prevention:** Try to avoid any substance that you think caused the hives.

❹ **Call Back If:**
- Severe hives or severe itching persists > 24 hours despite taking an antihistamine (e.g., Benadryl).
- Hives last > 1 week.
- You become worse.

Widespread Hives

❶ Widespread Hives:

- Remove allergens. For widespread hives, be certain to take a bath or shower, if triggered by pollens or animal contact. Change clothes.
- Take a cool bath for 10 minutes to relieve itching. Rub very itchy areas with an ice cube for 10 minutes.
- Hives normally come and go for 3 or 4 days, then disappear.

❷ Antihistamine Medicine for Widespread Hives:

- Take cetirizine (e.g., Zyrtec) or loratadine (e.g., Claritin) once each day for hives that itch. Continue taking it once a day until the hives are gone for 24 hours.
- **Cetirizine** (e.g., Zyrtec, Reactine): Adult dosage is 10 mg once each day.
- **Loratadine** (e.g., Alavert, Claritin): Adult dosage is 10 mg once each day. Alavert is not available in Canada.
- Cetirizine and loratadine are newer (second-generation) antihistamine medications that cause less sedation than diphenhydramine (Benadryl). They have the added advantage of being long acting (last up to 24 hours).
- If you do not have cetirizine or loratadine, you can instead take diphenhydramine (e.g., OTC Benadryl 25-50 mg orally) 4 times a day for hives that itch.
- *Read the instructions and warnings on the package insert for all medicines you take.*

❸ Caution—Antihistamines:

- Examples include diphenhydramine (Benadryl) and chlorpheniramine (Chlor-Trimeton, Chlor-Tripolon).
- May cause sleepiness. Do not drink alcohol, drive, or operate dangerous machinery while taking antihistamines.
- Do not take these medicines if you have prostate problems.

❹ Cool Bath for Itching: Take a cool bath for 10 minutes to relieve itching.
(Caution: Avoid any chill.)
Rub very itchy areas with an ice cube for 10 minutes.

❺ Prevention: If you identify a substance that causes hives, try to avoid that substance in the future.

❻ Prevention—Remove Allergens: Take a bath or shower if triggered by pollens or animal contact. Change clothes.

❼ Contagiousness: Hives are not contagious. You can return to work or school if the hives do not interfere with normal activities.

❽ Call Back If:

- Severe itching lasts > 24 hours while taking an antihistamine.
- Hives persist > 1 week.
- You become worse.

FIRST AID

First Aid Advice for Anaphylaxis—Epinephrine:

- If the patient has an epinephrine autoinjector, **give it now.** Do not delay.
- Use the autoinjector on the upper outer thigh. You may give it through clothing if necessary.
- Give epinephrine first, then call 911.
- Epinephrine is available in autoinjectors under trade names: EpiPen, EpiPen Jr, and Auvi-Q (Allerject in Canada). Auvi-Q has an audio chip and talks patients and caregivers through injection process.
- You may give a second (repeat) dose of epinephrine 10-15 minutes later, IF the person with anaphylaxis does not respond to the first dose AND ambulance arrival takes > 10 minutes.

First Aid Advice for Anaphylaxis—Benadryl:

- Give antihistamine by mouth **NOW** if able to swallow.
- Use Benadryl (diphenhydramine; adult dose: 50 mg) or any other available antihistamine medicine.

First Aid Advice for Anaphylactic Shock
(pending EMS arrival):
Lie down with the feet elevated.

BACKGROUND

Key Points

- The medical term for hives is urticaria.
- Hives are often an allergic skin reaction to something that the patient has eaten, touched, or in some other manner been exposed to. Hives are not contagious.
- Hives usually come and go for several days to a week. Sometimes they can reappear weeks or months later. Some individuals have chronic urticaria, and symptoms can be intermittently present for months.

Causes of Hives

Over-the-counter (OTC; nonprescription) medicines rarely, if ever, cause hives. They should only be suspected if the hives begin within 1 hour of taking the medicine and recur in this same pattern ≥ 2 times.

- **Localized Hives:** Localized hives are usually due to skin contact with plants, pollen, food, a chemical, or pet saliva. Dermographism is the term used to describe patients who have localized hives in response to firm stroking of the skin. Localized hives are not caused by drugs, infection, or swallowed foods. Localized hives usually resolve in < 4 hours.
- **Widespread Hives:** Widespread hives can be an allergic reaction to a food, cosmetic product, drug, insect bite, or other substance. Sometimes widespread hives show up after a viral infection. Stress may bring on or aggravate hives. Often the cause is not found (idiopathic).

Definitions

- **Anaphylactic Reaction:** Anaphylaxis is a serious allergic reaction that is rapid in onset and may cause death.
- **Severe Allergic Reaction:** Any associated symptoms besides skin findings: swollen tongue, shortness of breath, syncope, abdominal pain.
- **Localized Hives:** Hives on one area of the body only.
- **Widespread Hives:** Hives on multiple (≥ 2) areas of the body.

Anaphylactic Reactions and Hives

- **Onset:** Generally, the shorter the interval between the allergen exposure (e.g., food, drug, or sting) and the onset of the first systemic symptoms, the more serious the reaction will be. Anaphylaxis usually starts within 20 minutes and always by 2 hours. If no symptoms occur by 2 hours, the risk for anaphylaxis has passed.
- **Symptoms—Systemic:** By definition, an anaphylactic reaction must include respiratory (e.g., wheezing or stridor), cardiovascular (e.g., fainting), or CNS (e.g., confusion) symptoms.
- **Symptoms—Cutaneous:** Hives or another itchy rash is often present (> 80%). The appearance of cutaneous symptoms (hives or facial swelling) may be a precursor to anaphylaxis.
- **Causes:** Foods (especially peanuts, tree nuts, fish, and shellfish), drugs (especially antibiotics and NSAIDs), and stings are the most common causes of anaphylaxis.

IMMUNIZATION REACTIONS

Definition

- Patient believes they are having a reaction to a recent immunization.
- Reactions to anthrax; chickenpox (varicella); hepatitis A (HAV); hepatitis B (HBV); human papillomavirus (HPV); influenza; Japanese encephalitis; measles, mumps, rubella (MMR); meningococcal; pneumococcal; poliovirus; rabies; shingles (herpes zoster); smallpox (vaccinia); tetanus, diphtheria (Td); tetanus, diphtheria, pertussis (Tdap/DTaP); and yellow fever vaccines are covered.
- *Use this protocol only if the patient has symptoms that match Immunization Reaction.*

Symptoms

- **Minor, temporary adverse reactions are common.** Examples include local pain and swelling at the injection site, fever, headache, and muscle aches. Most local reactions at the injection site occur within 2 days. Fever with most vaccines begins within 24 hours and lasts 2-3 days. With live vaccines (MMR and chickenpox), fever and systemic reactions usually begin within 1-4 weeks.
- **Serious adverse reactions are rare.** Anaphylaxis can occur with any vaccine. Anaphylactic symptoms start within 2 hours (usually within 20 minutes) after injection.

TRIAGE ASSESSMENT QUESTIONS

Call EMS 911 Now

- Difficulty with breathing or swallowing starts within 2 hours after injection
  R/O: anaphylactic reaction
- Difficult to awaken or acting confused (e.g., disoriented, slurred speech)
  R/O: acute encephalopathy
- Unresponsive, passed out, or very weak
  R/O: acute encephalopathy
- Sounds like a life-threatening emergency to the triager

Go to ED/UCC Now
(or to Office With PCP Approval)

- Sounds like a severe, unusual reaction to the triager
  R/O: brachial neuritis, etc.

Go to Office Now

- Fever > 103° F (39.4° C)
  R/O: severe reaction, bacteremia
- Fever > 100.5° F (38.1° C) and > 60 years of age
- Fever > 100.0° F (37.8° C) and has diabetes mellitus or a weak immune system (e.g., HIV positive, cancer chemotherapy, organ transplant, splenectomy, chronic steroids)
- Fever > 100.0° F (37.8° C) and bedridden (e.g., nursing home patient, stroke, chronic illness, recovering from surgery)
  Reason: higher risk of bacterial infection
  Note: May need ambulance transport to ED.
- Measles vaccine and purple/blood-colored rash (onset day 6-12)
  R/O: purpura or petechiae, thrombocytopenia
- Redness or red streak around the injection site begins > 48 hours after shot
  R/O: cellulitis, lymphangitis

See Today in Office

- Fever present > 3 days (72 hours)
  R/O: bacterial superinfection
- Smallpox vaccine and eye pain, eye redness, or rash on eyelids
  R/O: inadvertent inoculation and resultant vaccinial keratitis

See Today or Tomorrow in Office

- Deep lump follows (in 2-8 weeks) Td or DTaP shot and becomes tender to the touch
  R/O: secondary bacterial infection
- Patient wants to be seen

Home Care

- Mild immunization reaction
- Painless lump at Td injection site
- Immunization reactions, questions about

HOME CARE ADVICE

General Home Care Advice

❶ Cold Pack for Local Reaction at Injection Site:
- Apply a cold pack or ice in a wet washcloth to the area for 20 minutes. Repeat in 1 hour.
- Then apply as needed for the first 48 hours after the injection.
  (Reason: Reduce the pain and swelling.)

❷ Pain and Fever Medicines:
- For pain or fever relief, take either acetaminophen or ibuprofen.
- They are over-the-counter (OTC) drugs that help treat both fever and pain. You can buy them at the drugstore.
- Treat fevers > 101° F (38.3° C). The goal of fever therapy is to bring the fever down to a comfortable level. Remember that fever medicine usually lowers fever 2° F (1-1½° C).

❸ Acetaminophen (e.g., Tylenol):
- **Regular Strength Tylenol:** Take 650 mg (two 325 mg pills) by mouth every 4-6 hours as needed. Each Regular Strength Tylenol pill has 325 mg of acetaminophen.
- **Extra Strength Tylenol:** Take 1,000 mg (two 500 mg pills) every 8 hours as needed. Each Extra Strength Tylenol pill has 500 mg of acetaminophen.
- The most you should take each day is 3,000 mg (10 Regular Strength or 6 Extra Strength pills a day).

Ibuprofen (e.g., Motrin, Advil):
- Take 400 mg (two 200 mg pills) by mouth every 6 hours.
- Another choice is to take 600 mg (three 200 mg pills) by mouth every 8 hours.
- The most you should take each day is 1,200 mg (six 200 mg pills), unless your doctor has told you to take more.

❹ Pain and Fever Medicines—Extra Notes:
- Use the lowest amount of medicine that makes your pain or fever better.
- Acetaminophen is thought to be safer than ibuprofen or naproxen in people > 65 years old. Acetaminophen is in many OTC and prescription medicines. It might be in more than one medicine that you are taking. You need to be careful and not take an overdose. An acetaminophen overdose can hurt the liver.

- McNeil, the company that makes Tylenol, has different dosage instructions for Tylenol in Canada and the United States. In Canada, the maximum recommended dose per day is 4,000 mg or 12 Regular Strength (325 mg) pills. In the United States, McNeil recommends a maximum dose of 10 Regular Strength (325 mg) pills.
- CAUTION: Do not take acetaminophen if you have liver disease.
- CAUTION: Do not take ibuprofen if you have stomach problems, have kidney disease, are pregnant, or have been told by your doctor to avoid this type of anti-inflammatory drug. Do not take ibuprofen for > 7 days without consulting your doctor.
- *Before taking any medicine, read all the instructions on the package.*

❺ Td or Tdap Vaccination Lump:
- A painless lump (or nodule) sometimes develops at the Td or Tdap injection site 1 or 2 weeks later.
- It is harmless and usually will disappear in about 2 months.

❻ Call Back If:
- Fever lasts > 3 days.
- Pain lasts > 3 days.
- Injection site starts to look infected.
- You become worse.

Common Harmless Reactions—Reassurance

❶ Anthrax Vaccine:
- A small lump at injection site (in 50%)
- Local pain, redness, swelling, and itching at injection site (in 30%-60%)
- Moderate local reactions 1-5" (2-13 cm) wide (in 1%-5%)
- Large local reactions (in < 1%)
- Muscle aches and joint aches (in 20%)
- Headaches (in 20%)
- Fever and chills (in 5%)

❷ **Chickenpox Vaccine:**
- Local pain at injection site (in 25%)
- Fever (in 10%-15%)
- Mild chickenpox-like rash (2-5 spots) occurring up to 1 month after vaccination (in 5%). There is minimal chance of transmission of the vaccine virus to others; only 3 cases of transmission in > 14 million vaccines. Adults with these vaccine rashes can go to work or school. Keep rash covered with clothing or Band-Aid. Avoid contact with immunocompromised individuals (e.g., HIV, cancer chemotherapy, transplant recipients).

❸ **Hepatitis A (HAV) Vaccine:**
- Local pain at injection site (in 50%).
- Headache (in 15%).
- Tiredness (in 7%).
- Fever is uncommon.

❹ **Hepatitis B (HBV) Vaccine:**
- Local pain at injection site (in 25%)
- Fever (in 1%)

❺ **Human Papillomavirus (HPV) Vaccine:**
- Pain and tenderness at the injection site (in 80%)
- Mild redness and mild swelling at the injection site (in 25%)
- Fever > 100.4° F (38.0° C) (in 10%) and > 102° F (38.9° C) (in 1%-2%)
- Malaise, nausea, headache, body aches

❻ **Influenza (TIV; Injection) Vaccine:**
- Local pain at injection site.
- Fever.
- Aches.
- If these symptoms occur, they usually last 1-2 days.

❼ **Influenza (LAIV; Intranasal) Vaccine:**
LAIV nasal spray is NOT RECOMMENDED for use during the 2017-2018 flu season in the United States. This vaccine is made from a weakened virus; it does not cause influenza but can cause mild symptoms in people who get it:
- Runny nose or nasal congestion
- Fever, chills, muscle aches, and feeling tired
- Headache
- Sore throat

❽ **Japanese Encephalitis Vaccine:**
- Pain, redness, or tenderness at the injection site (in 20%)
- Malaise, nausea, headache, abdominal pain, body aches (in 10%)

❾ **Measles, Mumps, Rubella (MMR) Vaccine:**
- Local pain at injection site (in 10%).
- Fever and rash occur within 7-12 days following the injection (in 5%). The fever is usually between 101° F and 103° F (38.3° C and 39.5° C) and lasts 2-3 days. The mild pink rash is mainly on the trunk and lasts 2-3 days. No treatment is necessary. You are not contagious.
- Temporary mild pain and stiffness in the joints. This typically occurs in women (in 25% of women).
- Temporary lymph node swelling.

❿ **Meningococcal Vaccine:**
- Mild local reaction (sore injection site) is common (50%-70%).
- Headache (40%).
- Joint pain (20%).
- Fever (1%).
- The vaccine does not cause meningitis.

⓫ **Pneumococcal Vaccine:**
- Mild pain, tenderness, swelling, OR redness at the injection site (in 50%)
- Fever, muscle aches lasting for 1-2 days (in 1%)

⓬ **Poliovirus Vaccine (IPV):**
- Tenderness at the injection site

⓭ **Rabies Vaccine:**
- Pain, redness, or tenderness at the injection site (in 30%-74%)
- Malaise, nausea, headache, abdominal pain, dizziness, body aches (in 5%-40%)

⓮ **Shingles (Herpes Zoster; Zostavax) Vaccine:**
- Redness, swelling, pain, or itching at the injection site (in 33%)
- Headache (in 10%)
- Fever > 100.4° F (38.0° C) (in 10%) and > 102° F (38.9° C) (in 1%-2%)
- Malaise, nausea, headache, body aches

⓯ **Smallpox Vaccine:**
- It is expected and desired that patients develop a red bump (papule) at the vaccination site at 2-5 days; this turns into a pustule and reaches its maximum size at 8-10 days; this scabs over by 14-21 days and leaves a permanent scar.
- Fever headache, muscle aches.
- Swelling of nearby lymph nodes.

⑯ **Tetanus, Diphtheria (Td) Vaccine:**
- Pain and tenderness at the injection site lasts for 24-48 hours (in 50%-85%).
- Mild redness and mild swelling at the injection site (in 20%-30%).
- Fever lasts for 24-48 hours (in 5%-10%).
- Malaise, nausea, headache.

⑰ **Tetanus, Diphtheria, Pertussis (Tdap/DTaP) Vaccine:**
- Pain and tenderness at the injection site (in 66%)
- Mild redness and mild swelling at the injection site (in 20%)
- Fever > 100.4° F (38.0° C) (in 1%) and > 102° F (38.9° C) (in 0.4%)
- Malaise, nausea, headache, body aches

⑱ **Yellow Fever Vaccine:**
- Pain, redness, or tenderness at the injection site.
- Malaise, nausea, headache, abdominal pain, body aches.
- These symptoms may occur in 25% of recipients; symptoms typically last 5-10 days.

Rare Adverse Reactions

❶ **Anthrax Vaccine:**
- Anaphylactic reaction (acute severe allergic reaction with wheezing, urticaria, shock). Very rare (1 person in 100,000).

❷ **Chickenpox Vaccine:**
- Anaphylactic reaction (acute severe allergic reaction with wheezing, urticaria, shock). Very rare.
- Pneumonia. Very rare.
- Seizure caused by fever (1 case per 1,000 doses of vaccine).
- Possible association with Guillain-Barré syndrome (1-2 cases per million doses of vaccine).

❸ **Hepatitis A (HAV) Vaccine:**
- Anaphylactic reaction (acute severe allergic reaction with wheezing, urticaria, shock). Very rare.

❹ **Hepatitis B (HBV) Vaccine:**
- Anaphylactic reaction (acute severe allergic reaction with wheezing, urticaria, shock). Estimated at 1 in 300,000 doses of vaccine.

❺ **Human Papillomavirus (HPV) Vaccine:**
- Anaphylactic reaction (acute severe allergic reaction with wheezing, urticaria, shock). Very rare.

❻ **H1N1 Influenza Vaccine (Inactivated; Injected):**
- Anaphylactic reaction (acute severe allergic reaction with wheezing, urticaria, shock). Very rare.
- In 1976, an earlier version of the swine flu vaccine was associated with cases of Guillain-Barré syndrome. Flu vaccines since that time have not been clearly linked to Guillain-Barré syndrome.

❼ **H1N1 Influenza Intranasal Vaccine (LAIV):**
- Anaphylactic reaction (acute severe allergic reaction with wheezing, urticaria, shock). Very rare.

❽ **Influenza (TIV; Injected) Vaccine:**
- Anaphylactic reaction (acute severe allergic reaction with wheezing, urticaria, shock). Very rare.
- Possible association with Guillain-Barré syndrome (1-2 cases per million doses of vaccine).

❾ **Influenza (LAIV; Intranasal) Vaccine:**
- Anaphylactic reaction (acute severe allergic reaction with wheezing, urticaria, shock). Very rare.

❿ **Japanese Encephalitis Vaccine:**
- Anaphylactic reaction (acute severe allergic reaction with wheezing, urticaria, shock). Rare.
- Severe allergic reactions with rash, hand and face swelling, breathing difficulty (about 60 per 10,000).
- Seizures and other nervous system problems (< 1 in 50,000).

⓫ **Measles, Mumps, Rubella (MMR) Vaccine:**
- Anaphylactic reaction (acute severe allergic reaction with wheezing, urticaria, shock)
- Encephalitis and encephalopathy
- Temporary low platelet count (1 in 30,000 vaccine doses)

⓬ **Meningococcal Vaccine:**
- Anaphylactic reaction (acute severe allergic reaction with wheezing, urticaria, shock). Extremely rare (1 person in 1,000,000).

⓭ **Pneumococcal Vaccine:**
- Anaphylactic reaction (acute severe allergic reaction with wheezing, urticaria, shock).

⓮ **Poliovirus Vaccine (IPV):**
- Severe allergic reaction. Very rare.

⓯ **Rabies Vaccine:**
- Hives, joint pain, fever (in 6%).
- Illness resembling Guillain-Barré syndrome, with complete recovery. Very rare.

⓰ **Shingles (Herpes Zoster; Zostavax) Vaccine:**
- No serious reactions have been reported with this vaccine.
- An anaphylactic reaction (acute severe allergic reaction with wheezing, urticaria, shock) is possible with any new medication.

⓱ **Smallpox Vaccine:**
- Inadvertent inoculation is the most common complication. This happens when the patient scratches the vaccine pustule and then spreads the vaccinia virus by touching another part of the body. Patients who develop eye pain or redness should see a physician.
  (Reason: possible vaccinia keratitis)
- Generalized vaccinia is a diffuse vesicular rash (blistering). Usually not serious (self-limited).
- Hives, erythema multiforme.
- The OVERALL RATE of these reactions is approximately 1,000 reactions for every 1 million doses of vaccine in patients receiving the vaccine for the first time. The rate is much less for patients being revaccinated.

⓲ **Tetanus, Diphtheria (Td) Vaccine:**
- Anaphylactic reaction (acute severe allergic reaction with wheezing, urticaria, shock)
- Brachial plexus neuropathy (deep ongoing upper arm pain with muscle atrophy and weakness)
- Guillain-Barré syndrome
- Sterile abscess

⓳ **Tetanus, Diphtheria, Pertussis (Tdap/DTaP) Vaccine:**
- Anaphylactic reaction (acute severe allergic reaction with wheezing, urticaria, shock)

⓴ **Yellow Fever Vaccine:**
- Anaphylactic reaction (acute severe allergic reaction with wheezing, urticaria, shock) (1 in 131,000)
- Nervous system reactions (approximately 1 in 200,000)

Rare Life-threatening Reactions

❶ **Smallpox Vaccine:**
- Encephalitis.
- Eczema vaccinatum, a serious diffuse rash seen in patients with underlying skin disorders (e.g., eczema).
- Progressive vaccinia (vaccinia necrosum) is a progressive necrosis (skin death) in the area of the vaccination.
- The OVERALL RATE of life-threatening reactions is approximately 14-52 reactions for every 1 million doses of vaccine in patients receiving the vaccine for the first time. The rate is less for patients being revaccinated. It is estimated that 1 patient in 1 million who receives the vaccine may die as a result; the death rate for revaccination has been estimated as 1 patient in 4 million.

FIRST AID

First Aid Advice for Anaphylaxis—Epinephrine:
- If the patient has an epinephrine autoinjector, **give it now.** Do not delay.
- Use the autoinjector on the upper outer thigh. You may give it through clothing if necessary.
- Give epinephrine first, then call 911.
- Epinephrine is available in autoinjectors under trade names: EpiPen, EpiPen Jr, and Auvi-Q (Allerject in Canada). Auvi-Q has an audio chip and talks patients and caregivers through injection process.
- You may give a second (repeat) dose of epinephrine 10-15 minutes later, IF the person with anaphylaxis does not respond to the first dose AND ambulance arrival takes > 10 minutes.

First Aid Advice for Anaphylaxis—Benadryl:
- Give antihistamine by mouth **NOW** if able to swallow.
- Use Benadryl (diphenhydramine; adult dose: 50 mg) or any other available antihistamine medicine.

BACKGROUND

Key Points

- Vaccines are generally safe and effective. Minor temporary adverse reactions are common. Serious adverse reactions are rare.
- Vaccinations are given in either the deltoid muscle of the upper arm (usually) or in the anterolateral thigh muscles (rarely). Vaccinations should not be given in the buttocks because studies have shown that such vaccination is not as effective because of the fatty tissue present.

Types of Reactions

- **Local Reaction:** Most local swelling, redness, and pain at the injection site begins within 24 hours of the shot (rarely 24-48 hours). It usually lasts 2 or 3 days. Occasionally, localized hives or itching occurs at the injection site; these usually last < 12 hours. Localized hives do not mean you are allergic to the vaccine.
- **Systemic Reaction:** Fever with most vaccines (e.g., DTaP) begins within 24 hours (rarely 24-48 hours). Headache, myalgias, malaise, and poor appetite can also be seen. Systemic symptoms usually last 1-3 days.

Vaccine Information Statements From the CDC

Vaccine Information Statements (VISs) are information sheets produced by the Centers for Disease Control and Prevention (CDC) that explain to vaccine recipients the benefits and risks of a vaccine. US federal law requires that a VIS be handed out at the time certain vaccinations are administered. Each VIS is available for viewing and downloading at: https://www.cdc.gov/vaccines/hcp/vis/index.html.

CDC US National Immunization Hotline

- Trained specialists provide vaccine information; available to patients, nurses, doctors
- Open 8:00 am-8:00 pm EST, Monday-Friday
- Toll-free phone number: 800/232-4636 (English)

Internet Resources—Recommended Adult Immunization Schedules:

- **Australia:** The 10th edition of the *Australian Immunisation Handbook* is available at: www.immunise. health.gov.au/internet/immunise/publishing.nsf/ Content/Handbook10-home.
- **Canada:** The National Advisory Committee on Immunization publishes vaccine recommendations. The *Canadian Immunization Guide* is available at: www.phac-aspc.gc.ca/publicat/cig-gci/index-eng. php.
- **New Zealand:** The *Immunisation Handbook 2017* is available at: www.health.govt.nz/publication/ immunisation-handbook-2017.
- **United States:** The Advisory Committee on Immunization Practices (ACIP) publishes vaccine recommendations. The most recent adult schedule is available at: www.cdc.gov/vaccines/schedules/hcp/adult. html.

US National Vaccine Injury Compensation Program

- In the rare event that a serious reaction has definitely occurred, a federal program has been created to help pay for the injury.
- Toll-free phone number: 800/338-2382.

Combination Vaccines

Combination vaccines are popular because they reduce the number of shots a person must receive. Knowing the names and content of combination vaccines allows the triage nurse to address the vaccine reactions of each ingredient:

- **MMR Vaccine:** Measles, mumps, rubella
- **Comvax:** *Haemophilus influenzae* type b and hepatitis B
- **Twinrix:** Hepatitis A and hepatitis B

Vaccine Reactions Versus Bacterial Infection of Injection Site

- Local vaccine reactions normally occur in > 25% of immunizations. This is a good sign that means the body is creating antibodies to the vaccine.
- Bacterial superinfections (e.g., cellulitis, lymphangitis, abscess) at the injection site are very rare. Usually they are due to a nonsterile injection technique.
- **Clues From Appearance:** Local vaccine reactions usually are blotchy red with indistinct borders. Cellulitis usually has confluent spreading redness with sharp borders. It also is very tender to the touch.
- **Clues From Onset:** Redness and fever from a vaccine reaction usually begin within 24 hours following the shot (rarely 24-48 hours). Redness and fever from a bacterial infection begin > 48 hours after the shot. *(Reason: It takes time for the bacteria to become established and multiply.)*

Anaphylactic Reactions From Vaccines

- **Definition:** A severe life-threatening reaction is called anaphylaxis.
- **Symptoms:** The main symptoms are difficulty breathing, difficulty swallowing, and hypotension (manifested by fainting or too weak to stand).
- **Onset:** Most serious anaphylactic reactions to vaccines occur in a physician's office because it's standard practice to observe the patient for 20 minutes following injection of a vaccine.
- **Incidence:** Anaphylactic reactions can occur with any vaccine, but they are very rare. Incidence is 1 per 500,000 doses of vaccine.

INFLUENZA, SEASONAL

Definition
- Influenza is a viral respiratory infection that affects the nose, throat, trachea, and bronchi. It is also called the flu.
- Adult thinks he/she has influenza because other family members have it.
- Adult thinks he/she has influenza and it's prevalent in the community.
- *Use this protocol only if the patient has symptoms that match Influenza.*

Symptoms
- **Fever** (≥ 100.0° F/37.8° C) or feeling feverish AND **one or more other influenza respiratory symptoms** from the following list: cough, sore throat, runny or stuffy nose.
- Patient may also have muscle or body aches, headaches, and fatigue.
- Respiratory symptoms are similar to a common cold: runny nose, sore throat, and a bad cough.
- The fever is usually higher (102° F-104° F; 38.9° C-40° C) with influenza than with a cold. Headaches and muscle aches are also worse with influenza.

The following groups of individuals are at higher risk for complications from influenza and therefore are considered HIGH RISK in this protocol. It is recommended that these individuals receive antiviral treatment for suspected or confirmed influenza.
- Persons ≥ 65 years
- Persons < 19 years who are receiving long-term aspirin therapy
  Reason: at risk for Reye syndrome
- Persons with immunosuppression, including that caused by medications (e.g., chemotherapy, chronic steroids) or by HIV infection
- Persons who are morbidly obese (i.e., BMI ≥ 40)
- Persons with chronic *pulmonary* (including asthma), *cardiovascular* (except hypertension alone), *renal, hepatic, hematological* (including sickle cell disease), or *metabolic* disorders (including diabetes mellitus)
- Persons with *neurologic* and neurodevelopment conditions (including disorders of the brain, spinal cord, peripheral nerve, and muscles such as cerebral palsy, epilepsy [seizure disorders], stroke, intellectual disability, moderate-severe developmental delay, muscular dystrophy, or spinal cord injury)

- Women who are pregnant or postpartum (up to 2 weeks)
- Nursing home residents and other persons residing in long-term care facilities
- American Indians and Alaskan Natives

TRIAGE ASSESSMENT QUESTIONS

Call EMS 911 Now
- ● SEVERE difficulty breathing (e.g., struggling for each breath, speaks in single words)
  R/O: respiratory failure, hypoxia
- ● Bluish (or gray) lips or face
  R/O: cyanosis and need for oxygen
- ● Shock suspected (e.g., cold/pale/clammy skin, too weak to stand)
  R/O: shock
  First Aid: Lie down with the feet elevated.
- ● Sounds like a life-threatening emergency to the triager

See More Appropriate Protocol
- ● Sounds like a cold and there is no fever
  Go to Protocol: Common Cold on page 79
- ● Cough and there is no fever
  Go to Protocol: Cough on page 95
- ● Severe cough
  Go to Protocol: Cough on page 95
- ● Throat pain and there is no fever
  Go to Protocol: Sore Throat on page 369
- ● Severe sore throat
  Go to Protocol: Sore Throat on page 369
- ● Influenza vaccine reaction is suspected
  Go to Protocol: Immunization Reactions on page 230

Go to ED Now
- ● Headache and stiff neck (can't touch chin to chest)
  R/O: meningitis
- ● Chest pain
  (Exception: MILD central chest pain, present only when coughing)
- ● R/O: pneumonia, pleurisy

Go to ED/UCC Now
(or to Office With PCP Approval)

● Difficulty breathing that is not severe and not relieved by cleaning out the nose
R/O: pneumonia

● Patient sounds very sick or weak to the triager
Reason: severe acute illness or serious complication suspected

Go to Office Now

● Fever > 104° F (40° C)
R/O: serious bacterial infection

● Fever > 100.5° F (38.1° C) and > 60 years of age
R/O: pneumonia

● Fever > 100.0° F (37.8° C) and diabetes mellitus or weak immune system (e.g., HIV positive, cancer chemotherapy, splenectomy, organ transplant, chronic steroids)
R/O: pneumonia

● Fever > 100.0° F (37.8° C) and bedridden (e.g., nursing home patient, stroke, chronic illness, recovering from surgery)
R/O: pneumonia
Note: May need ambulance transport to ED.

Discuss With PCP and Callback by Nurse Within 1 Hour

● HIGH RISK (e.g., age > 64 years, pregnant, HIV positive, chronic medical condition) and flu symptoms
Reason: treatment with antiviral medication should be considered, especially for symptoms present

See Today in Office

● Using nasal washes and pain medicine > 24 hours and sinus pain (lower forehead, cheekbone, or eye) persists
R/O: sinusitis

● Fever present > 3 days (72 hours)
R/O: bacterial sinusitis, bronchitis, pneumonia

● Fever returns after gone for > 24 hours and symptoms worse (or not improved)
R/O: bacterial sinusitis, bronchitis, pneumonia

● Earache
R/O: otitis media

See Today or Tomorrow in Office

● Patient wants to be seen

Discuss With PCP and Callback by Nurse Today

● Patient requests antiviral medicine for influenza and flu symptoms present < 48 hours
Note: Not a HIGH-RISK patient. Patients who are not high risk typically do not require treatment with antiviral medication.

See Within 3 Days in Office

● Nasal discharge present > 10 days
R/O: bacterial sinusitis, allergic rhinitis

● Cough present > 3 weeks

Home Care

○ Probable influenza (fever) with no complications and not HIGH RISK
Reason: not high risk; patients who are not high risk typically do not require treatment with antiviral medication

○ Probable mild influenza (no fever) or a common cold with no complications and not HIGH RISK

○ Influenza vaccine, questions about

HOME CARE ADVICE

General Care Advice

❶ **Reassurance:**
- For most healthy adults, influenza feels like a bad cold. The dangers of influenza for normal, healthy people (< 65 years of age) are overrated.
- The treatment of influenza depends on your main symptoms. Generally, treatment is the same as for other viral respiratory infections (colds). Bed rest is unnecessary.
- *Here is some care advice that should help.*

❷ **Influenza—Key Points:**
- Influenza is commonly known as the "flu."
- Influenza is a respiratory illness that is easily spread from person to person.
- The most common symptoms are the sudden onset of fever, muscle aches, cough, runny nose, sore throat, fatigue, and headache.
- The best way to prevent influenza is to get the vaccine every year.

❸ Influenza—How It Is Spread:
- Influenza is very contagious. That means it can spread very easily from person to person.
- The flu virus is spread via airborne droplet, from sneezing and coughing and even talking. It also can be transmitted by hands contaminated with secretions.
- A person is potentially contagious (virus may be in respiratory secretions) from 1 day prior to and for 7 days after the onset of symptoms (e.g., fever, cough). The CDC recommends that people with influenza-like illness remain at home until at least 24 hours after they are free of fever (100° F or 37.8°C).
- Symptoms usually start within 1-4 days after being exposed to a person with influenza (nearly always within 7 days). If > 7 days pass from exposure without developing symptoms, you should be safe and not get influenza.

❹ Influenza—Treating the Symptoms:
- **Cough:** Use cough drops.
- **Feeling Dehydrated:** Drink extra liquids. If the air in your home is dry, use a humidifier.
- **Fever:** For fever > 101° F (38.3° C), take acetaminophen every 4-6 hours (adults, 650 mg) OR ibuprofen every 6-8 hours (adults, 400-600 mg).
- **Muscle Aches, Headache, and Other Pains:** Often this comes and goes with the fever. Take acetaminophen every 4-6 hours (adults, 650 mg) OR ibuprofen every 6-8 hours (adults, 400-600 mg).
- **Sore Throat:** Try throat lozenges, hard candy, or warm chicken broth.

❺ Influenza—Treatment With Antiviral Drugs:
- There are 2 antiviral medications that are helpful in treating this infection: oseltamivir (brand name Tamiflu) and zanamivir (brand name Relenza).
- Treatment is recommended for HIGH-RISK patients (e.g., age > 64 years, pregnant, HIV positive, or chronic medical condition) with influenza or any patient with severe symptoms (per CDC).
- Treatment is typically not recommended for mild-moderate influenza illness that occurs in most healthy patients (per CDC). Most patients recover without taking antiviral medications.
- The benefits are limited. Antiviral medications may reduce the time you are sick by 1-1½ days. It helps reduce the symptoms but does not cure the disease.
- For best results, antiviral medications should be started within 48 hours of the onset of flu symptoms.

❻ Influenza—Prevention With Vaccine: The best way to prevent influenza is to get a flu vaccine every year.

❼ Expected Course: The fever lasts 2-3 days, the runny nose 5-10 days, and the cough 2-3 weeks.

❽ Call Back If:
- Fever lasts > 3 days.
- Runny nose lasts > 10 days.
- Cough lasts > 3 weeks.
- You become short of breath or worse.

Treating the Symptoms of Flu—Additional Information

❶ For a Runny Nose With Profuse Discharge: Blow the Nose
- Nasal mucus and discharge helps to wash viruses and bacteria out of the nose and sinuses.
- Blowing the nose is all that is needed.
- If the skin around your nostrils gets irritated, apply a tiny amount of petroleum ointment to the nasal openings once or twice a day.

❷ Nasal Washes for a Stuffy Nose:
- **Introduction:** Saline (salt water) nasal irrigation (nasal wash) is an effective and simple home remedy for treating stuffy nose and sinus congestion. The nose can be irrigated by pouring, spraying, or squirting salt water into the nose and then letting it run back out.
- **How It Helps:** The salt water rinses out excess mucus and washes out any irritants (dust, allergens) that might be present. It also moistens the nasal cavity.
- **Methods:** There are several ways to irrigate the nose. You can use a saline nasal spray bottle (available over the counter [OTC]), a rubber ear syringe, a medical syringe without the needle, or a neti pot.

❸ Nasal Washes—Step-by-step Instructions:
- **Step 1:** Lean over a sink.
- **Step 2:** Gently squirt or spray warm salt water into one of your nostrils.
- **Step 3:** Some of the water may run into the back of your throat. Spit this out. If you swallow the salt water, it will not hurt you.
- **Step 4:** Blow your nose to clean out the water and mucus.
- **Step 5:** Repeat steps 1-4 for the other nostril. You can do this a couple times a day if it seems to help you.

❹ How to Make Saline (Salt Water) Nasal Wash:
- You can make your own saline nasal wash.
- Add ½ tsp of table salt to 1 cup (8 oz; 240 mL) of warm water.
- You should use sterile, distilled, or previously boiled water for nasal irrigation.

❺ Coughing Spasms:
- Drink warm fluids. Inhale warm mist. *(Reason: Both relax the airway and loosen up the phlegm.)*
- Suck on cough drops or hard candy to coat the irritated throat.

❻ Nasal Decongestants for a Very Stuffy or Runny Nose:
- **Most people do not need to use these medicines.**
- If your nose feels blocked, you should try using nasal washes first.
- If you have a very stuffy nose, nasal decongestant medicines can shrink the swollen nasal mucosa and allow for easier breathing. If you have a very runny nose, these medicines can reduce the amount of drainage. They may be taken as pills by mouth or as a nasal spray.
- **Pseudoephedrine (Sudafed):** Available OTC in pill form. Typical adult dosage is two 30 mg tablets every 6 hours.
- **Oxymetazoline Nasal Drops (Afrin):** Available OTC. Clean out the nose before using. Spray each nostril once, wait 1 minute for absorption, and then spray a second time.
- **Phenylephrine Nasal Drops (Neo-Synephrine):** Available OTC. Clean out the nose before using. Spray each nostril once, wait 1 minute for absorption, and then spray a second time.
- *Before taking any medicine, read all the instructions on the package.*

❼ For All Fevers:
- Drink cold fluids to prevent dehydration.
- Dress in 1 layer of lightweight clothing and sleep with 1 light blanket.
- For fevers < 101° F (38.3° C), fever medicines are usually not needed.

❽ Pain and Fever Medicines:
- For pain or fever relief, take either acetaminophen or ibuprofen.
- They are over-the-counter (OTC) drugs that help treat both fever and pain. You can buy them at the drugstore.

- Treat fevers > 101° F (38.3° C). The goal of fever therapy is to bring the fever down to a comfortable level. Remember that fever medicine usually lowers fever 2° F (1-1½° C).

Acetaminophen (e.g., Tylenol):
- **Regular Strength Tylenol:** Take 650 mg (two 325 mg pills) by mouth every 4-6 hours as needed. Each Regular Strength Tylenol pill has 325 mg of acetaminophen.
- **Extra Strength Tylenol:** Take 1,000 mg (two 500 mg pills) every 8 hours as needed. Each Extra Strength Tylenol pill has 500 mg of acetaminophen.
- The most you should take each day is 3,000 mg (10 Regular Strength or 6 Extra Strength pills a day).

Ibuprofen (e.g., Motrin, Advil):
- Take 400 mg (two 200 mg pills) by mouth every 6 hours.
- Another choice is to take 600 mg (three 200 mg pills) by mouth every 8 hours.
- The most you should take each day is 1,200 mg (six 200 mg pills), unless your doctor has told you to take more.

❾ Pain and Fever Medicines—Extra Notes:
- Use the lowest amount of medicine that makes your pain or fever better.
- Acetaminophen is thought to be safer than ibuprofen or naproxen in people > 65 years old. Acetaminophen is in many OTC and prescription medicines. It might be in more than one medicine that you are taking. You need to be careful and not take an overdose. An acetaminophen overdose can hurt the liver.
- McNeil, the company that makes Tylenol, has different dosage instructions for Tylenol in Canada and the United States. In Canada, the maximum recommended dose per day is 4,000 mg or 12 Regular Strength (325 mg) pills. In the United States, McNeil recommends a maximum dose of 10 Regular Strength (325 mg) pills.
- CAUTION: Do not take acetaminophen if you have liver disease.
- CAUTION: Do not take ibuprofen if you have stomach problems, have kidney disease, are pregnant, or have been told by your doctor to avoid this type of anti-inflammatory drug. Do not take ibuprofen for > 7 days without consulting your doctor.
- *Before taking any medicine, read all the instructions on the package.*

🔟 **No Aspirin:** Do not use aspirin for treatment of fever or pain.
(Reason: There is an association between influenza and Reye syndrome.)

Inactivated Influenza Vaccine (TIV)—Flu Shot

❶ **General:**
- Given annually (in September-November) before the onset of influenza season.
- The vaccine is 70%-90% effective in preventing influenza. It is not 100% protective, as the influenza viruses change yearly.
- The Vaccine Information Statement (VIS) for influenza is available at: www.cdc.gov/vaccines/hcp/vis/vis-statements/flu.html.

❷ **Influenza Vaccine—Indications:** It is recommended that all adults receive an influenza vaccination.

❸ **Influenza Vaccine Indications:** People who can spread influenza to those at HIGH RISK:
- Health care workers
- Household contacts and caregivers of children from 0-59 months of age
- Household contacts and caregivers of persons with medical conditions that put them at higher risk for severe complications from influenza

Live Influenza Vaccine (LAIV)—Nasal Spray

❶ **General:**
- This is a live attenuated (weakened) virus vaccine to prevent influenza.
- It is sprayed in the nose.
- The Vaccine Information Statement (VIS) for the nasal spray flu vaccine is available at: www.cdc.gov/vaccines/hcp/vis/vis-statements/flulive.html.
- The nasal spray version of the flu vaccine is not recommended for the 2017-2018 flu season.
(Reason: not effective [CDC])

❷ **Indications:** If vaccination is indicated, the intranasal vaccine is an OPTION for vaccination of children and nonpregnant healthy adults from 5-49 years of age.

Additional Resources

❶ **Centers for Disease Control and Prevention:**
- www.cdc.gov/flu
- Influenza; general information and latest recommendations

BACKGROUND

Influenza—Key Points

- **Seasonal Epidemic:** Influenza viruses change (or mutate) yearly. This is why some people seem to get influenza every year. The influenza virus is spread via airborne droplet, from sneezing and coughing. Influenza epidemics occur commonly between November and March. During these months, 5%-40% of the population may be affected.
- **Expected Course:** The fever lasts 2-3 days, the runny nose 5-10 days, and the cough 2-3 weeks.
- **Incubation Period:** Spread is rapid because the incubation period is only 24-36 hours and the virus is very contagious. Symptoms usually start within 1-4 days after being exposed to a person with influenza (nearly always within 7 days).
- **Contagiousness:** A person is potentially contagious (virus may be in respiratory secretions) from 1 day prior to and for 7 days after the onset of symptoms (e.g., fever, cough). The CDC recommends that people with influenza-like illness remain at home until at least 24 hours after they are free of fever (100° F or 37.8°C).
- **Complications—Respiratory:** Viral and secondary bacterial pneumonia, COPD, and asthma exacerbations.
- **Complications—Other:** Heart failure, ECG abnormalities, Reye syndrome, poor diabetic control.
- **Internet Resource:** www.cdc.gov/flu.

Influenza Vaccine ("Flu Shot")

The influenza vaccine can help **prevent** influenza. For it to work it needs to be given prior to exposure.
- The best time to get the vaccine in the fall of every year (September-November) before the onset of influenza season.
- The vaccine is 70%-90% effective in preventing influenza. It is not 100% protective, as the influenza viruses change yearly.
- The Vaccine Information Statement (VIS) for influenza is available at: www.cdc.gov/vaccines/hcp/vis/vis-statements/flu.html. The VIS for the nasal spray flu vaccine is available at: www.cdc.gov/vaccines/hcp/vis/vis-statements/flulive.html.

Indications for Getting the Influenza Vaccine—Which Adults Should Get a Flu Shot?

- *It is recommended that all adults receive an influenza vaccination.*
- **Internet Resource:** https://www.cdc.gov/mmwr/preview/mmwrhtml/mm5931a4.htm.

When vaccine supplies are limited, the following caregivers, who can potentially spread influenza, should get preferential vaccination:
- Health care workers
- Household contacts and caregivers of children from 0-59 months of age
- Household contacts and caregivers of persons with medical conditions that put them at higher risk for severe complications from influenza

When vaccine supplies are limited, the following groups who are at higher risk for complications should get preferential vaccination:
- People ≥ 50 years.
- Patient populations at HIGH RISK for complications of influenza: chronic cardiopulmonary conditions (e.g., asthma), immunosuppression (e.g., chemotherapy), renal dysfunction, diabetes, women who will be pregnant during flu season.
- Patients with chronic medical conditions who reside in nursing home or chronic-care facilities.
- Healthy persons who could transmit influenza to high-risk patients: Health care workers, nursing home employees, and family members.
- Note that the indications for getting the nasal spray vaccine are slightly different than those for the shot since the nasal spray contains live virus. Refer to the VIS if additional information is needed.
- **Internet Resource:** www.cdc.gov/flu/protect/keyfacts.htm.

Antiviral Medications for Influenza

- Oseltamivir (Tamiflu) or zanamivir (Relenza) are the primary antiviral agents recommended for the treatment and prevention of influenza.
- **Treatment of Influenza:** Antiviral medications must be started within 48 hours of symptom onset for greatest benefit; after that, the benefit decreases substantially. It is recommended that individuals at HIGH RISK (see Definition) for influenza complications be treated with antiviral medications if antivirals can be started within 48 hours of symptom onset. Use of antiviral medications in individuals not at high risk is considered optional and clinical judgement is recommended. Antiviral medications have been shown to reduce the duration (by 1 day) and severity of flu symptoms.
- **Prevention of Influenza:** Antiviral medications can also be taken prophylactically during influenza epidemics to prevent illness in HIGH-RISK patients. However, they should not be used as a substitute for vaccination.
- **When to Call the PCP:** If callers ask for one of these drugs after being informed of their limited efficacy, recommend they call their PCP during office hours. If the office won't be open tomorrow and it is not the middle of the night (9:00 pm-9:00 am), transfer the call to the PCP.
- **Internet Resource:** www.cdc.gov/flu/professionals/antivirals/summary-clinicians.htm.

INFLUENZA EXPOSURE

Definition
- Exposure (close contact) to influenza.
- Patient has no respiratory symptoms (i.e., cough, runny or stuffy nose, sore throat).
- Questions about influenza.

Exposure (Close Contact)
- **Household Close Contact:** Living in the same house (household contacts) with a person with confirmed, probable, or suspected influenza.
- **Other close contact** (within 6 feet, 2 meters; touching distance) with a person with confirmed, probable, or suspected influenza. Examples of such close contact include kissing or hugging, sharing eating or drinking utensils, carpooling, close conversation, performing a physical examination (relevant to health care professionals), and any other direct contact with respiratory secretions of a person with influenza.

The following are not considered close contact exposures:
- Living in a community where there are ≥ 1 confirmed cases of influenza
- Being in the same school, church, workplace, or building as a person with influenza
- Walking by a person who has influenza

The following groups of individuals are at higher risk for complications from influenza and therefore are considered as HIGH RISK in this protocol. It is recommended that these individuals receive antiviral treatment for suspected or confirmed influenza.
- Persons ≥ 65 years
- Persons < 19 years who are receiving long-term aspirin therapy
  Reason: at risk for Reye syndrome
- Persons with immunosuppression, including that caused by medications (e.g., chemotherapy, chronic steroids) or by HIV infection
- Persons who are morbidly obese (i.e., BMI ≥ 40)
- Persons with chronic *pulmonary* (including asthma), *cardiovascular* (except hypertension alone), *renal*, *hepatic*, *hematological* (including sickle cell disease), or *metabolic* disorders (including diabetes mellitus)
- Persons with *neurologic* and neurodevelopment conditions (including disorders of the brain, spinal cord, peripheral nerve, and muscles such as cerebral palsy, epilepsy [seizure disorders], stroke, intellectual disability, moderate-severe developmental delay, muscular dystrophy, or spinal cord injury)
- Women who are pregnant or postpartum (up to 2 weeks)
- Nursing home residents and other persons residing in long-term care facilities
- American Indians and Alaskan Natives

TRIAGE ASSESSMENT QUESTIONS

See More Appropriate Protocol
- Influenza has been diagnosed by a health care professional
  Go to Protocol: Influenza Follow-up Call on page 249
- Influenza suspected (i.e., fever and respiratory symptoms; probable influenza exposure)
  Go to Protocol: Influenza, Seasonal on page 237
- Cough and begins > 7 days after influenza EXPOSURE
  Go to Protocol: Cough on page 95
- Influenza EXPOSURE (close contact) within the last 7 days and fever or any respiratory symptoms (i.e., cough, runny or stuffy nose, sore throat)
  Go to Protocol: Influenza, Seasonal on page 237
- Runny or stuffy nose and begins > 7 days after influenza EXPOSURE
  Go to Protocol: Common Cold on page 79
- Sore throat and begins > 7 days after influenza EXPOSURE
  Go to Protocol: Sore Throat on page 369

Go to ED/UCC Now (or to Office With PCP Approval)
- Patient sounds very sick or weak to the triager
  Reason: severe acute illness or serious complication suspected

Discuss With PCP and Callback by Nurse Within 1 Hour

● Influenza EXPOSURE within last 72 hours (3 days) and exposed person is HIGH RISK (e.g., age > 64 years, pregnant, HIV positive, chronic medical condition)
Reason: prophylaxis or early treatment with antiviral medication can be considered (CDC); PCP may wish to phone in a prescription to the pharmacy

● Influenza EXPOSURE within last 72 hours (3 days) and exposed person is a health care worker, public health worker, or first responder (EMS)
Reason: prophylaxis or early treatment with antiviral medication can be considered (CDC); PCP may wish to phone in a prescription to the pharmacy

See Today in Office

◐ Fever present > 3 days (72 hours)

Callback by PCP Today

◐ Influenza EXPOSURE (close contact) within last 72 hours (3 days) and NOT HIGH RISK and strongly requests antiviral medication
Note: Giving antiviral medication to people who are not high risk is considered optional and clinical judgment is recommended. PCP will need to decide if antiviral medication might be helpful.

See Within 3 Days in Office

◐ Patient wants to be seen

Home Care

○ Influenza EXPOSURE (close contact) within last 7 days and NO respiratory symptoms
Reason: not high risk; patients who are not high risk typically do not require prophylaxis with antiviral medication

○ Influenza EXPOSURE > 7 days ago and NO respiratory symptoms
Reason: asymptomatic and risk for transmission of influenza has passed

○ Influenza, questions about

○ Influenza prevention, questions about

○ Influenza Internet resources, questions about

○ Influenza and travel, questions about

○ Influenza and antiviral drugs, questions about

HOME CARE ADVICE

Influenza Exposure and Having No Symptoms

❶ **Reassurance—Influenza Exposure Within Past 7 Days:**
- Although you were exposed to flu (influenza), you do not have any symptoms.
- Symptoms usually develop within 1-4 days of exposure to another person with flu (7 days is an outer limit).
- There are some things that you can do to help prevent getting flu.
- *Here is some care advice that should help.*

❷ **Reassurance—Influenza Exposure > 7 Days Ago:**
- Although you were exposed to flu, you do not have any symptoms.
- Symptoms usually develop within 1-4 days of exposure to another person with flu (7 days is an outer limit).
- Since 7 days have passed, you should be safe and not get flu.
- There are some things that you can do to help prevent getting flu.
- *Here is some care advice that should help.*

❸ **Influenza—Key Points:**
- Influenza is commonly known as the "flu."
- Influenza is a respiratory illness that is easily spread from person to person.
- The most common symptoms are the sudden onset of fever, muscle aches, cough, runny nose, sore throat, fatigue, and headache.
- The best way to prevent flu is to get the vaccine every year.

❹ **Influenza—Symptoms:**
- Symptoms of flu are similar to a common cold: runny nose, sore throat, and a bad cough.
- However, the fever is usually higher (102° F-104° F; 38.9° C-40° C) with flu than with a cold. Headaches and muscle aches are also worse with flu.
- The symptoms often come on suddenly. One day a person can feel fine and the next day feel miserable.

❺ **Influenza—How It Is Spread:**
- Influenza is very contagious. That means it can spread very easily from person to person.
- The flu virus is spread from sneezing and coughing and even talking. It can also be spread from hands that are contaminated with nose and mouth secretions.
- A person can spread the virus (virus may be in respiratory secretions) from 1 day prior to and for 7 days after they start having flu symptoms (e.g., fever, cough). The CDC recommends that people with the flu remain at home until at least 24 hours after they are free of fever (100° F or 37.8°C).
- Flu symptoms usually start within 1-4 days of exposure to a person with flu (7 days is an outer limit). If it is > 7 days after you have been exposed to flu and you have not gotten any symptoms, you should be safe. It is unlikely that you will get the flu from that exposure.

❻ **Influenza—Treatment With Antiviral Drugs:**
- There are 2 antiviral medications that are helpful in treating this infection: oseltamivir (brand name Tamiflu) and zanamivir (brand name Relenza).
- Treatment is recommended for HIGH RISK patients (e.g., age > 64 years, pregnant, HIV positive, or chronic medical condition) with influenza or any patient with severe symptoms (per CDC).
- Treatment is usually not needed for most healthy people who have mild or moderate flu symptoms. Most patients recover without taking antiviral medications.
- The benefits are limited. Antiviral medications may reduce the time you are sick by 1-1½ days. It helps reduce the symptoms but does not cure the disease.
- For best results, antiviral medications should be started within 48 hours of the onset of flu symptoms.

❼ **Call Back If:**
- You have more questions.

Influenza and Prevention

❶ **How to Protect Yourself From Getting Sick:**
- Wash hands often with soap and water.
- Alcohol-based hand cleaners are also effective.
- Avoid touching the eyes, nose, or mouth. Germs on the hands can spread this way.
- Do not share eating utensils (e.g., spoon, fork).
- Try to avoid close contact with sick people.
- Try to avoid unnecessary visits to the ED and urgent care centers. You are more likely to be exposed to influenza in these places if you don't have it.

❷ **How to Protect Others—Stay Home When Sick:**
- Cover the nose and mouth with a tissue when coughing or sneezing.
- Wash hands often with soap and water, especially after coughing or sneezing. Alcohol-based hand cleaners are also effective.
- Limit contact with others to keep from infecting them.
- Stay home from school or work for at least 24 hours after the fever is gone.

❸ **Influenza—Prevention With Vaccine:** The best way to prevent flu is to get a flu vaccine every year.

❹ **Influenza—Prevention With Antiviral Drugs:**
- Antiviral drugs are prescription medicines that help fight viruses in your body. These drugs can be used to help prevent getting flu if you have been exposed to it. The 2 antiviral drugs that are used for preventing flu are zanamivir (Relenza) and oseltamivir (Tamiflu).
- **Who Should Get an Antiviral Drug?** An antiviral drug is recommended for HIGH-RISK patients (e.g., age > 64 years, pregnant, HIV positive, or chronic medical condition) who have been exposed to influenza, especially if the influenza exposure has been in the past 48 hours (2 days). An antiviral drug is considered optional for other people who have been exposed to influenza.
- **How Long Does the Antiviral Drug Work?** It is effective only while you are taking it and stops working as soon as you stop taking it.
- *You should take one of these antiviral medications only if your physician recommends it.*

❺ **Personal Storing or Stockpiling of Antiviral Drugs—Not Recommended:**
- Do NOT store or stockpile antiviral drugs (e.g., Relenza, Tamiflu) for future use.
- There are a few reasons why this is a bad idea.
- First, these are prescription medications. You should only take them if your doctor or qualified health care professional recommends doing so.
- Taking any drug when it is not needed helps a virus become resistant. This means that the virus can become stronger and the drug no longer works.
- All medications expire after a certain amount of time.
- And of course, if too many people stockpile these drugs, there will be less available for people who need the drugs the most.

❻ **Call Back If:**
- You have more questions.

Influenza and Travel

❶ **Do Not Travel if You Are Sick:** If you are sick with symptoms of influenza-like illness, you should not travel.

❷ **During Your Travels—If You Become Sick:**
- If you become seriously ill or injured abroad, an officer at the nearest consulate can assist you in locating appropriate medical services.
- **Canada:** Canadian citizens that are overseas can contact the Operations Center of Foreign Affairs at 613/996-8885.
- **United States:** The US Department of State toll-free number is 888/407-4747; if calling from overseas, the phone number is 202/501-4444.

❸ **Returning From Travels:**
- Monitor your health for 7 days after returning.
- Call your doctor if you develop a cough, runny nose, sore throat, fever, or shortness of breath.

❹ **Call Back If:**
- You have more questions.

Internet Resources

❶ **Internet Resources—Australia and New Zealand:**
- The Australian government provides influenza information at: www.immunise.health.gov.au/internet/immunise/publishing.nsf/content/home.
- The New Zealand Ministry of Health provides influenza information at: www.health.govt.nz/your-health/conditions-and-treatments/diseases-and-illnesses/influenza.

❷ **Internet Resources—Canada:**
- The Public Health Agency of Canada is the best source for influenza information: www.phac-aspc.gc.ca/influenza/index-eng.php.

❸ **Internet Resources—United States:**
- The Centers for Disease Control and Prevention (CDC) is the best source for influenza information: www.cdc.gov/flu/index.htm.
- Key facts about influenza and the flu vaccine are available at: www.cdc.gov/flu/keyfacts.htm.
- There is information about the flu vaccine at: www.cdc.gov/flu/protect/keyfacts.htm.
- Information is also available about antiviral drugs for the flu at: www.cdc.gov/flu/antivirals/whatyoushould.htm.

❹ **Internet Resources—Travel and Health:**
- **CDC:** The CDC has a Web site dedicated to traveler's health at: https://wwwnc.cdc.gov/travel.
- **World Health Organization (WHO):** WHO has a Web site about travel and health at: www.who.int/ith/en. WHO also has a section of its Web site devoted to influenza conditions in the world at: www.who.int/influenza/en.

❺ **Call Back If:**
- You have more questions.

BACKGROUND

Key Points

- Influenza is commonly known as the "flu."
- Influenza is a respiratory illness that is easily spread from person to person.
- The most common symptoms are the sudden onset of fever, muscle aches, cough, runny nose, sore throat, fatigue, and headache.
- The best way to prevent influenza is to get the vaccine every year.

Influenza

- **Seasonal Epidemic:** Influenza viruses change (or mutate) every year. This is the reason why some individuals seem to get influenza every year. The influenza virus is spread via airborne droplet, from sneezing and coughing. Influenza epidemics occur commonly between November and March. During these months 5%-40% of the population may be affected.
- **Expected Course:** The fever lasts 2-3 days, the runny nose 5-10 days, and the cough 2-3 weeks.
- **Incubation Period:** Spread is rapid because the incubation period is only 24-36 hours and the virus is very contagious. Symptoms usually start within 1-4 days after being exposed to a person with influenza (nearly always within 7 days).
- **Contagiousness:** A person is potentially contagious (virus may be in respiratory secretions) from 1 day prior to and for 7 days after the onset of symptoms (e.g., fever, cough). The CDC recommends that people with influenza-like illness remain at home until at least 24 hours after they are free of fever (100° F or 37.8°C).
- **Complications—Respiratory:** Viral and secondary bacterial pneumonia, COPD, and asthma exacerbations.
- **Complications—Other:** Heart failure, ECG abnormalities, Reye syndrome, poor diabetic control.

Prevention—Influenza Vaccine ("Flu Shot")

The influenza vaccine can help prevent influenza. For it to work it needs to be given prior to exposure.

- The best time to get the vaccine is in the fall of every year (September-November) before the onset of influenza season. However, patients should continue to be encouraged to get the vaccine throughout the flu season if they have not yet received one.
- The vaccine is 70%-90% effective in preventing influenza. It is not 100% protective, as the influenza viruses change yearly.
- A Vaccine Information Statement (VIS) for influenza is available at: www.cdc.gov/vaccines/hcp/vis/vis-statements/flu.html. A VIS for the nasal spray flu vaccine is available at: www.cdc.gov/vaccines/hcp/vis/vis-statements/flulive.html.

Which Adults Should Get a Flu Shot?

- *It is recommended that all adults receive an influenza vaccination.*
- **Internet Resource:** https://www.cdc.gov/mmwr/preview/mmwrhtml/mm5931a4.htm.

When vaccine supplies are limited, the following caregivers, who can potentially spread influenza, should get preferential vaccination:

- Health care workers
- Household contacts and caregivers of children from 0-59 months of age
- Household contacts and caregivers of persons with medical conditions that put them at higher risk for severe complications from influenza

When vaccine supplies are limited, the following groups who are at higher risk for complications should get preferential vaccination:

- People ≥ 50 years.
- Patient populations at high risk for complications of influenza: chronic cardiopulmonary conditions (e.g., asthma), immunosuppression (e.g., chemotherapy), renal dysfunction, diabetes, women who will be pregnant during flu season.
- Patients with chronic medical conditions who reside in nursing home or chronic care facilities.
- Healthy persons who could transmit influenza to high-risk patients: health care workers, nursing home employees, and family members.

- Note that the indications for getting the nasal spray vaccine are slightly different than those for the shot since the nasal spray contains live virus. Refer to the VIS if additional information is needed.
- **Internet Resource:** www.cdc.gov/flu/protect/keyfacts.htm.

Prevention—Antiviral Medications for Influenza

Oseltamivir (Tamiflu) or zanamivir (Relenza) are the primary antiviral agents recommended for the treatment and prevention of influenza.

- **Prevention of Influenza:** Antiviral medications can also be taken prophylactically during influenza epidemics to prevent illness in high-risk patients. However, they should not be used as a substitute for vaccination. Generally, postexposure chemoprophylaxis should only be used when antivirals can be started within 48 hours of the most recent exposure.
- **Treatment of Influenza:** Antiviral medications must be started within 48 hours of symptom onset for greatest benefit; after that, the benefit decreases substantially. It is recommended that individuals at HIGH RISK (see Definition) for influenza complications be treated with antiviral medications if antivirals can be started within 48 hours of symptom onset. Use of antiviral medications in individuals not at high risk is considered optional, and clinical judgment is recommended. Antiviral medications have been shown to reduce the duration (by 1 day) and severity of flu symptoms.
- **When to Call the PCP:** If callers ask for one of these drugs after being informed of their limited efficacy, recommend they call their PCP during office hours. If the office won't be open tomorrow and it is not the middle of the night (9:00 pm-9:00 am), transfer the call to the PCP.
- **Internet Resource:** www.cdc.gov/flu/professionals/antivirals/summary-clinicians.htm.

INFLUENZA FOLLOW-UP CALL

Definition
- Recently diagnosed as having "influenza" or "swine flu" in the last 2 weeks by a health care professional.
- All types of influenza (A, B, and H1N1) are included.
- Caller has concerns or questions, often about persistent symptoms.

Symptoms
- There is usually a sudden onset of fever, chills, feeling sick, muscle aches, and headache.
- Respiratory symptoms are similar to a common cold: runny nose, sore throat, and a bad cough.
- The fever is usually higher (102° F-104° F; 38.9° C-40° C) with influenza than with a cold. Headaches and muscle aches are also worse with influenza.

The following groups of individuals are at higher risk for complications from influenza and therefore are considered as HIGH RISK in this protocol. It is recommended that these individuals receive antiviral treatment for suspected or confirmed influenza.
- Persons ≥ 65 years
- Persons < 19 years who are receiving long-term aspirin therapy
  Reason: at risk for Reye syndrome
- Persons with immunosuppression, including that caused by medications (e.g., chemotherapy, chronic steroids) or by HIV infection
- Persons who are morbidly obese (i.e., BMI ≥ 40)
- Persons with chronic *pulmonary* (including asthma), *cardiovascular* (except hypertension alone), *renal, hepatic, hematological* (including sickle cell disease), or *metabolic* disorders (including diabetes mellitus)
- Persons with *neurologic* and neurodevelopment conditions (including disorders of the brain, spinal cord, peripheral nerve, and muscles such as cerebral palsy, epilepsy [seizure disorders], stroke, intellectual disability, moderate-severe developmental delay, muscular dystrophy, or spinal cord injury)
- Women who are pregnant or postpartum (up to 2 weeks)
- Nursing home residents and other persons residing in long-term care facilities
- American Indians and Alaskan Natives

TRIAGE ASSESSMENT QUESTIONS

Call EMS 911 Now
- SEVERE difficulty breathing (e.g., struggling for each breath, speaks in single words)
  R/O: respiratory failure, hypoxia
- Bluish (or gray) lips or face
  R/O: cyanosis and need for oxygen
- Shock suspected (e.g., cold/pale/clammy skin, too weak to stand, low BP, rapid pulse)
  R/O: shock
- Sounds like a life-threatening emergency to the triager

See More Appropriate Protocol
- Asthma attack (coughing, wheezing) is main concern and previously diagnosed with asthma OR using asthma medicines
  Go to Protocol: Asthma Attack on page 38

Go to ED Now
- Chest pain
  (Exception: MILD central chest pain, present only when coughing)
- R/O: pneumonia
- Headache and stiff neck (can't touch chin to chest)
  R/O: meningitis

Go to ED/UCC Now
(or to Office With PCP Approval)
- Difficulty breathing that is not severe and not relieved by cleaning out the nose
  R/O: pneumonia
- Patient sounds very sick or weak to the triager
  Reason: severe acute illness or serious complication suspected

Go to Office Now
- Fever > 104° F (40° C)
  R/O: serious bacterial infection

See Today in Office

● Fever present > 3 days (72 hours)
R/O: bacterial superinfection: sinusitis, bronchitis, pneumonia

● Fever returns after gone for > 24 hours and symptoms worse or not improved
R/O: bacterial sinusitis, bronchitis, pneumonia

● Using nasal washes and pain medicine > 24 hours and sinus pain (around cheekbone or eye) persists
R/O: sinusitis

● Earache
R/O: otitis media

See Today or Tomorrow in Office

● Patient wants to be seen

See Within 3 Days in Office

● Nasal discharge present > 10 days
R/O: sinusitis, allergic rhinitis

● Cough present > 3 weeks

Home Care

○ Influenza (diagnosed by health care professional) and no complications
Note: Caller probably needs additional care advice on symptom management.

○ Influenza and antiviral drugs, questions about

○ Influenza and breastfeeding, questions about

○ Influenza and Internet resources, questions about

HOME CARE ADVICE

Influenza—General Information

❶ **Reassurance:**
  • Influenza is commonly known as the "flu."
  • Influenza is a respiratory illness that is easily spread from person to person.
  • The most common symptoms are the sudden onset of fever, muscle aches, cough, runny nose, sore throat, fatigue, and headache. For healthy people, the symptoms of influenza are similar to those of the common cold. However, with influenza, the onset is more abrupt and fever is higher. Feeling very sick for the first 3 days is common.
  • The treatment of influenza depends on your main symptoms. It is usually no different from that used for other viral respiratory infections. Most people who get sick with influenza get better at home without special treatment.

  • There are things that you can do to feel better and decrease your symptoms.
  • *Here is some care advice that should help.*

❷ **Symptoms:**
  • Symptoms of influenza are similar to a common cold: runny nose, sore throat, and a bad cough.
  • However, the fever is usually higher (102° F-104° F; 38.9° C-40° C) with influenza than with a cold. Headaches and muscle aches are also worse with influenza.
  • The symptoms often come on suddenly. One day a person can feel fine and the next day feel miserable.

❸ **How It Is Spread:**
  • Influenza is very contagious. That means it can spread very easily from person to person.
  • The flu virus is spread by airborne droplet, from sneezing and coughing and even talking. It also can be transmitted by hands contaminated with secretions.
  • A person is potentially contagious (virus may be in respiratory secretions) from 1 day prior to and for 7 days after the onset of symptoms (e.g., fever, cough). The CDC recommends that people with the flu stay at home until at least 24 hours after they are free of fever (100° F or 37.8°C).
  • Symptoms usually start within 1-4 days after being exposed to a person with influenza (nearly always within 7 days). If > 7 days pass from exposure without you developing symptoms, you should be safe and not get influenza.

❹ **How to Protect Others—Stay Home When Sick:**
  • Cover the nose and mouth with a tissue when coughing or sneezing.
  • Wash hands often with soap and water, especially after coughing or sneezing. Alcohol-based hand cleaners are also effective.
  • Avoid sharing eating utensils (e.g., spoon, fork).
  • Limit contact with others to keep from infecting them.
  • Stay home from school or work for at least 24 hours after the fever is gone.

❺ How to Protect Others—Avoid People at HIGH RISK for Complications:
- Persons < 2 years
- Persons ≥ 65 years
- Persons < 19 years who are receiving long-term aspirin therapy
  Reason: at risk for Reye syndrome
- Pregnant women and women up to 2 weeks' postpartum
- Chronic medical conditions, including cardio-vascular (not hypertension), chronic pulmonary conditions (e.g., asthma, emphysema), renal failure, hepatic, hematologic (e.g., sickle cell disease), neurologic, neuromuscular, and diabetes mellitus
- Immunosuppression (e.g., chemotherapy, HIV)

❻ Isolation Is Needed Until After Fever Is Gone:
- If you have flu-like symptoms, please stay at home until at least 24 hours after you are free of fever.
- Do **not** go to work or school.
- Do **not** go to church, child care centers, shopping, or other public places.
- Do **not** shake hands.
- Do **not** share eating utensils (e.g., spoon, fork).
- Avoid close contact with others (hugging, kissing).

❼ Treating the Symptoms:
- **Cough:** Use cough drops.
- **Feeling Dehydrated:** Drink extra liquids. If the air in your home is dry, use a humidifier.
- **Fever:** For fever > 101° F (38.3° C), take acetaminophen every 4-6 hours (adults, 650 mg) OR ibuprofen every 6-8 hours (adults, 400-600 mg).
- **Muscle Aches, Headache, and Other Pains:** Often this comes and goes with the fever. Take acetaminophen every 4-6 hours (adults, 650 mg) OR ibuprofen every 6-8 hours (adults, 400-600 mg).
- **Sore Throat:** Try throat lozenges, hard candy, or warm chicken broth.

❽ No Aspirin: Do not use aspirin for treatment of fever or pain.
(Reason: There is an association between influenza and Reye syndrome.)

❾ Expected Course: The fever lasts 2-3 days, the runny nose 5-10 days, and the cough 2-3 weeks.

❿ Call Back If:
- Difficulty breathing.
- Fever lasts > 3 days.
- Runny nose lasts > 14 days.
- Cough lasts > 3 weeks.
- You become worse.

Influenza—Treating the Symptoms (More Detailed)

❶ Pain and Fever Medicines:
- For pain or fever relief, take either acetaminophen or ibuprofen.
- They are over-the-counter (OTC) drugs that help treat both fever and pain. You can buy them at the drugstore.
- Treat fevers > 101° F (38.3° C). The goal of fever therapy is to bring the fever down to a comfortable level. Remember that fever medicine usually lowers fever 2° F (1-1½° C).

Acetaminophen (e.g., Tylenol):
- **Regular Strength Tylenol:** Take 650 mg (two 325 mg pills) by mouth every 4-6 hours as needed. Each Regular Strength Tylenol pill has 325 mg of acetaminophen.
- **Extra Strength Tylenol:** Take 1,000 mg (two 500 mg pills) every 8 hours as needed. Each Extra Strength Tylenol pill has 500 mg of acetaminophen.
- The most you should take each day is 3,000 mg (10 Regular Strength or 6 Extra Strength pills a day).

Ibuprofen (e.g., Motrin, Advil):
- Take 400 mg (two 200 mg pills) by mouth every 6 hours.
- Another choice is to take 600 mg (three 200 mg pills) by mouth every 8 hours.
- The most you should take each day is 1,200 mg (six 200 mg pills), unless your doctor has told you to take more.

❷ For a Runny Nose—Blow Your Nose:
- Nasal mucus and discharge help wash viruses and bacteria out of the nose and sinuses.
- Blowing your nose helps clean out your nose. Use a handkerchief or a paper tissue.
- If the skin around your nostrils gets irritated, apply a tiny amount of petroleum ointment to the nasal openings once or twice a day.

❸ **For a Stuffy Nose—Use Nasal Washes:**
- **Introduction:** Saline (salt water) nasal irrigation (nasal wash) is an effective and simple home remedy for treating stuffy nose and sinus congestion. The nose can be irrigated by pouring, spraying, or squirting salt water into the nose and then letting it run back out.
- **How It Helps:** The salt water rinses out excess mucus, washes out any irritants (dust, allergens) that might be present, and moistens the nasal cavity.
- **Methods:** There are several ways to perform nasal irrigation. You can use a saline nasal spray bottle (available over the counter [OTC]), a rubber ear syringe, a medical syringe without the needle, or a neti pot.

Step-by-step Instructions:
- **Step 1:** Lean over a sink.
- **Step 2:** Gently squirt or spray warm salt water into one of your nostrils.
- **Step 3:** Some of the water may run into the back of your throat. Spit this out. If you swallow the salt water, it will not hurt you.
- **Step 4:** Blow your nose to clean out the water and mucus.
- **Step 5:** Repeat steps 1-4 for the other nostril. You can do this a couple times a day if it seems to help you.

How to Make Saline (Salt Water) Nasal Wash:
- You can make your own saline nasal wash.
- Add ½ tsp of table salt to 1 cup (8 oz; 240 mL) of warm water.
- You should use sterile, distilled, or previously boiled water for nasal irrigation.

❹ **Medicines for a Stuffy or Runny Nose:**
- Most cold medicines that are available OTC are not helpful.
- **Antihistamines:** Are only helpful if you also have nasal allergies.
- If you have a very runny nose and you really think you need a medicine, you can try using a nasal decongestant for a couple days.

❺ **Caution—Nasal Decongestants:**
- Do not take these medications if you have high blood pressure, heart disease, prostate problems, or an overactive thyroid.
- Do not take these medications if you are pregnant.
- Do not take these medications if you have used a monoamine oxidase (MAO) inhibitor such as isocarboxazid (Marplan), phenelzine (Nardil), rasagiline (Azilect), selegiline (Eldepryl, Emsam), or tranylcypromine (Parnate) in the past 2 weeks. Life-threatening side effects can occur.
- Do not use these medications for > 3 days. *(Reason: rebound nasal congestion)*

❻ **Cough Medicines:**
- **OTC Cough Syrups:** The most common cough suppressant in OTC cough medications is dextromethorphan. Often the letters DM appear in the name.
- **OTC Cough Drops:** Cough drops can help a lot, especially for mild coughs. They reduce coughing by soothing your irritated throat and removing that tickle sensation in the back of the throat. Cough drops also have the advantage of portability—you can carry them with you.
- **Home Remedy—Hard Candy:** Hard candy works just as well as medicine-flavored OTC cough drops. People who have diabetes should use sugar-free candy.
- **Home Remedy—Honey:** This old home remedy has been shown to help decrease coughing at night. The adult dosage is 2 teaspoons (10 mL) at bedtime. Honey should not be given to infants < 1 year of age.

❼ **OTC Cough Syrup—Dextromethorphan:**
- Cough syrups containing the cough suppressant DM may help decrease your cough. Cough syrups work best for coughs that keep you awake at night. They can also sometimes help in the late stages of a respiratory infection when the cough is dry and hacking. They can be used along with cough drops.
- **Examples:** Benylin, Robitussin DM, Vicks 44 Cough Relief.
- *Read the package instructions for dosage, contraindications, and other important information.*

❽ **Caution—Dextromethorphan:**
- Do not try to completely suppress coughs that produce mucus and phlegm. Remember that coughing is helpful in bringing up mucus from the lungs and preventing pneumonia.
- **Research Notes:** Dextromethorphan, in some research studies, has been shown to reduce the frequency and severity of cough in adults (≥ 18 years) without significant adverse effects. However, other studies suggest that DM is no better than placebo at reducing a cough.
- **Drug Abuse Potential:** It should be noted that DM has become a drug of abuse. This problem is seen most often in adolescents. Overdose symptoms can range from giggling and euphoria to hallucinations and coma.
- **Contraindicated:** Do not take DM if you are taking an MAO inhibitor now or in the past 2 weeks. Examples of MAO inhibitors include isocarboxazid (Marplan), phenelzine (Nardil), selegiline (Eldepryl, Emsam, Zelapar), and tranylcypromine (Parnate). Do not take DM if you are taking venlafaxine (Effexor).

❾ **Coughing Spasms:**
- Drink warm fluids. Inhale warm mist. *(Reason: Both relax the airway and loosen up the phlegm.)*
- Suck on cough drops or hard candy to coat the irritated throat.

❿ **For All Fevers:**
- Drink cold fluids to prevent dehydration.
- Dress in 1 layer of lightweight clothing and sleep with 1 light blanket.
- For fevers < 101° F (38.3° C), fever medicines are usually not needed.

⓫ **Pain and Fever Medicines—Extra Notes:**
- Use the lowest amount of medicine that makes your pain or fever better.
- Acetaminophen is thought to be safer than ibuprofen or naproxen in people > 65 years old. Acetaminophen is in many OTC and prescription medicines. It might be in more than one medicine that you are taking. You need to be careful and not take an overdose. An acetaminophen overdose can hurt the liver.
- McNeil, the company that makes Tylenol, has different dosage instructions for Tylenol in Canada and the United States. In Canada, the maximum recommended dose per day is 4,000 mg or 12 Regular Strength (325 mg) pills. In the United States, McNeil recommends a maximum dose of 10 Regular Strength (325 mg) pills.
- CAUTION: Do not take acetaminophen if you have liver disease.
- CAUTION: Do not take ibuprofen if you have stomach problems, have kidney disease, are pregnant, or have been told by your doctor to avoid this type of anti-inflammatory drug. Do not take ibuprofen for > 7 days without consulting your doctor.
- *Before taking any medicine, read all the instructions on the package.*

⓬ **Call Back If:**
- Difficulty breathing.
- Fever lasts > 3 days.
- Runny nose lasts > 14 days.
- Cough lasts > 3 weeks.
- You become worse.

Influenza and Antiviral Drugs

❶ **Influenza—Treatment With Antiviral Drugs:**
- There are 2 antiviral medications that are helpful in treating this infection: oseltamivir (brand name Tamiflu) and zanamivir (brand name Relenza).
- Treatment is recommended for HIGH-RISK patients (e.g., age > 64 years, pregnant, HIV positive, or chronic medical condition) with influenza or any patient with severe symptoms (per CDC).
- Treatment is typically not recommended for mild-moderate influenza illness that occurs in most healthy patients (per CDC). Most patients recover without taking antiviral medications.
- The benefits are limited. Antiviral medications may reduce the time you are sick by 1-1½ days. It helps reduce the symptoms but does not cure the disease.
- For best results, antiviral medications should be started within 48 hours of the onset of flu symptoms.

❷ **Persons at HIGH RISK of Complications:**
- Persons < 2 years
- Persons ≥ 65 years
- Persons < 19 years old who are receiving long-term aspirin therapy *(Reason: at risk for Reye syndrome)*
- Pregnant women
- Chronic medical conditions, including cardio-vascular (not hypertension), chronic pulmonary conditions (e.g., asthma, emphysema), renal failure, hepatic, hematologic (e.g., sickle cell disease), neurologic, neuromuscular, and diabetes mellitus
- Immunosuppression (e.g., chemotherapy, HIV)

Influenza and Breastfeeding

❶ **Breastfeeding When the Mother Has Influenza:** You should try to protect your baby from getting sick:
- If possible, ask someone who is not sick to feed and care for your baby. This person can give your baby expressed breast milk.
- If this is not possible, you should wear a face mask at all times when you are feeding or caring for your baby. You should also avoid sneezing or coughing around the baby. You should also wash your hands with soap and water before picking up the baby.

❷ **Breastfeeding and Taking Medications:**
- It is important to note that your doctor is the best source of information about breastfeeding and taking medications.
- It is better to take your medication at the end of a feeding.

❸ **Medicines That Are Safe to Take:**
- Acetaminophen (e.g., Tylenol)
- Ibuprofen (e.g., Motrin, Advil)
- Most antibiotics including penicillin (antibiotic), erythromycin (antibiotic), cephalosporins (antibiotic)
- *Before taking any medicine, read all the instructions on the package.*

❹ **Medications You Should Avoid:**
- Avoid pseudoephedrine because it can reduce milk production in some mothers.
- Avoid aspirin (Reason: concern about Reye syndrome).
- Avoid sulfa drugs (Septra and Bactrim) until baby is 4 weeks old.

❺ **Call Back If:**
- You have more questions.

Additional Resources

❶ **Internet Resources:**
- **LactMed:** LactMed is a drug/lactation Web site that provides information regarding the safety of medications while nursing. LactMed is located on TOXNET (the toxicology data Web site of the National Library of Medicine). It is available at: http://toxnet.nlm.nih.gov.
- **American Academy of Pediatrics (AAP):** The AAP published a clinical report, "The Transfer of Drugs and Therapeutics Into Human Breast Milk: An Update on Selected Topics" (*Pediatrics.* 2013;132[3]:e796–e809). Consider printing this document and having it readily available as a reference. It is available online at: http://pediatrics.aappublications.org/content/132/3/e796.

❷ **Internet Resources—Australia and New Zealand:**
- The Australian government provides influenza information at: www.immunise.health.gov.au/internet/immunise/publishing.nsf/content/home.
- The New Zealand Ministry of Health provides influenza information at: www.health.govt.nz/your-health/conditions-and-treatments/diseases-and-illnesses/influenza.

❸ **Internet Resources—Canada:**
- The Public Health Agency of Canada is the best source for influenza information: www.phac-aspc.gc.ca/influenza/index-eng.php.

❹ **Internet Resources—United States:**
- The Centers for Disease Control and Prevention (CDC) is the best source for influenza information: www.cdc.gov/flu/index.htm.
- Key facts about influenza and the flu vaccine are available at: www.cdc.gov/flu/keyfacts.htm.
- There is information about the flu vaccine at: www.cdc.gov/flu/protect/keyfacts.htm.
- Information is also available about antiviral drugs for the flu at: www.cdc.gov/flu/antivirals/whatyoushould.htm.

BACKGROUND

Seasonal Influenza—Key Points
- Influenza ("flu") is a viral infection of the nose, throat, trachea, and bronchi.
- **Seasonal Epidemic:** Influenza viruses change (or mutate) yearly. This is why some individuals seem to get influenza every year. Influenza epidemics occur commonly between November and March. During these months 5%-40% of the population may be affected.
- **Symptoms:** There is usually a sudden onset of fever, chills, feeling sick, muscle aches, and headache. Respiratory symptoms are similar to a common cold: runny nose, sore throat, and a bad cough. The fever is usually higher (102° F-104° F; 38.9° C-40° C) with influenza than with a cold. Headaches and muscle aches are also worse with influenza.
- **Treatment:** There are 4 antiviral medications licensed in the United States and 3 in Canada: amantadine (Symmetrel), rimantadine (Flumadine [not available in Canada]), zanamivir (Relenza), and oseltamivir (Tamiflu). These medications have been shown to reduce the duration (by 1 day) and severity of flu symptoms. They do not cure the disease or remove all the symptoms. They must be started within 48 hours of symptom onset.
- **Transmission:** The influenza virus is spread by airborne droplet, from sneezing and coughing. It also can be transmitted by hands contaminated with secretions.
- **Contagiousness:** Spread is rapid because the incubation period is only 24-36 hours and the virus is very contagious. Symptoms usually start within 1-4 days after being exposed to a person with influenza (nearly always within 7 days).
- **Expected Course:** The fever lasts 2-3 days, the runny nose 5-10 days, and the cough 2-3 weeks.
- **Internet Resource:** www.cdc.gov/flu.

Complications of Seasonal Influenza
- Otitis media
- Dehydration
- Exacerbation of asthma or COPD
- Worsening of chronic medical conditions like congestive heart failure and diabetes
- Pneumonia
- Hospitalization
- Death

Staying Home From Work and School
- The CDC recommends that people with influenza-like illness remain at home until at least 24 hours after they are free of fever (100° F [37.8°C]).
- More information on this is available at: www.cdc.gov/h1n1flu/guidance/exclusion.htm.

Dextromethorphan Cough Medicines for Cough
- The most common cough suppressant in OTC cough medications is dextromethorphan (DM). Usually the letters DM appear in the name. An example is Robitussin DM.
- **Research:** Dextromethorphan, in some research studies, has been shown to reduce the frequency and severity of cough in adults (≥ 18 years) without significant adverse effects. However, other studies suggest that DM is no better than placebo at reducing a cough.
- **Dextromethorphan and Adult Telephone Triage Protocols:** The care advice in these protocols continues to recommend DM-containing cough syrups. The rationale for this is: DM may reduce cough to some extent in adults, adult patients may benefit from the placebo effect of DM, many patients demand a recommendation for a cough syrup, there is no OTC medicine that works better than DM, and, generally, DM has no side effects.
- **Use Cough Drop or Hard Candy Instead:** Cough drops can often be used instead of cough syrup. While some would consider them a placebo similar to cough medicines, they may actually reduce coughing by soothing an irritated throat. In addition, they have the advantage of portability. Hard candy probably works just as well as an OTC cough drop.
- **Use Honey for Nocturnal Cough:** See Honey for Cough section.

- **Dextromethorphan—a Drug of Abuse:** It is important to note that DM has become a drug of abuse. This problem is seen most commonly in the adolescent population. Overdose symptoms can range from giggling and euphoria to hallucinations or coma.

Honey for Cough

- **Recent Research Study:** A recent research study (Paul) compared honey to either DM or no treatment for the treatment of nocturnal coughing. The study group contained 105 children aged 2-18 years. Honey consistently scored the best for reducing cough frequency and cough severity. It also scored best for improving sleep. Dextromethorphan did not score significantly better than no treatment (showing its lack of efficacy).
- **How Might Honey Work?** One explanation for how honey works is that sweet substances naturally cause reflex salivation and increased airway secretions. These secretions may lubricate the airway and remove the trigger (or tickle) that causes a dry, nonproductive cough.
- **Adult Dosage:** 2 teaspoons (10 mL) at bedtime.

Face Masks:

- Face masks refer to disposable masks labeled as surgical or dental masks.
- Sick people should wear a face mask if they must leave their home to seek medical care.
- For healthy people, face masks may help reduce the risk of getting flu in crowded settings. Avoiding sick people and frequent hand washing are more effective at preventing flu.

INSECT BITE

Definition
- Itching, pain, or swelling from an insect bite
- *This protocol excludes bedbugs, bees, ticks, mosquitoes, and spiders.*

Types of Insect Bites
- **Itchy Insect Bites:** Bites of chiggers (harvest mites), fleas, and bedbugs usually cause itchy, red bumps.
- **Painful Insect Bites:** Bites of horseflies, blackflies, deerflies, gnats, harvester ants, blister beetles, and centipedes usually cause a painful, red bump. Even though fire ants belong to the *Hymenoptera* or bee family, which have stingers on the back of their bodies, most people group them with other ants. Within a few hours, fire ant bites can change to blisters or pimples.

TRIAGE ASSESSMENT QUESTIONS

Call EMS 911 Now
- Passed out (i.e., fainted, collapsed and was not responding)
  R/O: anaphylaxis
  Use First Aid Advice for anaphylaxis.
- Wheezing or difficulty breathing
  R/O: anaphylaxis
  Use First Aid Advice for anaphylaxis.
- Hoarseness, cough, or tightness in the throat or chest
  R/O: anaphylaxis
  Use First Aid Advice for anaphylaxis.
- Swollen tongue or difficulty swallowing
- Life-threatening reaction (anaphylaxis) in the past to same insect bite and < 2 hours since bite
- Sounds like a life-threatening emergency to the triager

See More Appropriate Protocol
- Bee sting(s)
  Go to Protocol: Bee Sting on page 52
- Spider bite(s)
  Go to Protocol: Spider Bite on page 372
- Tick bite(s)
  Go to Protocol: Tick Bite on page 400
- Doesn't sound like an insect bite
  Go to Protocol: Rash or Redness, Localized on page 326

Go to ED/UCC Now
(or to Office With PCP Approval)
- Patient sounds very sick or weak to the triager
  Reason: severe acute illness or serious complication suspected

Go to Office Now
- SEVERE bite pain and not improved after 2 hours of pain medicine
- Fever and area is red
  R/O: cellulitis, lymphangitis
  Reason: fever and looks infected
- Fever and area is very tender to touch
  R/O: cellulitis, lymphangitis
  Reason: fever and looks infected.
- Red streak or red line and length > 2" (5 cm)
  R/O: lymphangitis
  Note: Lymphangitis looks like a red streak or line originating at the wound and ascending the arm or leg toward the heart.

See Today in Office
- Red or very tender (to touch) area, and started > 24 hours after the bite
  R/O: cellulitis
- Red or very tender (to touch) area, getting larger > 48 hours after the bite
  R/O: cellulitis

See Today or Tomorrow in Office
- Patient wants to be seen

See Within 3 Days in Office
- SEVERE local itching (i.e., interferes with work, school, activities) and not improved after 24 hours of hydrocortisone cream
- Scab drains pus or increases in size, and not improved after applying antibiotic ointment for 2 days
  R/O: infected sore, impetigo
- Bite starts to look bad (e.g., blister, purplish skin, ulcer)
  R/O: necrotic spider bite (brown recluse, hobo spider, or other cause of skin lesion)
- After 14 days the insect bite is not healed
  R/O: low-grade infection, misdiagnosis

Home Care

○ Itchy insect bite
○ Painful insect bite
○ Scab drains pus or increases in size
  R/O: infected sore, impetigo
○ West Nile virus, questions about
○ Preventing insect bites, questions about

HOME CARE ADVICE

Itchy Insect Bites

❶ **Reassurance:**
  • Insect bites often can be itchy.
  • Most insect bites look like a small red bump. Some are larger (like a hive) and some can have a small water blister in the center.
  • Here is some care advice that should help.

❷ **Four Simple Home Remedies for Itchy Mosquito Bites:**
  • Rub a bite with an ice cube for 30 seconds.
  • Try applying firm, direct, steady pressure to a bite for 10 seconds. A fingernail, pen cap, or other object can be used.
  • Apply calamine lotion to the bites.
  • Make baking soda paste by mixing baking soda with a small amount of water. Apply the paste to the bites.

❸ **Don't Scratch:**
  • Try not to scratch.
  • Scratching makes the itching worse (the "itch-scratch" cycle).
  • Cut your fingernails short. Wash hands frequently with an antibacterial soap. This will help prevent a bacterial skin infection.

❹ **Hydrocortisone Cream for Itching:**
  • You can use hydrocortisone for severe itching.
  • Put 1% hydrocortisone cream on the itchy area(s) 3 times a day. Use it for a couple days, until it feels better. This will help decrease the itching.
  • This is an over-the-counter (OTC) drug. You can buy it at the drugstore.
  • Some people like to keep the cream in the refrigerator. It feels even better if the cream is used when it is cold.
  • CAUTION: Do not use hydrocortisone cream for > 1 week without talking to your doctor.
  • *Read the instructions and warnings on the package insert for all medicines you take.*

❺ **Antihistamine Medicine for Severe Itching:**
  • Take an antihistamine by mouth to reduce the itching.
  • Diphenhydramine (Benadryl) is a good choice. The adult dosage of Benadryl is 25-50 mg by mouth and you can take it up to 4 times a day.
  • Another OTC antihistamine that causes less sleepiness is loratadine (e.g., Alavert or Claritin). Alavert is not available in Canada.
  • *Before taking any medicine, read all the instructions on the package.*

❻ **Caution—Antihistamines:**
  • Examples include diphenhydramine (Benadryl) and chlorpheniramine (Chlor-Trimeton, Chlor-Tripolon).
  • May cause sleepiness. Do not drink alcohol, drive, or operate dangerous machinery while taking antihistamines.
  • Do not take these medicines if you have prostate problems.

❼ **Expected Course:**
  • Most insect bites are itchy and puffy for several days.
  • Insect bites of the upper face can cause marked swelling around the eye, but this is harmless.
  • Any pinkness or redness usually lasts 3 days.

❽ **Call Back If:**
  • Severe pain persists > 2 hours after pain medicine.
  • Bite looks infected (pus, red streaks, increased tenderness).
  • Bite has not healed after 14 days.
  • Redness getting larger and > 48 hours after the bite.
  • You become worse.

Painful Insect Bites

❶ Reassurance:
- Some insect bites can be painful.
- Most insect bites look like a small red bump. Some are larger (like a hive) and some can have a small water blister in the center.
- *Here is some care advice that should help.*

❷ Two Simple Home Remedies for Painful Mosquito Bites:
- Rub a bite with an ice cube for 30 seconds.
- Make baking soda paste by mixing baking soda with a small amount of water. Apply the paste to the bites using a cotton ball or some gauze.

❸ Pain Medicines:
- For pain relief, you can take either acetaminophen, ibuprofen, or naproxen.
- They are over-the-counter (OTC) pain drugs. You can buy them at the drugstore.

Acetaminophen (e.g., Tylenol):
- **Regular Strength Tylenol:** Take 650 mg (two 325 mg pills) by mouth every 4-6 hours as needed. Each Regular Strength Tylenol pill has 325 mg of acetaminophen.
- **Extra Strength Tylenol:** Take 1,000 mg (two 500 mg pills) every 8 hours as needed. Each Extra Strength Tylenol pill has 500 mg of acetaminophen.
- The most you should take each day is 3,000 mg (10 Regular Strength or 6 Extra Strength pills a day).

Ibuprofen (e.g., Motrin, Advil):
- Take 400 mg (two 200 mg pills) by mouth every 6 hours.
- Another choice is to take 600 mg (three 200 mg pills) by mouth every 8 hours.
- The most you should take each day is 1,200 mg (six 200 mg pills), unless your doctor has told you to take more.

Naproxen (e.g., Aleve):
- Take 220 mg (one 220 mg pill) by mouth every 8 hours as needed. You may take 440 mg (two 220 mg pills) for your first dose.
- The most you should take each day is 660 mg (three 220 mg pills a day), unless your doctor has told you to take more.

❹ Pain Medicines—Extra Notes:
- Use the lowest amount of medicine that makes your pain better.
- Acetaminophen is thought to be safer than ibuprofen or naproxen in people > 65 years old. Acetaminophen is in many OTC and prescription medicines. It might be in more than one medicine that you are taking. You need to be careful and not take an overdose. An acetaminophen overdose can hurt the liver.
- McNeil, the company that makes Tylenol, has different dosage instructions for Tylenol in Canada and the United States. In Canada, the maximum recommended dose per day is 4,000 mg or 12 Regular Strength (325 mg) pills. In the United States, McNeil recommends a maximum dose of 10 Regular Strength (325 mg) pills.
- CAUTION: Do not take acetaminophen if you have liver disease.
- CAUTION: Do not take ibuprofen or naproxen if you have stomach problems, have kidney disease, are pregnant, or have been told by your doctor to avoid this type of anti-inflammatory drug. Do not take ibuprofen or naproxen for > 7 days without consulting your doctor.
- *Before taking any medicine, read all the instructions on the package.*

❺ Antibiotic Ointment: If the insect bite has a scab on it and the scab looks infected, apply an antibiotic ointment 4 times per day.
- Cover the scab with a Band-Aid to prevent scratching and spread.
- Repeat washing the sore, the antibiotic ointment, and the Band-Aid 4 times per day until healed.

❻ Expected Course:
- Most insect bites are itchy and puffy for several days.
- Insect bites of the upper face can cause marked swelling around the eye, but this is harmless.
- Any pinkness or redness usually lasts 3 days.

❼ Call Back If:
- Severe pain lasts > 2 hours after pain medicine.
- Bite looks infected (redness, red streaks, increased tenderness).
- Redness getting larger and > 48 hours after the bite.
- Infected scab doesn't look better after 48 hours of antibiotic ointment.
- You become worse.

Infected Sore or Scab

❶ Reassurance:
- Sometimes a small infected sore can develop at the site of a cut, scratch, insect bite, or sting.
- The typical appearance is a sore < 1" (2.5 cm) in diameter. It is often covered by a soft, honey-yellow or yellow-brown crust or scab. Sometimes the scab may drain a tiny amount of pus or yellow fluid. Usually there is minimal to no pain.
- Small infected sores usually get better with regular cleansing and use of an antibiotic ointment.
- *Here is some care advice that should help.*

❷ Cleaning:
- Wash the area 2-3 times daily with an antibacterial soap and warm water.
- Gently remove any scab. The bacteria live underneath the scab. You may need to soak the scab off by placing a warm, wet washcloth (or gauze) on the sore for 10 minutes.

❸ Antibiotic Ointment:
- Apply an antibiotic ointment 3 times per day.
- Cover the sore with a Band-Aid to prevent scratching and spread.
- Use bacitracin ointment (OTC in United States) or Polysporin ointment (OTC in Canada) or one that you already have.

❹ Avoid Picking: Avoid scratching and picking. This can spread a skin infection.

❺ Contagiousness:
- Infected sores can be spread by skin-to-skin contact.
- Wash your hands frequently and avoid touching the sore.
- **Work and School:** You can attend school or work if it is covered.
- **Contact Sports:** Generally, you need to receive antibiotic treatment for 3 days before you can return to the sport. There can be no pus or drainage. You should check with your trainer, if there is one for your sports team.

❻ Expected Course:
- The sore should stop growing in 1-2 days and it should begin improving within 2-3 days.
- The sore should be completely healed in 7-10 days.

❼ Call Back If:
- Fever occurs.
- Spreading redness or a red streak occurs.
- Sore increases in size.
- Sore not improving after 2 days using antibiotic ointment.
- Sore not completely healed in 7 days (1 week).
- New sore appears.
- You become worse.

Preventing Insect Bites

❶ Prevention:
- Wear long pants and long-sleeved shirts.
- Avoid being outside when the insect is most active. Many insects that cause itchy bites are most active at sunrise or sunset (e.g., chiggers, no-see-ums, mosquitoes).
- Insect repellents containing DEET are effective in preventing many itchy insect bites.

❷ DEET—an Insect Repellent:
- DEET is a very effective insect repellent. It also repels ticks.
- Higher concentrations of DEET do work better—but there appears to be no benefit in using DEET concentrations > 50%. For children and adolescents, the American Academy of Pediatrics recommends a maximum concentration of 30%. Health Canada recommends using a concentration of 5%-30% for adults.
- Apply to exposed areas of skin. Do not apply to eyes, mouth, or irritated areas of skin. Do not apply to skin that is covered by clothing.
- Remember to wash it off with soap and water when you return indoors.
- DEET can damage clothing made of synthetic fibers, plastics (e.g., eyeglasses), and leather.
- Breastfeeding women may use DEET. No problems have been reported (CDC).
- *Read and follow the package directions carefully.*

❸ Picaridin (also called KBR 3023):
- Picaridin (also known as KBR 3023, Bayrepel, and icaridin) is also on the CDC list of recommended insect repellents.
- It protects against mosquitoes. It may not be as effective against ticks and other bugs.
- It has been used in other countries for years, including Europe, Australia, Latin America, and Asia.

- Available in the United States (Cutter is one company). It is not yet available in Canada.
- *Read and follow the package directions carefully.*

West Nile Virus (WNV) Information

❶ **Symptoms of WNV:**
- **No Clinical Symptoms:** 80% of infections.
- **Mild Febrile Illness:** 20% of infections. Symptoms include fever, headache, body aches, and, occasionally, a skin rash. These symptoms last 3-6 days and resolve without any treatment (also called WNV fever).
- **Encephalitis or Viral Meningitis:** 0.7% (1:150) of infections. Symptoms are obvious: high fever, stiff neck, confusion, coma, convulsions, muscle weakness or paralysis. The muscle weakness is often unilateral.
- **Fatal Outcome:** 10% of those hospitalized.
- Pediatric cases are generally mild. Most deaths and encephalitis occur in people > age 60.

❷ **Diagnosis of WNV:**
- Mild cases do not need to be diagnosed.
- Severe cases (with encephalitis and viral meningitis) would all be hospitalized based on their symptoms, and the disease would be diagnosed by tests on the blood and spinal fluid. These tests are not available for the usual mild infections seen with this virus.

❸ **Treatment of WNV:**
- No special treatment is needed after a mosquito bite.
- There is no specific treatment or antiviral agent for WNV.
- Patients who require admission are treated supportively with IV fluids, airway management, and good nursing care.
- There is no vaccine available to prevent WNV in humans.

❹ **WNV—Spread by Mosquito:**
- WNV is spread by the bite of a mosquito. The reservoir for the virus is infected birds.
- Even in an area where WNV has been identified, < 1% of mosquitoes carry the virus.
- Transmission is mosquito to human.
- Person-to-person spread does not occur (e.g., from kissing, touching, sharing glassware, or sexual intercourse).

- Mothers with mosquito bites can continue breastfeeding (CDC).
- Incubation period: 3-14 days after the mosquito bite.

FIRST AID

First Aid Advice for Anaphylaxis—Epinephrine:
- If the patient has an epinephrine autoinjector, **give it now.** Do not delay.
- Use the autoinjector on the upper outer thigh. You may give it through clothing if necessary.
- Give epinephrine first, then call 911.
- Epinephrine is available in autoinjectors under trade names: EpiPen, EpiPen Jr, and Auvi-Q (Allerject in Canada). Auvi-Q has an audio chip and talks patients and caregivers through injection process.
- You may give a second (repeat) dose of epinephrine 10-15 minutes later, IF the person with anaphylaxis does not respond to the first dose AND ambulance arrival takes > 10 minutes.

First Aid Advice for Anaphylaxis—Benadryl:
- Give antihistamine by mouth **NOW** if able to swallow.
- Use Benadryl (diphenhydramine; adult dose: 50 mg) or any other available antihistamine medicine.

First Aid Advice for Anaphylactic Shock
(pending EMS arrival):
Lie down with the feet elevated.

BACKGROUND

Key Point
Tetanus vaccination after an insect bite is not necessary.

Anaphylactic Reaction With Insect Bites
- **Definition:** Anaphylaxis is a serious allergic reaction that is rapid in onset and may cause death.
- Anaphylaxis can occur following fire ant stings but rarely with other insects. It mainly occurs with bee, yellow jacket, or wasp stings. Onset usually begins within 20 minutes and almost always by 2 hours. If no symptoms occur by 2 hours, the risk for anaphylaxis is minimal.
- The systemic symptoms include: wheezing, hypotension, shock, generalized urticaria, and abdominal cramping.

No-see-ums

- No-see-ums are tiny bugs that are about 1/10-1/15 of an inch (0.16-0.25 cm). They can pass easily through screens. They are attracted to light. They are most active at sunset.
- **Other Names:** They are also called biting midges, punkies, or sand flies.
- **Habitat:** Adult no-see-ums live in wet sand. They are especially common along the seashore and shores of rivers and lakes. They lay their eggs near standing water (margins of ponds, ditches, lakes, muddy edges of a salt marsh).
- **Symptoms:** The initial bite is generally painless. But within 12 hours the bite mark becomes a small red spot that is intensely itchy. Some sensitive people can develop a larger reaction with a swollen itchy spot (hive) 1-2 inches in diameter (2-5 cm). Scratching makes the itching last longer.
- **OTC Treatment for Itching:** Topical hydrocortisone may help; antihistamines reduce the itching.
- **Prevention:** No-see-ums cannot bite through clothing; thus, good advice is to wear long pants and long-sleeved shirts. Insect repellents containing DEET also seem to be effective in preventing bites.

Chiggers

- Common chiggers are very tiny bugs that are about 1/150 of an inch (0.017 cm) in size.
- **Other Names:** They are also called harvest mites, red mites, jiggers, or red bugs. They can easily go through screens.
- **Habitat:** Tall grass, berry patches, edge of woods.
- **Symptoms:** The main symptom is intense itching, and this peaks on day 2. There are usually tiny red bumps or small hives. Tiny bumps may last for 1-2 weeks.
- **OTC Treatment:** Topical hydrocortisone may help; antihistamines reduce the itching.
- **Prevention:** Avoid areas where chiggers are known to be. Insect repellents containing DEET also seem to be effective in preventing bites.

Bedbugs

- Common bedbugs are small visible bloodsucking bugs that are about ¼" (7 mm) in length.
- **Habitat:** During the day bedbugs hide in the corners of mattresses, bed crevices, floors, and walls. At night the bedbugs come out of hiding and feed on their preferred host, humans. The common bedbug is found worldwide.

- **Symptoms:** There is no pain while the bedbug is biting. However, later, small red bumps or large itchy wheals (2-20 cm) may develop at the bite site. Occasionally blisters (bulla) can occur at the bite site.
- **OTC Treatment:** Topical hydrocortisone cream and oral antihistamines help reduce the itching. Watch for signs of infection.
- **Prevention:** Avoid hotels and hostels where bedbugs have been reported. Check along corners of bedding or mattresses for the presence of these bugs. Wash linens once a week in hot water. DEET and permethrin are effective against bedbugs.

Insect Repellent Precautions: The Environmental Protection Agency recommends the following precautions when using insect repellents:

- Repellents should be applied only to exposed skin and/or clothing (as directed on the product label). Do not use under clothing.
- Never use repellents over cuts, wounds, or irritated skin.
- Don't apply near eyes and mouth, and apply sparingly around ears. When using sprays do not spray directly onto face; spray on hands first and then apply to face.
- Do not allow children to handle these products, and do not apply to children's hands. When using on children, apply to your own hands and then put it on the child.
- Do not spray in enclosed areas. Avoid breathing a repellent spray, and do not use it near food.
- Use just enough repellent to cover exposed skin and/or clothing. Heavy application and saturation is unnecessary for effectiveness; if biting insects do not respond to a thin film of repellent, apply a bit more.
- After returning indoors, wash repellent off skin with soap and water or bathe. This is particularly important when repellents are used repeatedly in a day or on consecutive days. Also, wash treated clothing before wearing it again.
- If you suspect that you or your child are reacting to an insect repellent, discontinue use, wash treated skin, and then call your local Poison Center. If/when you go to a doctor, take the repellent with you.
- Specific medical information about the active ingredients in repellents and other pesticides can be obtained by calling the National Pesticide Information Center at 800/858-7378. The center operates from 9:30 am-7:30 pm ET/6:30 am-4:30 pm PT 7 days a week.

JOCK ITCH

Definition
- A fungus infection that grows on the warm, damp skin of the inner thigh. It is also referred to as tinea cruris.
- Causes an itchy, slowly expanding rash.
- *Use this protocol only if the patient has symptoms that match Jock Itch.*

Symptoms
- Slowly expanding pink-red rash of inner thigh near genital area; rash is usually symmetrical.
- Itchy and not painful.
- In men, does not involve penis or scrotum.
- In women, does not involve vulva.

TRIAGE ASSESSMENT QUESTIONS

See More Appropriate Protocol
- ● Pus or blood from end of penis
  Go to Protocol: Penis and Scrotum Symptoms on page 308
- ● Pain or burning with passing urine and female
  Go to Protocol: Urination Pain (Female) on page 418
- ● Pain or burning with passing urine and male
  Go to Protocol: Urination Pain (Male) on page 421
- ● Rash of penis or scrotum
  Go to Protocol: Penis and Scrotum Symptoms on page 308
- ● Rash of female genitalia (vulva)
  Go to Protocol: Vulvar Symptoms on page 437
- ● Pubic lice suspected
  Go to Protocol: Pubic Lice on page 317
- ● Poison ivy, oak, or sumac suspected as cause
  Go to Protocol: Poison Ivy/Oak/Sumac on page 310

Go to ED/UCC Now (or to Office With PCP Approval)
- ● Patient sounds very sick or weak to the triager
  Reason: severe acute illness or serious complication suspected

Go to Office Now
- ● Fever
  R/O: cellulitis

See Today in Office
- ● Rash is painful to touch
  R/O: cellulitis
- ● Boil, infected sore, deep ulcer present
  R/O: furuncle, abscess, impetigo, sexually transmitted infection

See Today or Tomorrow in Office
- ● Female
  Reason: jock itch is less common in women; see physician to confirm
- ● Diabetes mellitus or a weak immune system (e.g., HIV positive, cancer chemotherapy, transplant patient)
- ● After week on treatment and rash has not improved
- ● After 3 weeks on treatment and rash has not completely gone away
- ● Patient wants to be seen

Home Care
- ○ Mild jock itch in a male

HOME CARE ADVICE

❶ Genital Hygiene:
- Keep your penis and scrotal area clean. Wash this area once daily with unscented soap and water.
- After washing, dry the groin area before the feet. *(Reason: to prevent spread of tinea pedis to groin area)*
- Keep your penis and scrotal area dry.
- Wear cotton underwear. *(Reason: breathes and keeps area drier)* Avoid nylon or tight-fitting underwear.

❷ Antifungal Cream for Treatment of Jock Itch: Apply antifungal cream 2 times per day to the area of itching and rash. Apply it to the rash and 1" (2-3 cm) beyond its borders. Continue the cream for at least 7 days after the rash is cleared.
- Available over the counter in United States as clotrimazole (Lotrimin AF) or miconazole (Micatin, Monistat Derm).

- Available over the counter in Canada as clotrimazole (Clotrimazole cream) or miconazole (Micatin Cream, Micozole, Monistat Derm).

❸ **Expected Course:** The rash should clear up completely in 2-3 weeks.

❹ **Call Back If:**
- Rash is not improving after 1 week on treatment.
- Rash is not completely cleared by 3 weeks.
- Fever or pain occurs.
- You become worse.

BACKGROUND

Key Points

- Usually caused by the same organisms that cause athlete's foot.
- Jock itch, as the name implies, is much more common in men than women.
- Most individuals will be able to treat jock itch effectively using an over-the-counter antifungal cream.

KNEE INJURY

Definition

- Injuries to a bone, muscle, joint, or ligament of the knee.
- Associated skin and soft tissue injuries are also included.

TRIAGE ASSESSMENT QUESTIONS

Call EMS 911 Now

- ● Major bleeding (actively dripping or spurting) that can't be stopped
  First Aid: Apply direct pressure to the entire wound with a clean cloth.
- ● Bullet, stabbed by knife, or other serious penetrating wound
  First Aid: If penetrating object is still in place, don't remove it.
- ● Looks like a dislocated joint (crooked or deformed)
  R/O: fracture
- ● Sounds like a life-threatening emergency to the triager

See More Appropriate Protocol

- ● Wound looks infected
  Go to Protocol: Wound Infection on page 443

Go to ED/UCC Now
(or to Office With PCP Approval)

- ● Can't stand (bear weight) or walk
- ● Skin is split open or gaping (length > ½" or 12 mm)
  Reason: may need laceration repair (e.g., sutures)
- ● Bleeding won't stop after 10 minutes of direct pressure (using correct technique)
- ● Dirt in the wound and not removed after 15 minutes of scrubbing
  Reason: needs irrigation or debridement
- ● Sounds like a serious injury to the triager

Go to Office Now

- ● Looks infected (e.g., spreading redness, pus, red streak)
  R/O: cellulitis, lymphangitis

See Today in Office

- ● SEVERE pain (e.g., excruciating)
  R/O: fracture, joint effusion, severe sprain
- ● Patient wants to be seen

See Today or Tomorrow in Office

- ● Injury interferes with work or school
- ● A "snap" or "pop" was heard at the time of injury
  R/O: cruciate ligament tear
- ● Large swelling or bruise and size > palm of person's hand
  R/O: fracture, large contusion
- ● High-risk adult (e.g., age > 60, osteoporosis, chronic steroid use)
  Reason: greater risk of fracture in patients with osteoporosis
- ● Suspicious history for the injury
  R/O: domestic violence or elder abuse
- ● Wound and no tetanus booster in > 5 years (or > 10 years for clean cuts)
  Reason: may need a tetanus booster shot (vaccine)

See Within 3 Days in Office

- ● Injury and pain has not improved after 3 days
- ● Injury is still painful or swollen after 2 weeks
- ● Knee giving way (or buckling) when walking
  R/O: tear of anterior or posterior cruciate ligament, quadriceps tendon tear
- ● Knee feels like it is locking (i.e., joint gets stuck, catching)
  R/O: meniscal tear

Home Care

- ○ Minor knee injury
  R/O: minor bruise, strain, or sprain

HOME CARE ADVICE

Treatment of a Minor Bruise, Sprain, or Strain

❶ Reassurance—Direct Blow (Contusion, Bruise):
- A direct blow to your knee can cause a contusion. Contusion is the medical term for bruise.
- Symptoms are mild pain, swelling, and/or bruising.
- *Here is some care advice that should help.*

❷ Reassurance—Bending or Twisting Injury (Strain, Sprain):
- Strain and sprain are the medical terms used to describe overstretching of the muscles and ligaments of the knee. A twisting or bending injury can cause a strain or sprain.
- The main symptom is pain that is worse with movement and walking. Swelling can occur. Rarely there may be slight bruising.
- *Here is some care advice that should help.*

❸ Apply a Cold Pack:
- Apply a cold pack or an ice bag (wrapped in a moist towel) to the area for 20 minutes. Repeat in 1 hour, then every 4 hours while awake.
- Continue this for the first 48 hours after an injury.
- This will help decrease pain and swelling.

❹ Apply Heat to the Area:
- Beginning 48 hours after an injury, apply a warm washcloth or heating pad for 10 minutes 3 times a day.
- This will help increase blood flow and improve healing.

❺ Wrap With an Elastic Bandage:
- Wrap the injured part with a snug, elastic bandage for 48 hours.
- The pressure from the bandage can make it feel better and help prevent swelling.
- If you start to get numbness or tingling of your foot or toes, the bandage may be too tight. Loosen the bandage wrap.

❻ Elevate the Leg:
- Lay down and put your leg on a pillow. This puts (elevates) the knee above the heart.
- Do this for 15-20 minutes, 2-3 times a day, for the first 2 days.
- This can also help decrease swelling, bruising, and pain.

❼ Rest Versus Movement:
- Movement is generally more healing in the long term than rest.
- Continue normal activities (like walking) as much as your pain permits.
- Avoid running and active sports for 1-2 weeks or until the pain and swelling are gone.
- Complete rest should only be used for the first day or two after an injury. If it really hurts too much to walk, you will need to see the doctor.

❽ Expected Course:
- Pain, swelling, and bruising usually start to get better 2-3 days after an injury.
- Swelling most often is gone after 1 week.
- Bruises fade away slowly over 1-2 weeks.
- It may take 2 weeks for pain and tenderness of the injured area to go away.

❾ Call Back If:
- Pain becomes severe.
- Pain does not improve after 3 days.
- Pain or swelling lasts > 2 weeks.
- You become worse.

Treatment of a Small Cut or Scrape

❶ Reassurance—Superficial Laceration (Cut or Scratch) or Abrasion (Scrape):
- This sounds like a small cut or scrape that we can treat at home.
- *Here is some care advice that should help.*

❷ Bleeding: Apply direct pressure for 10 minutes with a sterile gauze to stop any bleeding.

❸ Cleaning the Wound:
- Wash the wound with soap and water for 5 minutes.
- For any dirt, scrub gently with a washcloth.
- For any bleeding, apply direct pressure with a sterile gauze or clean cloth for 10 minutes.

❹ Antibiotic Ointment:
- Apply an antibiotic ointment (e.g., OTC bacitracin), covered by a Band-Aid or dressing. Change daily or if it becomes wet.
- Option: A Telfa dressing won't stick to the wound when it is removed.
- Option: Another option is to use a liquid skin bandage that only needs to be applied once. Don't use antibiotic ointment if you use a liquid skin bandage.

❺ **Liquid Skin Bandage:**
- You can use a liquid skin bandage instead of antibiotic ointment and a dressing or a Band-Aid.
- **Benefits:** Liquid skin bandage has several benefits when compared with a regular bandage (e.g., a dressing or a Band-Aid). You only need to put a liquid bandage on once to minor cuts and scrapes. It helps stop minor bleeding. It seals the wound and may promote faster healing and lower infection rates. However, it also costs more.
- **How to Use It:** First clean and dry the wound. You put on the liquid as spray or with a swab. It dries in < 1 minute and usually lasts a week. You can get it wet.
- **Examples:** Liquid skin bandage is available over the counter. Examples are Band-Aid Liquid Bandage, New Skin, Curad Spray Bandage, and 3M No Sting Liquid Bandage Spray.

❻ **Call Back If:**
- Looks infected (pus, redness, increasing tenderness).
- Doesn't heal within 10 days.
- You become worse.

Over-the-counter Pain Medicines

❶ **Pain Medicines:**
- For pain relief, you can take either acetaminophen, ibuprofen, or naproxen.
- They are over-the-counter (OTC) pain drugs. You can buy them at the drugstore.

Acetaminophen (e.g., Tylenol):
- **Regular Strength Tylenol:** Take 650 mg (two 325 mg pills) by mouth every 4-6 hours as needed. Each Regular Strength Tylenol pill has 325 mg of acetaminophen.
- **Extra Strength Tylenol:** Take 1,000 mg (two 500 mg pills) every 8 hours as needed. Each Extra Strength Tylenol pill has 500 mg of acetaminophen.
- The most you should take each day is 3,000 mg (10 Regular Strength or 6 Extra Strength pills a day).

Ibuprofen (e.g., Motrin, Advil):
- Take 400 mg (two 200 mg pills) by mouth every 6 hours.
- Another choice is to take 600 mg (three 200 mg pills) by mouth every 8 hours.
- The most you should take each day is 1,200 mg (six 200 mg pills), unless your doctor has told you to take more.

Naproxen (e.g., Aleve):
- Take 220 mg (one 220 mg pill) by mouth every 8 hours as needed. You may take 440 mg (two 220 mg pills) for your first dose.
- The most you should take each day is 660 mg (three 220 mg pills a day), unless your doctor has told you to take more.

❷ **Pain Medicines—Extra Notes:**
- Use the lowest amount of medicine that makes your pain better.
- Acetaminophen is thought to be safer than ibuprofen or naproxen in people > 65 years old. Acetaminophen is in many OTC and prescription medicines. It might be in more than one medicine that you are taking. You need to be careful and not take an overdose. An acetaminophen overdose can hurt the liver.
- McNeil, the company that makes Tylenol, has different dosage instructions for Tylenol in Canada and the United States. In Canada, the maximum recommended dose per day is 4,000 mg or 12 Regular Strength (325 mg) pills. In the United States, McNeil recommends a maximum dose of 10 Regular Strength (325 mg) pills.
- CAUTION: Do not take acetaminophen if you have liver disease.
- CAUTION: Do not take ibuprofen or naproxen if you have stomach problems, have kidney disease, are pregnant, or have been told by your doctor to avoid this type of anti-inflammatory drug. Do not take ibuprofen or naproxen for > 7 days without consulting your doctor.
- *Before taking any medicine, read all the instructions on the package.*

❸ **Call Back If:**
- You have more questions.
- You become worse.

FIRST AID

First Aid Advice for Bleeding:

Apply direct pressure to the entire wound with a clean cloth.

First Aid Advice for Penetrating Object:

If penetrating object is still in place, don't remove it. *Reason: Removal could increase bleeding.*

First Aid Advice for Shock:

Lie down with the feet elevated.

First Aid Advice for Sprained Knee:

- Apply a cold pack or an ice bag (wrapped in a moist towel) to the area for 20 minutes.
- Wrap knee with an elastic bandage.

BACKGROUND

Types of Knee Injuries

- Fractures (broken bones).
- Dislocations (bone out of joint).
- Dislocation of patella (kneecap out of joint).
- **Sprains:** Stretches and tears of ligaments.
- **Strains:** Stretches and tears of muscles (e.g., pulled muscle).
- **Contusion:** A direct blow or crushing injury results in bruising of the skin, muscle, and underlying bone.
- **Quadriceps Tendon Rupture:** There is pain in the insertion of the quadriceps muscle into the patella (area just above kneecap). There is weakness or inability to extend the knee fully (e.g., while sitting down on chair, can't straighten knee).
- Cuts, abrasions.

What Cuts Need to Be Sutured?

- Any cut that is split open or gaping probably needs sutures (or staples or skin glue).
- Cuts > ½" (1 cm) usually need sutures.
- Any open wound that may need sutures should be evaluated by a physician regardless of the time that has passed since the initial injury.

When Does an Adult Need a Tetanus Booster (Tetanus Shot)?

- **Clean Cuts and Scrapes—Tetanus Booster Needed Every 10 Years:** Patients with clean minor wounds AND who have previously had ≥ 3 tetanus shots (full series) need a booster every 10 years. Examples of minor wounds include a superficial abrasion or a shallow cut from a clean knife blade. Obtain booster within 72 hours.
- **Dirty Wounds—Tetanus Booster Needed Every 5 Years:** Patients with dirty wounds need a booster if it has been > 5 years since the last booster. Examples of dirty wounds include those contaminated with soil, feces, and/or saliva and more serious wounds from deep punctures, crushing, and burns. Obtain booster within 72 hours.

KNEE PAIN

Definition
- Pain in the knee
- Not due to a traumatic injury

Pain Severity Scale
- **Mild (1-3):** Doesn't interfere with normal activities.
- **Moderate (4-7):** Interferes with normal activities (e.g., work or school), awakens from sleep, or limping.
- **Severe (8-10):** Excruciating pain, unable to do any normal activities, unable to walk.

TRIAGE ASSESSMENT QUESTIONS

Call EMS 911 Now
- ● Sounds like a life-threatening emergency to the triager

See More Appropriate Protocol
- ● Followed a knee injury
  Go to Protocol: Knee Injury on page 265

Go to ED Now
- ● Swollen knee joint and fever
  R/O: septic arthritis

Go to ED/UCC Now (or to Office With PCP Approval)
- ● Thigh or calf pain and only 1 side and present > 1 hour
  R/O: DVT
- ● Thigh or calf swelling and only 1 side
  R/O: DVT
- ● Patient sounds very sick or weak to the triager
  Reason: severe acute illness or serious complication suspected

Go to Office Now
- ● Can't move swollen joint at all
  R/O: unwitnessed trauma, severe joint effusion

See Today in Office
- ● SEVERE pain (e.g., excruciating, unable to walk)
  R/O: forgotten trauma, arthritis
- ● Very swollen joint
  R/O: forgotten trauma, arthritis
- ● Painful rash with multiple small blisters grouped together (i.e., dermatomal distribution or "band" or "stripe")
  R/O: herpes zoster (shingles)
- ● Looks like a boil, infected sore, deep ulcer, or other infected rash (spreading redness, pus)
  R/O: popliteal abscess, MRSA

See Within 3 Days in Office
- ● MODERATE pain (e.g., symptoms interfere with work or school, limping) and present > 3 days
- ● Swollen knee joint (no fever or redness)
  R/O: degenerative arthritis
- ● Fluid-filled sack just below kneecap (no fever or redness)
  R/O: prepatellar bursitis
- ● MILD knee pain persists > 7 days
- ● Patient wants to be seen

See Within 2 Weeks in Office
- ● Knee pain is a chronic symptom (recurrent or ongoing AND lasting > 4 weeks)
  R/O: arthritis, chondromalacia patellae
- ● Knee locking is a chronic symptom (recurrent or ongoing AND lasting > 4 weeks)
  R/O: meniscal cartilage tear, degenerative arthritis
- ● Knee giving way (or buckling) when walking is a chronic symptom (recurrent or ongoing AND lasting > 4 weeks)
  R/O: occult anterior or posterior cruciate ligament tear, patellar subluxation

Home Care
- ○ Knee pain
- ○ Caused by overuse from recent vigorous activity (e.g., aerobics, jogging/running, physical work, prolonged walking, sports)
  R/O: muscle strain, overuse

HOME CARE ADVICE

Knee Pain—General Care Advice

❶ Reassurance—Knee Pain:
- Usually knee pain is not serious. You have told me that there is no redness, fever, or swelling. You also told me that there has been no recent major injury.
- Knee pain can be caused by strained muscles, joint irritation, or arthritis.
- *Here is some care advice that should help.*

❷ Pain Medicines:
- For pain relief, you can take either acetaminophen, ibuprofen, or naproxen.
- They are over-the-counter (OTC) pain drugs. You can buy them at the drugstore.

Acetaminophen (e.g., Tylenol):
- **Regular Strength Tylenol:** Take 650 mg (two 325 mg pills) by mouth every 4-6 hours as needed. Each Regular Strength Tylenol pill has 325 mg of acetaminophen.
- **Extra Strength Tylenol:** Take 1,000 mg (two 500 mg pills) every 8 hours as needed. Each Extra Strength Tylenol pill has 500 mg of acetaminophen.
- The most you should take each day is 3,000 mg (10 Regular Strength or 6 Extra Strength pills a day).

Ibuprofen (e.g., Motrin, Advil):
- Take 400 mg (two 200 mg pills) by mouth every 6 hours.
- Another choice is to take 600 mg (three 200 mg pills) by mouth every 8 hours.
- The most you should take each day is 1,200 mg (six 200 mg pills), unless your doctor has told you to take more.

Naproxen (e.g., Aleve):
- Take 220 mg (one 220 mg pill) by mouth every 8 hours as needed. You may take 440 mg (two 220 mg pills) for your first dose.
- The most you should take each day is 660 mg (three 220 mg pills a day), unless your doctor has told you to take more.

❸ Pain Medicines—Extra Notes:
- Use the lowest amount of medicine that makes your pain better.
- Acetaminophen is thought to be safer than ibuprofen or naproxen in people > 65 years old. Acetaminophen is in many OTC and prescription medicines. It might be in more than one medicine that you are taking. You need to be careful and not take an overdose. An acetaminophen overdose can hurt the liver.
- McNeil, the company that makes Tylenol, has different dosage instructions for Tylenol in Canada and the United States. In Canada, the maximum recommended dose per day is 4,000 mg or 12 Regular Strength (325 mg) pills. In the United States, McNeil recommends a maximum dose of 10 Regular Strength (325 mg) pills.
- CAUTION: Do not take acetaminophen if you have liver disease.
- CAUTION: Do not take ibuprofen or naproxen if you have stomach problems, have kidney disease, are pregnant, or have been told by your doctor to avoid this type of anti-inflammatory drug. Do not take ibuprofen or naproxen for > 7 days without consulting your doctor.
- *Before taking any medicine, read all the instructions on the package.*

❹ Call Back If:
- Moderate pain (e.g., limping) lasts > 3 days.
- Mild pain lasts > 7 days.
- Signs of infection occur (e.g., spreading redness, warmth, fever).
- You become worse.

Muscle Strain and Overuse

❶ Reassurance—Muscle Strain:
- **Definition:** A muscle strain occurs from over-stretching or tearing a muscle. People often call this a "pulled muscle." This muscle injury can occur while exercising, while lifting something, or sometimes during normal activities.
- **Symptoms:** People often describe a sharp pain when the muscle strain occurs. The muscle pain worsens with movement of the knee (e.g., bending, going up stairs).
- *Here is some care advice that should help.*

❷ Reassurance—Overuse:
- **Definition:** Sore muscles are common following vigorous activity (overuse), especially when your body is not used to this amount of activity (e.g., running, sports, weight lifting, moving furniture).
- **Symptoms:** People often describe a diffuse soreness and aching in the overused muscles. Often the pain is present in in the same muscles of both knees.
- *Here is some care advice that should help.*

❸ Apply Cold to the Area for First 48 Hours:
- Apply a cold pack or an ice bag (wrapped in a moist towel) to the area for 20 minutes. Repeat in 1 hour, then every 4 hours while awake.
- Continue this for the first 48 hours after an injury. *(Reason: to reduce the swelling and pain)*

❹ Apply Heat to the Area:
- Beginning 48 hours after an injury, apply a warm washcloth or heating pad for 10 minutes 3 times a day.
- This will help increase blood flow and improve healing.

❺ Local Heat (bathtub option): If stiffness lasts > 48 hours, relax in a hot bath for 20 minutes twice a day and gently exercise the involved part underwater.

❻ Rest: You should try to avoid any exercise or activity that caused this pain for the next 3 days.

❼ Pain Medicines:
- For pain relief, you can take either acetaminophen, ibuprofen, or naproxen.
- They are over-the-counter (OTC) pain drugs. You can buy them at the drugstore.

Acetaminophen (e.g., Tylenol):
- **Regular Strength Tylenol:** Take 650 mg (two 325 mg pills) by mouth every 4-6 hours as needed. Each Regular Strength Tylenol pill has 325 mg of acetaminophen.
- **Extra Strength Tylenol:** Take 1,000 mg (two 500 mg pills) every 8 hours as needed. Each Extra Strength Tylenol pill has 500 mg of acetaminophen.
- The most you should take each day is 3,000 mg (10 Regular Strength or 6 Extra Strength pills a day).

Ibuprofen (e.g., Motrin, Advil):
- Take 400 mg (two 200 mg pills) by mouth every 6 hours.
- Another choice is to take 600 mg (three 200 mg pills) by mouth every 8 hours.
- The most you should take each day is 1,200 mg (six 200 mg pills), unless your doctor has told you to take more.

Naproxen (e.g., Aleve):
- Take 220 mg (one 220 mg pill) by mouth every 8 hours as needed. You may take 440 mg (two 220 mg pills) for your first dose.
- The most you should take each day is 660 mg (three 220 mg pills a day), unless your doctor has told you to take more.

❽ Pain Medicines—Extra Notes:
- Use the lowest amount of medicine that makes your pain better.
- Acetaminophen is thought to be safer than ibuprofen or naproxen in people > 65 years old. Acetaminophen is in many OTC and prescription medicines. It might be in more than one medicine that you are taking. You need to be careful and not take an overdose. An acetaminophen overdose can hurt the liver.

- McNeil, the company that makes Tylenol, has different dosage instructions for Tylenol in Canada and the United States. In Canada, the maximum recommended dose per day is 4,000 mg or 12 Regular Strength (325 mg) pills. In the United States, McNeil recommends a maximum dose of 10 Regular Strength (325 mg) pills.
- CAUTION: Do not take acetaminophen if you have liver disease.
- CAUTION: Do not take ibuprofen or naproxen if you have stomach problems, have kidney disease, are pregnant, or have been told by your doctor to avoid this type of anti-inflammatory drug. Do not take ibuprofen or naproxen for > 7 days without consulting your doctor.
- *Before taking any medicine, read all the instructions on the package.*

❾ Expected Course

- **Muscle Strain:** A minor muscle strain usually hurts for 2-3 days. The pain often peaks on day 2. A more severe muscle strain can hurt for 2-4 weeks.
- **Muscle Overuse:** Sore muscles from overuse usually hurt for 2-4 days. The pain often peaks on day 2.

❿ Call Back If:

- Moderate pain (e.g., limping) lasts > 3 days.
- Mild pain lasts > 7 days.
- You become worse.

BACKGROUND

Causes of Knee Pain

- Arthritis (e.g., degenerative, gouty, infectious, inflammatory, traumatic).
- **Baker Cyst** (popliteal cyst): This is a fluid collection in a cyst that bulges out from the knee joint. Symptoms include painful or painless swelling in the area behind the knee.
- **Bursitis:** Prepatellar bursitis is a fluid-filled sack localized on the inferior aspect of the anterior knee.
- Cellulitis.
- Overuse injury, tendonitis.
- Patellofemoral pain syndrome (chondromalacia patellae).
- Trauma (e.g., contusion, dislocation, fracture, sprain, strain).

Serious Signs and Symptoms

- Severe pain; even slight movement of the knee causes intense pain.
- Knee swelling with fever.
  R/O: septic arthritis
- Unilateral calf pain and/or swelling.
  R/O: deep vein thrombosis

LEG PAIN

Definition
- Pain in the leg(s).
- Not due to a traumatic injury.
- Minor muscle strain and overuse are covered in this protocol.

Pain Severity Scale
- **Mild (1-3):** Doesn't interfere with normal activities.
- **Moderate (4-7):** Interferes with normal activities (e.g., work or school), awakens from sleep, or limping.
- **Severe (8-10):** Excruciating pain, unable to do any normal activities, unable to walk.

TRIAGE ASSESSMENT QUESTIONS

Call EMS 911 Now
- Looks like a broken bone or dislocated joint (e.g., crooked or deformed)
  R/O: forgotten trauma, pathologic fracture or dislocation
- Sounds like a life-threatening emergency to the triager

See More Appropriate Protocol
- Followed a hip injury
  Go to Protocol: Hip Injury on page 222
- Followed a knee injury
  Go to Protocol: Knee Injury on page 265
- Followed an ankle or foot injury
  Go to Protocol: Ankle and Foot Injury on page 27
- Back pain radiating (shooting) into leg(s)
  Go to Protocol: Back Pain on page 48
- Foot pain is the main symptom
  Go to Protocol: Foot Pain on page 182
- Ankle pain is the main symptom
  Go to Protocol: Ankle Pain on page 31
- Knee pain is the main symptom
  Go to Protocol: Knee Pain on page 269
- Leg swelling is the main symptom
  Go to Protocol: Leg Swelling and Edema on page 279

Go to ED Now
- Chest pain
  R/O: DVT, pulmonary embolus
- Difficulty breathing
  R/O: DVT, pulmonary embolus
- Entire foot is cool or blue in comparison to other side
  R/O: iliofemoral arterial occlusion (ischemic foot)
- Unable to walk

Go to ED/UCC Now
(or to Office With PCP Approval)
- Fever and red area (or area very tender to touch)
  R/O: cellulitis, lymphangitis
  Note: It may be difficult to determine the rash color in people with darker-colored skin.
- Fever and swollen joint
  R/O: septic arthritis, acute rheumatic fever
- Thigh or calf pain in only one leg and present > 1 hour
  R/O: DVT
- Thigh, calf, or ankle swelling in only one leg
  R/O: DVT
- Thigh, calf, or ankle swelling in both legs, but one side is definitely more swollen
  R/O: DVT
- History of prior "blood clot" in leg or lungs (i.e., deep vein thrombosis, pulmonary embolism)
  Note: A "blood clot" typically would have required treatment with heparin or coumadin.
  Reason: increased risk of thromboembolism
  R/O: DVT
- History of inherited increased risk of blood clots (e.g., factor V Leiden, antithrombin III, protein C or protein S deficiency, prothrombin mutation)
  Note: Diagnosing such genetic blood disorders would have required prior blood testing.
  Reason: increased risk of thromboembolism
  R/O: pulmonary embolism
- Recent illness requiring prolonged bed rest (immobilization)
  R/O: DVT
- Hip or leg fracture in past 2 months (e.g., had cast on leg or ankle)
  R/O: DVT

- Major surgery in the past 2 months
  R/O: DVT
- Cancer treatment in the past 2 months
  (or has cancer now)
  R/O: DVT
- Recent long-distance travel with prolonged time
  in car, bus, plane, or train (i.e., within past 2 weeks;
  ≥ 6 hours' duration)
  *Reason: immobilization during prolonged travel
  increases risk of deep vein thrombosis*
- Patient sounds very sick or weak to the triager
  *Reason: severe acute illness or serious complication
  suspected*

Go to Office Now

- SEVERE pain (e.g., excruciating, unable to do any
  normal activities)
  Reason: inadequate analgesia
  R/O: sciatica, iliofemoral arterial occlusion
- Cast on leg or ankle and now has increasing pain
  R/O: swelling (cast may need to be bivalved) or DVT
- Red area or streak and large (> 2" or 5 cm)
  R/O: cellulitis, erysipelas, lymphangitis
  *Note: It may be difficult to determine the rash color in
  people with darker-colored skin.*

See Today in Office

- Painful rash with multiple small blisters grouped
  together (i.e., dermatomal distribution or "band"
  or "stripe")
  R/O: herpes zoster (shingles)
- Looks like a boil, infected sore, deep ulcer, or other
  infected rash (spreading redness, pus)
  R/O: abscess, venous stasis ulcer, cellulitis
- Localized rash is very painful (no fever)
  R/O: cellulitis, spider bite, bee sting

See Today or Tomorrow in Office

- Numbness in a leg or foot (i.e., loss of sensation)
  R/O: nerve root compression, herniated disk
- Localized pain, redness or hard lump along vein
  R/O: superficial thrombophlebitis
- Patient wants to be seen

See Within 3 Days in Office

- MODERATE pain (e.g., interferes with normal
  activities, limping) and present > 3 days
  R/O: sciatica, arthritis
- Swollen joint with no fever or redness
  R/O: degenerative arthritis
- Leg pain which occurs after walking a certain
  distance and disappears with rest, AND age > 50
  R/O: claudication
- Leg pain in shins (front of lower legs) and it
  occurs with running or jumping exercise
  (e.g., jogging, basketball)
  R/O: shin splints, stress fracture

See Within 2 Weeks in Office

- MILD pain persists > 7 days
  R/O: muscle strain, sciatica, arthritis, bursitis
- Leg pain or muscle cramp is a chronic symptom
  (recurrent or ongoing AND lasting > 4 weeks)
  *R/O: night muscle cramps, meralgia paresthetica,
  varicose veins*

Home Care

- Leg pain
- Caused by strained muscle
  R/O: muscle strain (pulled muscle)
- Caused by overuse from recent vigorous activity
  (e.g., aerobics, jogging/running, physical work,
  prolonged walking, sports)
  *R/O: muscle strain, overuse (sore muscles from
  overuse)*
- Caused by brief (now gone) muscle cramps in the
  thigh or calf
  R/O: muscle cramps, nocturnal cramps
- Caused by previously diagnosed varicose veins
  (same pain, worsened by prolonged standing,
  bulging veins in legs with wormlike appearance)
  R/O: varicose veins
- Caused by phantom leg pain
  *R/O: phantom limb pain or sensation
  after amputation*

HOME CARE ADVICE

Leg Pain—General Care Advice

❶ Reassurance—Leg Pain:

- Usually leg pain is not serious. You have told me that there is no redness, numbness, or swelling.
- Causes of leg pain can include a strained muscle, a forgotten minor injury, and tendinitis.
- *Here is some care advice that should help.*

❷ Pain Medicines:

- For pain relief, you can take either acetaminophen, ibuprofen, or naproxen.
- They are over-the-counter (OTC) pain drugs. You can buy them at the drugstore.

Acetaminophen (e.g., Tylenol):

- **Regular Strength Tylenol:** Take 650 mg (two 325 mg pills) by mouth every 4-6 hours as needed. Each Regular Strength Tylenol pill has 325 mg of acetaminophen.
- **Extra Strength Tylenol:** Take 1,000 mg (two 500 mg pills) every 8 hours as needed. Each Extra Strength Tylenol pill has 500 mg of acetaminophen.
- The most you should take each day is 3,000 mg (10 Regular Strength or 6 Extra Strength pills a day).

Ibuprofen (e.g., Motrin, Advil):

- Take 400 mg (two 200 mg pills) by mouth every 6 hours.
- Another choice is to take 600 mg (three 200 mg pills) by mouth every 8 hours.
- The most you should take each day is 1,200 mg (six 200 mg pills), unless your doctor has told you to take more.

Naproxen (e.g., Aleve):

- Take 220 mg (one 220 mg pill) by mouth every 8 hours as needed. You may take 440 mg (two 220 mg pills) for your first dose.
- The most you should take each day is 660 mg (three 220 mg pills a day), unless your doctor has told you to take more.

❸ Pain Medicines—Extra Notes:

- Use the lowest amount of medicine that makes your pain better.
- Acetaminophen is thought to be safer than ibuprofen or naproxen in people > 65 years old. Acetaminophen is in many OTC and prescription medicines. It might be in more than one medicine that you are taking. You need to be careful and not take an over-

dose. An acetaminophen overdose can hurt the liver.

- McNeil, the company that makes Tylenol, has different dosage instructions for Tylenol in Canada and the United States. In Canada, the maximum recommended dose per day is 4,000 mg or 12 Regular Strength (325 mg) pills. In the United States, McNeil recommends a maximum dose of 10 Regular Strength (325 mg) pills.
- CAUTION: Do not take acetaminophen if you have liver disease.
- CAUTION: Do not take ibuprofen or naproxen if you have stomach problems, have kidney disease, are pregnant, or have been told by your doctor to avoid this type of anti-inflammatory drug. Do not take ibuprofen or naproxen for > 7 days without consulting your doctor.
- *Before taking any medicine, read all the instructions on the package.*

❹ Call Back If:

- Moderate pain (e.g., limping) lasts > 3 days.
- Mild pain lasts > 7 days.
- Signs of infection occur (e.g., spreading redness, warmth, fever).
- You become worse.

Muscle Strain and Overuse

❶ Reassurance—Muscle Strain:

- **Definition:** A muscle strain occurs from overstretching or tearing a muscle. People often call this a "pulled muscle." This muscle injury can occur while exercising, while lifting something, or sometimes during normal activities.
- **Symptoms:** People often describe a sharp pain or popping when the muscle strain occurs. The muscle pain worsens with movement of the leg (e.g., bending, straightening).
- *Here is some care advice that should help.*

❷ Reassurance—Overuse:

- **Definition:** Sore muscles are common following vigorous activity (overuse), especially when your body is not used to this amount of activity (e.g., running, sports, weight lifting, moving furniture).
- **Symptoms:** People often describe a diffuse soreness and aching in the overused muscles. Often the pain is present in in the same muscles of both legs.
- *Here is some care advice that should help.*

❸ **Apply Cold to the Area for First 48 Hours:**
- Apply a cold pack or an ice bag (wrapped in a moist towel) to the area for 20 minutes. Repeat in 1 hour, then every 4 hours while awake.
- Continue this for the first 48 hours after an injury. *(Reason: to reduce the swelling and pain)*

❹ **Apply Heat to the Area:**
- Beginning 48 hours after an injury, apply a warm washcloth or heating pad for 10 minutes 3 times a day.
- This will help increase blood flow and improve healing.

❺ **Local Heat** (bathtub option): If stiffness lasts > 48 hours, relax in a hot bath for 20 minutes twice a day and gently exercise the involved part under water.

❻ **Rest:** You should try to avoid any exercise or activity that caused this pain for the next 3 days.

❼ **Pain Medicines:**
- For pain relief, you can take either acetaminophen, ibuprofen, or naproxen.
- They are over-the-counter (OTC) pain drugs. You can buy them at the drugstore.

Acetaminophen (e.g., Tylenol):
- **Regular Strength Tylenol:** Take 650 mg (two 325 mg pills) by mouth every 4-6 hours as needed. Each Regular Strength Tylenol pill has 325 mg of acetaminophen.
- **Extra Strength Tylenol:** Take 1,000 mg (two 500 mg pills) every 8 hours as needed. Each Extra Strength Tylenol pill has 500 mg of acetaminophen.
- The most you should take each day is 3,000 mg (10 Regular Strength or 6 Extra Strength pills a day).

Ibuprofen (e.g., Motrin, Advil):
- Take 400 mg (two 200 mg pills) by mouth every 6 hours.
- Another choice is to take 600 mg (three 200 mg pills) by mouth every 8 hours.
- The most you should take each day is 1,200 mg (six 200 mg pills), unless your doctor has told you to take more.

Naproxen (e.g., Aleve):
- Take 220 mg (one 220 mg pill) by mouth every 8 hours as needed. You may take 440 mg (two 220 mg pills) for your first dose.
- The most you should take each day is 660 mg (three 220 mg pills a day), unless your doctor has told you to take more.

❽ **Pain Medicines—Extra Notes:**
- Use the lowest amount of medicine that makes your pain better.
- Acetaminophen is thought to be safer than ibuprofen or naproxen in people > 65 years old. Acetaminophen is in many OTC and prescription medicines. It might be in more than one medicine that you are taking. You need to be careful and not take an overdose. An acetaminophen overdose can hurt the liver.
- McNeil, the company that makes Tylenol, has different dosage instructions for Tylenol in Canada and the United States. In Canada, the maximum recommended dose per day is 4,000 mg or 12 Regular Strength (325 mg) pills. In the United States, McNeil recommends a maximum dose of 10 Regular Strength (325 mg) pills.
- CAUTION: Do not take acetaminophen if you have liver disease.
- CAUTION: Do not take ibuprofen or naproxen if you have stomach problems, have kidney disease, are pregnant, or have been told by your doctor to avoid this type of anti-inflammatory drug. Do not take ibuprofen or naproxen for > 7 days without consulting your doctor.
- *Before taking any medicine, read all the instructions on the package.*

❾ **Expected Course:**
- **Muscle Strain:** A minor muscle strain usually hurts for 2-3 days. The pain often peaks on day 2. A more severe muscle strain can hurt for 2-4 weeks.
- **Muscle Overuse:** Sore muscles from overuse usually hurt for 2-4 days. The pain often peaks on day 2.

❿ **Call Back If:**
- Moderate pain (e.g., limping) lasts > 3 days.
- Mild pain lasts > 7 days.
- You become worse.

Muscle Cramp

❶ Reassurance—Muscle Cramps:
- Muscle cramps can occur in the calves and thighs.
- During attacks, you can break the muscle spasm by stretching the muscle in the direction opposite to how it is being pulled by the cramp or spasm. For example, for a calf cramp, pull the foot and toes backward as far as they will go.
- *Here is some care advice that should help.*

❷ Fluids for Heat Cramps (occurring during exercise on a hot day):
- Drink 1 cup (8 oz; 240 mL) of cold water every 15 minutes for the next 2 hours. Also eat some salty foods (e.g., potato chips or pretzels).
- OR drink a sports/rehydration drink (e.g., Gatorade or Powerade), which contains sugar and salt.

❸ Prevention: Future attacks may be prevented by daily stretching exercises of the heel cords. Stand with the knees straight and stretch the ankles by leaning forward against a wall.

❹ Expected Course:
- Muscle cramps usually last 5-30 minutes. Once the muscle cramp stops, the muscle returns to normal quickly. The pain should go away completely.
- If you have frequent muscle cramps, you should call your doctor (call us back) when the office is open. Sometimes the doctor can give medications to reduce the muscle cramps.

❺ Call Back If:
- Calf swelling or constant leg pain occurs.
- Signs of infection occur (e.g., spreading redness, warmth, fever).
- You become worse.

Varicose Veins

❶ Reassurance—Varicose Veins:
- Appear as bulging, winding (wormlike) blue blood vessels in the thigh and lower leg.
- Patients with varicose veins will sometimes report a mild aching in their legs after a prolonged day of standing or walking. The discomfort should go away with rest and leg elevation.
- *Here is some care advice that should help.*

❷ Varicose Veins—Treatment:
- Try to rest and elevate your legs above your heart a couple times each day for 15 minutes.
- Walking is good for your blood flow. *(Reason: helps pump the blood out of the veins)*
- Avoid prolonged standing in one place.
- Wear support hose.
- If you are overweight, talk with your doctor about a weight-loss program.

❸ Call Back If:
- Severe pain occurs.
- Calf swelling or constant calf pain occurs.
- Signs of infection occur (e.g., spreading redness, warmth, fever).
- You become worse.

Phantom Leg Pain

❶ Reassurance—Phantom Pain and Phantom Sensations:
- **Phantom Pain:** Phantom pain is pain that occurs in the part of the limb that is left after amputation. The pain can be aching, cramping, burning, sharp, or shooting. Most people experience phantom pain in the leg after an amputation. It seems that the worse the pain was in the leg prior to amputation, the more phantom pain a person will have.
- **Phantom Sensation:** There are a number of other phantom sensations that amputees can experience in the amputated part of the leg. These include tingling, numbness, cramping, cold, and warmth.
- Research has not shown a single best treatment for these pains and sensations.
- *Here is some care advice that may help.*

❷ Treatment—Phantom Pain:
- Try gently rubbing (massaging) or touching (tapping) your stump.
- Move or exercise other parts of your body.
- Do something to take your mind off the pain. Listen to music, read a book, watch a TV show.

❸ Treatment—Phantom Foot or Toes Feel Twisted or Cramped:
- Move the normal leg into a position of comfort.
- By doing this it may help the phantom leg feel better.

❹ **Expected Course:**
  • Usually, phantom pain and phantom sensation slowly get better over time.
  • You should speak with your doctor if you have more questions about this.
❺ **Call Back If:**
  • You become worse.

BACKGROUND

Causes

• **Deep Vein Thrombosis (DVT):** This is a serious and unfortunately common problem. The deep veins of the leg become obstructed with blood clots. Symptoms include calf pain and swelling, localized redness, and warmth. Risk factors for developing a DVT include: prolonged immobilization (e.g., recent surgery, prolonged travel), local injury (e.g., femur fracture), and an increased tendency to clot (e.g., pregnancy, cancer patients).

• **Muscle Cramps:** Brief pains (1-15 minutes) may be due to muscle spasms. Foot or calf muscles are especially prone to cramps that awaken from sleep. The pain should resolve completely after an episode of muscle spasm.

• **Muscle Strain (Pulled Muscle):** A muscle strain occurs from overstretching or tearing a muscle. This muscle injury can occur while exercising, while lifting something, and sometimes during normal activities. This is also referred to as a "pulled muscle."

• **Muscle Strain (Sore Muscles From Overuse):** Continuous acute pains (2-7 days) are often due to over-strenuous activities or forgotten muscle injuries from recent exercise or work-related activities.

• **Phantom Leg (Limb) Pain:** Phantom pain is pain that occurs in the part of the limb that is left after amputation. The pain can be aching, cramping, burning, sharp, or shooting. Most people experience phantom pain in the leg after an amputation. It seems that the worse the pain was in the leg prior to amputation, the more phantom pain a person will have.

• **Sciatica:** Sciatic pain is a common cause of leg pain in adults. Sciatic pain is pain that radiates from the back down into the leg, sometimes as far as the foot. It is cause by pressure on the spinal nerve roots from a herniated disk or from spinal arthritis.

• **Shin Splints:** This is an overuse injury typically from a jumping or running sport activity like jogging, aerobics, basketball, or gymnastics. Symptoms include pain in the shin area, especially during the sports activity.

• **Varicose Veins:** Appear as bulging, winding (wormlike) blue blood vessels in the thigh and lower leg. Patients with varicose veins will sometimes report a mild aching in their legs after a prolonged day of standing or walking. The discomfort usually subsides with rest and leg elevation. Sometimes a varicose vein can become thrombosed and inflamed (hard and red). This may cause localized pain but generally is not serious. Varicose veins occur more commonly in women.

• **Viral Illness:** Mild-moderate bilateral diffuse muscle aches can occur with many viral illnesses.

• **Other Causes:** Unwitnessed fracture, arthritis, arterial occlusion, skin infection (cellulitis, erysipelas), bursitis, and meralgia paresthetica.

Caution: Deep Vein Thrombosis (DVT)

• Consider the possibility of DVT in anyone with unexplained leg swelling and pain, especially if symptoms are predominantly unilateral.

• **Risk Factors:** Venous stasis (e.g., casting, long-distance travel, prolonged bed rest), leg/venous injury (e.g., fracture, prior DVT, leg surgery), and hypercoagulable states (e.g., pregnancy, cancer).

LEG SWELLING AND EDEMA

Definition
- Swelling of the leg(s) or generalized edema of body
- Pedal edema (bilateral swelling of feet and ankles)
- Not due to a traumatic injury

TRIAGE ASSESSMENT QUESTIONS

Call EMS 911 Now
- Sounds like a life-threatening emergency to the triager

See More Appropriate Protocol
- Chest pain
  Go to Protocol: Chest Pain on page 73
- Small area of swelling and followed an insect bite to the area
  Go to Protocol: Insect Bite on page 257
- Followed a knee injury
  Go to Protocol: Knee Injury on page 265
- Ankle or foot injury
  Go to Protocol: Ankle and Foot Injury on page 27

Go to ED Now
- Difficulty breathing at rest
  R/O: CHF, PE
- Entire foot is cool or blue in comparison to other side
  R/O: arterial occlusion

Go to L&D Now
- Pregnant > 20 weeks with blurred vision or visual change
  R/O: preeclampsia

Go to ED/UCC Now (or to Office With PCP Approval)
- SEVERE swelling (e.g., swelling extends above knee, entire leg is swollen, weeping fluid)
  Reason: severe edema (3-4+, evaluation needed)
- Thigh or calf pain and only 1 side and present > 1 hour
  R/O: DVT
- Thigh, calf, or ankle swelling in only one leg
  R/O: DVT

- Thigh, calf, or ankle swelling in both legs, but one side is definitely more swollen
  R/O: DVT
  Exception: long-standing difference between legs
- Cast on leg or ankle and has increasing pain
  R/O: cast swelling (may need it bivalved) or DVT
- Can't walk or can barely stand (new onset)
- Patient sounds very sick or weak to the triager
  Reason: severe acute illness or serious complication suspected

Go to Office Now
- Swelling of face, arm, or hands
  (Exception: slight puffiness of fingers during hot weather)
  R/O: renal disease, low protein state
- Pregnant > 20 weeks and sudden weight gain (i.e., > 2 lb, 1 kg in 1 week)
  R/O: preeclampsia

See Today in Office
- MODERATE swelling of both ankles (e.g., swelling extends up to the knees) AND new onset or worsening
  Reason: edema 2+, diagnostic evaluation or change in management may be needed
- Difficulty breathing with exertion AND worsening or new onset
  R/O: CHF
- Looks like a boil, infected sore, deep ulcer, or other infected rash (spreading redness, pus)
  R/O: abscess, MRSA
- Patient wants to be seen

See Within 3 Days in Office
- MILD swelling of both ankles (i.e., pedal edema) AND new onset or worsening

See Within 2 Weeks in Office
- MILD swelling of both ankles (i.e., pedal edema) and worsened by hot weather
  R/O: heat edema
- Mild swelling of both ankles and varicose veins
- Mild swelling of both ankles and chronic (unchanged)
  R/O: venous insufficiency

HOME CARE ADVICE

❶ **Heat Edema:** Many individuals experience heat edema during the first few days of hot weather or after traveling to a warmer climate. There may be mild swelling of the feet and ankles and some puffiness of the fingers. Typically, your body adjusts to the higher temperatures (acclimatizes) in a couple of days and the swelling resolves.

❷ **Varicose Veins:** Appear as bulging, winding (wormlike) blue blood vessels in the thigh and lower leg. Patients with varicose veins often report a mild swelling in their legs after a prolonged day of standing or walking. The swelling usually subsides with rest and leg elevation.

❸ **Varicose Veins—Treatment:**
- Try to rest and elevate your legs above your heart a couple times each day for 15 minutes.
- Walking is good for your blood flow. *(Reason: helps pump the blood out of the veins)*
- Avoid prolonged standing in one place.
- Support hose may be helpful. Put them on first thing in the morning when the swelling is least.

❹ **Expected Course:** If your leg swelling does not get better during the next week or if it recurs, make an appointment with your doctor.

❺ **Call Back If:**
- Swelling becomes worse.
- Swelling becomes red or painful to the touch.
- Calf pain occurs and becomes constant.
- You become worse.

BACKGROUND

Causes of Bilateral Swelling of the Leg
- Congestive heart failure (right-sided)
- Drugs, such as nifedipine
- Heat edema
- Idiopathic edema
- Liver failure and other low-protein conditions
- Lymphedema
- Pregnancy
- Renal failure
- Venous insufficiency or venous stasis

Causes of Unilateral Swelling of the Leg
- **Bypass Surgery:** After saphenous vein harvesting from leg for coronary artery bypass surgery
- **Cellulitis:** Localized swelling, redness, and tenderness
- **Deep Vein Thrombosis (DVT):** Calf swelling and tenderness
- **Insect Bites:** Localized swelling, often itchy
- **Leg Paralysis** (e.g., from stroke): Chronic swelling of extremity from disuse
- **Lymphedema:** Lymphatic obstruction from malignancy, radiation therapy, or surgery

Definition: Pitting Edema
- Press firmly with your thumb and hold for 5 seconds. If a visible indentation persists after the thumb is removed, pitting edema exists.
- Edema usually shows up first in the lower (dependent) extremities, where it is initially seen in the feet or ankles.

Caution: Deep Vein Thrombosis (DVT)
- Consider the possibility of DVT in anyone with unexplained leg swelling and pain, especially if symptoms are predominantly unilateral.
- **Risk Factors:** Immobility (e.g., casting, long-distance travel, prolonged bed rest), leg/venous injury (e.g., fracture, prior DVT, leg surgery), and hypercoagulable states (e.g., pregnancy, cancer).

LYMPH NODES, SWOLLEN

Definition
- Increased size of a lymph node in the neck, occipital area, armpit, or groin.
- Normal nodes are usually < ½" (1 cm) across (size of pea or pencil eraser).

Estimating Size:
- **Pea or Pencil Eraser:** ¼" or 6 mm
- **Marble:** ½" or 12 mm
- **Dime:** ¾" or 18 mm
- **Quarter:** 1" or 2.4 cm
- **Ping-pong Ball:** 1.6" or 4.0 cm
- **Golf Ball:** 1.7" or 4.3 cm
- **Tennis Ball:** 2.6" or 6.7 cm

TRIAGE ASSESSMENT QUESTIONS

Call EMS 911 Now
- Sounds like a life-threatening emergency to the triager

See More Appropriate Protocol
- Sore throat is the main symptom and has swollen node in the neck that is < 1" (2.5 cm) in size
  Go to Protocol: Sore Throat on page 369

Go to ED/UCC Now
(or to Office With PCP Approval)
- Node is in the neck and causes difficulty breathing
  R/O: impingement on airway
- Patient sounds very sick or weak to the triager
  Reason: severe acute illness or serious complication suspected

Go to Office Now
- Node is in the neck and can't swallow fluids
  R/O: retropharyngeal abscess
- Fever > 103° F (39.4° C)
  R/O: bacterial infection
- Lump or swelling in groin and pulsating (like heartbeat)
  R/O: femoral artery aneurysm
- Single large node and size > 1" (2.5 cm)
  R/O: bacterial adenitis
- Overlying skin is red
  R/O: bacterial adenitis

See Today in Office
- Rapid increase in size of node over several hours
  R/O: bacterial adenitis
- Tender node in the groin and has a sore, scratch, cut, or painful red area on that leg
  R/O: bacterial adenitis
- Tender node in the armpit and has a sore, scratch, cut, or painful red area on that arm
  R/O: bacterial adenitis
- Tender node in the neck and also has a sore throat with minimal/no runny nose or cough
  R/O: strep pharyngitis, mono (infectious mononucleosis)
- Fever present > 3 days (72 hours)
  R/O: bacterial adenitis, mono

See Today or Tomorrow in Office
- Large nodes at multiple locations
  R/O: malignancy, sarcoidosis, systemic illness
- Very tender to the touch but no fever
  R/O: low-grade bacterial adenitis
- Patient wants to be seen

See Within 2 Weeks in Office
- Large node present > 2 weeks
  R/O: malignancy, sarcoidosis
- Normal-sized node (i.e. < 1 cm, < ½") present > 2 weeks, but patient is worried about cancer
  R/O: malignancy

Home Care
- Mildly swollen lymph node present < 2 weeks, and has cold symptoms (e.g., runny nose, cough, sore throat)
- Normal-sized lymph node (i.e., < 1 cm, < ½")

HOME CARE ADVICE

❶ Swollen Lymph Nodes From a Viral Infection:
- Viral throat infections and colds can cause lymph nodes in the neck to double in size. Slight enlargement and mild tenderness means the lymph node is fighting the infection and doing a good job.
- **Treatment:** Usually no treatment is necessary.
- **Expected Course:** After the infection is gone, the nodes slowly return to normal size over 1-2 weeks. However, they will not ever completely disappear.
- **Contagiousness:** Swollen lymph nodes are not contagious.

❷ Normal Lymph Nodes:
- A pea-sized lymph node (< ½" or 1 cm) is usually a normal lymph node.
- **Expected Course:** Small normal-sized lymph nodes should not get any larger over time. Lymph nodes can temporarily swell and become tender when you have an infection. But after the infection is gone, the lymph node should shrink back to normal size.

❸ Pain and Fever Medicines:
- For pain or fever relief, take either acetaminophen or ibuprofen.
- They are over-the-counter (OTC) drugs that help treat both fever and pain. You can buy them at the drugstore.
- Treat fevers > 101° F (38.3° C). The goal of fever therapy is to bring the fever down to a comfortable level. Remember that fever medicine usually lowers fever 2° F (1-1½° C).

Acetaminophen (e.g., Tylenol):
- **Regular Strength Tylenol:** Take 650 mg (two 325 mg pills) by mouth every 4-6 hours as needed. Each Regular Strength Tylenol pill has 325 mg of acetaminophen.
- **Extra Strength Tylenol:** Take 1,000 mg (two 500 mg pills) every 8 hours as needed. Each Extra Strength Tylenol pill has 500 mg of acetaminophen.
- The most you should take each day is 3,000 mg (10 Regular Strength or 6 Extra Strength pills a day).

Ibuprofen (e.g., Motrin, Advil):
- Take 400 mg (two 200 mg pills) by mouth every 6 hours.
- Another choice is to take 600 mg (three 200 mg pills) by mouth every 8 hours.
- The most you should take each day is 1,200 mg (six 200 mg pills), unless your doctor has told you to take more.

❹ Pain and Fever Medicines—Extra Notes:
- Use the lowest amount of medicine that makes your pain or fever better.
- Acetaminophen is thought to be safer than ibuprofen or naproxen in people > 65 years old. Acetaminophen is in many OTC and prescription medicines. It might be in more than one medicine that you are taking. You need to be careful and not take an overdose. An acetaminophen overdose can hurt the liver.
- McNeil, the company that makes Tylenol, has different dosage instructions for Tylenol in Canada and the United States. In Canada, the maximum recommended dose per day is 4,000 mg or 12 Regular Strength (325 mg) pills. In the United States, McNeil recommends a maximum dose of 10 Regular Strength (325 mg) pills.
- CAUTION: Do not take acetaminophen if you have liver disease.
- CAUTION: Do not take ibuprofen if you have stomach problems, have kidney disease, are pregnant, or have been told by your doctor to avoid this type of anti-inflammatory drug. Do not take ibuprofen for > 7 days without consulting your doctor.
- *Before taking any medicine, read all the instructions on the package.*

❺ Call Back If:
- Node enlarges to > 1" (2.5 cm) in size.
- Overlying skin becomes red.
- Fever > 103° F (39.4° C) occurs.
- You become worse or are worried about a lymph node.

BACKGROUND

Key Points

- Lymph nodes are round, bean-shaped structures that assist the lymphatic system in fighting infection.
- Normally lymph nodes are < ½" (1 cm) in size. Lymph nodes enlarge and become tender when an infection is present.
- Children and adolescents generally have larger lymph nodes than adults.

Location of Lymph Nodes

- Occipital (posterior lower scalp)
- Cervical (neck)
- Supraclavicular (just above collarbone)
- Axillary (armpit)
- Epitrochlear (just above elbow)
- Inguinal (groin crease at top of thigh)

Causes of Lymph Node Swelling

- **Infection:** Viral, bacterial, or fungal infections can cause lymph nodes to become swollen and tender. Infection is the most common cause of lymph node swelling. The cervical (neck) nodes are most commonly involved because of respiratory and throat infections. Enlarged nodes in the armpit or groin are often reacting to a skin infection in the involved extremity. Lymph nodes in the groin can become swollen when there is a leg infection or an STI.
- **Malignancy:** Malignancy is a less common cause of lymph node enlargement. However, any persistently enlarged nontender lymph node could possibly be a sign of malignancy (cancer, lymphoma, leukemia).
- **Medications.**
- **Other:** e.g., collagen vascular disease, sarcoidosis, HIV.

Caution—Hernia: Groin hernias usually bulge out with straining (lifting, coughing, bowel movement) and subside with rest (lying down quietly). Painful swelling in this area requires immediate evaluation because of the possibility that the hernia is incarcerated (trapped) and strangulated (ischemic).

MENSTRUAL PERIOD, MISSED OR LATE

Definition
- **Late Menstrual Period:** ≥ 5 days overdue compared to usual menstrual cycle
- **Missed Menstrual Period:** No menstrual flow for > 6 weeks

TRIAGE ASSESSMENT QUESTIONS

Call EMS 911 Now
● Sounds like a life-threatening emergency to the triager

See More Appropriate Protocol
● Abdominal pain is present
  Go to Protocol: Abdominal Pain (Female) on page 1
● STI exposure and prevention, questions about
  Go to Protocol: STI Exposure and Prevention on page 377

Go to ED/UCC Now
(or to Office With PCP Approval)
● Patient sounds very sick or weak to the triager
  Reason: severe acute illness or serious complication suspected

See Today in Office
◐ Patient wants to be seen

See Within 3 Days in Office
◐ Pregnant and ANY of the following:
  – Has an IUD
  – Prior history of "ectopic pregnancy"
  – Previous tubal surgery (e.g., tubal ligation)
  – History of infertility
  Reason: higher risk for ectopic pregnancy
◐ Wants a pregnancy test done in the office

See Within 2 Weeks in Office
◐ Pregnant
◐ Weight loss > 10 lb (22 kg)
  R/O: excessive dieting, eating disorder, medical disorder
◐ Age > 40 years
  R/O: menopause
◐ Missed ≥ 2 periods in a row
  Reason: needs evaluation
◐ Missed period has occurred ≥ 2 times in the last year and cause is not known
  Reason: needs diagnosis determined, possible further workup

Home Care
○ Pregnancy suspected or possible
  Reason: needs a home pregnancy test
○ Recent stress (e.g., new school/job/home/ marriage, relationship problems)
  Reason: possible stress-related secondary amenorrhea
○ Menstrual period, missed or late

HOME CARE ADVICE

❶ Pregnancy Test, When in Doubt:
- If there is a chance that you might be pregnant, use a urine pregnancy test.
- You can buy a pregnancy test at the drugstore.
- It works best if you test your first urine in the morning.
- Call back if you are pregnant.
- *Follow the instructions included in the package.*

❷ Stress: Stress can interrupt normal menstrual periods. Try to reduce your stress by talking about it with a friend or family member. Try to avoid or decrease stressors. If this is not effective, seek help from a counselor or talk with your doctor.

❸ Call Back If:
- Pregnancy test is positive.
- You have difficulties with the home pregnancy test.
- New symptoms suggest pregnancy (e.g., morning sickness, breast tenderness/swelling).
- You need help coping with stress.
- You become worse.

BACKGROUND

Key Points
- The first day of menstrual bleeding is considered the first day of a new menstrual cycle.
- Menstrual bleeding typically lasts 3-7 days.
- Ovulation generally occurs 14 days before onset of menses.
- The length of the menstrual cycle varies from woman to woman. The range is from 24-35 days. The average is 28 days.

Causes
Pregnancy is the most important cause. This needs to be considered and ruled out in every woman who has a missed or late period. Other causes include:
- Birth control pills
- Depo-Provera injection
- Dieting, exercise, and weight loss
- Menopause
- Pituitary and other endocrine disorders
- Polycystic ovary syndrome
- Recent pregnancy
- Stress

Home Urine Pregnancy Tests
- Home urine pregnancy tests are inexpensive, accurate, and easy to use. Most drugstores sell these tests over the counter.
- Urine pregnancy tests can often diagnose pregnancy during the week after the first missed period (2 weeks after ovulation).
- Use of a first-morning urine specimen is recommended because the urine hCG concentration is highest in the morning.
- When a home pregnancy test is negative but there is still a high suspicion of pregnancy, the woman should either repeat the test in 3-5 days or go to her doctor's office for testing.
- The urine pregnancy test can sometimes be falsely negative if the urine specimen is grossly bloody. A small amount of blood (e.g., blood-tinged urine) should not interfere with the accuracy of the test.
- More information is available at: www.womenshealth.gov/publications/our-publications/fact-sheet/pregnancy-test.html.

MOUTH INJURY

Definition

- Injuries to the lip, frenulum (flap under the upper lip), tongue, buccal mucosa (inner cheeks), floor of the mouth, roof of the mouth (hard and soft palate), or back of the mouth (tonsils, oropharynx).
- Infected mouth wounds are covered here because they may look different from wound infections of the skin.

TRIAGE ASSESSMENT QUESTIONS

Call EMS 911 Now

- Major bleeding (actively dripping or spurting) that can't be stopped
  First Aid: Apply direct pressure to the entire wound with a clean cloth.
- Fainted or too weak to stand following large blood loss
  R/O: impending shock
  First Aid: Lie down with the feet elevated and apply pressure to the wound.
- Knocked out (unconscious) > 1 minute
  R/O: concussion
- Difficult to awaken or acting confused (e.g., disoriented, slurred speech)
  R/O: concussion, intoxication
- Difficulty breathing
  R/O: swelling occluding airway, aspiration of blood
- SEVERE neck pain (e.g., excruciating)
  R/O: cervical spine injury
  First Aid: Protect the neck from movement.
- Sounds like a life-threatening emergency to the triager

See More Appropriate Protocol

- Teeth or tooth injury is main concern
  Go to Protocol: Tooth Injury on page 408

Go to ED Now

- Can't open or close the mouth fully
  R/O: jaw fracture or TMJ dislocation
- Unable to swallow or new onset of drooling
  R/O: significant traumatic swelling, Ludwig angina

Go to ED/UCC Now
(or to Office With PCP Approval)

- Gaping cut of OUTER LIP (or length > ¼" or 6 mm)
  Reason: may need laceration repair (e.g., sutures)
- Gaping cut through border of the LIP where it meets the skin (or length > ¼" or 6 mm)
  Reason: cuts through vermillion border need precise approximation
- Cut of side or tip of TONGUE that gapes open (split tongue)
  Reason: may need laceration repair (e.g., sutures)
  Note: Tongue lacerations rarely need sutures.
- Cut on surface of TONGUE > 1" (24 mm) and that gapes open
  Reason: may need laceration repair (e.g., sutures)
  Note: Tongue lacerations rarely need sutures.
- Bleeding won't stop after 10 minutes of direct pressure (using correct technique)
  Reason: may need laceration repair (e.g., sutures)
- Injury to the back of the throat, tonsil, or soft palate (e.g., pencil or other sharp object placed in mouth)
  R/O: posterior pharynx injury needing close follow-up
- Sounds like a serious injury to the triager

Go to Office Now

- Looks infected (e.g., spreading redness, pus, red streak)
  Note: Healing wound in mouth is NORMALLY WHITE for several days.

See Today in Office

- SEVERE pain (e.g., excruciating)
  R/O: severe injury
- Closing the mouth and biting down does not feel normal
  R/O: tooth displacement, mandible or maxilla fracture
- Patient wants to be seen

See Today or Tomorrow in Office

- Wound and no tetanus booster in > 5 years (or > 10 years for clean cuts)
  Reason: may need a tetanus booster shot (vaccine)
- Suspicious history for the injury
  R/O: domestic violence or elder abuse

See Within 3 Days in Office

● Injury and pain has not improved after 3 days

Home Care

○ Minor mouth injury
  R/O: bruise, small cut or scrape
○ Minor mouth burn from hot food or drink
  (mouth pain or lip pain)

HOME CARE ADVICE

Minor Mouth Injury

❶ **Reassurance:**
  • It sounds like a minor injury that we can treat
    at home.
  • Here is some care advice that should help.

❷ **Stop Any Bleeding:**
  • **For Bleeding of the Outer Lip:** Apply direct
    pressure to the entire wound with a clean cloth
    or gauze.
  • **For Bleeding of the Inner Lip:** Press bleeding site
    against teeth or jaw for 10 minutes.
  • **For Bleeding From the Tongue:** Squeeze or press
    the bleeding site with a sterile gauze or piece of
    clean cloth for 10 minutes.
  • **For Bleeding From the Tissue That Connects
    the Upper Lip to the Gum** (i.e., torn frenulum):
    Apply pressure for 10 minutes.
  • CAUTION: Once bleeding from inside the lip
    stops, don't pull the lip out again to look at it.
    *(Reason: The bleeding will start up again; minor
    tears of the frenulum do not require sutures.)*

❸ **Treatment of Bruised Lip or Tongue:**
  • **Bruised Lip:** Apply a cold pack or an ice bag
    wrapped in a towel for 20 minutes each hour for
    4 consecutive hours (20 minutes of cold followed
    by 40 minutes of rest for 4 hours in a row).
  • **Bruised Tongue:** Put a piece of ice or Popsicle on
    the area that was injured for 20 minutes.
  • This helps reduce the pain and swelling.

❹ **Treatment of Minor Cuts or Scrapes
  (Abrasions) of Lip:**
  • Apply direct pressure for 10 minutes to stop
    any bleeding.
  • Wash the wound with soap and water for
    5 minutes.
  • Gently scrub out any dirt with a washcloth.
  • Apply an antibiotic ointment twice daily.

❺ **Treatment of Minor Cuts or Scrapes (Abrasions)
  of Tongue and Inner Cheek:**
  • Apply direct pressure for 10 minutes to stop
    any bleeding.
  • Rinse mouth or tongue wounds with warm water
    immediately after meals.

❻ **Diet:**
  • Eat a soft diet.
  • Avoid any spicy, hot, salty, or citrus foods that
    might sting.

❼ **Pain Medicines:**
  • For pain relief, you can take either acetaminophen,
    ibuprofen, or naproxen.
  • They are over-the-counter (OTC) pain drugs.
    You can buy them at the drugstore.

❽ **Acetaminophen (e.g., Tylenol):**
  • **Regular Strength Tylenol:** Take 650 mg
    (two 325 mg pills) by mouth every 4-6 hours
    as needed. Each Regular Strength Tylenol pill
    has 325 mg of acetaminophen.
  • **Extra Strength Tylenol:** Take 1,000 mg
    (two 500 mg pills) every 8 hours as needed.
    Each Extra Strength Tylenol pill has 500 mg
    of acetaminophen.
  • The most you should take each day is 3,000 mg
    (10 Regular Strength or 6 Extra Strength pills a day).
  Ibuprofen (e.g., Motrin, Advil):
  • Take 400 mg (two 200 mg pills) by mouth every
    6 hours.
  • Another choice is to take 600 mg (three 200 mg
    pills) by mouth every 8 hours.
  • The most you should take each day is 1,200 mg
    (six 200 mg pills), unless your doctor has told
    you to take more.
  Naproxen (e.g., Aleve):
  • Take 220 mg (one 220 mg pill) by mouth every
    8 hours as needed. You may take 440 mg
    (two 220 mg pills) for your first dose.
  • The most you should take each day is 660 mg
    (three 220 mg pills a day), unless your doctor
    has told you to take more.

❾ **Expected Course:**
  • Small cuts of the inner cheeks, inner lip, and
    tongue generally heal quickly and do not require
    suturing. They usually heal up in 3-7 days.
  • Bruised lips slowly get better over about a week.
  • Infections of mouth injuries are rare.

⓿ Call Back If:

- Severe pain lasts > 2 hours after pain medicine and ice.
- Area looks infected (mainly increasing pain or swelling after 48 hours).
  (Caution: Any healing wound in the mouth is normally white for several days.)
- Fever occurs.
- You become worse.

Minor Mouth Burn From Hot Food or Drink

❶ Reassurance:

- Burns of the mouth from hot food usually are painful for 2 days.
- They heal quickly because the lining of the mouth heals twice as fast as the skin.
- *Here is some care advice that should help.*

❷ Local Ice:

- Put a piece of ice in the mouth immediately for 10 minutes.
  (Reason: Reduce swelling and pain.)
- Rinse the mouth with ice water every hour for 4 hours.

❸ Call Back If:

- Difficulty with swallowing occurs.
- Difficulty with breathing occurs.
- Pain becomes severe.
- You become worse.

FIRST AID

First Aid Advice for Bleeding:

Apply direct pressure to the entire wound with a clean cloth.

First Aid Advice for Penetrating Object:

If penetrating object is still in place, don't remove it
Reason: Removal could increase bleeding.

First Aid Advice for Shock:

Lie down with the feet elevated.

BACKGROUND

Types of Mouth Injuries

- Cuts and bruises of the lips.
- Cuts inside of the cheeks.
- Cuts and bruises of the tongue.
- **Wounds of Posterior Pharynx:** Wounds can sometimes occur in the posterior pharynx. Usually this is the result of running and falling while having a sharp object in the mouth (e.g., pencil, fork). This occurs more commonly in children than in adults. Such wounds are potentially serious and nearly all require evaluation by a physician.

Causes

- **Altercations:** Direct blow from punch, kick, or object.
- Contact sports.
- Falls.
- Motor vehicle accidents.
- **Seizure:** After a generalized tonic-clonic (grand mal) seizure approximately 20%-30% of patients will awaken with bruising or a laceration of the tongue. These wounds nearly always occur on the side of the tongue.
- **Syncope:** Tongue lacerations occur only rarely from a syncopal (fainting) episode. When a cut does occur, it is usually a bite wound from suddenly falling and striking the chin on the ground.

Hot Food Burns of the Mouth

- **Definition:** Hot food or drink causes burn of the mouth's lining (mucous membrane).
- **Symptoms:** Immediate pain and redness. Sometimes causes small second-degree burn with area of white mucosa.
- **Causes:** Hot pizza burn is common because melted cheese sticks to roof of mouth. Hot chocolate or tea, hot soups or stews, etc. Microwaved foods also have increased risk.
- **Complications:** Mainly severe localized pain. Inability to swallow fluids (or drooling) and dehydration are very rare.
- **Treatment:** Immediate application of cold water or ice for 5-10 minutes. Then analgesics and soft diet for 2 days.

What Cuts Need to Be Sutured?

- **Outer Lip Lacerations:** Any wound of the lip that crosses the vermillion border (border of the lip where it meets the skin) needs to be sutured to ensure healing and for cosmetic reasons. A cut > ¼" (6 mm) of the outer lip or face may need sutures, especially if it is gaping.
- **Inner Lip and Cheek Lacerations:** Small cuts of the inner cheeks or inner lip generally heal quickly and do not require suturing. A gaping wound that is > ½" (12 mm) long may require sutures.
- **Tongue Lacerations:** Small cuts of the tongue generally heal quickly and do not require suturing. A gaping wound that is > ½" (12 mm) long may require sutures.
- Any open wound that may need sutures should be evaluated by a physician regardless of the time that has passed since the initial injury.

When Does an Adult Need a Tetanus Booster (Tetanus Shot)?

- **Clean Cuts and Scrapes—Tetanus Booster Needed Every 10 Years:** Patients with clean minor wounds AND who have previously had ≥ 3 tetanus shots (full series) need a booster every 10 years. Examples of minor wounds include a superficial abrasion or a shallow cut from a clean knife blade. Obtain booster within 72 hours.
- **Dirty Wounds—Tetanus Booster Needed Every 5 Years:** Patients with dirty wounds need a booster if it has been > 5 years since the last booster. Examples of dirty wounds include those contaminated with soil, feces, and/or saliva and more serious wounds from deep punctures, crushing, and burns. Obtain booster within 72 hours.

Caution—Associated Head and Neck Trauma

- Head trauma should be considered in all patients with a mouth injury. Signs of significant head injury include loss of consciousness, amnesia, unsteady walking, confusion, and slurred speech.
- Neck trauma should also be considered in all patients with a facial injury. Concerning findings include numbness, weakness, and neck pain.
- After using the Mouth Injury protocol, if the triager or caller has remaining concerns about head or neck trauma, the patient also should be triaged using the Head Injury and/or Neck Injury protocol on pages 201 and 290, respectively.

NECK INJURY

Definition
- Injuries to the neck.
- The anterior (front) neck extends from the lower edge of the mandible (jaw) to the clavicles (collarbones).
- The posterior (back) neck extends from the base of the skull to the first rib.

TRIAGE ASSESSMENT QUESTIONS

Call EMS 911 Now
- Dangerous mechanism of injury (e.g., MVA, contact sports, diving, fall on trampoline, fall > 10 feet or 3 m)
  (Exception: neck pain began > 1 hour after injury)
  First Aid: Protect the neck from movement.
  Don't move until a neck brace is applied.
- Weakness of arms or legs
  R/O: spinal cord injury
  First Aid: Protect the neck from movement.
  Don't move until a neck brace is applied.
- Numbness, tingling, or burning of arms, upper back/chest, or legs
  (Exception: brief, now gone)
  R/O: spinal cord injury
  First Aid: Protect the neck from movement.
  Don't move until a neck brace is applied.
- Major bleeding (actively dripping or spurting) that can't be stopped
  First Aid: Apply direct pressure to the entire wound with a clean cloth.
- Bullet, knife, or other serious penetrating wound
  First Aid: If penetrating object is still in place, don't remove it.
  Reason: removal could increase bleeding
- Difficulty breathing (e.g., choking or stridor)
  R/O: fractured larynx or other airway injury
- Knocked out (unconscious) > 1 minute
  First Aid: Protect the neck from movement.
  Don't move until a neck brace is applied.
- Direct blow to front of neck and cough, hoarseness, abnormal voice, or can't talk
  R/O: laryngeal or tracheal injury
- Sounds like a serious injury to the triager
- Sounds like a life-threatening emergency to the triager

See More Appropriate Protocol
- Neck pain not from an injury
  Go to Protocol: Neck Pain or Stiffness on page 294

Go to ED Now
- Dangerous mechanism of injury (e.g., MVA, contact sports, diving, fall on trampoline, fall > 10 feet or 3 m) and neck pain or stiffness began > 1 hour after injury
  R/O: muscle strain or whiplash injury
- Numbness, tingling, or burning of arms, upper back/chest, or legs and not present now (i.e., completely resolved)
  R/O: cord injury, "burners," "stingers"
- Coughing up blood
  R/O: laryngeal or tracheal injury
- Difficulty swallowing or drooling
  R/O: esophageal injury
- Skin is split open or gaping (length > ½" or 12 mm)
  Reason: may need laceration repair (e.g., sutures)
  R/O: deeper injury
- Puncture wound of neck
  R/O: injury to deeper neck structures
- Bleeding and won't stop after 10 minutes of direct pressure (using correct technique)
  R/O: need for sutures
- Large swelling or bruise (> 2" or 5 cm)
  R/O: expanding hematoma from vascular injury

Go to ED/UCC Now
(or to Office With PCP Approval)
- SEVERE neck pain (e.g., excruciating)

See Today in Office
- Patient is confused or is an unreliable provider of information (e.g., dementia, profound intellectual disability, alcohol intoxication)
- HIGH-RISK adult (e.g., rheumatoid arthritis, ankylosing spondylitis, cervical spine abnormalities)
- Patient wants to be seen

See Today or Tomorrow in Office
- Wound and no tetanus booster in > 5 years (or > 10 years for clean cuts)
  Reason: may need a tetanus booster shot (vaccine)
- Suspicious history for the injury
  R/O: domestic violence or elder abuse

See Within 3 Days in Office

- Injury and pain has not improved after 3 days
- Injury is still painful after 2 weeks

Home Care

○ Neck swelling, bruise, or pain from direct blow
to the neck
*Reason: minor neck injury and all triage questions
negative*

○ Neck pain or stiffness from lifting, bending,
or twisting injury
*Reason: minor neck injury and all triage questions
negative*

HOME CARE ADVICE

Treatment of a Minor Bruise, Sprain, or Strain

❶ **Reassurance—Bending or Twisting Injury
(Strain, Sprain):**
- Strain and sprain are the medical terms used
to describe overstretching of the muscles and
ligaments of the neck. A twisting or bending
injury can cause neck strain and sprain.
- The main symptom is pain that gets worse
with movement.
- *Here is some care advice that should help.*

❷ **Reassurance—Direct Blow (Contusion, Bruise):**
- A direct blow to your neck can cause a contusion.
Contusion is the medical term for bruise.
- Symptoms are mild pain, swelling, and/or bruising.
- *Here is some care advice that should help.*

❸ **Apply a Cold Pack:**
- Apply a cold pack or an ice bag (wrapped in a
moist towel) to the area for 20 minutes. Repeat
in 1 hour, then every 4 hours while awake.
- Continue this for the first 48 hours after an injury.
(Reason: to reduce the swelling and pain)

❹ **Apply Heat to the Area:**
- Beginning 48 hours after an injury, apply a warm
washcloth or heating pad for 10 minutes 3 times
a day.
- This will help increase blood flow and improve
healing.

❺ **Avoid:** Avoid heavy lifting and any sports activities
for the first week after an injury.

❻ **Rest Versus Movement:**
- Movement of the neck is generally more healing
in the long term than rest. Continue normal
activities as much as your pain permits.
- Rest should only be used for the first couple days
after an injury.

❼ **Call Back If:**
- Swelling or bruise becomes > 2" (5 cm).
- Pain not improving after 3 days.
- Pain or swelling lasts > 7 days.
- You become worse.

Treatment of a Small Cut or Scrape

❶ **Reassurance—Superficial Laceration
(Cut or Scratch) or Abrasion (Scrape):**
- This sounds like a small cut or scrape that we can
treat at home.
- *Here is some care advice that should help.*

❷ **Bleeding:** Apply direct pressure for 10 minutes with
a sterile gauze to stop any bleeding.

❸ **Cleaning the Wound:**
- Wash the wound with soap and water for 5 minutes.
- For any dirt, scrub gently with a washcloth.
- For any bleeding, apply direct pressure with a
sterile gauze or clean cloth for 10 minutes.

❹ **Antibiotic Ointment:**
- Apply an antibiotic ointment (e.g., OTC bacitracin),
covered by a Band-Aid or dressing. Change daily
or if it becomes wet.
- Option: A Telfa dressing won't stick to the wound
when it is removed.
- Option: Another option is to use a liquid skin
bandage that only needs to be applied once.
Don't use antibiotic ointment if you use a liquid
skin bandage.

❺ **Liquid Skin Bandage:**
- You can use a liquid skin bandage instead of
antibiotic ointment and a dressing or a Band-Aid.
- **Benefits:** Liquid skin bandage has several benefits
when compared with a regular bandage (e.g., a
dressing or a Band-Aid). You only need to put a
liquid bandage on once to minor cuts and scrapes.
It helps stop minor bleeding. It seals the wound
and may promote faster healing and lower
infection rates. However, it also costs more.

- **How to Use It:** First clean and dry the wound. You put on the liquid as spray or with a swab. It dries in < 1 minute and usually lasts a week. You can get it wet.
- **Examples:** Liquid skin bandage is available over the counter. Examples are Band-Aid Liquid Bandage, New Skin, Curad Spray Bandage, and 3M No Sting Liquid Bandage Spray.

❻ Call Back If:
- Looks infected (pus, redness, increasing tenderness).
- Doesn't heal within 10 days.
- You become worse.

Over-the-counter Pain Medicines

❶ Pain Medicines:
- For pain relief, you can take either acetaminophen, ibuprofen, or naproxen.
- They are over-the-counter (OTC) pain drugs. You can buy them at the drugstore.

Acetaminophen (e.g., Tylenol):
- **Regular Strength Tylenol:** Take 650 mg (two 325 mg pills) by mouth every 4-6 hours as needed. Each Regular Strength Tylenol pill has 325 mg of acetaminophen.
- **Extra Strength Tylenol:** Take 1,000 mg (two 500 mg pills) every 8 hours as needed. Each Extra Strength Tylenol pill has 500 mg of acetaminophen.
- The most you should take each day is 3,000 mg (10 Regular Strength or 6 Extra Strength pills a day).

Ibuprofen (e.g., Motrin, Advil):
- Take 400 mg (two 200 mg pills) by mouth every 6 hours.
- Another choice is to take 600 mg (three 200 mg pills) by mouth every 8 hours.
- The most you should take each day is 1,200 mg (six 200 mg pills), unless your doctor has told you to take more.

Naproxen (e.g., Aleve):
- Take 220 mg (one 220 mg pill) by mouth every 8 hours as needed. You may take 440 mg (two 220 mg pills) for your first dose.
- The most you should take each day is 660 mg (three 220 mg pills a day), unless your doctor has told you to take more.

❷ Pain Medicines—Extra Notes:
- Use the lowest amount of medicine that makes your pain better.
- Acetaminophen is thought to be safer than ibuprofen or naproxen in people > 65 years old. Acetaminophen is in many OTC and prescription medicines. It might be in more than one medicine that you are taking. You need to be careful and not take an overdose. An acetaminophen overdose can hurt the liver.
- McNeil, the company that makes Tylenol, has different dosage instructions for Tylenol in Canada and the United States. In Canada, the maximum recommended dose per day is 4,000 mg or 12 Regular Strength (325 mg) pills. In the United States, McNeil recommends a maximum dose of 10 Regular Strength (325 mg) pills.
- CAUTION: Do not take acetaminophen if you have liver disease.
- CAUTION: Do not take ibuprofen or naproxen if you have stomach problems, have kidney disease, are pregnant, or have been told by your doctor to avoid this type of anti-inflammatory drug. Do not take ibuprofen or naproxen for > 7 days without consulting your doctor.
- *Before taking any medicine, read all the instructions on the package.*

❸ Call Back If:
- You have more questions.
- You become worse.

FIRST AID

First Aid Advice for Bleeding:
Apply direct pressure to the entire wound with a clean cloth.

First Aid Advice for Penetrating Object:
If penetrating object is still in place, don't remove it.

First Aid Advice for Shock:
Lie down with the feet elevated.

First Aid Advice for Suspected Spinal Cord Injury:
Do not move until a spine board is applied.

BACKGROUND

History

- There are a number of historical pieces of information that should be obtained from a patient with a traumatic neck injury.
- Information that is valuable and may impact disposition include; mechanism of injury (e.g., auto accident, fall), associated injuries, date of injury, use of protective equipment (i.e., sports), and use of restraints (i.e., auto accident).

Dangerous Mechanisms of Injury

- Patients who have a dangerous mechanism of injury should be referred for medical evaluation immediately. Dangerous injuries include accidents involving autos, diving, trampoline, contact sports, and hanging. A forceful direct blow to the neck (e.g., baseball bat) should be considered serious.
- The mechanism of injury should also be considered dangerous if the patient has an associated significant injury of the head or other body part (e.g., fracture).

Types of Neck Injuries

- **Airway Injuries (Larynx and Trachea):** Can be caused by direct blow to the front of the neck. Examples are blow from high-speed object (e.g., baseball), hitting clothesline while running, strangulation, etc.
- **Cervical Spine Fracture:** The main risk from moving patients with cervical spine (bony) injuries is the potential for causing spinal cord injury.
- **Esophageal Injuries:** These are rare except with penetrating trauma.
- **Spinal cord injury.**
- **Strained Neck Muscles and "Whiplash":** Muscle strain is common from lifting, bending, or twisting injuries. Read Whiplash section for more information.
- **Vascular injuries (carotid artery, vertebral artery, jugular vein).**

Whiplash

- "Whiplash" is a term that refers to a cervical spine hyperextension injury followed by a flexing motion. The extension and flexion of the neck overstretches the muscles and ligaments of the cervical spine. Other terms which are used to describe this type of injury are neck strain and neck sprain. The most common cause of this type of injury is an auto accident. Patients may report neck pain beginning at the time of injury or developing slowly over the first 24 hours after the injury. The pain frequently increases during the first couple days after the injury. Patients may report associated symptoms of headache, paresthesia (tingling), neck stiffness, and dizziness.
- The pain from a "whiplash" injury often resolves within 1-2 weeks. However, some patients (10%-40%) may go on to have pain for weeks to months.

Strained Neck Muscles From Self-induced Twisting, Turning, or Overuse

- Self-induced strained or pulled neck muscles are a common cause of neck pain in adults.
- A strained neck is usually caused by sleeping in an awkward position, cradling telephone between neck and shoulder for extended conversation, painting a ceiling, reading in bed, reaching for something that was difficult to get, sitting in front row of movie theater, looking at something that requires extreme bending or turning of neck, prolonged typing, etc.

What Cuts Need to Be Sutured?

- Any cut that is split open or gaping probably needs sutures (or staples or skin glue).
- Cuts > ½" (1 cm) usually need sutures.
- Any open wound that may need sutures should be evaluated by a physician regardless of the time that has passed since the initial injury.

When Does an Adult Need a Tetanus Booster (Tetanus Shot)?

- **Clean Cuts and Scrapes—Tetanus Booster Needed Every 10 Years:** Patients with clean minor wounds AND who have previously had ≥ 3 tetanus shots (full series) need a booster every 10 years. Examples of minor wounds include a superficial abrasion or a shallow cut from a clean knife blade. Obtain booster within 72 hours.
- **Dirty Wounds—Tetanus Booster Needed Every 5 Years:** Patients with dirty wounds need a booster if it has been > 5 years since the last booster. Examples of dirty wounds include those contaminated with soil, feces, and/or saliva and more serious wounds from deep punctures, crushing, and burns. Obtain booster within 72 hours.

NECK PAIN OR STIFFNESS

Definition
- Complains of neck pain in the back, side, or front of the neck.
- Not due to a known traumatic injury.
- Minor muscle strain and overuse are covered in this protocol.

Pain Severity Scale
- **Mild (1-3):** Doesn't interfere with normal activities.
- **Moderate (4-7):** Interferes with normal activities or awakens from sleep.
- **Severe (8-10):** Excruciating pain, unable to do any normal activities.

TRIAGE ASSESSMENT QUESTIONS

Call EMS 911 Now
- Shock suspected (e.g., cold/pale/clammy skin, too weak to stand)
  R/O: shock
  First Aid: Lie down with the feet elevated.
- Similar pain previously and it was from "heart attack"
  R/O: myocardial infarction
- Similar pain previously from "angina" and not relieved by nitroglycerin
  R/O: cardiac ischemia, myocardial infarction
- Difficult to awaken or acting confused (e.g., disoriented, slurred speech)
  R/O: meningitis, encephalitis
- Sounds like a life-threatening emergency to the triager

See More Appropriate Protocol
- Followed an injury to neck (e.g., MVA, sports, impact, or collision)
  Go to Protocol: Neck Injury on page 290
- Chest pain
  Go to Protocol: Chest Pain on page 73
- Lymph node in the neck is swollen or painful to the touch
  Go to Protocol: Lymph Nodes, Swollen on page 281
- Sore throat is the main symptom
  Go to Protocol: Sore Throat on page 369

Go to ED/UCC Now (or to Office With PCP Approval)
- Difficulty breathing or unusual sweating (e.g., sweating without exertion)
  R/O: cardiac ischemia
- Chest pain lasting > 5 minutes
  Reason: chest pain is a high-risk complaint; referral for evaluation
- Stiff neck (can't touch chin to chest) and has headache
  R/O: meningitis or SAH
- Stiff neck (can't touch chin to chest) and fever
  R/O: meningitis
- Weakness of an arm or a hand
  R/O: nerve root compression
- Problems with bowel or bladder control
  R/O: cord compression
- Patient sounds very sick or weak to the triager
  Reason: severe acute illness or serious complication suspected

Go to Office Now
- SEVERE pain (e.g., excruciating, unable to do any normal activities)
- Head is twisting to one side (or ask, "Is it turning against your will?")
  R/O: acute dystonic reaction
  Note: Occurs as a side effect when taking medications like Compazine (prochlorperazine), Reglan (metoclopramide), Thorazine (chlorpromazine), Phenergan (promethazine), and Haldol (haloperidol).
- Fever > 103° F (39.4° C)
- Fever > 100.0° F (37.8° C) and IV drug abuse
  R/O: bacterial illness, epidural abscess
- Fever > 100.0° F (37.8° C) and has diabetes mellitus or a weak immune system (e.g., HIV positive, cancer chemotherapy, organ transplant, splenectomy, chronic steroids)

See Today in Office

- Numbness in an arm or hand (i.e., loss of sensation)
  R/O: nerve root compression
- Painful rash with multiple small blisters grouped together (i.e., dermatomal distribution or "band" or "stripe")
  R/O: herpes zoster (shingles)
- HIGH-RISK adult (e.g., history of cancer, HIV, or IV drug abuse)
  R/O: malignancy, metastasis, epidural abscess
- Patient wants to be seen

See Today or Tomorrow in Office

- Tenderness in front of neck over windpipe
  R/O: thyroiditis

See Within 3 Days in Office

- MODERATE neck pain (e.g., interferes with normal activities like work or school)
- Pain shoots (radiates) into arm or hand
  R/O: cervical radiculopathy, herniated cervical disk
- Neck pain persists > 2 weeks

See Within 2 Weeks in Office

- Neck pain is a chronic symptom (recurrent or ongoing AND lasting > 4 weeks)
- Age > 50 and no prior history of similar neck pain
  Reason: higher risk of pathology

Home Care

- ○ Neck pain or stiffness
- ○ Caused by twisting, bending, or lifting injury
  R/O: muscle strain, overuse

HOME CARE ADVICE

❶ **Reassurance—Neck Pain:**
  - Causes of unexplained neck pain and neck stiffness include: sleeping in an awkward position or forgotten twisting, muscle spasm and tension from stress, and poor posture.
  - Usually the pain will pass within several days.
  - *Here is some care advice that should help.*

❷ **Reassurance—Neck Pain From Twisting, Bending, or Lifting Injury:**
  - It sounds like an overstretched muscle. We can treat that at home.
  - For minor injuries, pain should improve over a 2- to 3-day period and disappear within 7 days.
  - *Here is some care advice that should help.*

❸ **Apply Cold to the Area or Heat:** During the first 2 days after a mild injury, apply a cold pack or an ice bag (wrapped in a towel) for 20 minutes 4 times a day. After 2 days, apply a heating pad or hot water bottle to the most painful area for 20 minutes whenever the pain flares up. Wrap hot water bottles or heating pads in a towel to avoid burns.

❹ **Sleep:**
  - Sleep on your back or side, not on your abdomen.
  - Sleep with a neck collar. Use a foam neck collar (from a pharmacy) OR a small towel wrapped around the neck.
    (Reason: Keep the head from moving too much during sleep.)

❺ **Stretching Exercises:**
  - After 48 hours of protecting the neck, begin gentle stretching exercises.
  - Improve the tone of the neck muscles with 2-3 minutes of gentle stretching exercises per day such as touching the chin to each shoulder, touching the ear to each shoulder, and moving the head forward and backward.
  - Don't apply any resistance during these stretching exercises.

❻ **Pain Medicines:**
- For pain relief, you can take either acetaminophen, ibuprofen, or naproxen.
- They are over-the-counter (OTC) pain drugs. You can buy them at the drugstore.

Acetaminophen (e.g., Tylenol):
- **Regular Strength Tylenol:** Take 650 mg (two 325 mg pills) by mouth every 4-6 hours as needed. Each Regular Strength Tylenol pill has 325 mg of acetaminophen.
- **Extra Strength Tylenol:** Take 1,000 mg (two 500 mg pills) every 8 hours as needed. Each Extra Strength Tylenol pill has 500 mg of acetaminophen.
- The most you should take each day is 3,000 mg (10 Regular Strength or 6 Extra Strength pills a day).

Ibuprofen (e.g., Motrin, Advil):
- Take 400 mg (two 200 mg pills) by mouth every 6 hours.
- Another choice is to take 600 mg (three 200 mg pills) by mouth every 8 hours.
- The most you should take each day is 1,200 mg (six 200 mg pills), unless your doctor has told you to take more.

Naproxen (e.g., Aleve):
- Take 220 mg (one 220 mg pill) by mouth every 8 hours as needed. You may take 440 mg (two 220 mg pills) for your first dose.
- The most you should take each day is 660 mg (three 220 mg pills a day), unless your doctor has told you to take more.

❼ **Pain Medicines—Extra Notes:**
- Use the lowest amount of medicine that makes your pain better.
- Acetaminophen is thought to be safer than ibuprofen or naproxen in people > 65 years old. Acetaminophen is in many OTC and prescription medicines. It might be in more than one medicine that you are taking. You need to be careful and not take an overdose. An acetaminophen overdose can hurt the liver.

- McNeil, the company that makes Tylenol, has different dosage instructions for Tylenol in Canada and the United States. In Canada, the maximum recommended dose per day is 4,000 mg or 12 Regular Strength (325 mg) pills. In the United States, McNeil recommends a maximum dose of 10 Regular Strength (325 mg) pills.
- CAUTION: Do not take acetaminophen if you have liver disease.
- CAUTION: Do not take ibuprofen or naproxen if you have stomach problems, have kidney disease, are pregnant, or have been told by your doctor to avoid this type of anti-inflammatory drug. Do not take ibuprofen or naproxen for > 7 days without consulting your doctor.
- *Before taking any medicine, read all the instructions on the package.*

❽ **Good Body Mechanics:**
- **Lifting:** Stand close to the object to be lifted. Keep your back straight and lift by bending your legs. Ask for help if needed.
- **Sleeping:** Sleep on a firm mattress.
- **Sitting:** Avoid sitting for long periods without a break. Avoid slouching. Place a pillow or towel behind your lower back for support.
- **Computer Screen:** Place at eye level.
- **Posture:** Maintain good posture.

❾ **Avoid:** Avoid triggers that overstress the neck such as working with the neck turned or bent backward, carrying heavy objects on the head, carrying heavy objects with one arm (instead of both arms), standing on the head, contact sports, or even friendly wrestling.

❿ **Call Back If:**
- Numbness or weakness occurs.
- Bowel or bladder problems occur.
- Pain lasts for > 2 weeks.
- You become worse.

BACKGROUND

Causes

- **Muscle Strain:** Acute neck pain is often from strained neck muscles caused by sleeping in an awkward position, cradling a telephone between neck and shoulder for extended conversation, painting a ceiling, reading in bed, reaching for something that was difficult to get, sitting in front of movie theater, looking at something that requires extreme bending or turning of neck, prolonged typing, etc.
- **Muscle Tension/Spasm:** Muscle tension neck pain is one of the most common causes of acute neck pain. It is seen in every age group and is related to stressful situations in the workplace and at home. The pain may radiate into the upper back and into the scalp. Frequently, patients with this type of tension neck pain will report that the discomfort is worse toward the end of the day. Therapy for this type of pain should be directed at stress reduction, good posture, and gentle neck exercises.
- **Pharyngitis:** Pain in the front or side of the neck is usually due to a sore throat (pharyngitis) or from swollen lymph nodes.
- **Degenerative arthritis.**
- **Inflammatory arthritis** (e.g., rheumatoid arthritis).
- **Muscle aches** (myalgia) from viral syndrome, URI.
- **Poor posture.**
- **Anxiety, stress, depression.**

Serious Causes

- Acute coronary syndrome
- Meningitis
- Subarachnoid hemorrhage
- Epidural abscess
- Epidural hematoma
- Thyroiditis
- Cancer

Stiff Neck

- Callers are frequently concerned about a "stiff neck" and the possibility of meningitis.
- The stiff neck that accompanies meningitis is the result of inflammation of the spinal cord membranes. Patients with meningitis are typically unable to touch the chin to their chest because of pain.
- Patients with muscle strain or myalgia may also describe some neck stiffness. However, such patients are usually able to touch their chin to their chest but have difficulty putting the chin to each shoulder (can't rotate the neck). In addition, the neck muscles are often painful to the touch.

Caution: Cardiac Ischemia

- The most life-threatening cause of acute neck pain is cardiac ischemia.
- Rarely, patients may present with anterior neck pain as the sole symptom of a myocardial infarction. Usually there will be other associated symptoms of cardiac ischemia: chest pain, shortness of breath, nausea, and/or diaphoresis.
- Cardiac ischemia should be suspected in any patients with risk factors for cardiac disease. These include: hypertension, smoking, diabetes, hyperlipidemia, a strong family history of heart disease, and age > 50.

NEUROLOGIC DEFICIT

Definition
- Weakness or paralysis of the face, arm, or leg
- Numbness of the face, arm, or leg
- Loss of speech; garbled or confused speech
- Not due to a known traumatic injury

TRIAGE ASSESSMENT QUESTIONS

Call EMS 911 Now
- Difficult to awaken or acting confused
  (e.g., disoriented, slurred speech)
  R/O: stroke, subarachnoid hemorrhage (SAH)
- New neurologic deficit that is present NOW,
  sudden onset of ANY of the following:
  – Weakness of the face, arm, or leg on one side
    of the body
  – Numbness of the face, arm, or leg on one side
    of the body
  – Loss of speech or garbled speech
    R/O: stroke
    *(Exception: Bell palsy suspected [i.e., weakness only
    one side of the face, developing over hours to days,
    no other symptoms])*
- Sounds like a life-threatening emergency to
  the triager

See More Appropriate Protocol
- Confusion, disorientation, or hallucinations are the
  main symptom
  Go to Protocol: Confusion (Delirium) on page 86
- Dizziness is the main symptom
  Go to Protocol: Dizziness on page 128
- Followed a head injury within last 3 days
  Go to Protocol: Head Injury on page 201

Go to ED/UCC Now
(or to Office With PCP Approval)
- Headache (with neurologic deficit)
  R/O: stroke, SAH
- Can't use hand normally (e.g., hold a glass of water)
  Reason: significant deficit requiring urgent evaluation
- Can't walk or can barely walk
  Reason: significant weakness or ataxia
- Back pain with numbness (loss of sensation) in
  groin or rectal area
  R/O: cauda equina syndrome

- Unable to urinate (or only a few drops) and bladder
  feels very full
  R/O: urinary retention, cauda equina syndrome
- Loss of control of bowel or bladder
  (i.e., incontinence) of new onset
  R/O: spinal cord lesion
- Patient sounds very sick or weak to the triager
  *Reason: severe acute illness or serious complication
  suspected*

Go to Office Now
- Neurologic deficit that was brief (now gone),
  ANY of the following:
  – Weakness of the face, arm, or leg on one side of
    the body
  – Numbness of the face, arm, or leg on one side of
    the body
  – Loss of speech or garbled speech
  *Note: Transient tingling from foot or hand "falling
  asleep" from prolonged sitting or lying on arm may
  best be triaged to Home Care Advice. Use nursing
  judgment.*
- Neurologic deficit of gradual onset, ANY of the
  following:
  – Weakness of the face, arm, or leg on one side of
    the body
  – Numbness of the face, arm, or leg on one side of
    the body
  – Loss of speech or garbled speech
  R/O: brain tumor, spinal cord lesion, TIA
- Bell palsy suspected (i.e., weakness only one side
  of the face, developing over hours to days, no
  other symptoms)
  *Reason: clinical evaluation; treatment with oral
  corticosteroids may be indicated*
- Tingling (e.g., pins and needles) of the face, arm, or
  leg on one side of the body, that is present now
  *(Exceptions: chronic/recurrent symptom lasting
  > 4 weeks or tingling from known cause [e.g.,
  bumped elbow, carpal tunnel syndrome,
  pinched nerve, frostbite])*

See Today in Office

- Neck pain (with neurologic deficit)
  R/O: herniated disk
- Back pain (with neurologic deficit)
  R/O: herniated disk
- Patient wants to be seen

See Within 3 Days in Office

- Loss of speech or garbled speech is a chronic symptom (recurrent or ongoing problem lasting > 4 weeks)
- Weakness of arm or leg is a chronic symptom (recurrent or ongoing problem lasting > 4 weeks)
- Numbness or tingling in one or both hands is a chronic symptom (recurrent or ongoing problem lasting > 4 weeks)
  R/O: peripheral neuropathy, carpal tunnel syndrome
- Numbness or tingling in one or both feet is a chronic symptom (recurrent or ongoing problem lasting > 4 weeks)
  R/O: peripheral neuropathy
- Numbness or tingling on both sides of body and is a new symptom lasting > 24 hours

Home Care

- ○ Brief (now gone) tingling in hand (e.g., pins and needles) after prolonged laying on arm
- ○ Brief (now gone) tingling in foot (e.g., pins and needles) after prolonged sitting with legs crossed
- ○ Brief (now gone) numbness (or tingling or burning) in hand and fingers after bumped elbow
  R/O: "bruised funny bone"

HOME CARE ADVICE

❶ Transient Tingling in Hand (e.g., Pins and Needles) After Prolonged Lying on Arm:

- **Description:** Many people note that if they lie down for a prolonged period on an arm, the hand becomes numb. People describe this as their "hand falling asleep." Direct pressure on one of the nerves in the arm is what causes this.
- **Expected Course:** Tingling should go away after several minutes of stretching and gentle movement of the arm.

❷ Transient Tingling in Foot (e.g., Pins and Needles) After Prolonged Sitting With Legs Crossed:

- **Description:** Many people note that if they sit for a prolonged period with legs crossed, their foot becomes numb. People describe this as their "foot falling asleep." Direct pressure on nerves in the leg from sitting in an unusual position is what causes this.
- **Expected Course:** Tingling should go away after several minutes of stretching and gentle movement of the leg.

❸ Bruised "Funny Bone":

- **Description:** A direct blow to the inner side of the posterior elbow can cause numbness, tingling, and burning in the hand. The involved fingers are usually the middle, ring, and little fingers (third, fourth, and fifth). Your "funny bone" is actually a nerve (ulnar) which wraps around the posterior part of your elbow.
- **Expected Course:** Symptoms from "bruising your funny bone" usually last only a few minutes. If the symptoms last > 30 minutes or if this problem seems to happen to you frequently, you should see the doctor for evaluation.

❹ Call Back If:

- Symptoms do not go away within 30 minutes.
- You become worse.

BACKGROUND

Causes

- **Bell Palsy:** Unilateral face weakness due to a facial nerve palsy. The main symptom is a crooked smile.
- Brain tumor.
- Guillain-Barré syndrome.
- Head trauma with intracranial bleeding (e.g., epidural or subdural hematoma).
- Hemiplegic or hemisensory migraine.
- Meningitis, encephalitis.
- Multiple sclerosis.
- Neuropathy.
- Spinal cord lesion (e.g., tumor, disc protrusion, epidural abscess).
- Stroke ("brain attack," cerebrovascular accident, CVA).
- Subarachnoid hemorrhage.
- Transient ischemic attack (TIA).
- **Todd Paralysis:** Temporary unilateral weakness after a seizure.
- Transverse myelitis.

Stroke ("Brain Attack")

- **"Brain attack"** is a new layperson term being used to describe a stroke. This term originated from the need to emphasize to patients the urgency of a stroke and the need for immediate evaluation.
- **Signs:** Signs of a brain attack include sudden onset of weakness or numbness of one side of the body, sudden loss of vision, sudden loss of speech, or sudden dizziness and unsteadiness. With thrombotic or embolic strokes there is usually minimal or no headache.
- **Cause:** A brain attack occurs when one of the blood vessels to the brain becomes blocked. This keeps blood from flowing to that part of the brain. Permanent damage can result.
- **Treatment—Thrombolytic (e.g., tPA, Alteplase):** There are thrombolytic medications ("clot-busters") that can be used to treat some patients with a brain attack. However, the thrombolytic must be given within 3-4½ hours of symptom onset. Because of this narrow window only about 2%-3% of all stroke patients qualify to receive this medication.

Transient Ischemic Attack (TIA)

- **Definition:** Some patients have a warning attack in which there are symptoms of a stroke, but the symptoms go away after a few minutes or hours.
- **Signs:** Signs of a TIA are the same as for a stroke. They include sudden onset of weakness or numbness of one side of the body, sudden loss of vision, sudden loss of speech, or sudden dizziness and unsteadiness.
- **Cause:** A TIA occurs when one of the blood vessels to the brain becomes temporarily blocked. This keeps blood from flowing to that part of the brain.
- **Triage:** These patients require urgent evaluation as they remain at risk for having a permanent stroke.

Bell Palsy

- **Definition:** Bell palsy is a paralysis of a facial nerve that results in muscle weakness on one side of the face.
- **Symptoms:** Individuals with Bell palsy describe the onset of weakness limited to one side of the face that develops over a couple hours to a couple days. Sometimes, just like a stroke, an individual may first notice the facial weakness on awakening in the morning when they look in the mirror. The eyelids

on the affected side may become weak and the person may not be able to close that eye completely. Individuals may also sometimes have problems with drooling from the corner of the mouth on the affected side.

- **Diagnosis:** There is no specific laboratory test or radiograph that can diagnose Bell palsy. Usually, it is a clinical diagnosis made by a physician after a careful history and examination.
- **Cause:** It is thought that Bell palsy is caused by an inflammation of the facial nerve. The cause of this inflammation is unknown. However, there has been some recent research suggesting the possibility that the herpes simplex virus (human herpesvirus type 1) may be the cause.
- **Expected Course:** The symptoms typically worsen over the first couple days and peak within 1 week. Approximately 75% of people will recover over 1-2 months. Unfortunately, some people are left with permanent facial weakness.
- **Treatment:** Treatment with corticosteroids (e.g., prednisone, prednisolone) appears to improve the outcome and the speed of recovery. Some doctors will also prescribe antiviral therapy with acyclovir (Zovirax) or valacyclovir (Valtrex). However, a recent Cochrane analysis concluded that antiviral therapy provided no additional benefit.
- **Triage:** These patients usually require urgent or emergent evaluation, as it is usually difficult over the phone to be able to clearly distinguish Bell palsy from a stroke.

The ABCD² Score and Risk of Stroke

- The **ABCD^2 score** is a clinical score that is used to determine the risk for a stroke within the first week following a TIA.
- **Age:** < 60 years (0 points), ≥ 60 years (1 point).
- **Blood Pressure:** Normal (0 points), > 139/89 (1 point).
- **Clinical Features:** Other (0 points), speech disturbance (1 point), unilateral weakness (2 points).
- **Duration of TIA:** < 10 minutes (0 points), 10-59 minutes (1 point), 60+ minutes (2 points).
- **Diabetes:** No diabetes (0 points), diabetes (1 point).
- **Interpretation:** 1-3 points (low; 1.2% risk of stroke), 4-5 points (moderate; 5.9%), 6-7 points (high; 11.7%).

NOSE INJURY

Definition
- Injuries to the inside or outside of the nose

TRIAGE ASSESSMENT QUESTIONS

Call EMS 911 Now
- ● Knocked out (unconscious) > 1 minute
  R/O: concussion
- ● Major bleeding (actively dripping or spurting) that can't be stopped
  First Aid: Apply direct pressure to the nose, lean forward.
- ● Sounds like a life-threatening emergency to the triager

See More Appropriate Protocol
- ● Wound looks infected
  Go to Protocol: Wound Infection on page 443
- ● Nosebleed not from trauma
  Go to Protocol: Nosebleed on page 305

Go to ED/UCC Now
(or to Office With PCP Approval)
- ● Nosebleed won't stop after 10 minutes of pinching the nostrils closed (applied twice)
- ● Black-and-blue skin around both eyes (bilateral periorbital ecchymosis)
  R/O: nasal fracture, ethmoid fracture, or raccoon eyes from basilar skull fracture
- ● Clear fluid is dripping from the nose
- ● Skin is split open or gaping (length > ¼" or 6 mm)
  Reason: may need laceration repair (e.g., sutures)
- ● Sounds like a serious injury to the triager

Go to Office Now
- ● Very deformed or crooked nose
  R/O: fracture
- ● Breathing through the nose is blocked on one side or both sides
  R/O: nasal septal hematoma, significant fracture
- ● Fever and increasing nose pain, ≥ 2 days after injury
  R/O: nasal septal abscess

See Today in Office
- ● SEVERE pain (e.g., excruciating)
- ● Tip of nose is very tender
- ● Nosebleed and taking Coumadin (warfarin) or other strong blood thinner, or known bleeding disorder (e.g., thrombocytopenia)
  Reason: higher risk of serious bleeding; may need testing of INR, prothrombin time, or platelet count
  Note: Besides Coumadin, other strong blood thinners include Arixtra (fondaparinux), Eliquis (apixaban), Pradaxa (dabigatran), and Xarelto (rivaroxaban).
- ● Patient wants to be seen

See Today or Tomorrow in Office
- ● Suspicious history for the injury
  R/O: domestic violence or elder abuse
- ● Wound and no tetanus booster in > 5 years (or > 10 years for clean cuts)
  Reason: may need a tetanus booster shot (vaccine)

See Within 3 Days in Office
- ● After 5 days and shape of the nose has not returned to normal
  R/O: fracture with deformity

Home Care
- ○ Minor nose injury
  R/O: bruise, superficial cut, or abrasion
  R/O: nondisplaced fracture

HOME CARE ADVICE

Treatment of a Minor Bruise

❶ **Reassurance—Direct Blow (Contusion, Bruise):**
- A direct blow to your nose can cause a contusion. Contusion is the medical term for bruise.
- Symptoms are pain, swelling, and/or bruising. Sometimes there can be a nosebleed.
- Sometimes after a nose injury there can be mild bruising around the eye. This is also called a black eye.
- *Here is some care advice that should help.*

❷ Nosebleed:
- Place your thumb and index finger over each side of the soft lower portion of the nose.
- Firmly pinch the nostrils together for 10-15 minutes.

❸ Apply a Cold Pack:
- Apply a cold pack or an ice bag (wrapped in a moist towel) to the area for 20 minutes. Repeat in 1 hour, then every 4 hours while awake.
- Continue this for the first 48 hours after an injury.
- This will help decrease pain and swelling.

❹ Concerns About a Broken (Fractured) Nose:
- Not all swollen noses are broken (have a fracture).
- Even if the nose is broken, in most cases, the only treatment that is needed is cold packs and pain medicine.
- Surgery to fix the nose is only needed when the nose is very deformed. It is common to delay fixing nose fractures until the swelling has decreased.
- Looking at the nose after the swelling is gone (day 5-7) is the best way to tell if it is broken and if it is deformed.
- X-rays are often not helpful because 1) minor fractures are treated the same as a bruise and 2) injuries to the cartilage do not show up on x-ray.

❺ Expected Course:
- Pain, swelling, and bruising usually start to get better 2-3 days after an injury.
- Swelling most often is gone after 1 week.
- Bruises fade away slowly over 1-2 weeks.
- It may take 2 weeks for the pain and tenderness to go away.

❻ Call Back If:
- Pain becomes severe.
- Shape of the nose has not returned to normal after 5 days.
- Signs of infection occur (a yellow discharge, increasing tenderness, or fever).
- You become worse.

Treatment of a Small Cut or Scrape

❶ Reassurance—Superficial Laceration (Cut or Scratch) or Abrasion (Scrape):
- This sounds like a small cut or scrape that we can treat at home.
- *Here is some care advice that should help.*

❷ Bleeding: Apply direct pressure for 10 minutes with a sterile gauze to stop any bleeding.

❸ Cleaning the Wound:
- Wash the wound with soap and water for 5 minutes.
- For any dirt, scrub gently with a washcloth.
- For any bleeding, apply direct pressure with a sterile gauze or clean cloth for 10 minutes.

❹ Antibiotic Ointment:
- Apply an antibiotic ointment (e.g., OTC bacitracin), covered by a Band-Aid or dressing. Change daily or if it becomes wet.
- Option: A Telfa dressing won't stick to the wound when it is removed.
- Option: Another option is to use a liquid skin bandage that only needs to be applied once. Don't use antibiotic ointment if you use a liquid skin bandage.

❺ Liquid Skin Bandage:
- You can use a liquid skin bandage instead of antibiotic ointment and a dressing or a Band-Aid.
- **Benefits:** Liquid skin bandage has several benefits when compared with a regular bandage (e.g., a dressing or a Band-Aid). You only need to put a liquid bandage on once to minor cuts and scrapes. It helps stop minor bleeding. It seals the wound and may promote faster healing and lower infection rates. However, it also costs more.
- **How to Use It:** First clean and dry the wound. You put on the liquid as spray or with a swab. It dries in < 1 minute and usually lasts a week. You can get it wet.
- **Examples:** Liquid skin bandage is available over the counter. Examples are Band-Aid Liquid Bandage, New Skin, Curad Spray Bandage, and 3M No Sting Liquid Bandage Spray.

❻ Call Back If:
- Dirt is still present in the wound after scrubbing.
- Looks infected (pus, redness).
- Doesn't heal within 10 days.
- You become worse.

Over-the-counter Pain Medicines

❶ Pain Medicines:

- For pain relief, you can take either acetaminophen, ibuprofen, or naproxen.
- They are over-the-counter (OTC) pain drugs. You can buy them at the drugstore.

Acetaminophen (e.g., Tylenol):

- **Regular Strength Tylenol:** Take 650 mg (two 325 mg pills) by mouth every 4-6 hours as needed. Each Regular Strength Tylenol pill has 325 mg of acetaminophen.
- **Extra Strength Tylenol:** Take 1,000 mg (two 500 mg pills) every 8 hours as needed. Each Extra Strength Tylenol pill has 500 mg of acetaminophen.
- The most you should take each day is 3,000 mg (10 Regular Strength or 6 Extra Strength pills a day).

Ibuprofen (e.g., Motrin, Advil):

- Take 400 mg (two 200 mg pills) by mouth every 6 hours.
- Another choice is to take 600 mg (three 200 mg pills) by mouth every 8 hours.
- The most you should take each day is 1,200 mg (six 200 mg pills), unless your doctor has told you to take more.

Naproxen (e.g., Aleve):

- Take 220 mg (one 220 mg pill) by mouth every 8 hours as needed. You may take 440 mg (two 220 mg pills) for your first dose.
- The most you should take each day is 660 mg (three 220 mg pills a day), unless your doctor has told you to take more.

❷ Pain Medicines—Extra Notes:

- Use the lowest amount of medicine that makes your pain better.
- Acetaminophen is thought to be safer than ibuprofen or naproxen in people > 65 years old. Acetaminophen is in many OTC and prescription medicines. It might be in more than one medicine that you are taking. You need to be careful and not take an overdose. An acetaminophen over-dose can hurt the liver.
- McNeil, the company that makes Tylenol, has different dosage instructions for Tylenol in Canada and the United States. In Canada, the maximum recommended dose per day is 4,000 mg or 12 Regular Strength (325 mg) pills. In the United States, McNeil recommends a maximum dose of 10 Regular Strength (325 mg) pills.
- CAUTION: Do not take acetaminophen if you have liver disease.
- CAUTION: Do not take ibuprofen or naproxen if you have stomach problems, have kidney disease, are pregnant, or have been told by your doctor to avoid this type of anti-inflammatory drug. Do not take ibuprofen or naproxen for > 7 days without consulting your doctor.
- *Before taking any medicine, read all the instructions on the package.*

❸ Call Back If:

- You have more questions.
- You become worse.

FIRST AID

First Aid Advice for Bleeding:

Apply direct pressure to the entire wound with a clean cloth.

First Aid Advice for Nosebleed:

- Placing your thumb and index finger over each side of the soft lower portion of the nose, firmly pinch the nostrils together. Pinch the nostrils together for 10-15 minutes.
- Lean slightly forward; this keeps the blood from trickling down the back of your throat.

First Aid Advice for Penetrating Object:

If penetrating object is still in place, don't remove it. *Reason: Removal could increase bleeding.*

First Aid Advice for Shock:

Lie down with the feet elevated.

BACKGROUND

Key Points

- Due to the prominence of the nose in the midface, it is commonly injured in individuals with facial trauma.
- Patients with > 1 site of injury may require you to use ≥ 2 Trauma protocols to ensure that you have recommended the safest disposition. Use your nursing judgment.

Types of Nose Injuries

- **Bloody nose** without a fracture.
- **Swelling and bruising of the nose** without a fracture.
- **Nasal septal hematoma.**
- **Fracture of the Nose:** Severe fractures of the nose (e.g., crooked nose) are usually reset the same day in the operating room. Most surgeons don't repair mild fractures until day 5-7 post-injury.

Nasal Septal Hematoma

- **Definition:** A blood clot that develops between the cartilage of the nasal septum and the perichondrium. It can be unilateral or bilateral. This is a rare but urgent ENT problem.
- **Symptoms:** Blockage of nasal passage on one side (or both sides) with inability to breathe through that side. Another clue is severe tenderness of the tip of the nose, especially when it is pressed upward.
- **Treatment:** Drainage using a needle or an incision, followed by nasal packing.
- **Complications:** A septal hematoma can cause pressure necrosis of the nasal cartilage, resulting in nasal deformity or perforated septum. This can occur if it is untreated for a period of days. A nasal septal abscess is a very rare complication; it is a superinfection of a septal hematoma. Symptoms are fever and increasing pain. This is an emergent ENT problem (ie, see within 4 hours).
- **Time After Presentation of Injury:** Immediately to 14 days (mean 5.9 days) (Savage). Therefore, the triage nurse needs to tell the caller to watch for symptoms of delayed onset of septal hematoma.

What Cuts Need to Be Sutured?

- Any cut that is split open or gaping probably needs sutures (or skin glue).
- Cuts on the nose > ¼" (6 mm) usually need sutures.
- Any open wound that may need sutures should be evaluated by a physician regardless of the time that has passed since the initial injury.

When Does an Adult Need a Tetanus Booster (Tetanus Shot)?

- **Clean Cuts and Scrapes—Tetanus Booster Needed Every 10 Years:** Patients with clean minor wounds AND who have previously had ≥ 3 tetanus shots (full series) need a booster every 10 years. Examples of minor wounds include a superficial abrasion or a shallow cut from a clean knife blade. Obtain booster within 72 hours.
- **Dirty Wounds—Tetanus Booster Needed Every 5 Years:** Patients with dirty wounds need a booster if it has been > 5 years since the last booster. Examples of dirty wounds include those contaminated with soil, feces, and/or saliva and more serious wounds from deep punctures, crushing, and burns. Obtain booster within 72 hours.

Caution: Associated Head and Neck Trauma

- Head trauma should be considered in all patients with a facial injury. Signs of significant head injury include loss of consciousness, amnesia, unsteady walking, confusion, and slurred speech.
- Neck trauma should also be considered in all patients with a facial injury. Concerning findings include numbness, weakness, and neck pain.
- After using the Nose Injury protocol, if the triager or caller has remaining concerns about head or neck trauma, the patient also should be triaged using the Head Injury and/or Neck Injury protocols on pages 201 and 290, respectively.

NOSEBLEED

Definition
- Bleeding from one or both nostrils
- Not due to a traumatic injury
- Includes follow-up calls about nasal packing placed by health care providers to control bleeding

TRIAGE ASSESSMENT QUESTIONS

Call EMS 911 Now
- ● Fainted (passed out) or too weak to stand following large blood loss
  R/O: impending shock
  First Aid: Lie down with the feet elevated.
- ● Sounds like a life-threatening emergency to the triager

See More Appropriate Protocol
- ● Nosebleed followed nose injury
  Go to Protocol: Nose Injury on page 301

Go to ED/UCC Now
(or to Office With PCP Approval)
- ● Bleeding present > 30 minutes and using correct method of direct pressure
  R/O: posterior nosebleed, coagulopathy
- ● Bleeding now and second call after being instructed in correct technique of direct pressure
  R/O: posterior nosebleed, coagulopathy
- ● Light-headedness or dizziness
  R/O: excessive blood loss
- ● Pale skin (pallor) of new onset or worsening
  R/O: excessive blood loss
- ● Has nasal packing (inserted by health care provider to control bleeding) and now has new rash
  R/O: toxic shock syndrome
- ● Has nasal packing and now has bleeding around the packing
  (Exception: few drops or ooze)
  Reason: may need to be repacked or have nasal cautery
- ● Patient sounds very sick or weak to the triager
  Reason: severe acute illness or serious complication suspected

Go to Office Now
- ● Large amount of blood has been lost (e.g., 1 cup)
  R/O: anemia

See Today in Office
- ◐ Bleeding recurs ≥ 3 times in 24 hours despite direct pressure
- ◐ Taking Coumadin (warfarin) or other strong blood thinner, or known bleeding disorder (e.g., thrombocytopenia)
  Reason: higher risk of serious bleeding; may need testing of INR, prothrombin time, or platelet count
  Note: Besides Coumadin, other strong blood thinners include Arixtra (fondaparinux), Eliquis (apixaban), Pradaxa (dabigatran), and Xarelto (rivaroxaban).
- ◐ Has skin bruises or bleeding gums that are not caused by an injury
  R/O: bleeding disorder
- ◐ Has nasal packing and now has fever > 100.5° F (38.1° C)
  R/O: sinusitis
- ◐ Patient wants to be seen

See Within 3 Days in Office
- ◐ Has nasal packing (inserted by health care provider to control bleeding)
  Reason: nasal packing needs removal 2-3 days after placement

See Within 2 Weeks in Office
- ◐ Hard-to-stop nosebleeds are a chronic symptom (recurrent or ongoing AND lasting > 4 weeks)
  R/O: bleeding disorder
- ◐ Easy bleeding present in other family members

Home Care
- ○ Mild-moderate nosebleed and bleeding has stopped now
- ○ Bleeding present < 30 minutes and using correct method of direct pressure
- ○ Nosebleed and needs instruction in correct technique of applying direct pressure

HOME CARE ADVICE

❶ Reassurance:
- Nosebleeds are common.
- It sounds like a routine nosebleed that we can treat at home.
- You should be able to stop the bleeding if you use the correct technique.
- Remember to sit up and lean forward to keep the blood from running down the back of your throat.

❷ Treating a Nosebleed—Pinch the Nostrils:
- First blow the nose to clear out any large clots.
- Sit up and lean forward.
  (Reason: Blood makes people choke if they lean backward.)
- Gently squeeze the soft parts of the lower nose (nostrils) together. Use your thumb and your index finger in a pinching manner. Do this for 15 minutes. Use a clock or watch to measure the time. Your goal is to apply continuous pressure to the bleeding point.
- If the bleeding does not stop after 15 minutes of squeezing, move your point of pressure and do this again for another 15 minutes.

❸ Treating a Nosebleed—Inserting a Gauze With Decongestant Nose Drops:
- If applying pressure fails, insert a gauze wet with decongestant nose drops (or petroleum jelly). *(Reason: The gauze helps to apply pressure and the nose drops shrink the blood vessels.)*
- Then repeat the process of gently squeezing the lower nose for 10 minutes.
- **Example Decongestant Medication:** Afrin (oxymetazoline) nasal spray is available over the counter and is a nasal decongestant.

❹ Caution—Nasal Decongestants:
- Do not take these medications if you have high blood pressure, heart disease, prostate problems, or an overactive thyroid.
- Do not take these medications if you are pregnant.
- Do not take these medications if you have used a monoamine oxidase (MAO) inhibitor such as isocarboxazid (Marplan), phenelzine (Nardil), rasagiline (Azilect), selegiline (Eldepryl, Emsam), or tranylcypromine (Parnate) in the past 2 weeks. Life-threatening side effects can occur.
- Do not use these medications for > 3 days. *(Reason: rebound nasal congestion)*

❺ Prevention:
- Dry air in your house or workplace can increase the chance of nosebleeds occurring. If the air is dry, use a humidifier in your bedroom to keep the nose from drying out. You can also apply petroleum jelly to the center wall (septum) inside the nose twice daily to reduce cracking and to promote healing.
- Bleeding can start again if you rub your nose or blow the nose too hard. Avoid touching your nose and nose picking. Avoid blowing the nose.
- Do not take aspirin or other anti-inflammatory medications (e.g., ibuprofen, naproxen) unless you have been instructed to by your physician.

❻ Expected Course:
- > 99% of nosebleeds will stop following 15 minutes of direct pressure if you press on the right spot.
- After swallowing blood from a nosebleed, you may feel nauseated because the blood can irritate your stomach. You may also later pass a dark stool that contains the blood.

❼ Call Back If:
- Nosebleed lasts > 30 minutes with using direct pressure.
- Light-headedness or weakness occurs.
- Nosebleeds become worse.
- You become worse.

FIRST AID

First Aid Advice for Nosebleed:

- First blow the nose to clear out any large blood clots.
- Placing your thumb and index finger over each side of the soft lower portion of the nose, firmly pinch the nostrils together. Pinch the nostrils together for 10-15 minutes.
- Lean slightly forward; this keeps the blood from trickling down the back of your throat.

BACKGROUND

Key Points

- Most nosebleeds (90%) originate from the anterior nasal septum.
- Most nosebleeds will stop with correctly applied pressure over the bleeding area. The correct method is to squeeze the soft parts of the nose using the thumb and index finger, thus applying pressure to the anterior nasal septum. Hold for 10-15 minutes.
- Leading risk factors for nosebleeds include upper respiratory infections (URIs) and nose picking.
- There is a higher incidence of nosebleeds in the 60- to 80-year-old age group. Individuals in this age group often have a couple risk factors for bleeding. A typical adult caller with a nosebleed might be 72, hypertensive, and exposed to the dry air of winter.

Risk Factors

- **Environmental:** Environmental factors include temperature and dryness of the air.
- **Local:** Local factors include URI, nasal drug inhalation, nasal tumors, septal deviation, too vigorous nose blowing, and nose picking.
- **Systemic:** Systemic factors include hypertension, arteriosclerosis, and coagulopathies.
- **Medications:** Certain medications can increase bleeding: aspirin, NSAIDs (e.g., ibuprofen, naproxen), heparin, Coumadin, Plavix (clopidogrel).

PENIS AND SCROTUM SYMPTOMS

Definition
- Penis symptoms include rash, pain, discharge, itching, and swelling.
- Scrotum symptoms include rash and itching.
- Not due to a traumatic injury.

TRIAGE ASSESSMENT QUESTIONS

Call EMS 911 Now
- Sounds like a life-threatening emergency to the triager

See More Appropriate Protocol
- Pain or burning with passing urine is the main symptom
  Go to Protocol: Urination Pain (Male) on page 421
- Pubic lice suspected
  Go to Protocol: Pubic Lice on page 317
- STI exposure and prevention, question about
  Go to Protocol: STI Exposure and Prevention on page 377

Go to ED/UCC Now
(or to Office With PCP Approval)
- Large amount of blood from end of penis
  R/O: urinary retention, UTI
- Foreskin pulled back and stuck (not circumcised)
  R/O: paraphimosis
- Fever > 100.5° F (38.1° C)
  R/O: UTI, epididymitis
- Unable to urinate (or only a few drops) and bladder feels very full
  R/O: acute urinary retention
- Painful erection present > 2 hours
  R/O: priapism
- Patient sounds very sick or weak to the triager
  Reason: severe acute illness or serious complication suspected

Go to Office Now
- SEVERE pain or burning with passing urine
  R/O: UTI, severe urethritis

- Entire penis is swollen (i.e., edema)
  R/O: CHF, anasarca
- Looks infected (e.g., draining sore, spreading redness)
  R/O: cellulitis

See Today in Office
- Pain or burning with passing urine
  R/O: UTI, urethritis
- Blood in urine (red, pink, or tea-colored)
  R/O: tumor, kidney stone
- Pus (white, yellow) or bloody discharge from end of penis
  R/O: Gonococcal or chlamydia urethritis, UTI
- Swollen foreskin (not circumcised)
  R/O: balanoposthitis
- Tiny water blisters rash, ≥ 3
  R/O: herpes simplex, pustules
- Antibiotic treatment > 3 days for STI (e.g., penile discharge from gonorrhea, chlamydia) and painful urination not improved
  R/O: resistant organism
- Patient wants to be seen

See Today or Tomorrow in Office
- SEVERE itching (i.e., interferes with work or school)
  R/O: poison ivy, pubic lice
- Painless rash (e.g., redness, tiny bumps, sore) present > 24 hours
  R/O: contact dermatitis, skin cancer, genital warts
- Patient is worried about an STI
  Reason: relieve fear and prevent spread of STI
- ALL other penis/scrotum symptoms
  (Exception: painless rash < 24 hours' duration)
  R/O: skin cancer, pubic lice

Home Care
- Painless rash (e.g., mild redness, tiny bumps, small sore) present < 24 hours
  R/O: contact dermatitis, abrasion

HOME CARE ADVICE

❶ Causes of Mild Rash:
- Irritation from a chemical product: perfumed soaps, latex condoms.
- Irritation from a plant (e.g., poison ivy, evergreen), chemicals (e.g., insecticides), fiberglass, detergents.
- Early finding of sexually transmitted infection (STI).
- Small friction burns can occur from intercourse (if inadequate lubrication).

❷ Cleaning: Wash the area once thoroughly with unscented soap and water to remove any irritants.

❸ Genital Hygiene:
- Keep your penis and scrotal area clean. Wash once daily with unscented soap and water.
- Keep your penis and scrotal area dry. Wear cotton underwear.

❹ Call Back If:
- Rash spreads or becomes worse.
- Rash lasts > 1 day.
- Fever occurs.
- You become worse.

BACKGROUND

Causes of Burning With Urination
- Bladder infection
- Blood in the urine
- Sexually transmitted infections (STIs) like gonorrhea, chlamydia

Causes of Discharge
- STIs (gonorrhea, chlamydia)

Causes of Itching
- Contact dermatitis (latex condoms)
- Irritation from a chemical product like perfumed soaps or spermicides
- Irritation from a plant, fiberglass, or detergent
- Poison ivy, oak, or sumac rash
- Skin cancer
- Skin disorders/rashes (psoriasis, eczema, and drug rashes)
- STIs (pubic lice)

Causes of Pain
- Bladder infection
- Injury
- Priapism
- STIs

Causes of Rash
- Contact dermatitis (latex condoms, lubricants, spermicides, and perfumed soaps)
- Poison ivy, oak, or sumac rash
- Rash after sex or masturbation (lack of lubrication)
- Skin cancer
- Skin disorders/rashes (psoriasis, eczema, and drug rashes)
- STIs (herpes)

Causes of Penis Swelling
- Priapism

Causes of Scrotal Swelling
- Cancer
- Edema, fluid retention (e.g., CHF)
- Hernia
- Orchitis (testicle infection)

What Is Priapism?
This is an erection that lasts > 4 hours. It is unwanted and often painful. It can be caused by sickle cell anemia. Certain drugs can also have this side effect. It may need to be treated in a hospital.

Erectile Dysfunction
- **Definition:** Erectile dysfunction is defined as an inability to achieve or maintain an erection. Approximately 40% of men between the ages of 40 and 70 have problems with erectile dysfunction.
- **Causes:** In most cases there is a medical (organic, non-psychiatric) cause. The main cause is atherosclerotic disease and, thus, risk factors are similar to those for heart disease (hypertension, obesity, smoking, diabetes). Other medical causes include neurological (spinal cord injury, cerebral disease), hormonal (e.g., hypothyroidism), and pharmacologic (especially antihypertensive medications).

PDE5 Inhibitor Drugs for Erectile Dysfunction
- There are 3 oral drugs that are now available by prescription for treatment of erectile dysfunction: Viagra (sildenafil), Levitra (vardenafil), and Cialis (tadalafil).
- These 3 medicines are in a class called phosphodiesterase (PDE5) inhibitors.
- **Side Effects:** Priapism (very rare), vision loss in one eye (very rare), vision changes (e.g., changes in color), headache, indigestion, flushing.
- **Warnings:** Using PDE5 drugs and nitrates at the same time can cause a sudden and possibly serious drop in blood pressure. Men who use PDE5 drugs should not take any medicines called "nitrates" or "nitroglycerin." For similar reasons, recreational drugs called "poppers," like amyl nitrate and butyl nitrate, must be avoided.

POISON IVY/OAK/SUMAC

Definition
- A very itchy, blistering rash caused by contact with the poison ivy plant or by contact with poison oak or poison sumac.
- *Use this protocol only if the patient has symptoms that match Poison Ivy.*

Symptoms
- The rash is extremely itchy.
- Localized redness, swelling, and weeping blisters.
- Rash is located on exposed body surfaces (e.g., hands) or areas touched by the hands (e.g., face or genitals).

TRIAGE ASSESSMENT QUESTIONS

See More Appropriate Protocol
- ● Doesn't match the SYMPTOMS of poison ivy, oak, or sumac
  Go to Protocol: Rash or Redness, Localized on page 326

Go to ED Now
- ● Difficulty breathing or severe coughing following exposure to burning weeds

Go to ED/UCC Now
(or to Office With PCP Approval)
- ● Patient sounds very sick or weak to the triager
  Reason: severe acute illness or serious complication suspected

Go to Office Now
- ● Fever and bright red area or streak (from open poison ivy sores)
  R/O: cellulitis, lymphangitis
- ● Increasing redness around poison ivy and > 2" (5 cm)
  R/O: cellulitis

See Today in Office
- ● SEVERE itching interferes with normal activities (e.g., work or school) or prevents sleep
  Reason: probably needs prednisone
- ● Rash involves > ¼ of the body
  Reason: probably needs prednisone

- ● Face, eyes, lips, or genitals are involved
  Reason: may need oral prednisone if more than a small area of rash
- ● Big blisters or oozing sores
- ● Severe poison ivy reaction in the past
- ● Taking oral steroids > 24 hours and rash becoming worse
  R/O: wrong diagnosis
- ● Patient wants to be seen

See Today or Tomorrow in Office
- ● Poison ivy rash lasts > 3 weeks
  R/O: wrong diagnosis

Home Care
- ○ Poison ivy, oak, or sumac with no complications

HOME CARE ADVICE

❶ Hydrocortisone Cream for Itching:
- Put 1% hydrocortisone cream on the itchy area(s) 3 times a day. Use it for 5 days. This will help decrease the itching.
- This is an over-the-counter (OTC) drug. You can buy it at the drugstore.
- Some people like to keep the cream in the refrigerator. It feels even better if the cream is used when it is cold.
- CAUTION: Do not use hydrocortisone cream for > 1 week without talking to your doctor.
- *Read the instructions and warnings on the package insert for all medicines you take.*

❷ Apply Cold to the Area: Soak the involved area in cool water for 20 minutes or massage it with an ice cube as often as necessary to reduce itching and oozing.

❸ Antihistamine Medicine for Itching:
- Take an antihistamine by mouth to reduce the itching.
- Diphenhydramine (Benadryl) is a good choice. The adult dosage of Benadryl is 25-50 mg by mouth and you can take it up to 4 times a day.
- Another OTC antihistamine that causes less sleepiness is loratadine (e.g., Alavert or Claritin). Alavert is not available in Canada.
- *Before taking any medicine, read all the instructions on the package.*

❹ Caution—Antihistamines:
- Examples include diphenhydramine (Benadryl) and chlorpheniramine (Chlor-Trimeton, Chlor-Tripolon).
- May cause sleepiness. Do not drink alcohol, drive, or operate dangerous machinery while taking antihistamines.
- Do not take these medicines if you have prostate problems.

❺ Avoid Scratching: Cut your fingernails short and try not to scratch so as to prevent a secondary infection from bacteria.

❻ New Blisters Appear: If new blisters occur several days after the first ones, you probably have had ongoing contact with the irritating plant oil. To prevent recurrences, bathe all dogs and wash all clothes and shoes that were with you on the day of exposure.

❼ Contagiousness: Poison ivy or oak is not contagious to others.

❽ Expected Course: Usually lasts 2 weeks. Treatment reduces the severity of the symptoms, not how long they last.

❾ Call Back If:
- Rash lasts > 3 weeks.
- It looks infected.
- You become worse.

BACKGROUND

Key Points
- Poison ivy, oak, and sumac are 3 plants that can cause an itchy red rash in sensitive individuals. The oil contained in the plant leaves irritates the skin. The redness and blistering from the rash are often arranged in streaks or lines, because the leaves brush across the body in a line as an individual walks past.
- **Onset:** Following a first-time exposure, the onset time for the rash is 1-2 weeks. For recurrences, the onset is 8-48 hours after the individual was in a forest or field.

Preventing the Rash
- **Avoid Exposure:** Avoid exposure to these plants, especially if you have had a bad reaction in the past.
- **Wash Skin:** If you are exposed, remove the irritating plant oil from your skin as soon as possible. Wash the exposed part of your body with soap and water within 30 minutes. Wash your clothes in warm soapy water.

Rule of 9s for Estimating Body Surface Area (BSA):
Each part of the body contributes a predictable portion of the total BSA:
- **Head and Neck:** 9%
- **Each Arm:** 9%
- **Anterior Chest and Abdomen:** 18%
- **Entire Back:** 18%
- **Each Leg:** 18%
- **Genital Region:** 1%

Wild Parsnip Photodermatitis
- **Definition:** The juice (sap) from broken stems and leaves of the wild parsnip can cause a photosensitivity rash in everyone. It is a 2-step reaction. First, the juice comes into contact with skin. Second, that area of skin is exposed to daylight (sun or cloudy day).
- **Symptoms:** Approximately 24-48 hours after wild parsnip juice and light exposure, a painful localized rash with blisters appears on the area of the skin that was exposed to the juice. Of note, while the rash of poison ivy is much itchier, the rash from wild parsnip is more painful and burning.
- **Expected Course:** Rash usually fades after a couple days.
- **Treatment:** None known.
- **Complications:** Can leave a scar at the site.
- **Prevention:** Learn what the plant looks like. Avoid contact. Wash exposed surfaces afterward. Avoid any sun exposure for 2 days after skin contact or wear sun-protecting clothing.
- **Internet Resources:** A nicely written article on this is available at: http://dnr.wi.gov/wnrmag/html/stories/1999/jun99/parsnip.htm.
- Photographs of wild parsnip are present on the Wisconsin Botanical Information System at: http://wisflora.botany.wisc.edu/cgi-bin/detail.cgi?SpCode=PASSAT.

POISONING

Definition
- Swallows a drug, chemical, plant, or other possibly poisonous substance.
- Occasionally, a poisonous gas is absorbed across the lungs or irritates the lungs (e.g., ammonia, chlorine).
- Rarely, a poisonous chemical is absorbed across the skin (e.g., organophosphates found in some insecticides).

Excluded:
- **Chemical in Eye:** Use Eye, Chemical In protocol on page 150.

TRIAGE ASSESSMENT QUESTIONS

Call EMS 911 Now
- SEVERE difficulty breathing (e.g., struggling for each breath, speaks in single words)
  R/O: respiratory failure, hypoxia
- Bluish (or gray) lips or face
  R/O: cyanosis and need for oxygen
- Seizure
- Difficult to awaken or acting confused (e.g., disoriented, slurred speech)
  R/O: overdose, shock
- Shock suspected (e.g., cold/pale/clammy skin, too weak to stand, low BP, rapid pulse)
  R/O: shock
  First Aid: Lie down with the feet elevated.
- Intentional overdose and suicidal thoughts or ideas
  Reason: suicidal ideation/gesture/attempt
- Suicide attempt, known or suspected
  Reason: suicidal ideation/gesture/attempt
- Sounds like a life-threatening emergency to the triager

See More Appropriate Protocol
- Chemical in eye
  Go to Protocol: Eye, Chemical In on page 150

Go to ED Now
- HARMFUL SUBSTANCE or ACID or ALKALI ingestion (e.g., toilet cleaners, drain cleaners, lye, Clinitest tablets, ammonia, bleaches) AND any symptoms (e.g., mouth pain, sore throat, breathing difficulty)
- PETROLEUM PRODUCT ingestion (e.g., kerosene, gasoline, benzene, furniture polish, lighter fluid) AND any symptoms (e.g., breathing difficulty, coughing, vomiting)
- Poison Center advised caller to go to ED and caller seeking second opinion
- Patient sounds very sick or weak to the triager
  Reason: harmful overdose suspected

Call Poison Center Now
- HARMFUL SUBSTANCE or ACID or ALKALI ingestion (e.g., toilet cleaners, drain cleaners, lye, Clinitest tablets, ammonia, bleaches) AND NO symptoms
- PETROLEUM PRODUCT ingestion (e.g., kerosene, gasoline, benzene, furniture polish, lighter fluid) AND NO symptoms
- Carbon monoxide exposure suspected
- Mercury spill (e.g., broken glass thermometer, broken spiral CFL)
- DOUBLE DOSE (an extra dose or lesser amount) of over-the-counter (OTC) drug and any symptoms (e.g., dizziness, nausea, pain, sleepiness)
- DOUBLE DOSE (an extra dose or lesser amount) of prescription drug and any symptoms (e.g., dizziness, nausea, pain, sleepiness)
- ALL OTHER POTENTIALLY HARMFUL SUBSTANCES (e.g., nearly all chemicals, plants, more than a double dose of a drug)
  (Exception: known harmless substances and asymptomatic double dose of OTC or prescription drug)
- Triager unable to answer question
- Patient or caller provides unclear information about type or amount of substance

Discuss With PCP and Callback by Nurse Within 1 Hour

● DOUBLE DOSE (an extra dose or lesser amount) of prescription drug and NO symptoms
(Exception: double dose of antibiotic [asymptomatic] can be handled with reassurance and self-care at home.)

● Diabetes drug overdose (e.g., insulin error or extra dose)
Note: Triager should consider medication, dose, and whether patient is alone. An upgrade to Go to ED Now (with friend or family) or EMS 911 may be indicated in some circumstances.

See Today in Office

◉ Patient wants to be seen

Discuss With PCP and Callback by Nurse Today

◉ Feces ingestion (e.g., patient with profound dementia or mental illness)
Reason: ingestion of a small amount of one's own stool is always harmless; ingestion of another human's stool has a small risk of causing diarrhea

Home Care

○ HARMLESS SUBSTANCE (nonpoisonous) ingestion
○ DOUBLE DOSE (an extra dose or lesser amount) of OTC drug and NO symptoms
○ DOUBLE DOSE (an extra dose or lesser amount) of antibiotic drug and NO symptoms
○ Poison-proofing your home, questions about

HOME CARE ADVICE

General Information

❶ **Accidental Ingestion of a Harmless Substance:**
  • You were lucky this time. What have you learned? What are you going to change?
  • It is time to poison-proof your home.

❷ **Accidental Harmless Overdose of OTC Drug or Antibiotic:** You have taken too much of this drug, but there shouldn't be any side effects. Think about ways that you can avoid this in the future. For example:
  • Use a form or a notepad to write down the names of your medicines, the amounts, and times you are supposed to take them.
  • Get a pill dispenser. You can obtain a plastic dispenser with compartments from the drugstore.
  • Throw away old pill bottles.

❸ **Avoid Vomiting:** Do not induce vomiting. Ipecac is unnecessary and should be disposed of.

❹ **Call Back If:**
  • You have any more questions.
  • You become worse.

Questions About Mercury Spills (e.g., Broken Glass Thermometer or Broken Spiral CFL)

❶ **Mercury Spills—What NOT to Do:**
  • DO NOT use a vacuum cleaner to clean up mercury. The vacuum cleaner will spread the mercury into the air.
  • DO NOT sweep up mercury with a broom. It will break the mercury into tiny drops and spread them apart.
  • DO NOT pour mercury down the drain. It is poisonous to the environment.

❷ **Internet Resource About Mercury Spills:**
  • The US EPA has a Web site on handling mercury spills: www.epa.gov/mercury/spills/index.htm. Information is provided on broken thermometers and broken compact fluorescent lightbulbs (CFLs).
  • Snopes.com has a brief information page on broken CFLs at: www.snopes.com/medical/toxins/cfl.asp.

Additional Poisoning Resources

❶ **Poison-Proofing Your Home:**
  • The American Association of Poison Control Centers has prepared a guide to preventing poisonings at home.
  • It is available online at www.1-800-222-1222.info/poisonPrevention/documents/homediag.pdf.

❷ **US Poison Center Number—1-800-222-1222:**
  • *This is the telephone number for every Poison Center in the United States.* It connects you automatically with the local Poison Center. You can call this number 24 hours a day, 7 days a week to talk to a poison expert.
  • **Reasons to Call:** Call right away if you have a poison emergency! You can also call this number if you have a question about a poison or about how to prevent poisoning.

FIRST AID

First Aid Advice for NARCOTIC OVERDOSE:

If narcotic overdose is known or suspected AND caller has Narcan nasal spray available, give Narcan nasal spray NOW:

- Peel back package and take out the nasal spray.
- Put the nozzle in one of the patient's nostrils.
- Press firmly down on the plunger to give the dose of Narcan.
- Turn patient on his or her side.
- Call 911. Emergency care is needed even if patient improves after Narcan is given.

Each package is a single dose of Narcan. If the patient does not respond by waking up or breathing normally, give another dose. If the patient gets worse after briefly getting better, give another dose.

First Aid Advice for Swallowed ACIDS OR ALKALIES:

- Remove any solid poisons out of the mouth (spit them out or rescuer can sweep them out with a finger).
- Drink ½ cup (120 mL) of water (or milk) to rinse out the esophagus.
- Avoid vomiting.
  (Reason: If these agents are vomited, additional damage can occur to the esophagus.)

First Aid Advice for Swallowed PETROLEUM PRODUCT:

- Do not eat or drink anything.
- Avoid vomiting.
  (Reason: If these hydrocarbon agents are vomited, additional damage can occur to the lungs from aspiration.)

First Aid Advice for Swallowed OTHER POISONOUS SUBSTANCES:

- Remove any solid poisons out of the mouth (spit them out or rescuer can sweep them out with a finger).
- Avoid vomiting (do not use syrup of ipecac).

US Poison Center Number—1-800-222-1222:

- This is the telephone number for every Poison Center in the United States.
- It connects you automatically with the local Poison Center.

BACKGROUND

Poisoning and Overdose—Telephone Triage Assessment and Disposition

Poisoning and overdose can be **accidental** or **intentional.** Accidental poisoning is more common in children. Children explore their world with enthusiastic curiosity. There is a natural tendency to put things in their mouth. In contrast, intentional poisoning or overdose is more common in adults. Sometimes adults take an overdose of a medicine on purpose to relieve pain or other symptoms. Sometimes adults take medicines or other substances to get high or feel better. Regardless, the triager should be always suspicious of the possibility of suicidality in adults with an intentional poisoning or overdose.

The triager should always be suspicious of the possibility of a **suicide gesture or attempt** in all adult poisonings and overdoses. It is appropriate for the triager to directly ask patients about their intent to harm themselves or end their own life. Such questions will not provoke a suicide attempt and may instead give patients a chance to unburden themselves. *Any patient who has attempted suicide or is threatening self-harm now needs to be seen immediately for evaluation.*

Poison Centers are cost-effective and prevent unnecessary visits to the ED. Most caller questions can be answered over the telephone. Research has shown that $1 invested in a Poison Center saves $7 on unnecessary health costs. The triager should have a very low threshold for referring or transferring poison calls to a Poison Center.

- **Australia:** The phone number 13 11 26 is available across New South Wales 24 hours a day and after-hours to the remainder of Australia.
- **Canada:** No nationwide number is available. Must contact local Poison Center directly. The phone number for the Ontario Poison Centre is 800/268-9017.
- **United States:** There is a nationwide toll-free phone number (1-800-222-1222) that will automatically connect a caller to the local Poison Center.

Based on the substance ingested, the triager should place the patient in one of the following **categories:**

- **Harmful Substances (e.g., Acid, Alkali, Petroleum Products):** Most of these patients will require a disposition of EMS 911 or Go to ED Now. If the person has no symptoms and is not suicidal, and the exposure sounds less concerning, a disposition of Call Poison Center may be appropriate.

- **Potentially Harmful Substances or Unknown:** The best disposition is Call Poison Center Now.
- **Harmless Substances:** Home Care is usually the appropriate disposition. When in doubt, the triager should refer the caller to a Poison Center.
- **Double Dose or Extra Dose of OTC Drugs and Prescription Antibiotics:** Home Care is usually the appropriate disposition. When in doubt, the triager should refer the caller to a Poison Center.

Harmful Substances—Acids, Alkalis, and Petroleum Products

Each of the substances in this category is extremely harmful. All individuals who have swallowed one of these substances and has any symptoms should be sent to the ED for evaluation and treatment.

Even individuals without symptoms will probably require ED evaluation. If the individual has no symptoms and is not suicidal, and the exposure sounds less concerning, a referral to a Poison Center may be appropriate.

- **Strong Acids and Alkalis:** Examples are toilet bowl cleaners, drain cleaners, lye, automatic dishwasher detergent, and Clinitest tablets.
- **Other Alkalis:** Examples are ammonia, bleaches, and chemical hair removers (e.g., Nair).
- **Petroleum Products:** Examples are kerosene, gasoline, benzene, furniture polish, and lighter fluid.

Potentially Harmful Substances or Unknown

This category includes nearly all prescription medicines, chemicals, and plants. Referral or call transfer to a Poison Center is recommended.

- **Prescription Medicines:** The following prescription drugs are especially dangerous if a person takes too much: barbiturates, clonidine, digoxin (Lanoxin), high blood pressure medicines, narcotics, tricyclic antidepressants, and warfarin (Coumadin).
- **Over-the-counter Medicines:** Two dangerous over-the-counter medicines are iron and aspirin. Acetaminophen (Tylenol) can also be dangerous if taken as an overdose.
- **Chemicals.**
- **Plants.**

Harmless Substances (Nonpoisonous)

The following substances are completely harmless if tasted or swallowed. A disposition of Home Care is appropriate, and the caller should be reassured. When in doubt, the triager should refer the caller to a Poison Center.

- **Cosmetics:** Lipstick, rouge, mascara. Deodorants and hair sprays are usually harmless, unless they contain alcohol. Perfumes always contain alcohol and can be harmful (see next section).
- **Glue:** White, arts and crafts.
- **Miscellaneous:** Candles, cooking lard or grease, dirt, glow products (glow sticks), mercury in glass thermometers (safe if swallowed but dangerous if inhaled), silica granules (in desiccant packets).
- **Mouth Products:** Breath mints, chewing gum, toothpaste.
- **Paints:** Watercolor paints and water-based paints.
- **Pet Products:** Dog or cat food, cat litter (earth or clay), stool.
- **Skin Care Products:** Corn starch baby powder (talcum powder can be harmful), hand lotions (creams or ointments), petroleum jelly, shaving cream, suntan lotion. Creams and ointments containing the following OTC medicines are safe: antibiotic, steroid, antifungal, anti-yeast, and diaper rash creams and ointments.
- **Soaps:** Hand soaps (liquid or bar), shampoo.
- **Writing Products:** Chalk, crayons, pen and marker ink, lead pencils (which are actually graphite).

The US National Capital Poison Center (Poison.org) maintains a list of nonpoisonous plants at: www.poison.org/prevent/plants.asp.

Double Dose or Extra Dose of OTC Drugs and Prescription Antibiotics

Taking one extra dose (double dose) of an over-the-counter (OTC) medicine or prescription antibiotic is harmless.

- **OTC Medicine:** Taking twice the recommended dose of an OTC medicine (e.g., cough or cold medicines, pain or fever medicines, vitamin pills) on a one-time basis is harmless.
- **Antibiotic:** Taking an extra dose of a prescription antibiotic is harmless.

When in doubt, the triager should refer the caller to a Poison Center.

Narcan Nasal Spray—Emergency Treatment for Narcotic Overdose

Deaths from drug overdose have risen greatly in the United States since 2000. In 2014, about 2 out of every 3 overdose deaths involved an opioid such as heroin or narcotic prescription pain medicine (Rudd et al). Narcan (naloxone) nasal spray is an emergency treatment that can help prevent deaths from narcotic overdose.

- **How does it work?** The medicine counteracts the life-threatening effects of a narcotic overdose. It is absorbed quickly across the nasal membranes into the bloodstream.
- **Who can give it?** It can be given by family members and friends.
- **When should someone give it?** It should be given right away if a narcotic overdose is suspected and the person is hard to arouse or wake up or has slow or shallow breathing.
- **What are symptoms of a narcotic overdose?** The main symptoms are severe sleepiness (or even coma) and slow or shallow breathing. The pupils are small (constricted).
- **What are the side effects?** People who use narcotics for a long time will likely develop sudden narcotic withdrawal symptoms after receiving Narcan. The symptoms may include nausea, vomiting, feeling anxious, shakes, and chills. If the person is using a narcotic to treat pain, after Narcan the pain will return until the Narcan wears off.
- **Should the caller call 911?** Yes. Narcan nasal spray is not a replacement for emergency care. Instruct callers to call 911 even if the patient's symptoms improve after Narcan is given. The medicine may wear off quickly and life-threatening symptoms may return.

If narcotic overdose is known or suspected AND caller has Narcan nasal spray available, give Narcan nasal spray NOW:

- Peel back package and take out the nasal spray.
- Put the nozzle in one of the patient's nostrils.
- Press firmly down on the plunger to give the dose of Narcan.
- Turn patient on his or her side.
- Call 911. Emergency care is needed even if patient improves after Narcan is given.

Each package is a single dose of Narcan. If the patient does not respond by waking up or breathing normally, give another dose. If the patient gets worse after briefly getting better, give another dose.

PUBIC LICE

Definition
- A genital area infection with tiny gray bugs called lice.
- *Use this protocol only if the patient has symptoms that match Pubic Lice.*

Symptoms
- Itching of the pubic area is the main symptom.
- Gray bugs (lice) are 1/16" (1-2 mm) long, move quickly, and are difficult to see.
- Nits (white or tan eggs) cemented to hair shafts near the skin (usually within ½" or 12 mm). Unlike dandruff or sand, nits can't be shaken off the hair shafts.

TRIAGE ASSESSMENT QUESTIONS

See More Appropriate Protocol
- ● Doesn't match the SYMPTOMS for lice, and insect bite suspected
  Go to Protocol: Insect Bite on page 257
- ● Doesn't match the SYMPTOMS for lice
  Go to Protocol: Rash or Redness, Localized on page 326

See Today in Office
- ● Looks infected (e.g., pus, soft scabs, open sores)
  R/O: superinfection with staph or strep
- ● New or unusual vaginal discharge (e.g., odorous, yellow, green, or foamy-white)
  Reason: patient also may have vaginitis from another sexually transmitted infection (STI)
- ● White or yellow discharge from penis
  Reason: sounds like patient also may have urethritis (another STI)

See Today or Tomorrow in Office
- ◐ Diagnosis of lice is uncertain
- ◐ Pubic lice or nits recurs within 1 month
  Reason: resistant pubic lice or reinfection
- ◐ > 3 hours since completing treatment and moving lice are seen in the pubic hair
  Reason: probably resistant lice
- ◐ Patient wants to be seen

See Within 3 Days in Office
- ◐ All other patients with pubic lice
  Reason: to make certain that the patient has no other STI

HOME CARE ADVICE

❶ **Nix Anti-Lice Creme Rinse:**
- *Buy Nix anti-lice creme rinse (permethrin).*
- Pour about 2 oz (60 mL) of the creme onto previously washed and towel-dried pubic hair. Add a little warm water to work up a lather. Be sure to work the creme into all the hair down to the roots.
- Leave the Nix on for a full 20 minutes or it won't kill all the lice (10 minutes is not enough).
- Rinse the hair thoroughly and dry it with a towel. Repeat the Nix treatment in 1 week to kill any nits that were missed.

❷ **Dead Nits:** Wait ≥ 3 hours after Nix treatment is completed before removing the dead nits. *(Reason: Let Nix permeate the nits.)* The nits can be loosened using a mixture of half vinegar and half warm water. After wetting the hair with this solution, cover the hair with a towel for 30 minutes. Then remove the dead nits by backcombing with a special nit comb or pull them out individually.

❸ **Pregnancy and Breastfeeding:** According to the Centers for Disease Control and Preventions, women who are pregnant or who are breastfeeding can be treated with products containing permethrin (e.g., Nix).

❹ **Contagiousness:** Pubic lice are very contagious. Pubic lice are transmitted by skin-to-skin contact during sexual intercourse (they cannot jump). You should have no sexual intercourse until 2 weeks after successful treatment.

❺ **Sexual Contacts:** Any sexual partners that you have had during the last month will also need treatment even if they don't see any obvious lice.

❻ **Expected Course:** With 2 treatments, all lice and nits should be killed. A recurrence usually means that there has been another contact with an infected person, the shampoo wasn't left on for 20 minutes, or the treatment wasn't repeated in 7 days. There are no lasting problems from having lice and they do not carry other diseases. Even after successful treatment, itching of the pubic area may persist for 1-2 weeks.

❼ **Other Shampoos:** If any of the pyrethrin anti-lice shampoos (A200 Clear, R&C, Pronto, or RID) are used, they must be applied to dry hair. Reapplication in 7 days to prevent reinfection is also required. Do not use these products if you are pregnant or breastfeeding.

❽ **Pregnancy Test, When in Doubt:**
- If there is a chance that you might be pregnant, use a urine pregnancy test.
- You can buy a pregnancy test at the drugstore.
- It works best if you test your first urine in the morning.
- *Follow the instructions included in the package.*
- Call back if you are pregnant.

❾ **Internet Resources**
- **Australia—Health Direct:** Information about sexually transmitted infections (STIs) is available at: https://www.healthdirect.gov.au/sexually-transmitted-infections-sti.
- **Canada—Public Health Agency of Canada:** Available on the Web at: www.phac-aspc.gc.ca/std-mts/faq-eng.php.
- **United States—AHSA: American Social Health Association.** Answers to questions about teen sexual health and STIs: www.ashasexualhealth.org/sexual-health.
- **United States—CDC:** *2015 Sexually Transmitted Diseases Treatment Guidelines:* https://www.cdc.gov/std/tg2015/default.htm.

❿ **Call Back If:**
- Pregnancy test is positive or if you have difficulties with the home pregnancy test.
- You become worse.

BACKGROUND

Key Points
- Slight redness may be present in the pubic area from scratching.
- Adult lice survive 3 weeks in the pubic area but only 24 hours once off the human body.
- The nits (eggs) are easier to see than the lice because they are white and very numerous.
- Nits hatch into lice in about 1 week. Off the body, they can survive up to 2 weeks.
- Nits that are > 1 cm from the skin are empty egg cases and very white in color.

Cause
- Pubic lice are tiny wingless insects which live only on human beings.
- The primary mode of transmission is via the skin-to-skin contact that occurs during sexual intercourse. Lice are very contagious. There is a 95% chance of transmission during a single episode of sexual intercourse.
- Rarely they may be transmitted via objects (i.e., fomites) such as infected bed linens or toilet seats.
- Pubic lice are annoying but cause no serious health problems.
- They are also referred to as "crabs."
- Up to 30% of individuals with pubic lice have another STI.

OTC Treatment of Pubic Lice: There are 2 medications that can be purchased OTC which are effective in treating pubic lice. The package instructions should be followed closely. They are:
- 1% permethrin (i.e., Nix)
- Pyrethrin with piperonyl butoxide (e.g., RID, A200 Clear, R&C, Pronto)

Prescription Medications for Treatment of Pubic Lice
- 5% permethrin (i.e., Elimite)
- Lindane (i.e., Kwell, Kwellada)
- Malathion (i.e., Ovide)

Pubic Lice in Pregnancy
- Women who are pregnant or breastfeeding can be treated with permethrin (Nix) (Workowski).
- Permethrin is considered a category B drug in pregnancy.

Internet Resources on Sexually Transmitted Infections
- **Australia—Health Direct:** Information about sexually transmitted infections (STIs) is available at: https://www.healthdirect.gov.au/sexually-transmitted-infections-sti.
- **Canada—Public Health Agency of Canada:** Available on the Web at: www.phac-aspc.gc.ca/std-mts/faq-eng.php.
- **United States—AHSA:** American Social Health Association. Answers to questions about teen sexual health and STIs: www.ashasexualhealth.org/sexual-health.
- **United States—CDC:** *2015 Sexually Transmitted Diseases Treatment Guidelines:* https://www.cdc.gov/std/tg2015/default.htm.

PUNCTURE WOUND

Definition
- Skin is punctured by a narrow, pointed object.

TRIAGE ASSESSMENT QUESTIONS

Call EMS 911 Now
- Shock suspected (e.g., cold/pale/clammy skin, too weak to stand)
  R/O: shock
  First Aid: Lie down with the feet elevated.
- Puncture wound of head, neck, chest, back, or abdomen that sounds life-threatening to triager
  First Aid: Apply direct pressure with a clean cloth.
- Sounds like a life-threatening emergency to the triager

See More Appropriate Protocol
- Caused by an animal bite
  Go to Protocol: Animal Bite on page 22
- Skin is cut or scraped, not punctured
  Go to Protocol: Skin Injury on page 361
- Puncture wound of eye or eyelid
  Go to Protocol: Eye Injury on page 161
- Foreign body is still in the skin
  (e.g., splinter, sliver, fishhook)
  Go to Protocol: Skin, Foreign Body on page 358

Go to ED Now
- Puncture wound of head, neck, chest, abdomen, or overlying a joint and it could be deep
  R/O: internal injury or penetration of joint
- Needlestick from used or discarded injection needle
  (Exception: clean, unused needle)
- High-pressure injection injury (e.g., from grease gun or paint gun, usually work related)
  Reason: deep tissue damage exceeds superficial injury

Go to ED/UCC Now
(or to Office With PCP Approval)
- Sounds like a serious injury to the triager

Go to Office Now
- SEVERE pain (e.g., excruciating)
  R/O: deep puncture or retained foreign body (FB)
- Puncture wound of foot and hurts too much to walk on (i.e., unable to bear weight, severe limp)
  R/O: retained FB, deep tissue injury
- Puncture wound of bare foot (no shoes) and setting was dirty
  Reason: need for wound irrigation or debridement
- Puncture wound of finger and entire finger swollen
  R/O: tenosynovitis
  Note: This serious infection typically develops 24-72 hours after wound occurs.
- Puncture wound from sharp object that was very dirty (e.g., barnyard)
  Reason: need for wound irrigation or debridement; depending on patient tetanus status, tetanus immune globulin (TIG) may be needed
- Dirt (debris) can be seen in the wound, not removed with 15-minute scrubbing
  Reason: additional scrubbing in ED, UCC, or office may be needed
- Tip of the object is broken off and missing
  R/O: retained FB
- Sensation of something still in the wound
  R/O: retained FB
  Note: Patients can nearly always feel if there is an FB in the wound.
- Looks infected (e.g., spreading redness, pus, red streak)
  R/O: cellulitis, lymphangitis

See Today in Office
- Pain or swelling present > 5 days
- No tetanus booster in > 5 years
  Reason: may need a tetanus booster shot (vaccine)
- No prior tetanus shots
  Reason: may need tetanus immune globulin (TIG)
  Note: Referral to the ED may likely be required as doctor's offices usually do not stock TIG.
- Patient wants to be seen

See Today or Tomorrow in Office

● After 14 days and wound isn't healed
R/O: low-grade infection
● Puncture wound on foot and patient has diabetes mellitus
Reason: increased risk of foot infection
● Puncture through shoe (e.g., tennis shoe) and into bottom of foot
Reason: wound check

Home Care

○ Minor puncture wound

HOME CARE ADVICE

❶ **Cleaning:**
- Wash the wound with soap and warm water for 15 minutes.
- If there is any dirt or debris, scrub the wound back and forth with a washcloth to remove it.

❷ **Trimming:** Cut off any flaps of loose skin that seal the wound and interfere with drainage or removing debris. Use fine scissors after cleaning them with rubbing alcohol.

❸ **Antibiotic Ointment:** Apply an antibiotic ointment and a Band-Aid to reduce the risk of infection. Resoak the area and reapply an antibiotic ointment every 12 hours for 2 days.

❹ **Pain Medicines:**
- For pain relief, you can take either acetaminophen, ibuprofen, or naproxen.
- They are over-the-counter (OTC) pain drugs. You can buy them at the drugstore.

Acetaminophen (e.g., Tylenol):
- **Regular Strength Tylenol:** Take 650 mg (two 325 mg pills) by mouth every 4-6 hours as needed. Each Regular Strength Tylenol pill has 325 mg of acetaminophen.
- **Extra Strength Tylenol:** Take 1,000 mg (two 500 mg pills) every 8 hours as needed. Each Extra Strength Tylenol pill has 500 mg of acetaminophen.
- The most you should take each day is 3,000 mg (10 Regular Strength or 6 Extra Strength pills a day).

Ibuprofen (e.g., Motrin, Advil):
- Take 400 mg (two 200 mg pills) by mouth every 6 hours.
- Another choice is to take 600 mg (three 200 mg pills) by mouth every 8 hours.
- The most you should take each day is 1,200 mg (six 200 mg pills), unless your doctor has told you to take more.

Naproxen (e.g., Aleve):
- Take 220 mg (one 220 mg pill) by mouth every 8 hours as needed. You may take 440 mg (two 220 mg pills) for your first dose.
- The most you should take each day is 660 mg (three 220 mg pills a day), unless your doctor has told you to take more.

❺ **Pain Medicines—Extra Notes:**
- Use the lowest amount of medicine that makes your pain better.
- Acetaminophen is thought to be safer than ibuprofen or naproxen in people > 65 years old. Acetaminophen is in many OTC and prescription medicines. It might be in more than one medicine that you are taking. You need to be careful and not take an overdose. An acetaminophen overdose can hurt the liver.
- McNeil, the company that makes Tylenol, has different dosage instructions for Tylenol in Canada and the United States. In Canada, the maximum recommended dose per day is 4,000 mg or 12 Regular Strength (325 mg) pills. In the United States, McNeil recommends a maximum dose of 10 Regular Strength (325 mg) pills.
- CAUTION: Do not take acetaminophen if you have liver disease.
- CAUTION: Do not take ibuprofen or naproxen if you have stomach problems, have kidney disease, are pregnant, or have been told by your doctor to avoid this type of anti-inflammatory drug. Do not take ibuprofen or naproxen for > 7 days without consulting your doctor.
- *Before taking any medicine, read all the instructions on the package.*

❻ **Expected Course:** Puncture wounds seal over in 1-2 hours. Pain should resolve within 2 days.

❼ Call Back If:
- Dirt is still present in the wound after scrubbing.
- It begins to look infected (redness, red streaks, tenderness, pus, fever).
- Pain becomes severe.
- You become worse.

FIRST AID

First Aid Advice for Bleeding:
Apply direct pressure to the entire wound with a clean cloth.

First Aid Advice for Shock:
Lie down with the feet elevated.

First Aid Advice for Puncture Wound:
Wash wound with soap and water.

BACKGROUND

Common Causes
- **Animal Bite:** See Animal Bite protocol on page 22.
- Fishhook.
- Nail.
- Needlestick.
- Pen.
- Pencil.
- Pin.
- Sewing needle.
- **Splinter:** See Skin, Foreign Body protocol on page 358.
- Toothpick.

Foot Punctures Through Athletic Shoes
- Puncture wounds of the plantar surface of the foot have a risk of infection of approximately 4%. This increases to 25% in patients with puncture wounds through athletic (tennis) shoes into the forefoot area of the plantar foot. Pain persisting > 4-5 days after the injury is suggestive of infection.
- *Pseudomonas* osteomyelitis is a rare complication (occurring in < 1% of punctures). *Pseudomonas* osteomyelitis or osteochondritis usually presents with localized pain and swelling that becomes worse after 5 days. Fever may be absent.
- The benefit of immediate physician evaluation and extra wound care (e.g., coring) for all athletic shoe punctures is unknown. Prophylactic antibiotics are recommended by some authors, but there is no convincing evidence that prophylactic antibiotics prevents *Pseudomonas* infection.

Pencil Lead Punctures
- Pencil lead is actually graphite (harmless), not poisonous lead. Even colored leads are nontoxic.
- They will cause a tattoo, however, and should be scrubbed out. If pigment remains, the ED, UCC, or office staff may scrub the wound again and be more successful. This should be done before the wound heals over.

When Does an Adult Need a Tetanus Booster (Tetanus Shot)?
- **Clean Puncture Wound—Every 10 Years:** Patients with clean puncture wounds and who have previously had ≥ 3 tetanus shots (full series) need a booster every 10 years. CLEAN punctures mean that both the skin and object were clean. Examples of clean punctures include a puncture wound from an unused injection needle, sewing needle, a thumbtack, or a safety pin. *Obtain tetanus booster within 72 hours.*
- **Dirty Puncture Wound—Every 5 Years:** Patients with dirty wounds need a booster every 5 years. Puncture wounds should be considered DIRTY if either the object or the skin was dirty. Examples of dirty puncture wounds include pencils (saliva), any sharp object on the floor, and if the punctured skin was contaminated with soil, saliva, or feces. *Obtain tetanus booster within 24 hours.*
- Persons with major or dirty wounds who have not received a full tetanus vaccination series (3 doses) also need tetanus immune globulin (TIG) when they get the tetanus booster (Td or Tdap).

RASH, WIDESPREAD ON DRUGS (DRUG REACTION)

Definition
- A widespread rash begins within 2 weeks of starting a new medication.
- The rash is most commonly red or pink spots that are smooth (macular) or slightly bumpy (papular).
- Other drug rashes that can occur include blisters (vesicles), skin redness (erythroderma), erythema nodosum, hives (urticaria), and pustules.
- May or may not be itchy.

Included:
- Drug rashes from prescription medications
- Drug rashes from nonsteroidal anti-inflammatory drugs (NSAIDs)
- Niacin flushing

Excluded:
- Do not use this protocol if the rash is thought to be caused by taking over-the-counter (OTC) medications like antihistamines, decongestants, cough/cold medicines, eye drops, or nose drops.
- Instead use the **Rash or Redness, Widespread** protocol on page 330.

TRIAGE ASSESSMENT QUESTIONS

Call EMS 911 Now
- Difficulty breathing or wheezing
  R/O: anaphylaxis, angioedema
- Hoarseness or cough that started soon after first dose of drug
  R/O: anaphylaxis, angioedema
- Swollen tongue that started soon after first dose of drug
- Fever and purple or blood-colored spots or dots
  R/O: meningococcemia, Rocky Mountain spotted fever
  Note: It may be difficult to determine the rash color in people with darker-colored skin.
- Too weak or sick to stand
  R/O: toxic shock syndrome or septic shock, meningitis
- Sounds like a life-threatening emergency to the triager

See More Appropriate Protocol
- Rash is only on one part of the body (localized)
  Go to Protocol: Rash or Redness, Localized on page 326
- Taking new nonprescription (OTC) antihistamine, decongestant, ear drops, eye drops, or other OTC cough/cold medicine
  Go to Protocol: Rash or Redness, Widespread on page 330
  Reason: these medicines rarely cause rashes
- Taking new prescription antihistamine, allergy medicine, asthma medicine, eye drops, ear drops, or nose drops
  Go to Protocol: Rash or Redness, Widespread on page 330
  Reason: these medicines rarely cause rashes
- Rash started > 3 days after stopping new prescription medicine
  Go to Protocol: Rash or Redness, Widespread on page 330

Go to ED Now
- Swollen tongue

Go to ED/UCC Now
(or to Office With PCP Approval)
- Widespread hives and onset < 2 hours of exposure to first dose of drug
  R/O: allergic reaction
  Reason: no history of life-threatening reaction and no anaphylactic symptoms
- Patient sounds very sick or weak to the triager
  Reason: severe acute illness or serious complication suspected

Go to Office Now
- Fever
  R/O: bacterial illness, DRESS syndrome
- Face or lip swelling
  Reason: may need steroids
- Purple or blood-colored spots or dots (no fever and sounds well to triager)
  R/O: purpura or petechiae, vasculitis
  Note: In comparison to other red rashes, petechiae and purpura do not temporarily blanch (fade) when pressure is applied to a spot. It may be difficult to determine the rash color in people with darker-colored skin.

● Joint pain or swelling
  R/O: gonococcemia
● Bloody crusts on lips or in mouth
  R/O: Stevens-Johnson syndrome
● Large or small blisters on skin (i.e., fluid-filled bubbles or sacs)
  R/O: Stevens-Johnson syndrome, TENS, disseminated herpes zoster, chickenpox

Callback by PCP Within 1 Hour
● Pregnant
● Rash beginning within 4 hours of a new prescription medication
  R/O: allergic drug reaction

See Today in Office
● Hives or itching
  R/O: allergic drug rash
● Patient wants to be seen

Callback by PCP Today
● Taking new prescription antibiotic
  (Exception: finished taking new prescription antibiotic)
  Reason: all triage questions negative and PCP may need to change antibiotic
● Taking new prescription medicine
  (Exceptions: finished taking new prescription antibiotic OR questions about flushing from niacin)
  R/O: cutaneous drug reaction
  Reason: all triage questions negative and PCP may need to change medicine

Discuss With PCP and Callback by Nurse Today
● Rash started within 3 days after antibiotic stopped
  R/O: allergic drug rash
● Niacin flush suspected

HOME CARE ADVICE

❶ **Reassurance:**
  • There are many causes of widespread rashes and most of the time they are not serious. Common causes include viral illness (e.g., cold viruses) and allergic reactions (to a food, medicine, or environmental exposure).
  • Here is some care advice that should help.

❷ **Stopping the Medication:**
  • **If Medication Is an Antibiotic:** Stop the medication
    (Reason: possible allergy).
  • **If Rash Is Hives or Is Very Itchy:** Stop the medication
    (Reason: possible allergy).
  • **If the Medication Is an OTC Drug:** Stop the medication
    (Reason: medicine is not essential).
  • **Other Rashes and Prescription Medications:** Continue the medication
    (Reason: lower likelihood of allergic drug reaction).

❸ **For Non-itchy Rashes:** No treatment is necessary.

❹ **For Itchy Rashes:** Wash the skin once with soap to remove any irritants. Use Benadryl or take an Aveeno bath to reduce the itching.

❺ **Antihistamine Medicine for Itching:**
  • Take an antihistamine by mouth to reduce the itching.
  • Diphenhydramine (Benadryl) is a good choice. The adult dosage of Benadryl is 25-50 mg by mouth and you can take it up to 4 times a day.
  • Another OTC antihistamine that causes less sleepiness is loratadine (e.g., Alavert or Claritin). Alavert is not available in Canada.
  • *Before taking any medicine, read all the instructions on the package.*

❻ **Oatmeal Aveeno Bath for Itching:**
  • Sprinkle contents of one Aveeno packet under running faucet with comfortably warm water. Bathe for 15-20 minutes, 1-2 times daily.
  • Pat dry with a towel. Do not rub the rash.

❼ **Contagiousness:** Avoid contact with pregnant women until a diagnosis is made. Most viral rashes are contagious (especially if a fever is present). Allergic drug rashes are not contagious.

❽ **Call Back If:**
  • You become worse.

FIRST AID

First Aid Advice for Anaphylaxis—Epinephrine:

- If the patient has an epinephrine autoinjector, **give it now.** Do not delay.
- Use the autoinjector on the upper outer thigh. You may give it through clothing if necessary.
- Give epinephrine first, then call 911.
- Epinephrine is available in autoinjectors under trade names: EpiPen, EpiPen Jr, and Auvi-Q (Allerject in Canada). Auvi-Q has an audio chip and talks patients and caregivers through injection process.
- You may give a second (repeat) dose of epinephrine 10-15 minutes later, IF the person with anaphylaxis does not respond to the first dose AND ambulance arrival takes > 10 minutes.

First Aid Advice for Anaphylaxis—Benadryl:

- Give antihistamine by mouth **NOW** if able to swallow.
- Use Benadryl (diphenhydramine; adult dose: 50 mg) or any other available antihistamine medicine.

BACKGROUND

Cutaneous Drug Reactions (Drug Rashes)

- Rashes are one of the most common adverse reactions to drugs.
- **Incidence:** Adults are more likely than children to have an allergic reaction to a medication. Of course, adults are more frequently taking multiple medications.
- **Onset:** Most drug rashes begin within 2 weeks of starting a medicine. In fact, if any new skin condition occurs within 2 weeks of starting a new medication, the medication should be considered as a possible cause. Occasionally, drug rashes begin after the drug is stopped. For example, a rash might appear 10 days after starting a 7-day course of antibiotic treatment.
- **Symptoms:** The rash is most commonly red or pink spots that are smooth (macular) or slightly bumpy (papular). Other drug rashes that can occur include blisters (vesicles), skin redness (erythroderma), erythema nodosum, hives (urticaria), and pustules. Most drug rashes have associated itching. Localized rashes are less likely to be caused by drugs.
- **Diagnosis:** Determining the cause of a rash is often very difficult. Rashes from a drug reaction often look similar to rashes from other causes (e.g., viral rashes). Usually the health care professional takes into consideration how likely a specific drug is to cause a rash and the rash appearance.

- **Treatment:** The patient should stop taking the drug that caused the rash. The patient can take oral antihistamine medications (e.g., diphenhydramine/Benadryl) if there is severe itching. Health care professionals may prescribe oral prednisone for severe drug rashes.
- **Expected Course:** A drug rash will almost always improve simply by stopping the drug that caused it. However, depending on the type of rash, it might take from a couple days (e.g., urticarial rash from ibuprofen) to 2-3 weeks (e.g., maculopapular rash from ampicillin) to get better.

Risk Factors for Developing a Drug Rash

- Older age; possibly from cumulative exposure
- Personal history of any prior drug allergy
- Family history of any drug allergy
- **Certain Concurrent Illnesses:** Cytomegalovirus or Epstein-Barr virus (mononucleosis) infections, AIDS, liver or renal disease

Drugs Most Likely to Cause Rashes

- **Angiotensin-converting Enzyme (ACE) Inhibitors:** Examples include enalapril (Vasotec, Renitec), lisinopril (Prinivil, Zestril), and benazepril (Lotensin).
- Allopurinol.
- **Antibiotics:** Examples include penicillins (e.g., amoxicillin, ampicillin) and sulfa antibiotics (e.g., trimethoprim-sulfamethoxazole/Bactrim).
- **Anticonvulsants:** Examples include phenytoin (Dilantin).
- Anti-lipids.
- Aspirin.
- **Diuretics:** Examples include hydrochlorothiazide (HCTZ) and furosemide (e.g., Lasix).
- **Nonsteroidal Anti-inflammatory Drugs (NSAIDs):** Examples include ibuprofen (e.g., Motrin, Advil), naproxen (e.g., Aleve, Naprosyn), and ketorolac (Toradol).
- Oral contraceptives.

Drugs Least Likely to Cause Rashes

Over-the-counter (OTC; nonprescription) medicines rarely cause a rash. Here is a list of drugs least likely to be the cause of a rash.

- Aminophylline
- Antacids (e.g., Mylanta)
- Acetaminophen (e.g., Tylenol)
- Ear drops, prescription and OTC
- Eye drops, prescription and OTC
- Meperidine

- Nitroglycerin
- Prednisone, prednisolone
- Propranolol
- Spironolactone

Types of Cutaneous Drug Reactions (Drug Rashes)

Maculopapular eruptions are the most common cutaneous drug reactions. The rash has widespread pink and red macules (smooth-flat spots) and papules (bumpy-raised spots).

- Acneiform (pustular) eruptions
- Alopecia
- Erythema multiform–like eruptions
- Erythema nodosum
- Erythroderma
- Fixed drug eruption
- Hypertrichosis
- Maculopapular (exanthematous) eruptions
- Photosensitivity
- Phototoxic
- Pityriasis rosea–like eruptions
- Serum sickness
- Skin pigmentation
- Stevens-Johnson syndrome
- Toxic epidermal necrolysis
- Vasculitis
- Vesicles and blisters

Definition of Hives

- Itchy, swollen patches that appear suddenly.
- Patches change shape and location frequently; any one patch generally only lasts for a few hours, then fades away.
- Sizes of patches vary from ½" (1.2 cm) to several inches (5-10 cm) across.

Niacin Flush

- Niacin (nicotinic acid) is used in the treatment of hyperlipidemia. Perhaps as many as 80% of people who take niacin experience skin flushing. It is a well-known side effect.
- **Symptoms:** Flushing (deep red coloration) of the face and upper body occurs approximately 20-60 minutes after taking niacin. Occasionally the skin flush spreads to the arms. Most people also report an accompanying sensation of warmth and itching. Usually the flushing lasts < 1 hour.

- **Treatment:** Taking an adult aspirin or other NSAID (e.g., ibuprofen) may help; however, the flushing goes away by itself within 1 hour.
- **Prevention:** Taking an adult aspirin or other NSAID (if there are no contraindications) 30 minutes before the niacin reduces the degree of flushing. Extended-release niacin causes less flushing than regular niacin. Individuals taking niacin should avoid alcohol, spicy foods, hot beverages, and hot baths/showers right after taking niacin, as these factors can increase the likelihood of flushing occurring.
- **Expected Course:** People who continue to take niacin for several weeks report that the flushing seems to happen less.

Anaphylaxis—Anaphylactic Reactions

- **Definition:** Anaphylaxis is a serious allergic reaction that is rapid in onset and may cause death.
- **Onset:** Generally, the shorter the interval between the allergen exposure (e.g., food, drug, or sting) and the onset of the first systemic symptoms, the more serious the reaction will be. Anaphylaxis usually starts within 20 minutes and always by 2 hours. If no symptoms occur by 2 hours, the risk for anaphylaxis has passed.
- **Symptoms—Systemic:** By definition, an anaphylactic reaction must include respiratory (e.g., wheezing or stridor), cardiovascular (e.g., fainting), or central nervous system (e.g., confusion) symptoms.
- **Symptoms—Cutaneous:** Hives or another itchy rashis often present (> 80%). The appearance of cutaneous symptoms (hives or facial swelling) may be a precursor to anaphylaxis.
- **Causes:** Foods (especially peanuts, tree nuts, fish, and shellfish), drugs (especially antibiotics and NSAIDs), and stings are the most common causes of anaphylaxis.

Caution—Fever:

- An adult with **fever and rash** should seek medical attention immediately. A number of serious infections present in this manner.

RASH OR REDNESS, LOCALIZED

Definition
- Rash or redness on one part of the body (localized or clustered).
- Cause of rash is unknown.

Includes:
- Localized areas of redness or skin irritation.
- Rash may be smooth (macular) or slightly bumpy (papular).
- Rash may look like small spots, large spots, or solid red.

TRIAGE ASSESSMENT QUESTIONS

Call EMS 911 Now
- Sounds like a life-threatening emergency to the triager

See More Appropriate Protocol
- Possible contact with poison ivy or oak
  Go to Protocol: Poison Ivy/Oak/Sumac on page 310
- Insect bite(s) suspected
  Go to Protocol: Insect Bite on page 257
- Athlete's foot suspected (i.e., itchy rash between the toes)
  Go to Protocol: Athlete's Foot on page 42
- Jock itch suspected (i.e., itchy rash on inner thighs near genital area)
  Go to Protocol: Jock Itch on page 263
- Wound infection suspected (i.e., pain, spreading redness, or pus; in a cut, puncture, scrape, or sutured wound)
  Go to Protocol: Wound Infection on page 443
- Rash of external female genital area (vulva)
  Go to Protocol: Vulvar Symptoms on page 437
- Rash of penis or scrotum
  Go to Protocol: Penis and Scrotum Symptoms on page 308
- Small spot, skin growth, or mole
  Go to Protocol: Skin Lesion (Moles or Growths) on page 367

Go to ED/UCC Now
(or to Office With PCP Approval)
- Fever and localized purple or blood-colored spots or dots that are not from injury or friction
  R/O: early meningococcemia
  Note: It may be difficult to determine the rash color in people with darker-colored skin.
- Fever and localized rash is very painful
  R/O: cellulitis
- Patient sounds very sick or weak to the triager
  Reason: severe acute illness or serious complication suspected

Go to Office Now
- Looks like a boil, infected sore, deep ulcer, or other infected rash (spreading redness, pus)
  R/O: cellulitis, erysipelas, abscess

See Today in Office
- Painful rash with multiple small blisters grouped together (i.e., dermatomal distribution or "band" or "stripe")
  R/O: herpes zoster (shingles)
- Localized rash is very painful (no fever)
  R/O: spider bite, bee sting
- Localized purple or blood-colored spots or dots that are not from injury or friction (no fever)
  R/O: bleeding disorder, petechiae, vasculitis
  Note: It may be difficult to determine the rash color in people with darker-colored skin.
- Lyme disease suspected (e.g., bull's-eye rash or tick bite/exposure)
  R/O: erythema chronicum migrans
- Patient wants to be seen

See Today or Tomorrow in Office
- Tender bumps in armpits
  R/O: hidradenitis suppurativa
- Pimples (localized) and no improvement after using Home Care Advice
- SEVERE local itching persists after 2 days of steroid cream
  R/O: poison ivy, contact dermatitis

Callback by PCP Today

● Applying cream or ointment and it causes severe itch, burning, or pain
R/O: severe contact dermatitis

See Within 3 Days in Office

● Localized rash present > 7 days
R/O: contact dermatitis, eczema, ringworm

See Within 2 Weeks in Office

● Red, moist, irritated area between skinfolds (or under larger breasts)
R/O: intertrigo
Note: See BACKGROUND information.

Home Care

○ Mild localized rash
○ Pimples (localized)
○ Redness or itching where jewelry (or metal) touches skin and jewelry contains nickel
Reason: probable nickel contact dermatitis

HOME CARE ADVICE

General Care Advice for Mild Localized Rash

❶ **Reassurance:** New rashes that are in one small (localized) area are usually due to skin contact with an irritating substance.

❷ **Find and Avoid the Cause:**
- Try to find the cause. The rash may be from irritants like a plant, chemicals, or fiberglass.
- A new makeup or jewelry can also cause contact dermatitis.
- A pet may carry the irritant in its fur. An example of this is poison ivy or poison oak.

❸ **Avoid Soap:** Wash the area once thoroughly with soap to remove any remaining irritants. Thereafter, avoid soaps to this area. Cleanse the area when needed with warm water.

❹ **Apply Cold to the Area:** Apply or soak in cold water for 20 minutes every 3-4 hours to reduce itching or pain.

❺ **Hydrocortisone Cream for Itching:**
- You can use hydrocortisone for very itchy spots.
- Put 1% hydrocortisone cream on the itchy area(s) 3 times a day. Use it for a couple days, until it feels better. This will help decrease the itching.
- This is an over-the-counter (OTC) drug. You can buy it at the drugstore.
- Some people like to keep the cream in the refrigerator. It feels even better if the cream is used when it is cold.
- CAUTION: Do not use hydrocortisone cream for > 1 week without talking to your doctor.
- *Before using any medicine, read all the instructions on the package.*

❻ **Avoid Scratching:** Try not to scratch. Cut your fingernails short.

❼ **Contagiousness:** Adults with localized rashes do not need to miss any work or school.

❽ **Expected Course:** Most of these rashes pass in 2-3 days.

❾ **Call Back If:**
- Rash spreads or becomes worse.
- Rash lasts > 1 week.
- You become worse.

General Care Advice for Pimples

❶ **Reassurance:**
- A pimple is a tiny, superficial infection without any redness. Pimples can occur with acne or friction.
- *Here is some care advice that should help.*

❷ **Cleaning:** Wash the infected area with an antibacterial soap and warm water 3 times a day.

❸ **Antibiotic Ointment:** Apply antibiotic ointment (OTC) to the infected area 3 times per day.

❹ **Call Back If:**
- Redness occurs.
- Fever occurs.
- More pimples occur.
- You become worse.

General Care Advice for Contact Dermatitis

❶ Nickel Contact Dermatitis:

- Some people have an allergy to nickel-containing metals. Nickel is often present in less-expensive jewelry.
- People with nickel allergy can get an itchy rash where the metal touches their skin: finger (rings), earlobes (earrings), neck (neck chains), lower abdomen (belt buckle, metal snap on jeans), wrist (bracelets and wrist watches).
- If you are uncertain if you have a nickel allergy, you may need to get checked by your doctor.

❷ Do Not Wear Nickel-Containing Jewelry.

❸ Hydrocortisone Cream for Itching:

- Put 1% hydrocortisone cream on the itchy red area 3 times a day. Use it for 5 days. This will help decrease the itching.
- This is an over-the-counter (OTC) drug. You can buy it at the drugstore.
- Some people like to keep the cream in the refrigerator. It feels even better if the cream is used when it is cold.
- CAUTION: Do not use hydrocortisone cream for > 1 week without talking to your doctor.
- *Before using any medicine, read all the instructions on the package.*

❹ Avoid Scratching: Try not to scratch. Cut your fingernails short.

❺ Expected Course:

- If you stop wearing the nickel-containing ring, the redness and itching should go away in 7-14 days.
- Make an appointment to see your doctor if it does not.

❻ Call Back If:

- Rash spreads or becomes worse.
- Rash lasts > 2 weeks.
- You become worse.

BACKGROUND

Key Points

- Four localized rashes that the patient may be able to recognize are: athlete's foot, insect bites, poison ivy, and ringworm. If present, go to that protocol. If not, use this protocol.
- **Main Cause of Acute-Onset Localized Rash:** Skin contact with some irritant.
- **Main Cause of Persistent Localized Rash:** Contact dermatitis.
- **Cellulitis:** Infection of the skin. There is spreading erythema (redness). The skin is also painful, tender to touch, and warm. There may or may not be any drainage or discharge.

Contact Dermatitis

Contact dermatitis is a common cause of persistent localized rashes. Contact dermatitis usually presents as localized raised red spots or a red area. Occasionally it progresses to localized blisters (e.g., poison ivy). The contact dermatitis rash is itchy.

Contact dermatitis is an allergic skin reaction that occurs after repeated contacts with the allergic substance. Once sensitized to a substance, however, reactions occur 12-24 hours after exposure. The location of the rash may suggest the cause.

- **Poison Ivy or Oak:** Exposed areas (e.g., hands, forearms)
- **Nickel (Metal):** Neck from necklaces, earlobe from earrings, belly button from metal snaps inside pants, wrist from wristwatch
- **Tanning Agents in Leather:** Tops of the feet from shoes or hands after wearing leather gloves
- **Preservatives in Creams, Lotions, Sunscreens, Shampoos:** Site of application
- **Neomycin in Antibiotic Ointment:** Site of application

Contact Dermatitis From Nickel

- **Definition:** > 10% of adults have an allergy to nickel-containing metals. Nickel is often present in less-expensive jewelry. Even gold posts should be avoided immediately after a piercing because even higher quality gold can contain trace amounts of nickel.
- **Symptoms:** People with nickel allergy can get an itchy rash where the metal touches their skin: finger (rings), earlobes (earrings), neck (neck chains), mid-abdomen (metal fasteners on jeans or belt buckle), wrist (bracelets and wristwatches), and face (eyeglass frames).
- **Diagnosis:** See doctor if diagnosis is uncertain.
- **Treatment:** Avoid further contact with nickel. Apply a small amount of hydrocortisone cream 3 times a day for 7 days to the red-itchy area.
- **Expected Course:** Once the person stops wearing the nickel-containing jewelry, the redness and itching should go away in 7-14 days.
- **Prevention:** Avoid nickel-containing jewelry. Piercing jewelry should be made of hypoallergenic metal. Examples of metals that cause the least amount of allergy are titanium, platinum, palladium, niobium, and nickel-free stainless steel. Significant amounts of nickel are present in white gold, yellow gold (≤ 12 karat), regular stainless steel, and "costume" jewelry.

Intertrigo

- **Symptoms:** Erythematous and macerated (moist) areas between skinfolds. Sometimes the patient may experience mild burning discomfort or itching.
- **Location:** The most common area is under the breasts. However, in obese individuals it can happen in multiple other areas of the body wherever skin folds over and creates a moist pocket. In obese individuals another common area is where the abdomen overlaps onto the upper thigh.
  - **Risk Factors:** Obesity, heat, humidity, sweating, occlusive clothing, and diabetes.
  - **Complications:** May become infected with yeast; a secondary bacterial infection of the skin can sometimes occur.
  - **Treatment:** Reducing the moisture in the area is the most important thing to do. Strategies for accomplishing this include wearing loose clothing, drying area with cool hair dryer or fan, keeping skinfolds open to the air with a towel, and losing weight. Sometimes antifungal cream is helpful.

RASH OR REDNESS, WIDESPREAD

Definition
- Rash over large area or most of the body (widespread or generalized).
- Occasionally just on hands, feet, and buttocks—but symmetrical.
- Cause of rash is unknown.
- Red or pink rash (erythema).
- Smooth (macular) or slightly bumpy (papular).
- Small spots, large spots, or solid red.

Excluded: Three widespread rashes that the patient may be able to recognize are: chickenpox, hives, and sunburn. If present, go to that protocol. If not, use this protocol.

TRIAGE ASSESSMENT QUESTIONS

Call EMS 911 Now
- Sudden onset of rash (within last 2 hours) and difficulty with breathing or swallowing
  R/O: anaphylaxis, angioedema
- Difficult to awaken or acting confused (e.g., disoriented, slurred speech)
  R/O: toxic shock syndrome or septic shock, meningitis
- Fever and purple or blood-colored spots or dots
  R/O: meningococcemia, Rocky Mountain spotted fever
  Note: It may be difficult to determine the rash color in people with darker-colored skin.
- Too weak or sick to stand
  R/O: meningococcemia
- Life-threatening reaction (anaphylaxis) in the past to similar substance (e.g., food, insect bite/sting, chemical, etc.) and < 2 hours since exposure
- Sounds like a life-threatening emergency to the triager

See More Appropriate Protocol
- Insect bites suspected
  Go to Protocol: Insect Bite on page 257
- Sunburn suspected
  Go to Protocol: Sunburn on page 392
- Hives suspected
  Go to Protocol: Hives on page 226
- Drug rash suspected and started taking new medicine within last 2 weeks
  (Exception: antihistamine, eye drops, ear drops, decongestant, or other OTC cough/cold medicines)
  Go to Protocol: Rash, Widespread on Drugs (Drug Reaction) on page 322

Go to ED/UCC Now (or to Office With PCP Approval)
- Bright red, sunburn-like rash and current tampon use
  R/O: toxic shock syndrome, staph or strep exotoxin rash
- Bright red, sunburn-like rash and current tampon use or nasal packing
  R/O: toxic shock syndrome, staph or strep exotoxin rash
  Note: It may be difficult to determine the rash color in people with darker-colored skin.
- Bright red, sunburn-like rash and wound infection or recent surgery
  R/O: toxic shock syndrome, staph or strep exotoxin rash
- Bright red skin that peels off in sheets
  R/O: TENS, scalded skin syndrome
- Stiff neck (can't touch chin to chest)
  R/O: meningitis
- Patient sounds very sick or weak to the triager
  Reason: severe acute illness or serious complication suspected

Go to Office Now

- Fever
  R/O: bacterial or rickettsial illness
- Face becomes swollen
  Reason: may need steroids
- Headache
  R/O: Rocky Mountain spotted fever
- Purple or blood-colored spots or dots
  (no fever and sounds well to triager)
  R/O: purpura or petechiae, vasculitis
  Note: In comparison to other red rashes, petechiae and purpura do not temporarily blanch (fade) when pressure is applied to a spot. It may be difficult to determine the rash color in people with darker-colored skin.
- Joint pain or swelling
  R/O: gonococcemia
- Sores in mouth
  R/O: Stevens-Johnson syndrome, chickenpox
- Rash looks like large or small blisters
  (i.e., fluid-filled bubbles or sacs on the skin)
  (Stevens-Johnson syndrome, erythema multiforme, TENS, disseminated herpes zoster)

Callback by PCP Within 1 Hour

- Pregnant
- Rash began within 4 hours of a new prescription medication
  R/O: allergic reaction

See Today in Office

- SEVERE itching
- Sore throat
  R/O: scarlet fever
- Ringlike appearance of rash (or ask, "Does it look like a 'target' or 'bull's-eye'?")
  R/O: target lesions of erythema multiforme
- Patient wants to be seen

See Today or Tomorrow in Office

- Mild widespread rash
  R/O: allergy, viral exanthem

HOME CARE ADVICE

❶ **Reassurance:**
  - There are many causes of widespread rashes and most of the time they are not serious. Common causes include viral illness (e.g., cold viruses) and allergic reactions (to a food, medicine, or environmental exposure).
  - *Here is some care advice that should help.*

❷ **For Non-itchy Rashes:** No treatment is necessary, except for heat rashes, which respond to cool baths.

❸ **For Itchy Rashes:**
  - Wash the skin once with gentle non-perfumed soap to remove any irritants. Rinse the soap off thoroughly.
  - You may also take an oatmeal (Aveeno) bath or take an antihistamine medication by mouth to help reduce the itching.

❹ **Oatmeal Aveeno Bath for Itching:**
  - Sprinkle contents of one Aveeno packet under running faucet with comfortably warm water. Bathe for 15-20 minutes, 1-2 times daily.
  - Pat dry with a towel. Do not rub the rash.

❺ **Oral Antihistamine Medication for Itching:**
  - Take an antihistamine like diphenhydramine (Benadryl) for widespread rashes that itch. The adult dosage of Benadryl is 25-50 mg by mouth 4 times daily.
  - An over-the-counter antihistamine that causes less sleepiness is loratadine (e.g., Alavert or Claritin).
  - CAUTION: This type of medication may cause sleepiness. Do not drink alcohol, drive, or operate dangerous machinery while taking antihistamines. Do not take these medications if you have prostate problems.
  - *Before taking any medicine, read all the instructions on the package.*

❻ **Caution—Antihistamines:**
  - Examples include diphenhydramine (Benadryl) and chlorpheniramine (Chlor-Trimeton, Chlor-Tripolon).
  - May cause sleepiness. Do not drink alcohol, drive, or operate dangerous machinery while taking antihistamines.
  - Do not take these medicines if you have prostate problems.

❼ **Contagiousness:** Avoid contact with pregnant women until a diagnosis is made. Most viral rashes are contagious (especially if a fever is present). You can return to work or school after the rash is gone or when your doctor says it is safe to return with the rash.

❽ **Expected Course:** Most viral rashes disappear within 48 hours.

❾ **Call Back If:**
- You become worse.

FIRST AID

First Aid Advice for Anaphylaxis—Epinephrine:

- If the patient has an epinephrine autoinjector, **give it now.** Do not delay.
- Use the autoinjector on the upper outer thigh. You may give it through clothing if necessary.
- Give epinephrine first, then call 911.
- Epinephrine is available in autoinjectors under trade names: EpiPen, EpiPen Jr, and Auvi-Q (Allerject in Canada). Auvi-Q has an audio chip and talks patients and caregivers through injection process.
- You may give a second (repeat) dose of epinephrine 10-15 minutes later, IF the person with anaphylaxis does not respond to the first dose AND ambulance arrival takes > 10 minutes.

First Aid Advice for Anaphylaxis—Benadryl:

- Give antihistamine by mouth NOW if able to swallow.
- Use Benadryl (diphenhydramine; adult dose: 50 mg) or any other available antihistamine medicine.

BACKGROUND

Key Points
- Adult patients with fever and rash require urgent evaluation. There are a number of serious infections which can present in this manner. Examples of serious infections include meningococcemia, gonococcemia, endocarditis, and Rocky Mountain spotted fever.
- It is difficult to assess rash color in people with darker-colored skin. When this situation occurs, simply ask the caller to describe what he/she sees.

Fever and Rash
- **Toxic Shock Syndrome:** The rash is a widespread erythroderma (painless "sunburn") that usually fades in 72 hours. It is followed by skin desquamation (peeling), especially of the palms and soles. Other signs and symptoms of the syndrome include fever, muscle aches, vomiting or diarrhea, multiorgan dysfunction (liver, kidney), confusion, shock, and death. Those at risk include menstruating women using tampons, postsurgical patients, and patients with nasal packings.
- **Rocky Mountain Spotted Fever:** This is a tick-borne disease most commonly seen along the south Atlantic seaboard and in the south-central states. The rash usually starts as red spots on the hands and wrists and then becomes petechial (does not blanch with pressure). The rash occurs 2-14 days after a tick bite. Associated symptoms include headache and muscle aches.
- **Meningococcemia:** A rapidly fatal infectious disease that presents with fever, rash, headache, and stiff neck.
- **Gonococcemia:** The skin rash may first appear on the hands and feet as red pales (small raised spots) that then become pus-filled. Associated symptoms include fever and joint pain.
- **Endocarditis:** Bacterial infection of the heart. Risk factors for developing endocarditis include IV drug abuse, valvular heart disease, artificial heart valves, and indwelling IV catheters.

RECTAL BLEEDING

Definition

- Blood-colored material mixed in with the stool or passed separately
- Bloody or maroon-colored stools
- Tarry-black stools (melena)
- Includes calls about blood just on toilet paper, few drops into toilet water, or streaks on surface of normal formed bowl movement (BM)

Rectal Bleeding Severity:

- **Drops, Spots, Streaks:** Blood on toilet paper or a few drops in toilet bowl; streaks or drops of blood on surface of BM.
- **Mild:** More than just a few drops or streaks.
- **Moderate:** Small blood clots, passing blood without stool, or toilet water turns red.
- **Severe:** Large blood clots; on-and-off or constant bleeding.

TRIAGE ASSESSMENT QUESTIONS

Call EMS 911 Now

- Passed out (i.e., fainted, collapsed and was not responding)
  R/O: shock
  First Aid: Lie down with the feet elevated.
- Shock suspected (e.g., cold/pale/clammy skin, too weak to stand)
  R/O: shock
  First Aid: Lie down with the feet elevated.
- Vomiting red blood or black (coffee-ground) material
- Sounds like a life-threatening emergency to the triager

See More Appropriate Protocol

- Diarrhea is the main symptom
  Go to Protocol: Diarrhea on page 123
- Rectal symptoms
  Go to Protocol: Rectal Symptoms on page 336

Go to ED Now

- SEVERE rectal bleeding (large blood clots; on-and-off or constant bleeding)
  R/O: significant blood loss, anemia
- Severe dizziness (e.g., unable to stand, requires support to walk, feels like passing out now)
  R/O: significant blood loss, anemia
- MODERATE rectal bleeding (small blood clots, passing blood without stool, or toilet water turns red) > 1 a day
- Bloody, black, or tarry BMs
  R/O: GI bleed
  (Exception: chronic-unchanged black-gray BMs and is taking iron pills or Pepto-Bismol)
- HIGH-RISK adult (e.g., prior surgery on aorta, abdominal aortic aneurysm)
  R/O: aortoenteric fistula
- Rectal foreign body (inserted or swallowed)

Go to ED/UCC Now
(or to Office With PCP Approval)

- SEVERE abdominal pain (e.g., excruciating)
- Constant abdominal pain lasting > 2 hours
  R/O: ischemic colitis, acute abdomen
- Pale skin (pallor) of new onset or worsening
  R/O: anemia from GI bleeding
- Patient sounds very sick or weak to the triager
  Reason: severe acute illness or serious complication suspected

See Today in Office

- MODERATE rectal bleeding (small blood clots, passing blood without stool, or toilet water turns red)
  R/O: polyp, diverticulosis
- Taking Coumadin (warfarin) or other strong blood thinner, or known bleeding disorder (e.g., thrombocytopenia)
  Reason: higher risk of serious bleeding; may need testing of INR, prothrombin time, or platelet count
  Note: Besides Coumadin, other strong blood thinners include Arixtra (fondaparinux), Eliquis (apixaban), Pradaxa (dabigatran), and Xarelto (rivaroxaban). Plavix (clopidogrel; antiplatelet drug) also increases risk in head injury.

- Colonoscopy in past 72 hours
  R/O: post-polypectomy bleeding
- Known cirrhosis of the liver (or history of liver failure or ascites)
- Patient wants to be seen

See Within 3 Days in Office

- MILD rectal bleeding (more than just a few drops or streaks)
- Cancer of rectum or intestines (colon)
  R/O: possibility of recurrence
- Radiation therapy to lower abdomen or pelvis
  R/O: radiation proctitis

See Within 2 Weeks in Office

- Normal formed BM with a few streaks or drops of blood on surface of BM
  R/O: hemorrhoids, anal fissure
- Rectal bleeding is minimal (e.g., blood just on toilet paper, a few drops in toilet bowl)
  R/O: hemorrhoids, anal fissure

HOME CARE ADVICE

❶ **Reassurance:**
  - You have told me that there is only mild bleeding.
  - Often this can be caused by hemorrhoids or a small tear (fissure) in the skin of the anus (rectal opening).
  - There are several things that you can do to make this better.

❷ **Warm Saline Sitz Baths—Twice Daily for Rectal Symptoms:**
  - Sit in a warm sitz bath for 20 minutes twice a day. This will decrease swelling and irritation, keep the area clean, and help with healing.
  - Afterward, pat area dry with unscented toilet paper.

❸ **Warm Saline Sitz Bath—How to Make a Sitz Bath:**
  - Here is how you can make a saline sitz bath.
  - Fill the tub with warm water until it is 3-4" (7-10 cm) deep.
  - Add ¼ cup (80 g) of table salt or baking soda to a tub of warm water. Stir the water until it dissolves.

❹ **High-Fiber Diet:**
  - A high-fiber diet will help improve your intestinal function and soften your BMs. The fiber works by holding more water in your stools.
  - Try to eat fresh fruit and vegetables at each meal (peas, prunes, citrus, apples, beans, corn).
  - Eat more grain foods (bran flakes, bran muffins, graham crackers, oatmeal, brown rice, and whole wheat bread). Popcorn is a source of fiber.

❺ **Hydrocortisone Ointment for Rectal Itching:**
  - After sitz bath and drying your rectal area, put hydrocortisone ointment on the area 2 times a day. This will help decrease the itching.
  - This is an over-the-counter (OTC) drug. You can buy it at the drugstore. It can be found in a number of OTC hemorrhoid medicines (e.g., Anusol HC, Preparation H Hydrocortisone, Analpram-HC Cream).
  - Some people like to keep the ointment in the refrigerator. It feels even better if the cream is used when it is cold.
  - CAUTION: Do not use this medicine for > 1 week without talking to your doctor.
  - *Before using any medicine, read all the instructions on the package.*

❻ **Call Back If:**
  - Bleeding increases in amount.
  - Bleeding occurs ≥ 3 times after treatment begins.
  - You become worse.

FIRST AID

First Aid Advice for Shock:

Lie down with the feet elevated.

BACKGROUND

Causes

Some common causes of rectal bleeding are:

- **Anal Fissure:** This is a small crack or tear in the skin of the anus. It may result from passing hard stools or from having many diarrhea stools. Symptoms include pain during and right after passing a stool, mild rectal bleeding, and rectal itching.
- **Hemorrhoids:** Another name for these is piles. These are enlarged veins that are just inside ("internal") or outside ("external") the rectal opening (anus). Two top reasons why people get hemorrhoids are chronic constipation and pregnancy. People with hemorrhoids often see blood in the toilet water or small amounts of blood on the stool.

Some less common causes of rectal bleeding include:

- Angiodysplasia
- Cancer of colon (intestines)
- Cancer of rectum (anus)
- Colon polyps
- Crohn disease
- Diarrhea
- Proctitis
- Pseudomembranous colitis
- Radiation treatment
- Rectal foreign body
- Rectal varices due to portal hypertension
- Ulcerative colitis

Types of Rectal Bleeding

- **Bright Red Blood Just on Toilet Paper:** This is least serious. It often means that the bleeding is coming from the rectal opening (anus). The 2 most common causes of this type of bleeding are hemorrhoids and anal fissures.
- **Bright Red Blood on the Surface of a Stool:** This often means that the bleeding is from the anus or just inside. This can be caused by hemorrhoids or anal fissures. It can also be caused by more serious problems like cancer and polyps.
- **Blood Mixed With a Stool:** This usually means that there is a disease or problem inside the rectum or higher up in the colon (intestines). Examples are colon cancer, colon polyps, diverticulosis, and ulcerative colitis.

- **Blood Mixed With Diarrheal Stool:** With some more severe colon infections there can be blood mixed in with the stool.
- **Tarry-Black Stool:** Rarely, a person can have such severe bleeding from the stomach or esophagus that it passes all the way through and comes out the rectum. The stool can look black, tarry, or bloody. Stomach acid breaks down the blood and turns it black.

What Can Cause Red or Black Stools That Is *Not* Blood?

Causes of black-colored stools (not blood) include:

- Bismuth (Pepto-Bismol).
- Black licorice.
- Blueberries.
- Dark green stools may sometimes look like black. Put stool on white paper and hold under bright light. Is it green or black? Spinach and other dark vegetables can make stool look dark green.

Causes of red-colored stools (not blood) include:

- Beets
- Cranberries
- Medicines (Omnicef)
- Red food coloring dyes (red gelatin/Jell-O, red Kool-Aid)
- Red licorice
- Tomato juice or soup

RECTAL SYMPTOMS

Definition
- Rash, pain, itching, swelling, and other symptoms of the rectal area (anus)

TRIAGE ASSESSMENT QUESTIONS

Call EMS 911 Now
- ● Sounds like a life-threatening emergency to the triager

See More Appropriate Protocol
- ● Diarrhea is the main symptom
  Go to Protocol: Diarrhea on page 123
- ● Constipation is the main symptom
  (e.g., pain or discomfort caused by passage of hard bowel movements [BMs])
  Go to Protocol: Constipation on page 89
- ● Blood in or on BM is the main symptom
  Go to Protocol: Rectal Bleeding on page 333

Go to ED/UCC Now
(or to Office With PCP Approval)
- ● Sexual assault
  R/O: sexual assault, rectal injury from foreign body (FB)
- ● Injury to rectum
  R/O: sexual assault, rectal injury from FB
- ● Patient sounds very sick or weak to the triager
  Reason: severe acute illness or serious complication suspected

Go to Office Now
- ● Severe rectal pain
  R/O: abscess, herpes
- ● Rectal pain or redness and fever > 100.5° F (38.1° C)
  R/O: cellulitis, abscess
- ● Acute onset rectal pain and constipation (straining with rectal pressure or fullness), which is not relieved by sitz bath or suppository
  R/O: fecal impaction

See Today in Office
- ● MODERATE-SEVERE rectal pain
  (i.e., interferes with school, work, or sleep)
  R/O: thrombosed hemorrhoid, abscess, sexually transmitted infection (STI)
- ● MODERATE-SEVERE rectal itching
  (i.e., interferes with school, work, or sleep)
  R/O: contact dermatitis, poison ivy, pinworms
- ● Last BM > 4 days ago
  R/O: fecal impaction
- ● Rectal area looks infected
  (e.g., draining sore, spreading redness)
  R/O: abscess, cellulitis, STI
- ● Rash of rectal area (e.g., open sore, painful tiny water blisters, unexplained bumps)
  R/O: STI
- ● Caller is worried about an STI
  Reason: prevent spread of STI or relieve fear

See Today or Tomorrow in Office
- ● Home treatment > 3 days for rectal pain and not improved
  R/O: thrombosed hemorrhoid, anal fissure, abscess
- ● Home treatment for > 3 days for rectal itching and not improved
  R/O: pruritus ani, contact dermatitis, cancer, STI
- ● Patient wants to be seen

See Within 2 Weeks in Office
- ● Recurrent episodes of unexplained rectal pain, but NO rectal symptoms now
  R/O: proctalgia fugax
- ● Painless lump in rectal area
  R/O: hemorrhoid, condyloma, anal cancer

Home Care
- ○ Mild rectal pain
  R/O: hemorrhoids, fissure
- ○ Mild rectal itching
  R/O: contact dermatitis
- ○ Acute onset rectal pain and constipation
  (i.e., straining with rectal pressure or fullness) that is untreated
  R/O: fecal impaction

HOME CARE ADVICE

Rectal Pain

❶ Reassurance:
- Rectal pain and irritation can often be caused by either hemorrhoids or a tiny tear in the rectal opening (anal fissure). Home treatment can usually make the discomfort feel better.
- Small drops of blood can sometimes be seen on the toilet paper or stool in people with hemorrhoids or rectal irritation from hard bowel movements (BMs).

❷ Warm Saline Sitz Baths—Twice Daily for Rectal Symptoms:
- Sit in a warm sitz bath for 20 minutes twice a day. This will decrease swelling and irritation, keep the area clean, and help with healing.
- Afterward, pat area dry with unscented toilet paper.

❸ Warm Saline Sitz Bath—How to Make a Sitz Bath:
- Here is how you can make a saline sitz bath.
- Fill the tub with warm water until it is 3-4" (7-10 cm) deep.
- Add ¼ cup (80 g) of table salt or baking soda to a tub of warm water. Stir the water until it dissolves.

❹ Stool Softener (Colace) for Hard BMs:
- Stool softeners help reduce rectal pain during BMs.
- Colace (docusate sodium) is available OTC. Adult dosage 100 mg by mouth each day.
- *Before taking any medicine, read all the instructions on the package.*

❺ Caution—Colace:
- If you are pregnant or nursing, speak with your physician before using.
- *Before taking any medicine, read all the instructions on the package.*

❻ Preventing Constipation:
- Eat a high-fiber diet.
- Drink adequate liquids.
- Exercise regularly (even a daily 15-minute walk!).
- Get into a rhythm—try to have a BM at the same time each day.
- Don't ignore your body's signals regarding having a BM.
- Avoid enemas and stimulant laxatives.

❼ Expected Course: Rectal pain should be completely relieved by these instructions over the next couple days. If the discomfort does not go away, you should be seen by your PCP.

❽ Call Back If:
- Severe rectal pain.
- Rectal pain not improved after 3 days.
- Rectal bleeding is more than minor (e.g., more than just blood on toilet paper or few drops).
- Rectal bleeding is minor but is ongoing (e.g., occurs > 2 times).
- You become worse.

Rectal Pain or Fullness From Fecal Impaction

❶ Warm Saline Sitz Bath—Twice Daily for Rectal Pain Due to Constipation:
- Sit in a warm sitz bath for 20 minutes twice a day.
- A sitz bath may help relax the muscles around your rectum and make it easier to have a BM.
- Afterward, pat area dry with unscented toilet paper.

❷ Warm Saline Sitz Bath—How to Make a Sitz Bath:
- Here is how you can make a saline sitz bath.
- Fill the tub with warm water until it is 3-4" (7-10 cm) deep.
- Add ¼ cup (80 g) of table salt or baking soda to a tub of warm water. Stir the water until it dissolves.

❸ Suppository: If the sitz bath doesn't work, use 1 or 2 glycerin suppositories (OTC).

❹ Fleet Enema: If the sitz bath and suppository do not relieve the rectal pain, a Fleet phosphate enema may be helpful.

❺ Caution—Fleet Enema:
- Do not use if there is fever, abdominal pain, or rectal bleeding.
- Do not use if you have heart disease, kidney disease, or inflammatory bowel disease.
- Do not use if you have neutropenia (very low white cell count).
- Do not use if you are pregnant.

❻ **Preventing Constipation:**
- Eat a high-fiber diet.
- Drink adequate liquids.
- Exercise regularly (even a daily 15-minute walk!).
- Get into a rhythm—try to have a BM at the same time each day.
- Don't ignore your body's signals regarding having a BM.
- Avoid enemas and stimulant laxatives.

❼ **Expected Course:**
- Rectal pain should be completely relieved by these instructions.
- If the discomfort does not go away, you should be seen right away.

❽ **Call Back If:**
- Rectal pain is not relieved.
- Constant or increasing abdominal pain.
- Abdominal swelling or vomiting occur.
- You become worse.

Rectal Itching

❶ **Reassurance:** The main treatment for rectal itching is to keep the rectal area clean and dry and to avoid excessive rubbing or scratching.

❷ **Cleansing After BM:**
- Clean the anus with warm water after each BM. Use wet cotton or tissue.
- Pat the area dry using unscented toilet paper. Avoid rubbing area with toilet paper.

❸ **Warm Saline Sitz Baths—Twice Daily for Rectal Symptoms:**
- Sit in a warm sitz bath for 20 minutes twice a day. This will decrease swelling and irritation, keep the area clean, and help with healing.
- Afterward, pat area dry with unscented toilet paper.

❹ **Warm Saline Sitz Bath—How to Make a Sitz Bath:**
- Here is how you can make a saline sitz bath.
- Fill the tub with warm water until it is 3-4" (7-10 cm) deep.
- Add ¼ cup (80 g) of table salt or baking soda to a tub of warm water. Stir the water until it dissolves.

❺ **Hydrocortisone Ointment for Rectal Itching:**
- After sitz bath and drying your rectal area, put hydrocortisone ointment on the area 2 times a day. This will help decrease the itching.
- This is an over-the-counter (OTC) drug. You can buy it at the drugstore. It can be found in a number of OTC hemorrhoid medicines (eg, Anusol HC, Preparation H Hydrocortisone, Analpram-HC Cream).
- Some people like to keep the ointment in the refrigerator. It feels even better if the cream is used when it is cold.
- CAUTION: Do not use this medicine for > 1 week without talking to your doctor.
- *Before using any medicine, read all the instructions on the package.*

❻ **Preventing Itching:**
- Wear cotton underwear.
- Avoid perfumed or colored toilet papers.
- Avoid perfumed soap. Even regular soap can be irritating.
- Avoid foods that worsen your rectal itching. For some people this may include tomatoes, spices (pepper), coffee, and citrus fruits.

❼ **Call Back If:**
- Itching not improved after 3 days.
- You become worse.

BACKGROUND

Some Basics

- The anus and skin have rich nerve supplies. Pain or itching in this area can be intense.
- Passing of large hard stools or diarrhea stools causes most rectal symptoms. Dried stool left on the skin is irritating and can cause itching.

Common Causes of Rectal Pain

- Anal fissure
- Fecal impaction
- Hemorrhoids—thrombosed (clotted)
- Perirectal abscess and fistula
- Proctalgia fugax (severely painful muscle spasm of rectal area)
- Sexually transmitted infection (e.g., herpes simplex)

Common Causes of Rectal Itching (Pruritus Ani)

- Contact dermatitis (scented toilet products)
- Foods (citrus fruit, coffee, spices, tomatoes)
- Hemorrhoids
- Pinworms
- Poison ivy
- Pruritus ani (itching with no other cause found)
- Skin disorders (psoriasis, seborrhea, skin cancer)

What Are Hemorrhoids (Piles)?

- **Definition:** Large veins at the rectal opening (anus).
- **Internal Hemorrhoids:** Are located just inside the rectum. Symptoms include pain, bleeding, and itching. Sometimes internal hemorrhoids can bulge (prolapse) out of the rectal opening. People have a fullness in this area after a BM.
- **External Hemorrhoids:** Found just outside the rectal opening. Symptoms include pain, bleeding, and itching. They can be thrombosed (clotted, hard, painful tense blue lump) or not thrombosed (soft flesh-colored lump).
- **Causes:** Constipation, obesity, pregnancy, sitting for long periods, diarrhea, straining to lift heavy objects.
- **Treatment:** Sitz baths, hemorrhoid cream, stool softeners. Thrombosed hemorrhoids sometimes need surgery.
- **Prevention:** Good bowel habits include drinking enough fluids (6-8 glasses of water daily) and regular exercise. Other good habits are a high-fiber diet and having a BM at same time each day.

What Is Pruritus Ani?

- **Definition:** A term meaning anal itching. It is a common and bothersome symptom. This term is used when there is no other medical cause for the itching.
- **Causes:** In most cases itching is caused by irritation of the sensitive rectal nerve endings from stool or scented toilet products. Hemorrhoids can also cause itching. Sometimes certain foods can cause itching. Rarely, long-standing itching can be caused by skin disorders or rectal cancer.
- **Treatment:** The main treatment for rectal itching is to keep the rectal area clean and dry. Avoid rubbing or scratching this area. Loose cotton underwear helps keep the area dry. Over-the-counter hydrocortisone cream can also reduce itching.
- **Prevention:** Avoid scented toilet products. Keep rectal area clean and dry.

SEIZURE

Definition
- A seizure (convulsion) occurs.

Symptoms
- During a generalized seizure, the victim loses consciousness, becomes stiff, and has jerking of the arms and legs.
- During a partial (focal) seizure, jerking of an arm or leg on one side occurs.
- Most seizures last < 5 minutes.

TRIAGE ASSESSMENT QUESTIONS

Call EMS 911 Now
- ● First seizure ever
  R/O: stroke, brain tumor
- ● Epileptic seizure (in adult with known epilepsy) and continues > 5 minutes
  Reason: increased risk of status epilepticus
- ● ≥ 2 seizures and stays confused between seizures
  R/O: status epilepticus
- ● Bluish (or gray) lips or face
  First Aid: Begin mouth-to-mouth breathing if breathing stops.
  Note: Most adults breathe adequately during a seizure; a red-purple coloration of face is common.
- ● Head injury caused the seizure
  R/O: concussion, cerebral contusion, subdural/ epidural, or intracerebral hemorrhage
- ● Pregnant or postpartum
  Reason: higher-risk situation (mother and fetus); consider eclampsia if third trimester
- ● Known poisoning or overdose
- ● Seizure in a swimming pool
  R/O: aspiration
  First Aid: Remove victim from swimming pool.
- ● Has diabetes (diabetes mellitus)
  R/O: hypoglycemia
- ● Unresponsive (can't be awakened) after the seizure stops and persists > 5 minutes
  R/O: stroke, head trauma, overdose
- ● Acting confused (e.g., disoriented, slurred speech) after the seizure stops and persists > 30 minutes
  R/O: stroke, head trauma, overdose
- ● Sounds like a life-threatening emergency to the triager

Go to ED Now
- ● Second seizure occurs on the same day
  R/O: low anticonvulsant drug level
- ● Fever > 99.5° F (37.5° C)
  R/O: meningitis
- ● Severe headache
  R/O: meningitis, intracerebral hemorrhage
  Note: Most seizure victims will have a headache after a seizure.
- ● HIGH-RISK adult (e.g., alcohol or drug abuse)
  R/O: alcohol withdrawal seizure.

Go to ED/UCC Now
(or to Office With PCP Approval)
- ● Wants to sleep after the seizure and persists much longer than usual
  Reason: prolonged postictal sleepiness
- ● Patient sounds very sick or weak to the triager
  Reason: severe acute illness or serious complication suspected

See Today in Office
- ◐ Not on or ran out of seizure medicines (anticonvulsants)
  Reason: needs to be on anticonvulsant medications

See Today or Tomorrow in Office
- ◐ Stopped taking seizure medicines (anticonvulsants)
  Reason: patient education
  Note: Needs to resume anticonvulsant medications.
- ◐ Epileptic seizures occur frequently (several per week)
  R/O: low anticonvulsant drug level
- ◐ Patient wants to be seen

Home Care
- ○ Seizure lasting < 5 minutes with a history of prior seizure(s), and taking anticonvulsants
  Reason: brief seizure in patient on anticonvulsants

HOME CARE ADVICE

❶ **Reassurance:**
- This seizure did not last very long and there is a history of prior seizures. There is no need to go to the ED for every seizure.
- *Here is some care advice that should help.*

❷ **Anticonvulsant Medication:** If the seizure victim missed a dose of seizure medicine in the last 2 days, he/she should take that missed dose now.

❸ **Anticonvulsant Medication Levels:** If patient takes phenytoin (Dilantin), carbamazepine (Tegretol), valproic acid (Depakene, Depakote), or phenobarbital:
- You should have the blood levels of your seizure medication(s) checked periodically.
- If it has been > 1 month, we should arrange to get your medication levels checked this week.

❹ **Headache:**
- Most people after a seizure will have a headache.
- If the seizure has stopped and the person is now awake and alert, it is OK to treat the headache with acetaminophen (Tylenol; 650-1,000 mg by mouth).

❺ **Postictal Period:**
- Most seizure victims will be confused and groggy for a period after the seizure stops.
- Immediately after the seizure, the seizure victim will be very sleepy and may have noisy breathing.
- Gradually, the seizure victim will become more and more alert.
- Usually, the seizure victim is fully alert within 1-2 hours.

❻ **Sleep:**
- Let the seizure victim sleep if he/she wishes. *(Reason: The brain is temporarily exhausted, and sleep is restorative.)*
- Check the individual frequently for any breathing problems.

❼ **Expected Course:** After a brief seizure, most people feel normal within 1-2 hours.

❽ **Call Back If:**
- Another seizure occurs.
- Fever or severe headache.
- Stays confused (e.g., disoriented or slurred speech) > 30 minutes.
- Wants to sleep > 2 hours (or longer than usual).
- Patient becomes worse or you have more questions.

FIRST AID

First Aid Advice for Seizure:
DO PROTECT the VICTIM:
- Lay the seizing person on the ground, preferably on his/her side.
- Place a pillow or soft item under the head.
- Remove glasses.
- Move lamps, chairs, etc., away from person to prevent injury.
- Stay with victim until help arrives.

First Aid Advice for Seizure:
DO NOT:
- DO NOT put your finger or any object into the victim's mouth. This is unnecessary and can cut the mouth, injure a tooth, cause vomiting, or result in a serious bite of your finger.
- DO NOT try to restrain or hold the patient down.
- DO NOT try to resuscitate the victim just because breathing stops momentarily for 5-10 seconds. Breathing never looks normal during the seizure, but it's adequate if the color is not bluish.

First Aid Advice for Breathing Stopped or Cardiac Arrest
Hands-Only CPR
- Call 911.
- Push hard and fast on the center of the chest.

Special Notes:
- **High-quality CPR:** Rescuers should push hard to a depth of at least 2" (5 cm), at a rate of at least 100 compressions per minute; allow full chest recoil; and minimize interruptions in chest compressions. The disco song "Stayin' Alive" has the right beat for CPR.
- The American Heart Association (AHA) provides a 1-minute instructional video on Hands-Only CPR at: http://handsonlycpr.org. Be prepared. Watch it now, before you need it!
- Answers to frequently asked questions about Hands-Only CPR are available here: www.heart.org/HEARTORG/CPRAndECC/HandsOnlyCPR/LearnMore/Learn-More_UCM_440810_FAQ.jsp.
- You are strongly encouraged to get training in CPR from the American Red Cross or the AHA.
- Hands-Only CPR is a trademark of the AHA.

"All rescuers, regardless of training, should provide chest compressions to all cardiac arrest victims. Because of their importance, chest compressions should be the initial CPR action for all victims regardless of age. Rescuers who are able should add ventilations to chest compressions. Highly trained rescuers working together should coordinate their care and perform chest compressions as well as ventilations in a team-based approach." Source: 2010 AHA Guidelines for Cardiopulmonary Resuscitation and Emergency Cardiovascular Care

CPR by Trained Rescuers

Trained (confident) rescuers should add ventilations to chest compressions while waiting for paramedics to arrive:

- Call 911.
- Perform chest compressions and mouth-to-mouth breathing in cycles of 30 compressions and then 2 breaths.

Special Notes:

- Rescuers should push hard to a depth of at least 2" (5 cm), at a rate of at least 100 compressions per minute; allow full chest recoil; and minimize interruptions in chest compressions.

BACKGROUND

Types of Seizures

- **Generalized:** A generalized seizure involves the whole brain. The victim loses consciousness, becomes stiff, and has bilateral jerking of the arms and legs.
- **Partial:** A partial (focal) seizure involves only part of the brain. Jerking of an arm or leg on one side of the body occurs, with no loss of consciousness.
- **Complex:** A complex seizure is characterized by a period of abnormal behavior with associated confusion. There are no jerking movements.
- **Febrile:** Seen in children, not in adults.
- **Status Epilepticus:** The victim has a prolonged seizure (> 30 minutes) or does not awaken between 2 separate seizures.

Causes

- Alcohol withdrawal.
- Brain tumor.
- **Eclampsia:** Women in their third trimester of pregnancy can develop hypertension (preeclampsia) and, rarely, seizures (eclampsia).
- **Epilepsy:** Most seizures occur in adults already known to have epilepsy (recurrent seizure disorder).
- Head injury.
- Heatstroke.
- **Hypoxia:** Cerebral hypoxia can cause seizures.
- **Infection:** Examples include meningitis, encephalitis.
- **Low Drug Levels:** The most common cause of a seizure in a person with epilepsy is noncompliance with drug regimen of anticonvulsant medications.
- **Metabolic:** Examples include hypoglycemia and hyponatremia.
- **Stroke:** This can be either cerebral infarction or hemorrhage.

Epilepsy

- **Definition:** Epilepsy is a recurrent seizure disorder.
- Many individuals with epilepsy wear medical identification (e.g., medical alert bracelet). If there is no medical ID and no other information available to confirm epilepsy, the triager should assume that a seizure is a first seizure.
- **Triage Disposition:** A person with epilepsy does not need to come into the ED if the following conditions are met: seizure < 5 minutes AND returns to consciousness AND is not pregnant or diabetic AND there is no injury.
- **Treatment:** Anticonvulsant medications can reduce the frequency of seizures.

Postictal Symptoms

After experiencing a brief generalized (grand mal) seizure lasting < 5 minutes, many adults with epilepsy will have postictal symptoms for up to 2 hours afterward. During the initial several minutes of this postictal period the patient will be in a postictal coma; the patient is unresponsive to painful stimuli and has loud snoring respirations. For up to 15-30 minutes after a seizure the patient may have postictal confusion; the patient should demonstrate gradually improving alertness and orientation. For up to 2 hours after a seizure the patient may have postictal sleepiness; with verbal stimuli, the patient can be awakened and is not confused but may return to sleep when left alone. A headache is a common complaint. A patient whose postictal symptoms last longer than these periods may have a complication (e.g., head trauma, drug overdose, stroke, status epilepticus). Because of potential complications, the following cutoffs are used in this protocol for seeing postictal adults following a brief generalized seizure:

- **Postictal Coma:** > 5 minutes
- **Postictal Confusion:** > 30 minutes
- **Postictal Sleepiness:** > 2 hours, or longer than usual

SEXUAL ASSAULT OR RAPE

Definition
- Sexual intercourse or activity occurs without freely given consent.
- **Note:** Consent is when someone agrees, gives permission, or says "yes" to sexual activity with another person. Consent must be given voluntarily. Consent may be withdrawn at any point, including during the sexual activity.

TRIAGE ASSESSMENT QUESTIONS

Call EMS 911 Now
- In immediate danger now
  Reason: police involvement needed
- Major blood loss and has fainted or too weak to stand
  R/O: impending shock
- Major bleeding (actively dripping or spurting) that can't be stopped
  First Aid: Apply direct pressure to the entire wound with a clean cloth.
- Sounds like a life-threatening emergency to the triager

Go to ED Now
- Sexual assault (sexual intercourse or activity occurs without freely given consent)
  Reason: perform a medical forensic history and evidence collection (semen, DNA), counseling (Exception: patient refusal; patient does not want to have a sexual assault exam with evidence collection)
- Attempted sexual assault
  Reason: perform a medical forensic history and evidence collection (semen, DNA), counseling (Exception: patient refusal; patient does not want to have a sexual assault exam with evidence collection)
- Injury (or injuries) that need medical care
- Suspected victim of rape drug (e.g., GHB, ketamine, Rohypnol)
  Reason: blood or urine drug testing, counseling (Exception: patient refusal; patient does not want to undergo blood or testing)
  Note: Drug tests work best if done right away; 120 hours (5 days) is the outside time limit for detecting most drugs.

See Today in Office
- Requesting testing for sexually transmitted infection (STI) and does not want a sexual assault exam performed with evidence collection
  Reason: refer for evaluation and counseling
- Patient wants to be seen

Call Local Agency Today
- Requesting emergency contraception and does not want a sexual assault exam performed with evidence collection
  Reason: refer for counseling
  Note: Emergency contraception pills are available over the counter to women ≥ 17 years.

Home Care
- Emergency contraceptive pills, over-the-counter, questions about
- Sexual assault on a college campus and Title IX reporting, questions about
- Sexual assault in the US military (Department of Defense) and victim assistance, question about

HOME CARE ADVICE

General Information
❶ **Note to Triager—Provide Support:**
  - "I'm glad you called."
  - Encourage the victim to seek medical evaluation and help.
  - Encourage the victim to bring a family member or friend for support.

❷ **Note to Triager—Notifying Law Enforcement (Police):**
  - *Encourage the caller to call the police now. Give the caller the phone number.*
  - The quality of the evidence from a sexual assault exam decreases the longer the victim delays reporting.
  - Except in situations covered by mandatory reporting laws, **the victim, not the health care worker, makes the decision** to report a sexual assault to law enforcement.

❸ **Note to Triager—Referral for Counseling:**
- A sexual assault victim often benefits from counseling.
- The victim should be referred to a local sexual advocacy support clinic (Rape Crisis Center) during daytime hours. Give the caller the number.
- **United States:** If there is not an available local clinic, there is a National Sexual Assault Online Hotline: 800/656-HOPE (4673). Available at: https://ohl.rainn.org/online.

❹ **Note to Triager—Sexual Assault on Campus and Title IX Reporting (United States):**
- Title IX is a 1972 law that protects people from discrimination based on sex in education programs or activities which receive federal financial assistance.
- Title IX also protects people from sexual harassment and sexual violence.
- **A person (the victim) has the right file a complaint under Title IX.** This is not mandatory. It is up to the victim. It is completely separate from making a police report.
- A victim can file a complaint with his/her school's Title IX coordinator. If a Title IX coordinator is not available, a victim can instead file a complaint with the US Office for Civil Rights.

❺ **Note to Triager—Sexual Assault in the US Military:**
- A victim of sexual assault should be offered the assistance of a sexual assault response coordinator (SARC) or victim advocate (VA). More information is available at: www.sapr.mil/index.php/victim-assistance.
- The US Department of Defense provides a 24-hour-a-day Safe Helpline to members of the service who have been sexually assaulted. The phone number is 877/995-5247. Available at: https://www.safehelpline.org.

❻ **Data:** Obtain the patient's name, address, phone number, and city/county in which the sexual assault occurred.

❼ **Helpful Telephone Numbers:**
- Police department:

  — — — - — — — - — — — —
- Rape Crisis Center:

  — — — - — — — - — — — —
- Rape, Abuse & Incest National Network (RAINN) National Sexual Assault Telephone Hotline: 800/656-HOPE (4673)

❽ **Call Back If:**
- You have any other question or if I can help you in any way.
- You become worse.

Instructions for Patients Being Sent to ED for Sexual Assault Examination

❶ **Preserve the Evidence:**
- Do not bathe or wash.
- Do not change clothes.
- Do not brush your hair.
- Following vaginal intercourse, do not douche or change your tampon.
- Following oral intercourse, do not eat, drink, or brush teeth.
- Bring any articles of clothing that may contain blood or semen.

❷ **Bring Clothes:**
- If the victim has not changed clothes since the assault, bring a change of clothes to put on at the hospital.

❸ **Support:**
- "I'm glad you called."
- Encourage the victim to seek medical evaluation and help.
- Encourage the victim to bring a family member or friend for support.

Emergency Contraceptive Pill (ECP)

❶ **ECP:**
- ECPs are very effective in preventing pregnancy after unprotected sexual intercourse. They can reduce the pregnancy rate by 75%-88%.
- They are also sometimes called "morning-after pills," but you do not have to take them just in the morning.
- The sooner the pills are started, the better they work. The pills must be started within 120 hours (5 days) and ideally within 72 hours (3 days) of the unprotected sexual intercourse.
- ECPs do not prevent sexually transmitted infections.

❷ **ECP—Effectiveness** (statistics for women in second or third week of cycle):
- **No Treatment:** 8 out of 100 women will get pregnant.
- **Treatment 72-120 Hours After Intercourse:** 3-4 out of 100 women will get pregnant.
- **Treatment Within 72 hours After Intercourse:** 1-2 out of 100 women will get pregnant.

❸ **ECP—Side Effects:**
- **Nausea:** 30%-60%
- **Vomiting:** 5%-20%
- **Abdominal Pain:** 10%-20%
- **Fatigue and Headache:** 10%-20%
- **Change in Menstrual Bleeding Onset or Amount:** 50%

❹ **ECP—Contraindications:**
- Pregnancy known or suspected.
- Abnormal vaginal bleeding and cause is unknown.

❺ **ECP—No Increased Risk of Birth Defects:**
- ECPs do not cause any birth defects.

❻ **ECP—Dosage for Plan B (Levonorgestrel):**
- **Availability:** You can get Plan B without a prescription at most pharmacies. Contact your local pharmacy to determine if it has and provides this pill.
- **Dosage:** Take one pill now and one pill in 12 hours.
- **Cost:** The typical cost of ECP is $20-$30.

Military Service Members Who Are Victims of Sexual Assault

❶ **Victims of Sexual Assault and US Department of Defense Sexual Assault Prevention and Response (SAPR) Policy:**
- Each person covered under the US Department of Defense SAPR policy who reports a sexual assault must be offered the assistance of a sexual assault response coordinator (SARC) or victim advocate (VA).
- SARCs and VAs address safety needs, explain the reporting options and services available, and assist with navigating the military criminal justice process.

- SARCs and VAs offer expertise to prepare victims for the road ahead and will advocate on behalf of a victim along the way. They will provide professional assistance with obtaining medical care, counseling services, legal and spiritual support, and off-base resources, if so desired.
- **Source:** www.sapr.mil/index.php/victim-assistance.

❷ **Offer Assistance of a Sexual Assault Response Coordinator (SARC) or Victim Advocate (VA):**
- If you approve, I would like to arrange for you to get help from a SARC or VA.
- They can help make sure you are safe, get the right medical care, and explain what services are available for you.
- They can be your advocate and make suggestions for counseling services, legal and spiritual support, and obtaining off-base resources, if desired.

Additional Internet Resources:

❶ *National Protocol for Sexual Assault Medical Forensic Examinations of Adults/Adolescents.* U.S. Department of Justice. Available online at: https://www.ncjrs.gov/pdffiles1/ovw/241903.pdf.

❷ **National Sexual Violence Resource Center:** 877/739-3895 or 717/909-0710. Available at: www.nsvrc.org.

❸ **Rape, Abuse & Incest National Network (RAINN)** has a hotline that victims of sexual assault can call: 800/656-HOPE (4673). Available at: www.rainn.org.
- Rape, Abuse & Incest National Network (RAINN) has a search engine for locating a local counseling center for a victim of sexual assault: www.rainn.org.

❹ **US Department of Defense Sexual Assault Prevention and Response Office:** www.sapr.mil/index.php/victim-assistance.

BACKGROUND

Key Points

- The victim is usually female (96%).
- Between 60% and 80% of the time, the victim knows the assailant.
- Approximately 40% of the time, the assault occurs in the victim's or assailant's home.
- It is essential to respond to individuals disclosing sexual assault in a timely, appropriate, sensitive, and respectful way.
- Except in situations covered by mandatory reporting laws, **patients, not health care workers, make the decision to report a sexual assault** to law enforcement.
- **Physical Examination:** General body trauma is more commonly found than genital trauma. General body injuries are usually minor and include contusions, abrasions, and lacerations.
- **Evidence Collection:** Many jurisdictions currently use 72 hours after the assault as the standard cutoff time for collecting evidence. Evidence collection beyond that point is still possible, especially with recent advances in DNA testing. Because of this, some jurisdictions have extended the standard cutoff time (e.g., up to 5 days).
- **Pregnancy Risk After Sexual Assault:** The risk of pregnancy after sexual assault is between 2% and 5%. Emergency (morning-after) contraceptive pills can prevent pregnancy. The sooner the pills are started, the better they work. The pills must be started within 120 hours (5 days) and ideally within 72 hours (3 days) of the unprotected sexual intercourse. It can reduce the risk of pregnancy by 75%-88%.

Sexual Assault and Patient Concerns and Fears

- Becoming pregnant.
- Bringing shame to family.
- Costs of medical care.
- Cultural factors, including loss of virginity and acceptability for a marriage.
- Getting a sexually transmitted infection (STI).
- Getting HIV.
- Law enforcement involvement might result in a report to immigration authorities and deportation.
- Loss of home, children, citizenship, income— especially if assault by an intimate partner.
- Physical injury.

Emergency Contraceptive Pills—History, Legislation, and Over-the-counter (OTC) Availability

- **Australia:** Emergency contraceptive pills became available OTC in 2004.
- **Canada:** On April 19, 2005, the Canadian Ministry of Health approved the sale of Plan B (levonorgestrel) without prescription in pharmacies in Canada.
- **United States:** On August 24, 2006, Plan B (levonorgestrel) was approved by the US Food and Drug Administration (FDA) for nonprescription sale in pharmacies to women and men ≥ 18 years in the United States. On April 22, 2009, Plan B was approved by the FDA for nonprescription sale in pharmacies to women ≥ 17 years.

Emergency Contraceptive Pills— How the Pills Work

The exact mode of action of ECPs in any given case cannot be known. The mode of action depends on where you are in your menstrual cycle. There are 4 ways ECPs prevent pregnancy:

❶ ECPs can stop ovulation for a few days.

❷ ECPs can slow the movements of the egg or the sperm in the tubes between the ovaries and the uterus.

❸ ECPs may prevent a sperm from fertilizing an egg.

❹ ECPs can change the lining of the uterus, which may prevent a fertilized egg from attaching properly.

Emergency Contraceptive Pills— Over-the-counter Availability

- **Plan B—Available in Canada and the United States:** Plan B comes in a package of 2 tablets (each tablet contains 0.75 mg levonorgestrel). While the package instructions recommend taking 1 pill now and 1 pill 12 hours later, it is better to take both pills at the same time. Research supports this because the pills are more effective the sooner that they are used. The pills should be taken within 120 hours (5 days) of unprotected sexual intercourse. Levonorgestrel causes less nausea and vomiting than prescription birth control pills and appears to be more effective at preventing pregnancy. Further information is available at the Emergency Contraception Website (http://ec.princeton.edu).

- **Plan B One-Step—Available in the United States:** Plan B One-Step is becoming available in pharmacies in the United States. It is a single 1.5 mg tablet of levonorgestrel. The pill should be taken within 120 hours (5 days) of unprotected intercourse. Further information is available at the Emergency Contraception Website (http://ec.princeton.edu).
- **Next Choice—Available in the United States:** While the package instructions recommend taking 1 pill now and 1 pill 12 hours later, it is better to take both pills at the same time. The pills should be taken within 120 hours (5 days) of unprotected intercourse. Further information is available at the Emergency Contraception Website (http://ec.princeton.edu).
- **NorLevo 0.75 mg—Available in Canada:** While the package instructions recommend taking 1 pill now and 1 pill 12 hours later, it is better to take both pills at the same time. The pills should be taken within 120 hours (5 days) of unprotected intercourse.
- **Levonelle-1, NorLevo 1.5 mg, Postinor 1— Available in Australia:** Package instructions are to take 1 pill within 120 hours (5 days) of unprotected sexual intercourse.

Emergency Contraceptive Pills— Important Internet Resources

- **The Emergency Contraception Website:** http://ec.princeton.edu. This is a very useful Web site with answers to many frequently asked questions. This Web site also lists physicians and clinics in the United States and Canada that provide emergency contraceptive pills.
- **Canadian Paediatric Society Adolescent Health Committee** position statement: www.cps.ca/en/ documents/position/emergency-contraception.

Rape Drugs

- **Definition:** There are several drugs that are referred to as "rape drugs" because they are used by rapists to make a victim confused or unconscious. The drugs are typically put into the victim's drink without the victim's knowledge or consent. The drugs can be tasteless, colorless, and odorless; the victim does not know that she (or he) is being drugged.
- **Alternate Term:** Drug-facilitated sexual assault.
- **Symptoms:** Victims report waking up feeling drugged or more hungover than expected. Victims sometimes report amnesia; they may remember taking a drink but then can't remember what

happened after that. Sometimes victims report that they feel like someone had sex with them but they cannot remember anything more.
- **Examples of Rape Drugs:** GHB, ketamine, Rohypnol (flunitrazepam).
- **Urine Testing for Rape Drugs:** Date rape drugs can be detected in the urine. However, the body metabolizes these drugs very quickly and the drug may be difficult to detect in as little as 12 hours.
- **Alcohol and Alcohol-Facilitated Sexual Assault:** Approximately 30%-75% of victims of sexual assault have been drinking alcohol. Thus, there is a correlation between alcohol intoxication and the risk of sexual assault.

Internet Resources—United States

- **The National Sexual Violence Resource Center (NSVRC):** 877/739-3895 or 717/909-0710. Available at: www.nsvrc.org.
- **Rape, Abuse & Incest National Network (RAINN)** has a hotline that victims of sexual assault can call: 800/656-4673 (HOPE). Available at: www.rainn.org.
- **Rape, Abuse & Incest National Network (RAINN)** has a search engine for locating a local counseling center for a victim of sexual assault: www.rainn.org.
- **US Department of Justice:** *A National Protocol for Sexual Assault Medical Forensic Examinations:* www.safeta.org.
- **US Department of Defense (DoD) Sexual Assault Prevention and Response (DoD SAPR):** *"Each person covered under DoD SAPR policy who reports a sexual assault is offered the assistance of a Sexual Assault Response Coordinator (SARC) or Victim Advocate (VA) who addresses safety needs, explains the reporting options, services available, and assists with navigating the military criminal justice process. SARCs and SAPR VAs offer expertise to prepare victims for the road ahead and will advocate on behalf of a victim along the way."* Available at: www.sapr.mil/index.php/ victim-assistance.
- **US DoD Safe Helpline:** The Safe Helpline provides confidential crisis intervention, support, and information to service members of the US DoD community who have been sexually assaulted. The 24-hour-a-day phone number is 877/995-5247. Available at: https://www.safehelpline.org.
- **US Office for Civil Rights and Title IX Reporting:** www2.ed.gov/about/offices/list/ocr/docs/ tix_dis.html.

SHOULDER INJURY

Definition
- Injuries to a bone, muscle, joint, or ligament in the shoulder.
- Associated skin and soft tissue injuries are also included.

TRIAGE ASSESSMENT QUESTIONS

Call EMS 911 Now
- Major bleeding (actively dripping or spurting) that can't be stopped
  First Aid: Apply direct pressure to the entire wound with a clean cloth.
- Amputation or bone sticking through the skin
- Bullet, stabbed by knife, or other serious penetrating wound
  First Aid: If penetrating object is still in place, don't remove it.
- Sounds like a life-threatening emergency to the triager

See More Appropriate Protocol
- Wound looks infected
  Go to Protocol: Wound Infection on page 443

Go to ED Now
- Looks like a broken bone or dislocated joint (crooked or deformed)
  R/O: fracture, dislocation

Go to ED/UCC Now (or to Office With PCP Approval)
- Can't move injured shoulder at all
  R/O: fracture
- Collar bone is painful or tender to touch
  R/O: clavicle fracture
- Skin is split open or gaping (length > ½" or 12 mm)
  Reason: may need laceration repair (e.g., sutures)
- Bleeding won't stop after 10 minutes of direct pressure (using correct technique)
- Dirt in the wound and not removed after 15 minutes of scrubbing
  Reason: needs irrigation or debridement
- Sounds like a serious injury to the triager

See Today in Office
- SEVERE pain (e.g., excruciating)
  R/O: fracture, strain, rotator cuff tear
- Can't move injured shoulder normally (e.g., full range of motion, able to touch top of head)
  R/O: strain, sprain, rotator cuff tear
- Large swelling or bruise and size > palm of person's hand
  R/O: fracture, large contusion
- Patient wants to be seen

See Today or Tomorrow in Office
- Injury interferes with work or school
- HIGH-RISK adult (e.g., age > 60, osteoporosis, chronic steroid use)
  Reason: greater risk of fracture in patients with osteoporosis
- Wound and no tetanus booster in > 5 years (or > 10 years for clean cuts)
  Reason: may need a tetanus booster shot (vaccine)
- Suspicious history for the injury
  R/O: domestic violence or elder abuse

See Within 3 Days in Office
- Injury and pain has not improved after 3 days
- Injury is still painful or swollen after 2 weeks

Home Care
○ Minor shoulder injury
  R/O: minor bruise, strain, or sprain

HOME CARE ADVICE

Treatment of a Minor Bruise, Sprain, or Strain

❶ Reassurance—Direct Blow (Contusion, Bruise):
- A direct blow to your shoulder can cause a contusion. Contusion is the medical term for bruise.
- Symptoms are mild pain, swelling, and/or bruising.
- *Here is some care advice that should help.*

❷ Reassurance—Bending or Twisting Injury (Strain, Sprain):
- Strain and sprain are the medical terms used to describe overstretching of the muscles and ligaments of the shoulder. A twisting or bending injury can cause a strain or sprain.
- The main symptom is pain that is worse with movement.
- *Here is some care advice that should help.*

❸ Apply a Cold Pack:
- Apply a cold pack or an ice bag (wrapped in a moist towel) to the area for 20 minutes. Repeat in 1 hour, then every 4 hours while awake.
- Continue this for the first 48 hours after an injury.
- This will help decrease pain and swelling.

❹ Apply Heat to the Area:
- Beginning 48 hours after an injury, apply a warm washcloth or heating pad for 10 minutes 3 times a day.
- This will help increase blood flow and improve healing.

❺ Rest Versus Movement:
- Movement is generally more healing in the long term than rest.
- Continue normal activities as much as your pain permits.
- Avoid heavy lifting and active sports for 1-2 weeks or until the pain and swelling are gone.
- Complete rest should only be used for the first day or two after an injury. If it really hurts to use the arm at all, you will need to see the doctor.

❻ Expected Course:
- Pain, swelling, and bruising usually start to get better 2-3 days after an injury.
- Swelling most often is gone after 1 week.
- Bruises fade away slowly over 1-2 weeks.
- It may take 2 weeks for pain and tenderness of the injured area to go away.

❼ Call Back If:
- Pain becomes severe.
- Pain does not improve after 3 days.
- Pain or swelling lasts > 2 weeks.
- You become worse.

Treatment of a Small Cut or Scrape

❶ Reassurance—Superficial Laceration (Cut or Scratch) or Abrasion (Scrape):
- This sounds like a small cut or scrape that we can treat at home.
- *Here is some care advice that should help.*

❷ Bleeding: Apply direct pressure for 10 minutes with a sterile gauze to stop any bleeding.

❸ Cleaning the Wound:
- Wash the wound with soap and water for 5 minutes.
- For any dirt, scrub gently with a washcloth.
- For any bleeding, apply direct pressure with a sterile gauze or clean cloth for 10 minutes.

❹ Antibiotic Ointment:
- Apply an antibiotic ointment (e.g., OTC bacitracin), covered by a Band-Aid or dressing. Change daily or if it becomes wet.
- Option: A Telfa dressing won't stick to the wound when it is removed.
- Option: Another option is to use a liquid skin bandage that only needs to be applied once. Don't use antibiotic ointment if you use a liquid skin bandage.

❺ Liquid Skin Bandage:
- You can use a liquid skin bandage instead of antibiotic ointment and a dressing or a Band-Aid.
- **Benefits:** Liquid skin bandage has several benefits when compared with a regular bandage (e.g., a dressing or a Band-Aid). You only need to put a liquid bandage on once to minor cuts and scrapes. It helps stop minor bleeding. It seals the wound and may promote faster healing and lower infection rates. However, it also costs more.

- **How to Use It:** First clean and dry the wound. You put on the liquid as spray or with a swab. It dries in < 1 minute and usually lasts a week. You can get it wet.
- **Examples:** Liquid skin bandage is available over the counter. Examples are Band-Aid Liquid Bandage, New Skin, Curad Spray Bandage, and 3M No Sting Liquid Bandage Spray.

❻ **Call Back If:**
- Looks infected (pus, redness, increasing tenderness).
- Doesn't heal within 10 days.
- You become worse.

Over-the-counter Pain Medicines

❶ **Pain Medicines:**
- For pain relief, you can take either acetaminophen, ibuprofen, or naproxen.
- They are over-the-counter (OTC) pain drugs. You can buy them at the drugstore.

Acetaminophen (e.g., Tylenol):
- **Regular Strength Tylenol:** Take 650 mg (two 325 mg pills) by mouth every 4-6 hours as needed. Each Regular Strength Tylenol pill has 325 mg of acetaminophen.
- **Extra Strength Tylenol:** Take 1,000 mg (two 500 mg pills) every 8 hours as needed. Each Extra Strength Tylenol pill has 500 mg of acetaminophen.
- The most you should take each day is 3,000 mg (10 Regular Strength or 6 Extra Strength pills a day).

Ibuprofen (e.g., Motrin, Advil):
- Take 400 mg (two 200 mg pills) by mouth every 6 hours.
- Another choice is to take 600 mg (three 200 mg pills) by mouth every 8 hours.
- The most you should take each day is 1,200 mg (six 200 mg pills), unless your doctor has told you to take more.

Naproxen (e.g., Aleve):
- Take 220 mg (one 220 mg pill) by mouth every 8 hours as needed. You may take 440 mg (two 220 mg pills) for your first dose.
- The most you should take each day is 660 mg (three 220 mg pills a day), unless your doctor has told you to take more.

❷ **Pain Medicines—Extra Notes:**
- Use the lowest amount of medicine that makes your pain better.
- Acetaminophen is thought to be safer than ibuprofen or naproxen in people > 65 years old. Acetaminophen is in many OTC and prescription medicines. It might be in more than one medicine that you are taking. You need to be careful and not take an overdose. An acetaminophen overdose can hurt the liver.
- McNeil, the company that makes Tylenol, has different dosage instructions for Tylenol in Canada and the United States. In Canada, the maximum recommended dose per day is 4,000 mg or 12 Regular Strength (325 mg) pills. In the United States, McNeil recommends a maximum dose of 10 Regular Strength (325 mg) pills.
- CAUTION: Do not take acetaminophen if you have liver disease.
- CAUTION: Do not take ibuprofen or naproxen if you have stomach problems, have kidney disease, are pregnant, or have been told by your doctor to avoid this type of anti-inflammatory drug. Do not take ibuprofen or naproxen for > 7 days without consulting your doctor.
- *Before taking any medicine, read all the instructions on the package.*

❸ **Call Back If:**
- You have more questions.
- You become worse.

FIRST AID

First Aid Advice for Bleeding:
Apply direct pressure to the entire wound with a clean cloth.

First Aid Advice for Penetrating Object:
If penetrating object is still in place, don't remove it. *Reason: Removal could increase bleeding.*

First Aid Advice for Shock:
Lie down with the feet elevated.

First Aid Advice for Suspected Fracture or Dislocation of the Shoulder:
- Use a sling to support the arm. Make the sling with a triangular piece of cloth.
- Or, at the very least, the patient can support the injured arm with the other hand or a pillow.

BACKGROUND

Types of Shoulder Injuries

- Fractures (broken bones)
- Dislocations (bone out of joint)
- **Sprains:** Stretches and tears of ligaments
- **Strains:** Stretches and tears of muscles (e.g., pulled muscle)
- Muscle overuse injuries from sports or exercise (e.g., strain, bursitis, tendonitis)
- Muscle bruise from a direct blow (e.g., contusion)
- **Causes Extrinsic to Shoulder (Referred Pain):** Examples include neck pain, cardiac disease, abdominal disorders, spleen injury

What Cuts Need to Be Sutured?

- Any cut that is split open or gaping probably needs sutures (or staples or skin glue).
- Cuts > ½" (1 cm) usually need sutures.
- Any open wound that may need sutures should be evaluated by a physician regardless of the time that has passed since the initial injury.

When Does an Adult Need a Tetanus Booster (Tetanus Shot)?

- **Clean Cuts and Scrapes—Tetanus Booster Needed Every 10 Years:** Patients with clean minor wounds AND who have previously had ≥ 3 tetanus shots (full series) need a booster every 10 years. Examples of minor wounds include a superficial abrasion or a shallow cut from a clean knife blade. Obtain booster within 72 hours.
- **Dirty Wounds—Tetanus Booster Needed Every 5 Years:** Patients with dirty wounds need a booster if it has been > 5 years since the last booster. Examples of dirty wounds include those contaminated with soil, feces, and/or saliva and more serious wounds from deep punctures, crushing, and burns. Obtain booster within 72 hours.

Caution: Cardiac Ischemia

- The most life-threatening cause of acute shoulder pain is cardiac ischemia.
- Rarely, patients may present with shoulder pain as the sole symptom of a myocardial infarction. Usually there will be other associated symptoms of cardiac ischemia: chest pain, shortness of breath, nausea, and/or diaphoresis.
- Cardiac ischemia should be suspected in any patients with risk factors for cardiac disease. These include: hypertension, smoking, diabetes, hyperlipidemia, a strong family history of heart disease, male gender, and age > 60.

SINUS PAIN AND CONGESTION

Definition
- Sensation of fullness, pressure, and pain on the face overlying a sinus cavity (e.g., above the eyebrow, behind the eye, around the eye, or over the cheekbone).
- Pain or pressure may be bilateral but more often is unilateral (on one side of the face).
- Associated symptoms are a blocked nose, nasal discharge, and/or postnasal drip.

Pain Severity Scale
- **Mild (1-3):** Doesn't interfere with normal activities.
- **Moderate (4-7):** Interferes with normal activities (e.g., work or school) or awakens from sleep.
- **Severe (8-10):** Excruciating pain, unable to do any normal activities.

TRIAGE ASSESSMENT QUESTIONS

Call EMS 911 Now
- Sounds like a life-threatening emergency to the triager

Go to ED Now
- Difficulty breathing, and not from stuffy nose (e.g., not relieved by cleaning out the nose)
  R/O: pneumonia

Go to ED/UCC Now
(or to Office With PCP Approval)
- SEVERE headache and has fever
  R/O: bacterial frontal sinusitis, cavernous sinus thrombosis, meningitis
- Patient sounds very sick or weak to the triager
  Reason: severe acute illness or serious complication suspected

Go to Office Now
- SEVERE sinus pain
  R/O: bacterial sinusitis
- Severe headache
  R/O: cavernous sinus thrombosis, meningitis
- Redness or swelling on the cheek, forehead, or around the eye
  R/O: sinusitis with overlying cellulitis, osteomyelitis, preseptal cellulitis

- Fever > 103° F (39.4° C)
  R/O: sinusitis, pneumonia
- Fever > 100.5° F (38.1° C) and > 60 years of age
  R/O: pneumonia, sinusitis.
- Fever > 100.0° F (37.8° C) and has diabetes mellitus or a weak immune system (e.g., HIV positive, cancer chemotherapy, organ transplant, splenectomy, chronic steroids)
  R/O: pneumonia, sinusitis
- Fever > 100.0° F (37.8° C) and bedridden (e.g., nursing home patient, stroke, chronic illness, recovering from surgery)
  R/O: pneumonia, sinusitis
  Note: May need ambulance transport to ED.

See Today in Office
- Fever present > 3 days (72 hours)
  R/O: bacterial sinusitis
- Fever returns after gone for > 24 hours and symptoms worse or not improved
  R/O: bacterial sinusitis, bronchitis, pneumonia
- Sinus pain (not just congestion) and fever
  R/O: bacterial sinusitis
- Earache
  R/O: ear infection

See Today or Tomorrow in Office
- Sinus congestion (pressure, fullness) present > 10 days
  R/O: bacterial sinusitis, allergic rhinitis
- Nasal discharge present > 10 days
  R/O: bacterial sinusitis, allergic rhinitis
- Using nasal washes and pain medicine > 24 hours and sinus pain (lower forehead, cheekbone, or eye) persists
  R/O: bacterial sinusitis, allergic rhinitis
- Lots of coughing
  R/O: cough triggered by sinusitis
- Patient wants to be seen

Home Care
- Sinus congestion as part of a cold, present < 10 days

HOME CARE ADVICE

General Care Advice for Mild Sinus Pain and Congestion

❶ **Reassurance:**
- Sinus congestion is a normal part of a cold.
- Usually, home treatment with nasal washes can prevent an actual bacterial sinus infection.
- Antibiotics are not helpful for the sinus congestion that occurs with colds.
- *Here is some care advice that should help.*

❷ **For a Runny Nose With Profuse Discharge— Blow the Nose:**
- Nasal mucus and discharge helps to wash viruses and bacteria out of the nose and sinuses.
- Blowing the nose is all that is needed.
- If the skin around your nostrils gets irritated, apply a tiny amount of petroleum ointment to the nasal openings once or twice a day.

❸ **Nasal Washes for a Stuffy Nose:**
- **Introduction:** Saline (salt water) nasal irrigation (nasal wash) is an effective and simple home remedy for treating stuffy nose and sinus congestion. The nose can be irrigated by pouring, spraying, or squirting salt water into the nose and then letting it run back out.
- **How It Helps:** The salt water rinses out excess mucus and washes out any irritants (dust, allergens) that might be present. It also moistens the nasal cavity.
- **Methods:** There are several ways to irrigate the nose. You can use a saline nasal spray bottle (available over the counter), a rubber ear syringe, a medical syringe without the needle, or a neti pot.

❹ **Nasal Washes—Step-by-Step Instructions:**
- **Step 1:** Lean over a sink.
- **Step 2:** Gently squirt or spray warm salt water into one of your nostrils.
- **Step 3:** Some of the water may run into the back of your throat. Spit this out. If you swallow the salt water, it will not hurt you.
- **Step 4:** Blow your nose to clean out the water and mucus.
- **Step 5:** Repeat steps 1-4 for the other nostril. You can do this a couple times a day if it seems to help you.

❺ **How to Make Saline (Salt Water) Nasal Wash:**
- You can make your own saline nasal wash.
- Add ½ tsp of table salt to 1 cup (8 oz; 240 mL) of warm water.
- You should use sterile, distilled, or previously boiled water for nasal irrigation.

❻ **Medicines for a Stuffy or Runny Nose:**
- Most cold medicines that are available over the counter (OTC) are not helpful.
- **Antihistamines:** Are only helpful if you also have nasal allergies.
- If you have a very runny nose and you really think you need a medicine, you can try using a nasal decongestant for a couple days.

❼ **Hydration:** Drink plenty of liquids (6-8 glasses of water daily). If the air in your home is dry, use a cool mist humidifier.

❽ **Expected Course:**
- Sinus congestion from viral upper respiratory infections (colds) usually lasts 5-10 days.
- Occasionally, a cold can worsen and turn into bacterial sinusitis. Clues to this are sinus symptoms lasting > 10 days, fever lasting > 3 days, and worsening pain. Bacterial sinusitis may need antibiotic treatment.

❾ **Call Back If:**
- Severe pain lasts > 2 hours after pain medicine.
- Sinus pain lasts > 1 day after starting treatment using nasal washes.
- Sinus congestion (fullness) lasts > 10 days.
- Fever lasts > 3 days.
- You become worse.

Over-the-counter Medicines for Sinus Symptoms

❶ **Pain or Fever Medicines:**
- For pain and fever relief, take acetaminophen or ibuprofen.
- Treat fevers > 101° F (38.3° C).
- The goal of fever therapy is to bring the fever down to a comfortable level. Remember that fever medicine usually lowers fever 2° F-3° F (1° C-1.5° C).

Acetaminophen (e.g., Tylenol):
- Take 650 mg (two 325 mg pills) by mouth every 4-6 hours as needed. Each Regular Strength Tylenol pill has 325 mg of acetaminophen. The most you should take each day is 3,250 mg (10 Regular Strength pills a day).

- Another choice is to take 1,000 mg (two 500 mg pills) every 8 hours as needed. Each Extra Strength Tylenol pill has 500 mg of acetaminophen. The most you should take each day is 3,000 mg (6 Extra Strength pills a day).

Ibuprofen (e.g., Motrin, Advil):
- Take 400 mg (two 200 mg pills) by mouth every 6 hours as needed.
- Another choice is to take 600 mg (three 200 mg pills) by mouth every 8 hours as needed.
- The most you should take each day is 1,200 mg (six 200 mg pills a day), unless your doctor has told you to take more.

Naproxen (e.g., Aleve):
- Take 220 mg (one 220 mg pill) by mouth every 8 hours as needed. You may take 440 mg (two 220 mg pills) for your first dose.
- The most you should take each day is 660 mg (three 220 mg pills a day), unless your doctor has told you to take more.

Extra Notes:
- Acetaminophen is thought to be safer than ibuprofen or naproxen for people > 65 years old. Acetaminophen is in many OTC and prescription medicines. It might be in more than one medicine that you are taking. You need to be careful and not take an overdose. An acetaminophen overdose can hurt the liver.
- McNeil, the company that makes Tylenol, has different dosage instructions for Tylenol in Canada and the United States. In Canada, the maximum recommended dose per day is 4,000 mg or 12 Regular Strength (325 mg) pills. In the United States, McNeil recommends a maximum dose of 10 Regular Strength (325 mg) pills.
- *Before taking any medicine, read all the instructions on the package.*

❷ Caution—NSAIDs (e.g., Ibuprofen, Naproxen):
- Do not take nonsteroidal anti-inflammatory drugs (NSAIDs) if you have stomach problems, kidney disease, heart failure, or other contraindications to using this type of medication.
- Do not take NSAIDs for > 7 days without consulting your PCP.
- Do not take NSAIDs if you are pregnant.

- You may take this medicine with or without food. Taking it with food or milk may lessen the chance the drug will upset your stomach.
- **Gastrointestinal Risk:** There is an increased risk of stomach ulcers, GI bleeding, and perforation.
- **Cardiovascular Risk:** There may be an increased risk of heart attack and stroke.

❸ Nasal Decongestants for a Very Stuffy Nose:
- **Most people do not need to use these medicines.**
- If your nose feels blocked, you should try using nasal washes first.
- If you have a very stuffy nose, nasal decongestant medicines can shrink the swollen nasal mucosa and allow for easier breathing. If you have a very runny nose, these medicines can reduce the amount of drainage. They may be taken as pills by mouth or as a nasal spray.
- **Pseudoephedrine (Sudafed):** Available over the counter in pill form. Typical adult dosage is two 30 mg tablets every 6 hours.
- **Oxymetazoline Nasal Drops (Afrin):** Available over the counter. Clean out the nose before using. Spray each nostril once, wait 1 minute for absorption, and then spray a second time.
- **Phenylephrine Nasal Drops (Neo-Synephrine):** Available over the counter. Clean out the nose before using. Spray each nostril once, wait 1 minute for absorption, and then spray a second time.
- *Before taking any medicine, read all the instructions on the package.*

❹ Caution—Nasal Decongestants:
- Do not take these medications if you have high blood pressure, heart disease, prostate enlargement, or an overactive thyroid.
- Do not take these medications if you are pregnant.
- Do not take these medications if you have used a monoamine oxidase (MAO) inhibitor such as isocarboxazid (Marplan), phenelzine (Nardil), rasagiline (Azilect), selegiline (Eldepryl, Emsam), or tranylcypromine (Parnate) in the past 2 weeks. Life-threatening side effects can occur.
- Do not use these medications for > 3 days. *(Reason: rebound nasal congestion)*

❺ Call Back If:
- You have more questions.

Neti Pot for Sinus Symptoms

❶ Neti Pot:

- The neti pot is a small ceramic or plastic pot with a narrow spout. It looks like a small teapot. Two manufacturers of the neti pot are the Himalayan Institute in Pennsylvania and SinuCleanse in Wisconsin.
- **How It Helps:** The neti pot performs nasal washing (also called nasal irrigation or "jala neti"). The salt water rinses out excess mucus and washes out any irritants (dust, allergens) that might be present. It also moisturizes the nasal cavity.
- **Indications:** The neti pot is widely used as a home remedy to relieve conditions such as colds, sinus infections, and hay fever (nasal allergies).
- **Adverse Reactions:** None. However, some people do not like how it feels to pour water into their nose.
- **YouTube Instructional Video:** There are instructional videos on how to use a neti pot on both manufacturers' Web sites and also on YouTube: www.youtube.com/watch?v=j8sDIbRAXIg.

❷ Neti Pot Step-by-Step Instructions:

- **Step 1:** Follow the directions on the salt package to make warm salt water.
- **Step 2:** Lean forward and turn your head to one side over the sink. Keep your forehead slightly higher than your chin.
- **Step 3:** Gently insert the spout of the neti pot into the higher nostril. Put it far enough so that it forms a comfortable seal.
- **Step 4:** Raise the neti pot gradually so the salt water flows in through your higher nostril and out of the lower nostril. Breathe through your mouth.
- **Step 5:** When the neti pot is empty, blow your nose to clean out the water and mucus.
- **Step 6:** Some of the water may run into the back of your throat. Spit this out. If you swallow the salt water, it will not hurt you.
- **Step 7:** Refill the neti pot and repeat on the other side. Again, blow your nose to clear the nasal passages.

❸ How to Make Saline (Salt Water) Nasal Wash:

- You can make your own saline nasal wash.
- Add ½ tsp of table salt to 1 cup (8 oz; 240 mL) of warm water.
- You should use sterile, distilled, or previously boiled water for nasal irrigation.

❹ Neti Pot and Primary Amebic Meningoencephalitis (PAM):

- Primary amebic meningoencephalitis (PAM) is caused by *Naegleria fowleri,* the so-called "brain-eating ameba." This is an extremely rare infection. There were 32 cases in the United States between 2001 and 2010.
- The majority of the cases of PAM have occurred in the southern United States and were linked to swimming or bathing in freshwater lakes, rivers, and ponds containing this ameba. The ameba can also be found in hot springs, geothermal water sources, and poorly maintained swimming pools.
- In 2011 there were 2 cases of PAM in Louisiana that occurred after nasal irrigation with a neti pot. These 2 cases suggest—but are not definite proof—that the nasal irrigation fluid that the individuals used was somehow contaminated with the *N fowleri* ameba.
- The Centers for Disease Control and Prevention recommends that you should use distilled, sterile, or previously boiled water for nasal irrigation. It is also important to rinse the irrigation device after each use and leave it open to air-dry.

❺ Call Back If:

- You have more questions.

BACKGROUND

Causes of Sinus Pain and Congestion

- Sinus opening(s) becomes blocked by an infection or nasal allergy.
- **Viral Sinusitis:** Sinusitis can occur as part of a viral upper respiratory infection (e.g., rhinosinusitis or the "common cold"). The viral infection and inflammation of the lining of the nose can also affect the lining of all the paranasal sinuses.
- **Bacterial Sinusitis:** Approximately 1%-2% of viral sinusitis cases progress to become bacterial sinusitis; ≥ 1 of the sinuses affected with viral sinusitis becomes secondarily infected with bacteria. Distinguishing symptoms are symptoms lasting > 10 days, increasing sinus pain, and the return of fever.
- **Allergic Sinusitis:** When an allergen (e.g., pollen) activates the lining of the nose (allergic rhinitis), sinus congestion may occur due to swelling of the sinus passage openings (ostia). Symptoms suggesting an allergic etiology include sneezing, itchy nose, clear nasal discharge, and itchy, watery eyes.

- **Rhinitis Medicamentosa:** Prolonged continuous use (> 5 days) of decongestant nose drops can lead to "rebound" congestion where the nose becomes even more stuffy.

Treatment of Sinusitis

- **Viral Sinusitis:** Saline nasal washes. Antibiotics are not helpful.
- **Bacterial Sinusitis:** Saline nasal washes. Oral antibiotics may be needed.
- **Allergic Sinusitis (Hay Fever):** Oral antihistamines can relieve mild-moderate symptoms. Examples include diphenhydramine (Benadryl), loratadine (Claritin, Alavert), fexofenadine (Allegra), and cetirizine (Zyrtec). Nasal corticosteroid sprays are probably the most effective treatment for allergic rhinitis. Saline nasal washes are also helpful.

Site of Pain and Sinus Involved

- Ethmoid sinusitis causes pain between or behind the eyes.
- Maxillary sinusitis causes pain in the area of the zygomatic arch, cheek, or upper teeth.
- Frontal sinusitis causes pain above the eyebrow or frontal headaches.

Color of Nasal Discharge With Colds

- The nasal discharge normally changes color during different stages of a cold.
- It starts as a clear discharge and later becomes cloudy.
- Sometimes it becomes yellow or green colored for a few days, and this is still normal.
- Intermittent yellow or green discharge is more common with sleep, antihistamines, or low humidity. *(Reason: All of these events reduce the production of normal nasal secretions.)*
- Yellow or green nasal secretions suggest the presence of a bacterial sinusitis ONLY if they occur in combination with (1) sinus pain OR (2) drainage that persists > 10 days without improvement.
- Nasal secretions only need treatment with nasal washes when they block the nose and interfere with breathing through the nose. During a cold, if nasal breathing is noisy but the caller can't see blockage in the nose, it usually means the dried mucus is farther back. Nasal washes can remove it.

Nasal Washes (Nasal Irrigation) for Sinus Symptoms

- **Introduction:** Saline (salt water) nasal irrigation is an effective and simple home remedy for treating cold symptoms and other conditions involving the nasal and sinus passages. Nasal irrigation consists of pouring, spraying, or squirting salt water into the nose and then letting it run back out.
- **How It Helps:** The salt water rinses out excess mucus, washes out any irritants (dust, allergens) that might be present, and moisturizes the nasal cavity.
- **Indications:** Nasal irrigation appears to be an effective treatment for chronic sinusitis. It may also help reduce sinus symptoms from acute viral upper respiratory infection (colds), irritant rhinitis (e.g., dust from the workplace), and allergic rhinitis (hay fever). Some doctors recommend it for rhinitis of pregnancy.
- **Adverse Reactions:** Nasal irrigation is safe and there are no serious adverse effects. However, not everyone likes the sensation of having water in their nose.
- **Methods:** There are several ways to perform nasal irrigation. None has been proven to be better than any other. Methods include use of a nasal spray bottle (available over the counter), a rubber ear syringe, a Waterpik set on "low," a 5-20 mL medical syringe without the needle, or a neti pot.
- **How to Make Salt Water for Nasal Irrigation:** Add ½ teaspoon of table salt to 1 cup (8 oz; 240 mL) of warm water.

Neti Pot for Sinus Symptoms

- The neti pot is a small ceramic or plastic pot with a narrow spout. It looks like a small teapot. Two manufacturers of the neti pot are the Himalayan Institute in Pennsylvania and SinuCleanse in Wisconsin.
- **How It Helps:** The neti pot performs nasal washing (also called nasal irrigation or "jala neti"). The salt water rinses out excess mucus, washes out any irritants (dust, allergens) that might be present, and moisturizes the nasal cavity.
- **Indications:** The neti pot is widely used as a home remedy to relieve conditions such as colds, sinus infections, and hay fever (nasal allergies).
- **Adverse Reactions:** None. Nasal irrigation with a neti pot is safe and there are no serious adverse effects. However, not everyone likes the sensation of having salt water poured into their nose.
- **YouTube Instructional Video:** www.youtube.com/watch?v=j8sDIbRAXlg.

Neti Pot and Primary Amebic Meningoencephalitis (PAM)

- Primary amebic meningoencephalitis (PAM) is caused by *Naegleria fowleri,* the so-called "brain-eating ameba." This is an extremely rare infection. There were 32 cases in the United States between 2001 and 2010.
- The majority of the cases of PAM have occurred in the southern United States and were linked to swimming or bathing in freshwater lakes, rivers, and ponds containing this ameba. The ameba can also be found in hot springs, geothermal water sources, and poorly maintained swimming pools.
- In 2011 there were 2 cases of PAM in Louisiana that occurred after nasal irrigation with a neti pot. These 2 cases suggest—but are not definite proof—that the nasal irrigation fluid that the individuals used was somehow contaminated with the *N fowleri* ameba.
- The Centers for Disease Control and Prevention recommends that individuals should use distilled, sterile, or previously boiled water for nasal irrigation. It's also important to rinse the irrigation device after each use and leave open to air-dry.

Nasal Decongestants: Use only if the sinus is still blocked after nasal washes.
- CAUTION: These medications should not be taken by individuals with high blood pressure, heart disease, or prostate enlargement. These medications should not be used for > 3 days. (*Reason: rebound nasal congestion*)
- CAUTION: The individual may currently be taking a decongestant medication and not know it or not have told the triager.
- Commonly used decongestants include Allegra D, Benadryl Allergy and Congestion, Claritin D, Dimetapp, Duratuss, Entex, ephedrine, pseudoephedrine, Rondec, Semprex-D, Sudafed, Triaminic, and many others.

SKIN, FOREIGN BODY

Definition
- Patient reports a foreign body (e.g., splinter, fishhook, sliver of glass) embedded in the skin.

Symptoms:
- **Pain:** Most tiny slivers (e.g., cactus spine, stinging nettles, fiberglass spicules) are in the superficial skin and do not cause much pain. Deeper or perpendicular foreign bodies are usually painful to pressure.
- **Foreign Body Sensation:** Often adult patients may report the sensation of something being in the skin ("I feel something there").

TRIAGE ASSESSMENT QUESTIONS

Call EMS 911 Now
- Sounds like a life-threatening emergency to the triager

See More Appropriate Protocol
- Puncture wound (and no current foreign body)
  Go to Protocol: Puncture Wound on page 319

Go to ED/UCC Now
(or to Office With PCP Approval)
- SEVERE pain (e.g., excruciating)
  Reason: home attempts to remove may push it in deeper; ultrasound may be needed for locating foreign body (FB)
- Deeply embedded FB (e.g., needle or toothpick in foot)
  Reason: home attempts to remove may push it in deeper; ultrasound may be needed for locating FB
- FB has a barb (e.g., fishhook)
  Reason: need special technique to remove
- Sounds like a serious injury to the triager

Go to Office Now
- Caller can't get FB out and it's causing pain
- Caller reluctant to take out FB and it's causing pain
- FB is clear (glass or plastic)
  Reason: difficult to see for removal
- FB is a BB
  Reason: needs incision to remove
- Wound looks infected (e.g., spreading redness, red streak, pus)
  R/O: cellulitis, lymphangitis
- Dirt (debris) can be seen in the wound, not removed with 15-minute scrubbing
  Reason: additional scrubbing in the ED, UCC, or office may be needed

See Today in Office
- Patient wants to be seen

See Today or Tomorrow in Office
- No tetanus booster in > 5 years (or > 10 years for clean wounds)
  Reason: may need a tetanus booster shot (vaccine)
- No prior tetanus shots
  Reason: may need a tetanus booster shot (vaccine)

See Within 3 Days in Office
- Minor sliver, splinter, or thorn (removable) and patient has diabetes mellitus
  Reason: diabetic neuropathy and decreased resistance to infection
  Note: More urgent evaluation is needed if the FB is not removable.

Home Care
- ○ Minor sliver, splinter, or thorn that needs removal
  Reason: patient should be able to remove this FB at home
- ○ Tiny plant stickers (e.g., cactus spines, stinging nettles) or fiberglass spicules that need removal
  Reason: patient should be able to remove this FB at home
- ○ Tiny, superficial, pain-free slivers
  Reason: do not need removal

HOME CARE ADVICE

Removing Slivers, Splinters, and Thorns

❶ **Needle and Tweezers:**
- You can remove slivers, splinters, or thorns with a needle and tweezers.
- Check the tweezers beforehand to be certain the ends (pickups) meet exactly (If they do not, bend them).
- Sterilize the tools with rubbing alcohol or a flame.
- Clean the skin surrounding the sliver briefly with rubbing alcohol before trying to remove it. Be careful not to push the splinter in deeper. If you don't have rubbing alcohol, use soap and water, but don't soak the area if FB is wood. *(Reason: can cause swelling of the splinter)*

❷ **Step-by-Step Instructions:**
- **Step 1:** Use the needle to completely expose the end of the sliver. Use good lighting. A magnifying glass may help.
- **Step 2:** Then grasp the end firmly with the tweezers and pull it out at the same angle that it went in. Getting a good grip the first time is especially important with slivers that go in perpendicular to the skin or those trapped under the fingernail.

❸ **Additional Instructions:**
- For slivers under a fingernail, sometimes a wedge of the nail must be cut away with fine scissors to expose the end of the sliver.
- Superficial horizontal slivers (where you can see all of it) usually can be removed by pulling on the end. If the end breaks off, open the skin with a sterile needle along the length of the sliver and flick it out.

❹ **Antibiotic Ointment:** Apply an antibiotic ointment (OTC) to the area once after removal to reduce the risk of infection.

❺ **Tetanus Booster:**
- If your last tetanus shot was given > 10 years ago, you need a booster.
- You should try to get this booster shot within the next couple days.

❻ **Call Back If:**
- Can't get it all out.
- Removed it, but pain becomes worse.
- Starts to look infected.
- You become worse.

Removing Tiny Plant Stickers (e.g., Cactus Spines, Stinging Nettles) or Fiberglass Spicules

❶ **Tiny Plant Stickers:** Plant stickers (e.g., stinging nettles), cactus spines, or fiberglass spicules are difficult to remove. Usually they break when pressure is applied with tweezers.

❷ **Tape:** First try to remove the small spines or spicules by touching the area lightly with packaging tape or another very sticky tape.

❸ **Wax Hair Remover** (if tape does not work):
- Warm up the wax in your microwave for 10 seconds and apply a layer over the spicules (or fiberglass). Cover it with the cloth strip that came in the hair remover package. Let it air-dry for 5 minutes or accelerate the process with a hair dryer. Then peel it off with the spicules. Most will be removed. The others will usually work themselves out with normal shedding of the skin.
- You can also try all-purpose white glue, but it's far less effective.

❹ **Tetanus Booster:**
- If your last tetanus shot was given > 10 years ago, you need a booster.
- You should try to get this booster shot within the next couple days.

❺ **Call Back If:**
- Can't get it all out and it's painful.
- Starts to look infected.
- You become worse.

Tiny, Superficial, Pain-Free Slivers

❶ **Tiny, Pain-Free Slivers:** If superficial slivers are numerous, tiny, and pain free, they can be left in. Eventually they will work their way out with normal shedding of the skin or the body will reject them by forming a tiny little pimple.

❷ **Tetanus Booster:**
- If your last tetanus shot was given > 10 years ago, you need a booster.
- You should try to get this booster shot within the next couple days.

❸ **Call Back If:**
- Starts to look infected.
- You become worse.

BACKGROUND

Types of Foreign Bodies (FBs)

- Fiberglass spicules
- **Fishhooks:** May have a barbed point that make removal difficult
- Glass
- **Metallic FBs:** Bullets, BBs, nails, sewing needles, pins, tacks
- Pencil lead (graphite)
- Plastic
- **Wood/Organic:** Splinters, cactus spines, thorns, toothpicks
- Other

Pencil Punctures

- There's no danger of lead poisoning. Pencil leads are made of graphite and clay, not lead.
- Sometimes the graphite dust can leave a tiny black stain (tattoo) in the puncture wound.

Diagnosis—FBs With X-ray Films

- **Metal:** X-ray films are helpful in localization of metallic FBs. Even tiny pieces of metal will usually show up on x-rays.
- **Glass:** Glass is radiopaque (meaning visible on x-ray), so x-ray films can be helpful. However, tiny pieces of glass (< 2 mm) cannot usually be seen on x-ray.
- **Wood/Organic:** Organic materials like wood are radiolucent and usually do not show up on x-ray.

Treatment—Need for Removal

- A general principle is that if an FB needs to be removed in a medical setting, it's better for the patient to get seen sooner, before the FB becomes hidden by swelling or pushed in more deeply by the patient.
- Most small, superficially located skin FBs can be removed at home. Examples include splinters, cactus spines, fiberglass spicules, and pieces of glass.
- **BBs:** BBs from an air gun usually lodge superficially and generally need to be removed by making a tiny incision (with local anesthesia).
- **Bullets:** Of course anyone with an acute bullet wound needs to be evaluated on an emergency basis! Interestingly, though, most bullets and bullet fragments are not removed unless they are interfering with bodily function or causing ongoing pain.
- **Glass and Metal FBs:** Glass and metal are inert, which means that they do not react with human tissue and generally do not become infected. If the FB is causing pain it will need to be removed. Sometimes a tiny (< 2 mm) painless glass or metal FB is not removed by the treating physician because removal would cause more problems than leaving the FB where it is.
- **Wood/Organic:** Organic FBs like wood splinters or thorns can cause infection if they are not removed.

SKIN INJURY

Definition
- Cuts, lacerations, gashes, and tears

TRIAGE ASSESSMENT QUESTIONS

Call EMS 911 Now
- Shock suspected (e.g., cold/pale/clammy skin, too weak to stand)
  R/O: shock
  First Aid: Lie down with the feet elevated.
- Cut on the neck, chest, back, or abdomen that may go deep (e.g., stab wound or other suspicious penetrating injury)
- Major bleeding (actively dripping or spurting) that can't be stopped
  First Aid: Apply direct pressure to the entire wound with a clean cloth.
- Amputation
  First Aid: Apply direct pressure to the entire wound with a clean cloth.
- Sounds like a life-threatening emergency to the triager

See More Appropriate Protocol
- Animal bite and broken skin
  Go to Protocol: Animal Bite on page 22
- Injury is a puncture wound
  Go to Protocol: Puncture Wound on page 319
- Splinter in the skin
  Go to Protocol: Skin, Foreign Body on page 358
- Wound looks infected
  Go to Protocol: Wound Infection on page 443
- Burn
  Go to Protocol: Burns on page 61

Go to ED Now
- High-pressure injection injury (e.g., from paint gun, usually work-related)
  Reason: deep tissue damage may exceed superficial injury
- Skin loss involves > 10% of surface area
  Note: The palm of the hand = 1%.
  R/O: need for burn care

Go to ED/UCC Now
(or to Office With PCP Approval)
- Skin is split open or gaping (length > ½" or 12 mm on the skin, ¼" or 6 mm on the face)
  Reason: may need laceration repair (e.g., sutures)
- Bleeding won't stop after 10 minutes of direct pressure (using correct technique)
- Cut or scrape is very deep (e.g., can see bone or tendons)
  R/O: tendon injury
- Dirt in the wound and not removed after 15 minutes of scrubbing
  Reason: needs irrigation or debridement
- Wound causes numbness (i.e., loss of sensation)
  R/O: nerve injury
- Wound causes weakness (i.e., decreased ability to move hand, finger, toe)
  R/O: nerve injury
- Sounds like a serious injury to the triager

Go to Office Now
- Looks infected (fever, spreading redness, pus, or red streak)
  R/O: cellulitis, lymphangitis
- Expanding raised bruise with size > 2" (5 cm)
  R/O: progressive hematoma

See Today in Office
- SEVERE pain (e.g., excruciating)
- Patient wants to be seen

See Today or Tomorrow in Office
- Suspicious history for the injury
  R/O: domestic violence or elder abuse
- Has diabetes (diabetes mellitus) and has minor cut or scratch on foot
  Reason: increased risk of foot infection or ulcer
- No tetanus booster in > 5 years (or > 10 years for clean wounds)
  Reason: may need a tetanus booster shot (vaccine)
- No prior tetanus shots
  Reason: needs to get full tetanus vaccination (a series of 3 shots)

See Within 3 Days in Office
- After 14 days and wound isn't healed
  R/O: low-grade infection

Home Care

○ Swelling, bruise, or pain from a direct blow
  R/O: contusion

○ Superficial cut (scratch) or abrasion (scrape)

HOME CARE ADVICE

Minor Contusion (Bruise From Direct Blow)

❶ **Reassurance:**

- This sounds like a minor contusion of that area. Contusion is the medical term for bruise. Any type of direct blow to your skin can cause a bruise.
- Symptoms are mild pain, swelling, and bruising.
- *Here is some care advice that should help.*

❷ **Apply a Cold Pack:**

- Apply a cold pack or an ice bag (wrapped in a moist towel) to the area for 20 minutes. Repeat in 1 hour, then every 4 hours while awake.
- Continue this for the first 48 hours after an injury. *(Reason: to reduce the swelling and pain)*

❸ **Apply Heat to the Area:**

- Beginning 48 hours after an injury, apply a warm washcloth or heating pad for 10 minutes 3 times a day.
- This will help increase blood flow and improve healing.

❹ **Pain Medicines:**

- For pain relief, you can take either acetaminophen, ibuprofen, or naproxen.
- They are over-the-counter (OTC) pain drugs. You can buy them at the drugstore.

  Acetaminophen (e.g., Tylenol):
- **Regular Strength Tylenol:** Take 650 mg (two 325 mg pills) by mouth every 4-6 hours as needed. Each Regular Strength Tylenol pill has 325 mg of acetaminophen.
- **Extra Strength Tylenol:** Take 1,000 mg (two 500 mg pills) every 8 hours as needed. Each Extra Strength Tylenol pill has 500 mg of acetaminophen.
- The most you should take each day is 3,000 mg (10 Regular Strength or 6 Extra Strength pills a day).

  Ibuprofen (e.g., Motrin, Advil):
- Take 400 mg (two 200 mg pills) by mouth every 6 hours.
- Another choice is to take 600 mg (three 200 mg pills) by mouth every 8 hours.

- The most you should take each day is 1,200 mg (six 200 mg pills), unless your doctor has told you to take more.

  Naproxen (e.g., Aleve):
- Take 220 mg (one 220 mg pill) by mouth every 8 hours as needed. You may take 440 mg (two 220 mg pills) for your first dose.
- The most you should take each day is 660 mg (three 220 mg pills a day), unless your doctor has told you to take more.

❺ **Pain Medicines—Extra Notes:**

- Use the lowest amount of medicine that makes your pain better.
- Acetaminophen is thought to be safer than ibuprofen or naproxen in people > 65 years old. Acetaminophen is in many OTC and prescription medicines. It might be in more than one medicine that you are taking. You need to be careful and not take an overdose. An acetaminophen overdose can hurt the liver.
- McNeil, the company that makes Tylenol, has different dosage instructions for Tylenol in Canada and the United States. In Canada, the maximum recommended dose per day is 4,000 mg or 12 Regular Strength (325 mg) pills. In the United States, McNeil recommends a maximum dose of 10 Regular Strength (325 mg) pills.
- CAUTION: Do not take acetaminophen if you have liver disease.
- CAUTION: Do not take ibuprofen or naproxen if you have stomach problems, have kidney disease, are pregnant, or have been told by your doctor to avoid this type of anti-inflammatory drug. Do not take ibuprofen or naproxen for > 7 days without consulting your doctor.
- *Before taking any medicine, read all the instructions on the package.*

❻ **Expected Course:**

- Pain and swelling usually begin to get better 2-3 days after an injury.
- Swelling is usually gone in 1 week
- Pain may take 2 weeks to go away.

❼ **Call Back If:**

- Swelling or bruise becomes > 2" (5 cm).
- Pain not improved after 72 hours.
- Pain or swelling lasts > 7 days.
- You become worse.

Superficial Laceration (Cut or Scratch) or Abrasion (Scrape)

❶ Reassurance:
- It sounds like a small cut or scrape that we can treat at home.
- *Here is some care advice that should help.*

❷ Bleeding: Apply direct pressure for 10 minutes with a sterile gauze to stop any bleeding.

❸ Cleaning the Wound:
- Wash the wound with soap and water for 5 minutes.
- For any dirt, scrub gently with a washcloth.
- For any bleeding, apply direct pressure with a sterile gauze or clean cloth for 10 minutes.

❹ Antibiotic Ointment:
- Apply an antibiotic ointment (e.g., OTC bacitracin), covered by a Band-Aid or dressing. Change daily or if it becomes wet.
- Option: A Telfa dressing won't stick to the wound when it is removed.
- Option: Another option is to use a liquid skin bandage that only needs to be applied once. Don't use antibiotic ointment if you use a liquid skin bandage.

❺ Liquid Skin Bandage:
- You can use a liquid skin bandage instead of antibiotic ointment and a dressing or a Band-Aid.
- **Benefits:** Liquid skin bandage has several benefits when compared with a regular bandage (e.g., a dressing or a Band-Aid). You only need to put a liquid bandage on once to minor cuts and scrapes. It helps stop minor bleeding. It seals the wound and may promote faster healing and lower infection rates. However, it also costs more.
- **How to Use It:** First clean and dry the wound. You put on the liquid as spray or with a swab. It dries in < 1 minute and usually lasts a week. You can get it wet.
- **Examples:** Liquid skin bandage is available over the counter. Examples are Band-Aid Liquid Bandage, New Skin, Curad Spray Bandage, and 3M No Sting Liquid Bandage Spray.

❻ Pain Medicines:
- For pain relief, you can take either acetaminophen, ibuprofen, or naproxen.
- They are over-the-counter (OTC) pain drugs. You can buy them at the drugstore.

Acetaminophen (e.g., Tylenol):
- **Regular Strength Tylenol:** Take 650 mg (two 325 mg pills) by mouth every 4-6 hours as needed. Each Regular Strength Tylenol pill has 325 mg of acetaminophen.
- **Extra Strength Tylenol:** Take 1,000 mg (two 500 mg pills) every 8 hours as needed. Each Extra Strength Tylenol pill has 500 mg of acetaminophen.
- The most you should take each day is 3,000 mg (10 Regular Strength or 6 Extra Strength pills a day).

Ibuprofen (e.g., Motrin, Advil):
- Take 400 mg (two 200 mg pills) by mouth every 6 hours.
- Another choice is to take 600 mg (three 200 mg pills) by mouth every 8 hours.
- The most you should take each day is 1,200 mg (six 200 mg pills), unless your doctor has told you to take more.

Naproxen (e.g., Aleve):
- Take 220 mg (one 220 mg pill) by mouth every 8 hours as needed. You may take 440 mg (two 220 mg pills) for your first dose.
- The most you should take each day is 660 mg (three 220 mg pills a day), unless your doctor has told you to take more.

❼ Pain Medicines—Extra Notes:
- Use the lowest amount of medicine that makes your pain better.
- Acetaminophen is thought to be safer than ibuprofen or naproxen in people > 65 years old. Acetaminophen is in many OTC and prescription medicines. It might be in more than one medicine that you are taking. You need to be careful and not take an overdose. An acetaminophen overdose can hurt the liver.
- McNeil, the company that makes Tylenol, has different dosage instructions for Tylenol in Canada and the United States. In Canada, the maximum recommended dose per day is 4,000 mg or 12 Regular Strength (325 mg) pills. In the United States, McNeil recommends a maximum dose of 10 Regular Strength (325 mg) pills.
- CAUTION: Do not take acetaminophen if you have liver disease.

- CAUTION: Do not take ibuprofen or naproxen if you have stomach problems, have kidney disease, are pregnant, or have been told by your doctor to avoid this type of anti-inflammatory drug. Do not take ibuprofen or naproxen for > 7 days without consulting your doctor.
- *Before taking any medicine, read all the instructions on the package.*

❽ Call Back If:
- Looks infected (pus, redness, increasing tenderness).
- Doesn't heal within 10 days.
- You become worse.

When Does an Adult Need a Tetanus Booster?

❶ Dirty Wounds—Tetanus Booster Needed Every 5 Years:
- People with dirty wounds need a booster every 5 years.
- Examples of dirty wounds include any cut contaminated with soil, feces, and saliva. It also includes more serious wounds from deep punctures, crushing, and burns.
- You should try to get the tetanus booster as soon as possible. Make certain you get the booster within 3 days of the injury.

❷ Clean Cuts and Scrapes—Tetanus Booster Needed Every 10 Years:
- People with clean minor wounds AND who have previously had ≥ 3 tetanus shots (full series) need a booster every 10 years.
- Examples of minor wounds include a minor scrape or scratch, a shallow cut from a clean knife blade, or a small glass cut that happened while washing dishes.
- You should try to get the tetanus booster within 3 days of the injury.

❸ Call Back If:
- You have more questions.

FIRST AID

First Aid Advice for Bleeding:
Apply direct pressure to the entire wound with a clean cloth.

First Aid Advice for Severe Bleeding:
- Place 2 or 3 sterile dressings (or a clean towel or washcloth) over the wound immediately.
- Apply direct pressure to the wound, using your entire hand.
- If bleeding continues, apply pressure more forcefully or move the pressure to a slightly different spot.
- Act quickly because ongoing blood loss can cause shock.
- Do not use a tourniquet.

First Aid Advice for Penetrating Object:
If penetrating object is still in place, don't remove it. *Reason: Removal could increase bleeding.*

First Aid Advice for Shock:
Lie down with the feet elevated.

First Aid Advice for Transport of an Amputated Finger or Toe:
- Briefly rinse amputated part with water (to remove any dirt).
- Place amputated part in plastic bag (to protect and keep clean).
- Place plastic bag containing part in a cup of ice water (to keep cool and preserve tissue).

BACKGROUND

Types of Skin Injury

- **Abrasion:** An abrasion (scrape) is an area of superficial skin that has been scraped off. It commonly occurs on the knees, elbows, and palms.
- **Bruise:** A bruise (contusion) usually is the result of a direct blow from a blunt object. There is bleeding under the skin from damaged blood vessels.
- **Cut—Superficial:** Superficial cuts (scratches) only extend partially through the skin and rarely become infected.
- **Cut—Deep:** Deep cuts (lacerations) go through the skin (dermis). Cuts > ½" (12 mm) or ¼" (6 mm) on the face usually need sutures.
- **Hematoma:** A hematoma is a collection of blood in the soft tissues.
- **Puncture Wound:** A puncture wound is the result of the skin being penetrated by a sharp, pointed object.
- **Skin Tear:** A skin tear is a separation of the epidermis from the underlying dermis. It is primarily seen in the elderly and in chronically ill individuals. The most common location is the arms.

Lacerations—Methods of Repairing (Closing)

- **Suturing (Stitches):** This is the most common method for closing lacerations.
- **Stapling (Staples):** Wound staples work best in uncomplicated lacerations overlying flat areas of the body surface; for this reason, they are mostly used in cuts on the scalp, torso, arms, and legs.
- **Skin Glue (Tissue Adhesives):** Skin glue works well on small, straight lacerations where there is little skin tension. Skin glue is often used to close small cuts on the face. Dermabond (2-octyl cyanoacrylate, Ethicon) is the name of the skin glue used by doctors in the United States and Canada.
- **Tissue Tapes (e.g., 3M, Steri-Strips):** Tissue tapes can be used for very superficial cuts. They are available over the counter and can be applied at home. They do not work well over joints and tend to fall off if they become wet.

Lacerations—What to Repair

- Cuts that are gaping open and > ½" (12 mm) usually need repair (e.g., sutures).
- On the face, cuts > ¼" (6 mm) need repair.
- Any open wound that may need sutures should be evaluated by a physician regardless of the time that has passed since the initial injury.

Lacerations—Timing of Repair

❶ **Primary closure** is the repair of a new wound. The sooner a wound is closed, the lower the infection rate. Generally, lacerations on most parts of the body should be repaired (e.g., sutured) within 12 hours; lacerations of the face and scalp should be repaired within 24 hours.
(Reason: highly vascular area, less prone to infection)
Clean wounds can wait longer than dirty wounds.

❷ **Secondary closure** is having a wound heal over without suturing it or using another method of repair. This leaves a wider scar. Secondary closure is needed for infected wounds and abscesses.

❸ **Delayed primary closure** is suturing a wound on day 4 or 5, after watching it to make certain it is not infected. This approach is used for contaminated wounds, many animal bites, and wounds that are brought in after 12-24 hours. All of these individuals need to be seen initially, however, for wound irrigation, debridement, and possibly antibiotics.

Liquid Skin Bandage for Minor Cuts and Scrapes

- Liquid skin bandage has several benefits when compared with a regular bandage (e.g., a dressing or a Band-Aid). Liquid bandage only needs to be applied once to minor cuts and scrapes. It helps stop minor bleeding. It seals the wound and may promote faster healing and lower infection rates. However, it is also more expensive.
- After the wound is washed and dried, the liquid is applied by spray or with a swab. It dries in < 1 minute and usually lasts a week. It's resistant to bathing.
- **Examples:** Band-Aid Liquid Bandage, New Skin, Curad Spray Bandage, and 3M No Sting Liquid Bandage Spray.

What Is Tetanus?

- **Definition:** Tetanus is a rare infection caused by bacteria that are found in many places, especially in dirt and soil. The tetanus bacteria enter through a break in the skin and then spread through the body.
- **Symptoms:** Tetanus is commonly called "lockjaw" because the first symptom is a tightening of the muscles of the face. However, the final stage of the infection is much more serious. All of the muscles of the body go into severe spasm, including the muscles that control breathing. Eventually a person with a tetanus infection loses the ability to breath and may die in spite of intense treatment in the hospital.

- **Prevention:** A tetanus booster protects you from getting a tetanus infection. It does not prevent other kinds of wound infection.

Tetanus Booster—When Does an Adult Need a Tetanus Shot?

- **Clean Cuts and Scrapes—Tetanus Booster Needed Every 10 Years:** Patients with clean minor wounds AND who have previously had ≥ 3 tetanus shots (full series) need a booster every 10 years. Examples of minor wounds include a superficial knee abrasion, a small cut from a clean knife blade, or a glass cut sustained while washing dishes. All wounds need wound care and cleaning right away. A tetanus booster (Td or Tdap) should be given within 72 hours.
- **Dirty Wounds—Tetanus Booster Needed Every 5 Years:** Patients with dirty wounds need a booster every 5 years. Examples of dirty wounds include any cut contaminated with soil, feces, and/or saliva and more serious wounds from deep punctures, crushing, and burns. All wounds need to be cleaned right away. Dirty wounds usually need immediate care in a doctor's office, urgent care, or ED. A tetanus booster (Td or Tdap) should be given as soon as possible, preferably at the time of wound care, and definitely within 72 hours.
- Contaminated major wounds (e.g., crush injuries, amputations, avulsions, gaping cuts, larger burns, or any other wound that needs debridement or irrigation) are all referred in immediately for wound care. For these patients, if a tetanus booster is required, it will be given on the day of the injury. Persons with major or dirty wounds who have not received a full tetanus vaccination series (3 doses) also need tetanus immune globulin (TIG) when they get the tetanus booster (Td or Tdap).

Skin Tear

- **Definition:** A skin tear is a separation of the epidermis from the underlying dermis. The most common location for skin tears is the arms.
- **Causes:** Minor trauma is the most frequently listed cause of skin tears. The trauma can be as little as bumping into an object like a counter, transferring from bed to wheelchair, and tape removal. However, it is reported that for nearly half of skin tears that occur, the cause is unknown—the person does not recall hurting himself/herself.

- **Risk Factors:** Skin tears are primarily seen in the elderly and in chronically ill individuals. They occur commonly in patients who reside in nursing home patients and long-term care facilities. One can recognize individuals at risk; their skin looks paper thin and like it could tear easily.
- **Classification of Skin Tears:** Category I tears have no loss of skin or tissue; the torn skin edges can be pulled together (approximated). Category II tears have some tissue loss. Category III tears have complete loss of tissue loss; the torn skin covering the dermis has been completely ripped off.
- **Prevention:** There are a number of measures that can be done to reduce skin tears, though no way to completely prevent them from happening in at-risk individuals. Preventive measures include wearing shirts with sleeves, education of caregivers, application of skin lotion, padding side rails in hospital beds, and using gentle skin cleansers.
- **Treatment—Category I Tears:** Treatment should begin with gentle washing of the skin tear with 0.9% saline (or a nontoxic wound cleanser) and then gently blotting the skin dry (or letting it air-dry). Category I skin tears can be closed by pulling ("approximating") the skin edges together and then using either Steri-Strips (skin tapes) or skin glue (e.g., octyl cyanoacrylate adhesives, Dermabond).
- **Treatment—Category II and III Tears:** Treatment should begin with gentle washing of the skin tear with 0.9% saline (or a nontoxic wound cleanser) and then gently blotting the skin dry (or letting it air-dry). There are a variety of approaches that are recommended for Category II and III tears (e.g., hydrogel sheets, hydrocolloids, Steri-Strips). Transparent occlusive films like Tegaderm are contraindicated because they promote accumulation of fluid. Recent research suggests that skin glue (e.g., octyl cyanoacrylate adhesives) is effective—it can be applied to the open areas of a skin tear; an extra benefit is decreased pain and bleeding in comparison with other dressings.
- **Triage:** Small Category I skin tears could potentially be managed at home with the treatment described herein. However, triagers often find it difficult to confidently elicit a description from a caller that allows the triager to distinguish a laceration from a skin tear.

SKIN LESION (MOLES OR GROWTHS)

Definition
- Small bump, lump, spot, growth, or pigmented area of skin
- Moles, skin tags, warts included
- Questions about skin cancer included

TRIAGE ASSESSMENT QUESTIONS

Go to ED/UCC Now
(or to Office With PCP Approval)
● Patient sounds very sick or weak to the triager
Reason: severe acute illness or serious complication suspected

Go to Office Now
● Fever and bump is tender to touch
R/O: abscess

See Today in Office
◉ Looks infected (e.g., spreading redness, pus, red streak)
R/O: cellulitis, lymphangitis
◉ Looks like a boil, infected sore, or deep ulcer
R/O: abscess, boil/furuncle, impetigo, ulcer

See Today or Tomorrow in Office
◉ Caller can't describe it clearly

See Within 3 Days in Office
◉ Patient wants to be seen

See Within 2 Weeks in Office
◉ Skin growth or mole and 2 sides do not look the same (it is asymmetric)
R/O: skin cancer
◉ Skin growth or mole and border is irregular or blurry
R/O: skin cancer
◉ Skin growth or mole and changes color or it has more than one color
R/O: skin cancer
◉ Skin growth or mole and it is larger than a pencil eraser or increasing in size
R/O: skin cancer
◉ Skin growth or mole and bleeds
R/O: skin cancer

◉ Sticks up out of the skin (elevated) and feels rough to the touch
R/O: skin cancer, wart, skin tag, seborrheic keratosis
◉ Flat waxy-yellow patch near eyelids
R/O: xanthelasma
◉ Scar that is growing larger
R/O: keloid
◉ Caller is uncertain what it is
Reason: obtain diagnosis

Home Care
○ Freckles
○ Small growth or mole that is unchanged in size or appearance

HOME CARE ADVICE

❶ **Freckles:**
- Tend to be inherited and are more common in individuals with fair skin.
- Increase with sun exposure.

❷ **Monthly Skin Self-examination:**
- Some doctors recommend that you perform a skin self-examination once a month.
- Stand in front of a mirror. Examine every inch of your skin for new moles or changes in old ones.

❸ **Skin Health:**
- Avoid sun exposure. Use sunscreen or wear protective clothing (eg, long-sleeved shirts).
- Stay in the shade during the middle of the day. Wear a wide-brimmed hat to keep the sun off your face and neck.
- Do not go to tanning salons. Tanning booths also cause skin damage.

❹ **Call Back If:**
- Fever or pain occurs.
- Any change in the mole or growth.
- You become worse.

BACKGROUND

Causes

- Abscess, boils (furuncles or carbuncles)
- Birthmarks
- Freckles
- Keloid
- Lipoma
- Moles
- Sebaceous cysts
- Seborrheic keratosis
- **Skin Cancer:** Malignant melanoma, basal cell, squamous cell
- Skin tags
- Warts
- Xanthelasma

Is It a Mole or Could It Be Melanoma? The following are signs of possible malignant melanoma (skin cancer):

- **A—Symmetry:** The shape of the mole is not round, and 2 sides of a mole do not look the same.
- **B—Border:** The borders of the mole are irregular or blurry or look like they are "leaking" pigment into the adjacent skin.
- **C—Color:** A mole that changes color or contains > 1 color.
- **D—Diameter:** Size larger than a pencil eraser (> 6 mm or > 0.25").
- **E—Elevation:** Moles that are rough and are raised above the skin surface.

Other Possible Signs of Skin Cancer

- A new skin growth or mole
- A skin growth or mole that bleeds or feels irritated
- An enlarging skin lesion in sun-damaged areas of skin—possible basal cell cancer or squamous cell cancer

SORE THROAT

Definition
- Pain, discomfort, or raw feeling of the throat, especially when swallowing

Pain Severity Scale
- **Mild (1-3):** Doesn't interfere with eating or normal activities.
- **Moderate (4-7):** Interferes with eating some solids and normal activities.
- **Severe (8-10):** Excruciating pain, interferes with most normal activities.
- **Severe Dysphagia:** Can't swallow liquids, drooling.

TRIAGE ASSESSMENT QUESTIONS

Call EMS 911 Now
- ● SEVERE difficulty breathing (e.g., struggling for each breath, speaks in single words)
  R/O: airway obstruction
- ● Sounds like a life-threatening emergency to the triager

See More Appropriate Protocol
- ● Productive cough is the main symptom
  Go to Protocol: Cough on page 95
- ● Runny nose is the main symptom
  Go to Protocol: Common Cold on page 79

Go to ED/UCC Now
(or to Office With PCP Approval)
- ● Drooling or spitting out saliva (because can't swallow)
  R/O: epiglottitis
- ● Unable to open mouth completely
  R/O: peritonsillar abscess
- ● Drinking very little and has signs of dehydration (e.g., no urine > 12 hours, very dry mouth, very light-headed)
- ● Patient sounds very sick or weak to the triager
  Reason: severe acute illness or serious complication suspected

Go to Office Now
- ● Difficulty breathing (per caller) but not severe
  R/O: swollen tonsils that are touching
- ● Fever > 103° F (39.4° C)
- ● Refuses to drink anything for > 12 hours
  R/O: tonsillitis, abscess

See Today in Office
- ● SEVERE sore throat pain
  R/O: strep pharyngitis
- ● Pus on tonsils (back of throat) and swollen neck lymph nodes ("glands")
  R/O: strep pharyngitis
- ● Earache also present
  R/O: peritonsillar abscess, tonsillitis
- ● Widespread rash (especially chest and abdomen)
  R/O: scarlet fever
- ● Diabetes mellitus or weak immune system (e.g., HIV positive, cancer chemotherapy, splenectomy, organ transplant, chronic steroids)
  R/O: candidal pharyngitis
- ● History of rheumatic fever
- ● Patient wants to be seen

See Today or Tomorrow in Office
- ● Fever present > 3 days (72 hours)

Strep Test Only Visit Today or Tomorrow
- ● Patient requesting a strep throat test
  R/O: strep pharyngitis
- ● Strep exposure within last 10 days
- ● Sore throat is the main symptom and persists > 48 hours
- ● Sore throat with cough/cold symptoms present > 5 days

Home Care
- ○ Sore throat
  Reason: probably viral pharyngitis

HOME CARE ADVICE

❶ For Relief of Sore Throat Pain:
- Sip warm chicken broth or apple juice.
- Suck on hard candy or a throat lozenge (over the counter).
- Gargle warm salt water 3 times daily (1 teaspoon of salt in 8 oz or 240 mL of warm water).
- Avoid cigarette smoke.

❷ Pain and Fever Medicines:
- For pain or fever relief, take either acetaminophen or ibuprofen.
- They are over-the-counter (OTC) drugs that help treat both fever and pain. You can buy them at the drugstore.
- Treat fevers > 101° F (38.3° C). The goal of fever therapy is to bring the fever down to a comfortable level. Remember that fever medicine usually lowers fever 2° F (1-1½° C).

Acetaminophen (e.g., Tylenol):
- **Regular Strength Tylenol:** Take 650 mg (two 325 mg pills) by mouth every 4-6 hours as needed. Each Regular Strength Tylenol pill has 325 mg of acetaminophen.
- **Extra Strength Tylenol:** Take 1,000 mg (two 500 mg pills) every 8 hours as needed. Each Extra Strength Tylenol pill has 500 mg of acetaminophen.
- The most you should take each day is 3,000 mg (10 Regular Strength or 6 Extra Strength pills a day).

Ibuprofen (e.g., Motrin, Advil):
- Take 400 mg (two 200 mg pills) by mouth every 6 hours.
- Another choice is to take 600 mg (three 200 mg pills) by mouth every 8 hours.
- The most you should take each day is 1,200 mg (six 200 mg pills), unless your doctor has told you to take more.

❸ Pain and Fever Medicines—Extra Notes:
- Use the lowest amount of medicine that makes your pain or fever better.
- Acetaminophen is thought to be safer than ibuprofen or naproxen in people > 65 years old. Acetaminophen is in many OTC and prescription medicines. It might be in more than one medicine that you are taking. You need to be careful and not take an overdose. An acetaminophen overdose can hurt the liver.
- McNeil, the company that makes Tylenol, has different dosage instructions for Tylenol in Canada and the United States. In Canada, the maximum recommended dose per day is 4,000 mg or 12 Regular Strength (325 mg) pills. In the United States, McNeil recommends a maximum dose of 10 Regular Strength (325 mg) pills.
- CAUTION: Do not take acetaminophen if you have liver disease.
- CAUTION: Do not take ibuprofen if you have stomach problems, have kidney disease, are pregnant, or have been told by your doctor to avoid this type of anti-inflammatory drug. Do not take ibuprofen for > 7 days without consulting your doctor.
- *Before taking any medicine, read all the instructions on the package.*

❹ Soft Diet: Cold drinks and milk shakes are especially good.
(Reason: Swollen tonsils can make some foods hard to swallow.)

❺ Drink Plenty of Liquids:
- Drink plenty of liquids. This is important to prevent dehydration.
- A healthy adult should drink 6-8 cups (240 mL) or more of liquid each day.
- **How can you tell if you are drinking enough liquids?** The goal is to keep the urine clear or light yellow in color. If your urine is bright yellow or dark yellow, you are probably not drinking enough liquids.
- CAUTION: Some medical problems require fluid restriction.

❻ Contagiousness: You can return to work or school after the fever is gone and you feel well enough to participate in normal activities. If your doctor determines that you have strep throat, you will need to take an antibiotic for 24 hours before you can return.

❼ Expected Course: Sore throats with viral illnesses usually last 3 or 4 days.

❽ Call Back If:
- Sore throat is the main symptom and it lasts > 24 hours.
- Sore throat is mild but lasts > 4 days.
- Fever lasts > 3 days.
- You become worse.

BACKGROUND

Key Points

- Sore throat is one of the most common reasons why patients go to the doctor's office.
- The medical term for a throat infection is pharyngitis or tonsillopharyngitis.

Causes

- **Colds:** Most sore throats are from a cold or other viral infection. The presence of a cough, hoarseness, or nasal symptoms points to a cold or viral infection as the cause of the sore throat.
- **Strep:** In adults, approximately 10%-20% of sore throats are caused by the *Streptococcus* (strep) bacteria. Streptococcal pharyngitis is the only commonly occurring bacteria for which antibiotic therapy is definitely indicated.
- **Mono:** Infectious mononucleosis is primarily seen in young adults, causing 5%-10% of the sore throats in this population. It should be suspected in young adults with fever, sore throat, cervical adenopathy, and a negative strep throat culture. A blood test called a "monospot" can help make the diagnosis. There is no antibiotic treatment.
- **Other:** Other common causes include dry air, smoking, postnasal drip, allergies, singing, and yelling. Sexually transmitted infections (e.g., gonorrhea) can also cause pharyngitis.

Streptococcal Pharyngitis (Strep Throat)

- **Cause:** Strep throat is a type of bacterial pharyngitis caused by group A beta-hemolytic *Streptococcus*.
- **Symptoms:** The main symptom is sore throat and pain with swallowing. Other symptoms can include fever, headache, swollen lymph nodes, nausea, and malaise. Cough, hoarseness, conjunctivitis, and rhinorrhea are usually not seen with strep throat and are more suggestive of a viral pharyngitis.
- **Physical Examination:** Examination of the throat typically shows redness and exudate (pus) on the tonsils.
- **Diagnosis:** Strep throat culture and/or rapid strep test. In adults the diagnosis is sometimes made by health care providers clinically, without testing.
- **Treatment:** Since this is caused by bacteria, antibiotic treatment is needed. Penicillin, amoxicillin, and erythromycin are the first-line antibiotics used for treatment of this infection.
- **Complications:** Complications are rare; they include peritonsillar abscess, acute rheumatic fever, and poststreptococcal glomerulonephritis.

Antibiotic Prescription for Presumed Strep Pharyngitis Over the Phone

- Some physicians are willing to initiate empiric antibiotic therapy for presumed strep pharyngitis over the telephone. Remember, most sore throats are not caused by strep.
- **Should Be Present:** (1) Pus on tonsils (back of throat) AND (2) fever > 101°F (38.3°C) AND (3) swollen neck lymph nodes ("glands").
- **Should Be Absent (or Minimal):** Cough, runny nose, hoarseness.
- **Typical Antibiotic Prescription:** Penicillin (penicillin-VK 500 mg by mouth twice a day for 10 days). If allergic to penicillin, erythromycin (e.g., erythromycin base 500 mg by mouth 4 times a day for 10 days) can be used. The dosage of erythromycin depends on the type prescribed.

Testing

- Throat cultures aren't urgent. Rapid strep tests also aren't urgent. Treating a strep infection within 9 days of onset will still prevent rheumatic fever.
- Both of these tests can usually be done in the doctor's office.
- Sometimes a patient requests a rapid strep test now because they are leaving on a trip or have other urgent needs.

What Patients Really Want: Pain Relief

A study was performed with 298 patients (adolescents and adults) who saw their PCP for chief complaint of "sore throat." They were asked to rank the importance of 13 reasons for visiting the PCP. Here are the pertinent results:

- #1 reason was to establish the cause of the sore throat.
  (Note: Pharyngitis as part of a cold can usually be determined by telephone.)
- #2 was pain relief.
  (Note: can absolutely be provided by telephone)
- #3 was information on the expected course of the illness.
  (Note: can usually be provided by telephone)
- **Surprise:** Hopes for an antibiotic was #11.
- **Summary:** If we meet the caller's request for pain relief, we may be able to prevent unnecessary ED and office visits.
- **Reference:** *Ann Fam Med.* 2006;4(6):494–499.

SPIDER BITE

Definition

- Bite from a spider seen on the skin.
- Onset of spider bite symptoms (redness, pain, swelling) and a spider is seen in close proximity.

TRIAGE ASSESSMENT QUESTIONS

Call EMS 911 Now

- Difficulty breathing or swallowing
  R/O: anaphylactic shock
- Difficult to awaken or acting confused (e.g., disoriented, slurred speech)
  R/O: anaphylactic shock
- Pale cold skin and very weak (can't stand)
  R/O: shock
- Sounds like a life-threatening emergency to the triager

See More Appropriate Protocol

- Not a spider bite
  Go to Protocol: Insect Bite on page 257

Go to ED Now

- Black widow (or brown widow) spider bite and local skin changes
- Abdominal pain, chest tightness, or other muscle cramps
  R/O: black or brown widow spider
- Urine is brown, black, or red in color
  R/O: brown recluse spider bite with hemolysis
- Vomiting
  R/O: systemic venom reaction

Go to ED/UCC Now
(or to Office With PCP Approval)

- Patient sounds very sick or weak to the triager
  Reason: severe acute illness or serious complication suspected

Go to Office Now

- SEVERE bite pain and not improved after 2 hours of pain medicine
- Rash elsewhere on body that developed after spider bite
  R/O: hives, systemic venom reaction

- Fever and area is red
  R/O: cellulitis, lymphangitis
  Reason: fever and looks infected
- Fever and area is very tender to touch
  R/O: cellulitis, CA-MRSA, abscess
  Reason: fever and looks infected
- Red streak or red line and length > 2" (5 cm)
  R/O: lymphangitis
  Note: Lymphangitis looks like a red streak or line originating at the wound and ascending the arm or leg toward the heart.

See Today in Office

- Red or very tender (to touch) area, and started > 24 hours after the bite
  R/O: cellulitis
- Red or very tender (to touch) area, getting larger > 48 hours after the bite
  R/O: cellulitis
- Eye irritation after handling or touching a tarantula
  R/O: foreign body (hairs) keratoconjunctivitis or ophthalmia nodosa
- Patient wants to be seen

See Today or Tomorrow in Office

- Has diabetes with spider bite wound on foot
  Reason: diabetic neuropathy and decreased resistance to infection

See Within 3 Days in Office

- Scab drains pus or increases in size, and not improved after applying antibiotic ointment for 2 days
  R/O: infected sore, impetigo
- Bite starts to look bad (e.g., blister, purplish skin, ulcer)
  R/O: necrotic spider bite (brown recluse, hobo spider) or other cause of skin lesion

Home Care

- Nonserious spider bite
- Scab drains pus or increases in size
  R/O: infected sore, impetigo
- Prevention of spider bites, questions about

HOME CARE ADVICE

Nonserious Spider Bite

❶ Cleaning: Wash the bite with antibacterial soap and warm water.

❷ Pain Medicines:
- For pain relief, you can take either acetaminophen, ibuprofen, or naproxen.
- They are over-the-counter (OTC) pain drugs. You can buy them at the drugstore.

Acetaminophen (e.g., Tylenol):
- **Regular Strength Tylenol:** Take 650 mg (two 325 mg pills) by mouth every 4-6 hours as needed. Each Regular Strength Tylenol pill has 325 mg of acetaminophen.
- **Extra Strength Tylenol:** Take 1,000 mg (two 500 mg pills) every 8 hours as needed. Each Extra Strength Tylenol pill has 500 mg of acetaminophen.
- The most you should take each day is 3,000 mg (10 Regular Strength or 6 Extra Strength pills a day).

Ibuprofen (e.g., Motrin, Advil):
- Take 400 mg (two 200 mg pills) by mouth every 6 hours.
- Another choice is to take 600 mg (three 200 mg pills) by mouth every 8 hours.
- The most you should take each day is 1,200 mg (six 200 mg pills), unless your doctor has told you to take more.

Naproxen (e.g., Aleve):
- Take 220 mg (one 220 mg pill) by mouth every 8 hours as needed. You may take 440 mg (two 220 mg pills) for your first dose.
- The most you should take each day is 660 mg (three 220 mg pills a day), unless your doctor has told you to take more.

❸ Pain Medicines—Extra Notes:
- Use the lowest amount of medicine that makes your pain better.
- Acetaminophen is thought to be safer than ibuprofen or naproxen in people > 65 years old. Acetaminophen is in many OTC and prescription medicines. It might be in more than one medicine that you are taking. You need to be careful and not take an overdose. An acetaminophen overdose can hurt the liver.
- McNeil, the company that makes Tylenol, has different dosage instructions for Tylenol in Canada and the United States. In Canada, the maximum recommended dose per day is 4,000 mg or 12 Regular Strength (325 mg) pills. In the United States, McNeil recommends a maximum dose of 10 Regular Strength (325 mg) pills.
- CAUTION: Do not take acetaminophen if you have liver disease.
- CAUTION: Do not take ibuprofen or naproxen if you have stomach problems, have kidney disease, are pregnant, or have been told by your doctor to avoid this type of anti-inflammatory drug. Do not take ibuprofen or naproxen for > 7 days without consulting your doctor.
- *Before taking any medicine, read all the instructions on the package.*

❹ Expected Course: Some swelling and pain for 1-2 days. It shouldn't be any worse than a bee sting.

❺ Call Back If:
- Severe bite pain lasts > 2 hours after pain medicine.
- Abdominal pains or muscle spasms occur.
- Local pain lasts > 2 days (48 hours).
- Bite begins to look infected.
- You become worse.

Infected Sore or Scab

❶ Reassurance:
- Sometimes a small infected sore can develop at the site of a cut, scratch, insect bite, or sting.
- The typical appearance is a sore < 1" (2.5 cm) in diameter. It is often covered by a soft, "honey-yellow" or yellow-brown crust or scab. Sometimes the scab may drain a tiny amount of pus or yellow fluid. Usually there is minimal to no pain.
- Small infected sores usually get better with regular cleansing and use of an antibiotic ointment.
- *Here is some care advice that should help.*

❷ Cleaning:
- Wash the area 2-3 times daily with an antibacterial soap and warm water.
- Gently remove any scab. The bacteria live underneath the scab. You may need to soak the scab off by placing a warm, wet washcloth (or gauze) on the sore for 10 minutes.

❸ **Antibiotic Ointment:**
- Apply an antibiotic ointment 3 times per day.
- Cover the sore with a Band-Aid to prevent scratching and spread.
- Use bacitracin ointment (OTC in United States) or Polysporin ointment (OTC in Canada) or one that you already have.

❹ **Avoid Picking:** Avoid scratching and picking. This can spread a skin infection.

❺ **Contagiousness:**
- Infected sores can be spread by skin-to-skin contact.
- Wash your hands frequently and avoid touching the sore.
- **Work and School:** You can attend school or work if it is covered.
- **Contact Sports:** Generally, you need to receive antibiotic treatment for 3 days before you can return to the sport. There can be no pus or drainage. You should check with your trainer, if there is one for your sports team.

❻ **Expected Course:**
- The sore should stop growing in 1-2 days and it should begin improving within 2-3 days.
- The sore should be completely healed in 7-10 days.

❼ **Call Back If:**
- Fever occurs.
- Spreading redness or a red streak occurs.
- Sore increases in size.
- Sore not improving after 2 days using antibiotic ointment.
- Sore not completely healed in 7 days (1 week).
- New sore appears.
- You become worse.

Preventing Spider Bites

❶ **Prevention—Outdoors:**
- Be especially careful around woodpiles and when clearing brush.
- Wear long pants with the pants tucked into your socks.
- Wear long-sleeved shirts and use gloves.
- DEET is a very effective insect repellent. It also repels spiders.

❷ **Prevention—Indoors:**
- Remove spiderwebs.
- Make certain that doorways and windows are effectively sealed and insulated.

❸ **Using DEET-Containing Insect Repellents When Outdoors:**
- DEET is a very effective insect repellent. It also repels spiders.
- Higher concentrations of DEET do work better—but there appears to be no benefit in using DEET concen-trations > 50%. For children and adolescents, the American Academy of Pediatrics recommends a maximum concentration of 30%. Health Canada recommends using a concentration of 5%-30% for adults.
- Apply to exposed areas of skin. Do not apply to eyes, mouth, or irritated areas of skin. Do not apply to skin that is covered by clothing.
- Remember to wash it off with soap and water when you return indoors.
- DEET can damage clothing made of synthetic fibers, plastics (e.g., eyeglasses), and leather.
- Breastfeeding women may use DEET. No problems have been reported (CDC).
- *Read and follow the package directions carefully.*

FIRST AID

First Aid Advice for Shock:
Lie down with the feet elevated.

First Aid Advice for Spider Bite (localized symptoms only):
- Wash bite wound with soap and water.
- Apply a cold pack to the area of the bite for 10-20 minutes.

First Aid Advice for Black Widow Spider Bite:
- Wash bite wound with soap and water.
- Apply a cold pack to the area of the bite for 10-20 minutes.
- If possible, capture the spider and place it in a jar (for spider identification).

Special Notes:
- Do not apply heat.
  (Reason: It may increase the pain.)
- Do not apply a tourniquet or pressure bandage.
  (Reason: There is no evidence that this helps.)

First Aid Advice for Brown Recluse Spider Bite:
- Wash bite wound with soap and water.
- Apply a cold pack to the area of the bite for 10-20 minutes.
- If possible, capture the spider and place it in a jar (for spider identification).

BACKGROUND

Key Points

- There are approximately 20,000+ species of spiders in the world.
- In the United States and Canada, there are 2 species of medical importance that cause bites in humans: the black widow (*Latrodectus*) and the brown recluse (*Loxosceles*).
- Patients sometimes incorrectly believe that they sustained a spider bite, when instead a minor break in the skin simply became infected with *Staphylococcus aureus*. An infection with CA-MRSA must be considered as a possible cause of any infected-appearing "spider bite."

Types of Spider Bites

❶ Black Widow Spider Bite

- **Description:** A shiny, jet-black spider with long legs. Size is about 1" (2.5 cm). A red (or orange) hourglass-shaped marking may be on its underside (not present in all *Latrodectus* species).
- **Habitat:** Found throughout North America, except Alaska and the far North.
- **Symptoms—Bite Wound:** The black widow spider produces one of nature's most potent neurotoxic venoms. The bite causes immediate moderate-severe pain; there is usually minimal to no local reaction.
- **Symptoms—Systemic:** Severe muscle cramps are present by 1-6 hours and last 24-48 hours. Other possible symptoms include abdominal pain, vomiting, restlessness, hypertension, and weakness.
- **Treatment—Local Wound Care:** Wash bite with soap and water. Apply an ice pack.
- **Treatment—Medications:** Tetanus prophylaxis should be provided. Parenteral analgesics may be needed for pain and benzodiazepines for muscle spasms. There is a *Latrodectus* antivenin that is indicated for severe symptoms, seizures, or uncontrolled hypertension.
- **Expected Course:** All symptoms usually resolve over 2-3 days. Death may occur rarely; a bite is more serious in a small child; and multiple spider bites are also more serious.
- **Special Note:** Many bite wounds are "dry bites" (no venom injected into skin) because the fangs are small.

❷ Brown Widow Spider Bite

- The brown widow spider is related to the black widow and is also a member of *Latrodectus* (*Latrodectus geometricus*).
- **Habitat:** First appeared in North America in 1980. Has been reported in the southern United States (Florida, Georgia, Louisiana, Texas, California).
- **Symptoms:** Brown widow spider bites are thought to be less serious than those from black widows.
- **Treatment:** Same as for black widow spiders.

❸ Brown Recluse Spider Bite

- Also known as the "violin" or "fiddleback" spider.
- **Description:** A brown spider with long legs. Size is about ½" (1.2 cm). Dark violin-shaped marking on top of its head (not present in all *Loxosceles* species).
- **Habitat:** Found in the southern, southwestern, and midwestern United States.
- **Symptoms—Bite Wound:** The spider produces a venom that causes cell destruction and blood cell breakdown. The bite is initially painless or there is mild stinging discomfort. Localized aching, itching, and blister formation develops in 4-8 hours. The center becomes bluish and depressed (craterlike) over 2-3 days. A deep necrotic ulcer may develop.
- **Symptoms—Systemic:** Systemic symptoms include fever, vomiting, and myalgias (but no life-threatening symptoms).
- **Red, White, and Blue Sign:** These bites have some distinguishing features. They are very painful. The puncture mark left by the spider's fangs is off-center. The bite progresses to 3 concentric red, white, and blue zones. The outer zone is red (erythema). The middle zone is white (ischemia). The inner zone is blue, suggesting impending necrosis. By contrast, the necrotic lesion of cutaneous anthrax is painless and does not have the red, white, and blue sign (Source: Dr Edwin Masters, Cape Girardeau, MO).
- **Treatment—Local Wound Care:** Cleansing of wound with soap and water, cold pack.
- **Treatment—Medications:** Tetanus prophylaxis should be provided.
- **Expected Course:** Most necrotic ulcers heal over 1-8 weeks. Permanent scarring occurs in 10%-15%. Skin damage sometimes requires skin grafting.

❹ Tarantulas

- **Habitat:** Tarantulas are found in the southern United States (e.g., desert southwest).
- **Symptoms—Bite Wound:** Mild stinging with minimal local inflammation. No skin necrosis occurs.
- **Symptoms—Eye:** Some genera of tarantula have "urticating" hairs that can come off. Like a little piece of fiberglass, they can penetrate human skin and cause itching and redness. If they lodge in the cornea they can cause foreign body keratoconjunctivitis or ophthalmia nodosa.
- **Symptoms—Systemic:** None.
- **Treatment—Local Wound Care:** Cleansing of bite wound with soap and water, cold pack, oral analgesics. Obtaining a tetanus booster is appropriate if it has been > 10 years.
- **Treatment—Eye Irritation:** Individuals with eye irritation or redness after handling a tarantula should be referred to an ophthalmologist for a slit lamp examination of the eye.
- **Expected Course:** Bite wounds heal completely. Eye problems generally resolve under the close follow-up care of an ophthalmologist.

❺ Minor (Non-dangerous) Spider Bites

- > 50 spiders in the United States and Canada have venom and can cause minor, localized, nonserious reactions. Many single, unseen, and unexplained painful bites that occur during the night can be from spiders.
- **Symptoms—Bite Wound:** The bites are painful and mildly swollen for 1 or 2 days (much like a bee sting).
- **Symptoms—Systemic:** None.
- **Treatment—Local Wound Care:** Cleansing of bite wound with soap and water, cold pack, oral analgesics. Obtaining a tetanus booster is appropriate if it has been > 10 years.
- **Expected Course:** Bite wounds heal completely.

Brown Recluse Spider Versus Anthrax

- **Brown Recluse Spider and the Red, White, and Blue Sign:** Brown recluse bites have some distinguishing features. Initially there may be mild stinging pain or no discomfort. The puncture mark left by the spider's fangs is off-center. The bite progresses to 3 concentric red, white, and blue zones. The outer zone is red (erythema). The middle zone is white (ischemia). The inner zone is blue, suggesting impending necrosis.
- **Anthrax:** By contrast, the necrotic lesion of cutaneous anthrax is painless and does not have the red, white, and blue sign.
- **Source:** Dr Edwin Masters, Cape Girardeau, MO.

Community Acquired Methicillin-Resistant *Staphylococcus aureus* (CA-MRSA)

- *Staphylococcus aureus* is bacteria that can cause a variety of skin infections, including pimples, boils, abscesses, cellulitis, wound infections, and impetigo. It can also cause more serious infections like staphylococcal pneumonia, sepsis, and toxic shock syndrome.
- In the 1960s strains of *S aureus* that were resistant to penicillin-type antibiotics started appearing in hospitals and health care settings. These were referred to as methicillin-resistant *S aureus* (MRSA) infections.
- More recently, strains of penicillin-resistant *S aureus* have increasingly become the cause of skin infections in healthy individuals in the community. These are now being referred to as community acquired methicillin-resistant *S aureus* (CA-MRSA) infections. There have been outbreaks in athletes (e.g., wrestling teams) and in prison populations.
- CA-MRSA requires treatment with specific types of antibiotics.
- More information about CA-MRSA is available at: www.cdc.gov/mrsa/index.html.

STI EXPOSURE AND PREVENTION

Definition
- Exposure to someone with proven sexually transmitted infection (STI)
- Questions about STIs

Exposure:
- Sexual intercourse (oral, vaginal, or anal) with someone who was diagnosed with an STI

TRIAGE ASSESSMENT QUESTIONS

See More Appropriate Protocol
- ● Rash or sores on penis or scrotum
  Go to Protocol: Penis and Scrotum Symptoms on page 308
- ● Rash or sores on female genital area (vulvar area)
  Go to Protocol: Vulvar Symptoms on page 437

Go to ED Now
- ● Forced to have sex (sexual assault or rape) in the past 3 days

Go to ED/UCC Now
(or to Office With PCP Approval)
- ● Sexual intercourse (in the past 72 hours) with someone who was diagnosed with HIV
- ● Female and ANY of the following:
  - Fever and burning (pain) with urination
  - Constant lower abdominal pain lasting > 2 hours
  - Unable to urinate for > 4 hours and bladder feels very full
- ● Male and ANY of the following:
  - Fever and burning (pain) with urination
  - Fever and testicle pain or swelling
  - Unable to urinate for > 4 hours and bladder feels very full

See Today in Office
- ● Forced to have sex (sexual assault or rape) > 3 days ago
- ● Female and ANY of the following:
  - Burning (pain) with urination
  - Unexplained lower abdominal pain
  - Abnormal color of vaginal discharge (i.e., yellow, green, gray)
  - Bad-smelling vaginal discharge
- ● Male with ANY of the following:
  - Burning (pain) with urination
  - Pus (white, yellow) or bloody discharge from end of penis
  - Testicle pain or swelling
- ● Rectal discharge or unusual rectal pain or itching
- ● Patient wants to be seen

See Within 3 Days in Office
- ● Patient is worried about an STI
  Reason: relieve fear and prevent spread of STI
- ● Sexual intercourse (oral, vaginal, or anal) with someone who was diagnosed with an STI
  Reason: will need to be tested and treated

Home Care
- ○ Questions about preventing STIs

HOME CARE ADVICE

❶ General Condom Information:
- *Latex condoms are the only effective way to prevent STIs during sexual intercourse.*
- You can also use condoms during oral sex.

❷ Obtaining a Condom:
- Buy latex rubber condoms. Persons who are allergic to latex can use a polyurethane (plastic) condom. Never use condoms made from animal skins; they can leak.
- You can get condoms at public health clinics (often free), drugstores, supermarkets, and via the Internet. You do not need a prescription.

❸ **Storing Condoms**
- Store condoms at room temperature. Avoid extreme heat, extreme cold, or sunlight.
- You might want to keep a condom in your wallet or purse; this way it is ready and available.

❹ **Putting on a Condom—Instructions:**
- Hold the condom at the tip to squeeze out the air.
- Roll the condom all the way down the erect penis (do not try to put a condom on a soft penis).
- If you use a lubricant during sex, make sure it is water-based (e.g., K-Y Liquid, Astroglide). Do not use petroleum jelly (Vaseline), vegetable oil (Crisco), or baby oil; these can cause a condom to break.

❺ **Taking Off a Condom—Instructions:**
- After sex, hold onto the condom while the penis is being pulled out.
- The penis should be pulled out while still erect, so that sperm (semen) doesn't leak out of the condom.

❻ **Female Condoms:**
- There are female condoms (e.g., Reality) that you can also buy without a prescription.
- A female condom is a polyurethane (plastic) sheath that is placed inside the vagina.

❼ **United States—STI Hotline:**
- American Sexual Health Association STD Hotline provides information on sexually transmitted infections (STIs), such as chlamydia, gonorrhea, HPV/genital warts, herpes, and HIV/AIDS. Specialists can provide general information, referrals to local clinics, and written materials about STIs and disease prevention.
- Toll-free number (English): **800/227-8922.**
- Toll-free number (Spanish): **800/344-7432.**
- Web site: www.ashastd.org.

❽ **Pregnancy Test, When in Doubt:**
- If there is a chance that you might be pregnant, use a urine pregnancy test.
- You can buy a pregnancy test at the drugstore.
- It works best if you test your first urine in the morning.
- *Follow the instructions included in the package.*
- Call back if you are pregnant.

❾ **Call Back If:**
- Pregnancy test is positive or if you have difficulties with the home pregnancy test.
- You become worse.

BACKGROUND

Some Basics
- A sexually transmitted infection (STI) is an infection that is spread through vaginal, anal, and oral sex. It is also sometimes called a sexually transmitted disease (STD).
- Examples of STIs include chlamydia, gonorrhea, genital herpes, HIV, pubic lice, and *Trichomonas*.
- Some STIs can be cured with antibiotics (gonorrhea, chlamydia).
- Some STIs cannot be cured, but the symptoms can be reduced (herpes, HIV) by taking prescription medications.

How Are STIs Spread?
- Most STIs are spread through body fluids during vaginal, anal, and oral sex. Some of these fluids are vaginal fluids, semen, and blood.
- They can also be spread through contact with sores during sex.
- A latex condom works well to stop STIs from spreading during sex.

How Can a Person Avoid Getting an STI?
There are only two 100% effective means of avoiding STIs:
- Not having sex or oral sex (abstinence)
- Having one long-term sexual partner who you know does not have any STIs

There are some sexual acts that most often do not spread STIs. Some of these are holding hands, hugging, and touching. Kissing is generally safe. Make sure there are no sores on the lips or in the mouth. Touching semen during mutual masturbation is often safe.

What Things Don't Work to Prevent an STI?
- Douching the vagina or taking a shower after sex does not prevent STIs.
- Withdrawal is not a way to prevent STIs or pregnancy. This is when a man pulls his penis out before he ejaculates.
- Having an STI one time does not stop you from getting it again.
- Using birth control pills, patches, or shots will not prevent you from getting an STI. You still need to protect yourself with condoms.

STREP THROAT TEST FOLLOW-UP CALL

Definition
- Strep throat culture or rapid strep test done and results called to triage nurse by the laboratory, PCP, or adult caller.
- Patient has been previously triaged by triage nurse or examined by PCP.
- In most cases, the triage nurse needs to call the patient.

TRIAGE ASSESSMENT QUESTIONS

See More Appropriate Protocol
● Sore throat symptoms are much worse
Go to Protocol: Sore Throat on page 369

Go to ED/UCC Now
(or to Office With PCP Approval)
● Patient sounds very sick or weak to the triager
Reason: severe acute illness or serious complication suspected

See Today or Tomorrow in Office
◐ Patient wants to be seen

Discuss With PCP and Callback by Nurse Today
◐ Positive throat culture or rapid strep test (according to lab, PCP, caller, etc.) AND NO standing order to call in prescription for antibiotic
Reason: antibiotic prescription needed

Home Care
○ Positive throat culture or rapid strep test (according to lab, PCP, caller, etc.) AND standing order to call in prescription for antibiotic
Reason: antibiotic prescription needed
○ Rapid strep test negative and symptoms not worse
○ Strep throat culture negative and symptoms not worse

HOME CARE ADVICE

POSITIVE Rapid Strep Test or Strep Throat Culture
❶ **Strep Throat Culture POSITIVE:** Your throat culture was positive. You have strep throat. Strep throat is treated with antibiotics.
❷ **Rapid Strep Test POSITIVE:** Your rapid strep test was positive. You have strep throat. Strep throat is treated with antibiotics.
❸ **Antibiotic Prescription for Strep Throat:**
- Penicillin (penicillin-VK 500 mg by mouth twice a day for 10 days).
- **Penicillin Allergy:** If allergic to penicillin, erythromycin (erythromycin base 500 mg by mouth 4 times a day for 10 days). Erythromycin can cause nausea and vomiting in some people. Another alternative for penicillin allergic patients is Zithromax (a 5-day Z-Pak).
❹ **Contagiousness:** After taking antibiotics for 24 hours, the disease is no longer considered contagious and you can return to work or school.
❺ **Expected Course:** Antibiotic treatment should make you feel much better within 48 hours.
❻ **Call Back If:**
- Fever lasts > 2 days on antibiotics.
- Symptoms last > 3 days on antibiotics.
- You become worse.

NEGATIVE Rapid Strep Test or Strep Throat Culture
❶ **Strep Throat Culture NEGATIVE:** Your throat culture was negative, so you don't have strep. Most sore throats are caused by a virus and are just part of a cold.
❷ **Rapid Strep Test NEGATIVE:** Your rapid strep test was negative. Most sore throats are caused by a virus and are just part of a cold.
❸ **No Antibiotics:** Antibiotics are not helpful for viral sore throats.
❹ **Expected Course:** Sore throats with viral illnesses usually last 3 or 4 days.
❺ **Contagiousness:** You can return to work or school after the fever is gone and you feel well enough to participate in normal activities.
❻ **Call Back If:**
- Fever lasts > 3 days.
- You become worse.

General Care Advice for Sore Throat

❶ For Relief of Sore Throat Pain:
- Sip warm chicken broth or apple juice.
- Suck on hard candy or a throat lozenge (over the counter).
- Gargle warm salt water 3 times daily (1 teaspoon of salt in 8 oz or 240 mL of warm water).
- Avoid cigarette smoke.

❷ Pain and Fever Medicines:
- For pain or fever relief, take either acetaminophen or ibuprofen.
- They are over-the-counter (OTC) drugs that help treat both fever and pain. You can buy them at the drugstore.
- Treat fevers > 101° F (38.3° C). The goal of fever therapy is to bring the fever down to a comfortable level. Remember that fever medicine usually lowers fever 2° F (1-1½° C).

Acetaminophen (e.g., Tylenol):
- **Regular Strength Tylenol:** Take 650 mg (two 325 mg pills) by mouth every 4-6 hours as needed. Each Regular Strength Tylenol pill has 325 mg of acetaminophen.
- **Extra Strength Tylenol:** Take 1,000 mg (two 500 mg pills) every 8 hours as needed. Each Extra Strength Tylenol pill has 500 mg of acetaminophen.
- The most you should take each day is 3,000 mg (10 Regular Strength or 6 Extra Strength pills a day).

Ibuprofen (e.g., Motrin, Advil):
- Take 400 mg (two 200 mg pills) by mouth every 6 hours.
- Another choice is to take 600 mg (three 200 mg pills) by mouth every 8 hours.
- The most you should take each day is 1,200 mg (six 200 mg pills), unless your doctor has told you to take more.

❸ Pain and Fever Medicines—Extra Notes:
- Use the lowest amount of medicine that makes your pain or fever better.
- Acetaminophen is thought to be safer than ibuprofen or naproxen in people > 65 years old. Acetaminophen is in many OTC and prescription medicines. It might be in more than one medicine that you are taking. You need to be careful and not take an overdose. An acetaminophen overdose can hurt the liver.
- McNeil, the company that makes Tylenol, has different dosage instructions for Tylenol in Canada and the United States. In Canada, the maximum recommended dose per day is 4,000 mg or 12 Regular Strength (325 mg) pills. In the United States, McNeil recommends a maximum dose of 10 Regular Strength (325 mg) pills.
- CAUTION: Do not take acetaminophen if you have liver disease.
- CAUTION: Do not take ibuprofen if you have stomach problems, have kidney disease, are pregnant, or have been told by your doctor to avoid this type of anti-inflammatory drug. Do not take ibuprofen for > 7 days without consulting your doctor.
- *Before taking any medicine, read all the instructions on the package.*

❹ Soft Diet: Cold drinks and milkshakes are especially good.
(Reason: Swollen tonsils can make some foods hard to swallow.)

❺ Drink Plenty of Liquids:
- Drink plenty of liquids. This is important to prevent dehydration.
- A healthy adult should drink 8 cups (240 mL) or more of liquid each day.
- **How can you tell if you are drinking enough liquids?** The goal is to keep the urine clear or light yellow in color. If your urine is bright yellow or dark yellow, you are probably not drinking enough liquids.
- CAUTION: Some medical problems require fluid restriction.

❻ Call Back If:
- Fever lasts > 3 days.
- You become worse.

BACKGROUND

Key Points

- Sore throat is one of the most common reasons why patients go to the doctor's office.
- The medical term for a throat infection is pharyngitis or tonsillopharyngitis.

Causes of a Sore Throat

- **Colds:** Most sore throats are from a cold or other viral infection.
- **Strep:** In adults, approximately 10%-20% of sore throats are caused by the strep bacteria. Streptococcal pharyngitis is the only commonly occurring bacteria for which antibiotic therapy is definitely indicated.
- **Mono:** Infectious mononucleosis is primarily seen in young adults, causing 5%-10% of the sore throats in this population. It should be suspected in young adults with fever, sore throat, cervical adenopathy, and a negative strep throat culture. A blood test called a "monospot" can help make the diagnosis. There is no antibiotic treatment.
- **Other:** Other common causes include dry air, smoking, postnasal drip, allergies, singing, and yelling. Sexually transmitted infections (e.g., gonorrhea) can also cause pharyngitis.

Streptococcal Pharyngitis (Strep Throat)

- **Cause:** Strep throat is a type of bacterial pharyngitis caused by group A beta-hemolytic *Streptococcus.*
- **Symptoms:** The main symptom is sore throat and pain with swallowing. Other symptoms can include fever, headache, swollen lymph nodes, nausea, and malaise.
- **Physical Examination:** Examination of the throat typically shows redness and exudate (pus) on the tonsils.
- **Diagnosis:** Strep throat culture and/or rapid strep test. In adults the diagnosis is often made by health care professionals clinically, without testing.
- **Treatment:** Since this is caused by bacteria, antibiotic treatment is needed. Penicillin, amoxicillin, and erythromycin are the first-line antibiotics used for treatment of this infection.
- **Complications:** Complications are rare; they include peritonsillar abscess, acute rheumatic fever, and poststreptococcal glomerulonephritis.

Strep Throat—Return to Work or School

Adults can return to work or school after taking antibiotics for 24 hours and the fever is gone.

Strep Throat—Risk of Secondary Cases in the Family

- A recent research study from Australia followed 202 families who had a child with acute strep pharyngitis. A secondary case of strep pharyngitis occurred in 43% of these families.
- **Significance:** Strep pharyngitis is readily transmitted to siblings and even parents.
- **Reference:** Danchin, *Pediatrics* 2007.

SUBSTANCE ABUSE AND DEPENDENCE

Definition
- Caller has questions or concerns about substance abuse (drug abuse).
- Substance abuse is using (huffing, ingesting, injecting, smoking, snorting) any drug or alcohol with the intention of experiencing euphoria or other mind-altering sensations.

TRIAGE ASSESSMENT QUESTIONS

Call EMS 911 Now
- Coma (e.g., not moving, not talking, not responding to stimuli)
  R/O: overdose, occult head trauma
- Difficult to awaken or acting confused (e.g., disoriented, slurred speech)
  R/O: overdose, occult head trauma
- Seeing or hearing or feeling things that are not there (i.e., auditory, visual, or tactile hallucinations)
  R/O: hallucinations
- Slow, shallow, and weak breathing
  R/O: impending respiratory arrest
- Seizure
  R/O: overdose, hypoxia
- Violent behavior or threatening to kill someone
  R/O: homicidal ideation
- Sounds like a life-threatening emergency to the triager

See More Appropriate Protocol
- Suicide thoughts, threats, and attempts, questions or concerns about
  Go to Protocol: Suicide Concerns on page 387
- Other significant medical symptom is present, see that protocol (e.g., chest pain, headache, vomiting)
  Go to that specific symptom protocol (e.g., Chest Pain, Headache, Vomiting)
- Alcohol use, abuse, or dependence, question or problem related to
  Go to Protocol: Alcohol Abuse and Dependence on page 12
- Depression is main problem or symptom (e.g., feelings of sadness or hopelessness)
  Go to Protocol: Depression on page 103

Go to ED Now
- Very strange, paranoid, or confused behavior
  R/O: drug-induced psychosis, current drug intoxication
  Note: Factors that the nurse triager should consider in selecting the best disposition include risk of harm to self or others, how this compares to normal (baseline) behavior, and the patient's support systems (available family and friends).
- Feeling very shaky (i.e., visible tremors of hands)
  R/O: withdrawal
- Pregnant and symptoms of narcotic withdrawal (e.g., vomiting, severe muscle cramps)
  Reason: effect of withdrawal on fetus

Go to ED/UCC Now
(or to Office With PCP Approval)
- Fever > 100.0° F (37.8° C) and IV drug abuse
  R/O: bacterial endocarditis from IV drug abuse
- Patient sounds very anxious or agitated
  R/O: anxiety, drug intoxication, withdrawal symptoms
- Patient sounds very sick or weak to the triager
  Reason: severe acute illness or serious complication suspected

See Today in Office
- White of the eyes have turned yellow (i.e., jaundice)
  R/O: hepatitis, cirrhosis of the liver
- Fever > 101° F (38.3° C)
  R/O: bacterial illness

See Today or Tomorrow in Office
- Patient wants to be seen

Callback by PCP Today
- Pregnant and admits to substance abuse problem
  Reason: risk to fetus

Call Local Agency Today
- Alcohol or drug abuse, known or suspected
  Reason: needs evaluation and counseling
- Inhalant abuse (e.g., huffing), known or suspected
  Note: Examples include adhesives (glue, rubber cement), aerosols (spray paint, hair spray), solvents (nail polish remover) and cleaning agents (spot remover); see Background.
- Requesting admission for substance (drug) abuse
- Requesting to talk with a counselor (mental health worker, psychiatrist, etc.)
- Drug use interferes with work or school

Home Care

○ Substance abuse, questions about

○ Urine drug tests, questions about

○ Finding a substance abuse treatment center, questions about

HOME CARE ADVICE

General Information

❶ Local Substance Abuse Treatment Program:

- If available, local alcohol treatment program:

  __ __ __ - __ __ __ - __ __ __ __

- If available, local psychiatric crisis service at _____ hospital:

  __ __ __ - __ __ __ - __ __ __ __

❷ Urine Drug Testing:

- Urine drug tests may be helpful in 3 situations: (1) Where a drug's identity is needed to treat an acutely intoxicated adult (i.e., with symptoms); (2) as part of an ongoing drug rehabilitation program; (3) as a required drug screening evaluation for work.
- **Positive Tests:** False-positive tests are possible. A physician should be involved in the interpretation of positive drug screen results.
- **Negative Tests:** Negative tests do not mean there is not a drug problem; they simply mean that no drugs are detected at the time of the test, or that someone has tampered with the urine sample.

❸ Urine Drug Testing—Time Detectable:

- **Alcohol:** 1 day
- **Amphetamines:** 8-24 hours
- **Barbiturates:** 2-10 days
- **Benzodiazepines:** 2-7 days
- **Cocaine:** 1-4 days
- **Codeine:** 1-2 days
- **Gamma-hydroxybutyrate (GHB; Rohypnol):** 1-3 days; special test required
- **Heroin:** 1-4 days
- **Inhalants:** Not detected
- **LSD:** 8 hours
- **Marijuana:** Single use, 1-7 days; chronic use, 1-4 weeks
- **MDMA (ecstasy):** Not detected
- **Methamphetamines:** 1-2 days
- **Morphine:** 1-3 days
- **Phencyclidine (PCP):** 1-7 days

❹ Call Back If:

- You have more questions about substance abuse.
- You become worse.

Additional Resources

❶ Canada—Hotlines and Helplines:

- The Canadian Centre on Substance Use and Addiction provides a list of addiction treatment helplines at: www.ccsa.ca/Eng/Pages/Addictions-Treatment-Helplines-Canada.aspx.
- **Alberta:** Addiction Helpline—866/332-2322, 780/427-7164.
- **New Brunswick:** Department of Health and Wellness Addiction Services: www2.gnb.ca/content/gnb/en/departments/health/Addiction.html. Offered by region.
- **Newfoundland and Labrador:** Newfoundland and Labrador Addictions Services: www.health.gov.nl.ca/health/addictions/services.html. Services offered by region.
- **Northwest Territories:** Nats'ejée K'éh Treatment Centre crisis line—800/661-0846.
- **Ontario:** ConnexOntario: Provides access to addiction, mental health, and problem gambling services. Available at: www.connexontario.ca. The phone number for the helpline is 866/531-2600.
- **Ontario:** Centre for Addiction and Mental Health (CAMH)—800/463-6273.

❷ Narcotics Anonymous:

- Narcotics Anonymous is *"a nonprofit fellowship or society of men and women for whom drugs had become a major problem. We…meet regularly to help each other stay clean….We are not interested in what or how much you used…but only in what you want to do about your problem and how we can help."*
- Membership is open to any drug addict, regardless of the particular drug or combination of drugs used.
- Chapters of Narcotics Anonymous are present in every state in the United States and in many countries of the world. Each has a local contact phone number.
- More information is available at: www.na.org.

❸ United States—National Institute on Drug Abuse (NIDA):

- There is extensive information on drug abuse provided on the NIDA Web site: www.drugabuse.gov.
- There is a useful and well-organized chart of commonly abused drugs at: www.drugabuse.gov/drugs-abuse/commonly-abused-drugs/commonly-abused-drugs-chart.

❹ **United States—Substance Abuse and Mental Health Services Administration (SAMHSA):**
- This governmental agency works to improve the quality and availability of substance abuse prevention, alcohol and drug addiction treatment, and mental health services.
- More information is available at: www.samhsa.gov.

❺ **United States—SAMHSA National Helpline:**
- The SAMHSA National Helpline (http://samhsa.gov/treatment) is a *"confidential, free, 24-hour-a-day, 365-day-a-year, information service, in English and Spanish, for individuals and family members facing substance abuse and mental health issues. This service provides referrals to local treatment facilities, support groups, and community-based organizations. Callers can also order free publications and other information in print on substance abuse and mental health issues."*
- The phone number is 800/662-HELP (4357).

❻ **United States—SAMHSA Substance Abuse Treatment Facility Locator:**
- SAMHSA has an Internet tool for finding local drug abuse treatment programs.
- This locator is available at: http://findtreatment.samhsa.gov.

FIRST AID

First Aid Advice for Narcotic Overdose:

If narcotic overdose is known or suspected AND caller has Narcan nasal spray available, give Narcan nasal spray NOW:
- Peel back package and take out the nasal spray.
- Put the nozzle in one of the patient's nostrils.
- Press firmly down on the plunger to give the dose of Narcan.
- Turn patient on his or her side.
- Call 911. Emergency care is needed even if patient improves after Narcan is given.

Each package is a single dose of Narcan. If the patient does not respond by waking up or breathing normally, give another dose. If the patient gets worse after briefly getting better, give another dose.

BACKGROUND

Key Points
- Chemical dependency/addiction is a disease and can be treated. Medical detox followed by 12-step/educational services can be successful in helping a patient to recover.
- Addiction can occur to legal/prescription drugs.

Priorities in Substance Abuse Triage
- *The triager should first evaluate the drug abuse patient for medical life threats, suicidal ideation, physical injuries, and any active medical complaints. If this evaluation is negative, the triager should refer the patient for substance abuse counseling.*
- On average, addicts have been wanting to seek help for ≥ 7 years. It is important to acknowledge this and provide support while helping them with the next step. The next step is often referring the caller to a local substance abuse program, the SAMHSA Center for Substance Abuse Treatment hotline (240/276-1660), or a local chapter of Narcotics Anonymous.
- Families and friends often call with questions and concerns. Generally, treatment will not be effective unless the addict himself/herself wants help. Encourage the family to seek supportive services for themselves.
- Names and content of street drugs are ever-changing. Do not focus on the name of the drug. Instead, engage the caller to determine symptoms and the impact of the drug on day-to-day living.

Common Illegal Drugs of Abuse, Their Street Names, and Route of Use
- **Cocaine** (coke, crack, rock): Inject/smoke/snort
- **Heroin** (smack, horse, junk): Inject/smoke/snort
- **LSD** (acid, microdot, blotter): Ingest
- **Marijuana** (grass, pot, reefer, weed, blunts): Smoke/ingest
- **Methamphetamine** (crank, crystal, ice, glass, meth): Inject/smoke/ingest/snort
- **PCP** (phencyclidine) (angel dust, embalming fluid, rocket fuel): Inject/ingest/smoke

Types of Drugs

- **Anabolic Steroids:** Used to enhance athletic performance, strength, or physical appearance. May cause mania, delusions, hallucinations, or overaggressiveness ("roid rage").
- **Designer Drugs:** Designer drugs are synthetic chemical modifications of commonly abused drugs. The most well-known one is Ecstasy (MDMA), a designer amphetamine. It is a stimulant and a hallucinogen. Users describe initial anxiety and nausea, followed by relaxation, euphoria, and feelings of enhanced emotional insight. Very popular in the dance-club setting. Can lead to death associated with hyperthermia.
- **Dextromethorphan (DM):** Can cause a LSD-like picture (visual hallucinations, confusion, excitation). It can also cause coma and death. DM is present in OTC cough medicines.
- **Dissociative** (ketamine, phencyclidine/PCP): Causes perceptual alterations and hallucinations.
- **Hallucinogens/Psychedelics** (LSD, mescaline): Cause visual hallucinations, perceptual alterations, and a dreamlike state.
- **Inhalants** (toluene/glue, gasoline, butane, trichloroethane/typewriter correction fluid): Can cause giddiness or euphoria. Can also rarely cause sudden death from cardiac arrhythmias.
- **Marijuana (Cannabis):** Marijuana is the most commonly used illegal drug. > 40% of high school seniors have tried marijuana. It's the only illegal drug with virtually no lethal potential except from secondary accidents. Hence, patients with mild symptoms (mellow euphoria) don't need to be seen on an emergency basis. Marijuana sold on the streets today is much stronger than it was in the 1960s/1970s. Marijuana causes euphoria and in higher concentrations can be associated with paranoia, delusions, and hallucinations.
- **Narcotics/Opiates** (heroin, morphine, codeine, pentazocine, methadone): Cause sedation and euphoria. Overdose can cause profound respiratory depression, coma, and death. Withdrawal from opiates is not life-threatening. However, the withdrawal symptoms are extremely uncomfortable (i.e., yawning, nausea, vomiting, diarrhea, muscle cramps).
- **Sedative-Hypnotics/Depressants** (barbiturates, benzodiazepines, tranquilizers): Cause sedation, drowsiness, and euphoria. Can cause coma and death.
- **Stimulants** (cocaine, crack cocaine, amphetamine, methamphetamine): Causes hyperalertness, stimulation, restlessness, and euphoria. Can cause stroke, coma, arrhythmias, and death.

Marijuana (Cannabis)

- Marijuana is the most commonly used illegal drug in the world.
- Laws and policies are changing. As of early 2016, 4 states (Colorado, Washington, Oregon, and Alaska) and the District of Columbia in the United States have passed laws legalizing cannabis for recreational use by adults. Many US states now permit cannabis use for medical purposes.
- **Symptoms:** Marijuana can have positive and negative effects on a person's senses, mood, and thinking.
- **Altered Senses:** Colors may seem brighter; time passes differently.
- **Altered Mood:** Feel more relaxed or happy; feel sad or depressed.
- **Altered Thinking:** Impaired thought, problem-solving, and memory; decreased ability to focus.
- **Physical Symptoms:** Dry mouth, feeling hungry, increased breathing rate, increased heart rate ("heart racing"), increased blood pressure. Just like smoking cigarettes, smoking marijuana can also sometimes cause breathing problems and cough.
- **Cause:** Marijuana is the dried leaves, flowers, stems, and seeds from the plant *Cannabis sativa*. The plant contains the mind-altering chemical delta-9-tetrahydrocannabinol (THC) and other related compounds.
- **Testing:** The active chemical in marijuana, THC, can be found in a person's blood, hair, or urine. Urine testing is the least costly and easiest way to test for marijuana.

Inhalant Abuse

- Inhaling (huffing) chemical vapors is the most common form of substance abuse from age 12-15 years. The reason is that solvents are cheap and are readily available.
- **Types of Inhalants:** Toluene from glue, butane from lighters, gasoline, paints, paint thinners, hair spray, air fresheners, and hundreds more. The latest dangerous fad is "dusting": inhaling the Freon propellants in computer keyboard cleaners.
- **Symptoms:** Inhaling these substances from a rag soaked with them (often in a plastic bag) can give a 3-minute "high" (dizziness, giddiness, even euphoria). Acute neurologic symptoms are common: altered mental status, slurred speech, ataxia.
- **Complications:** Chronic inhalant use can permanently damage the white matter of the brain (memory, etc). On rare occasions, inhalants have caused sudden death from cardiac arrhythmias, sometimes even the first time they are used.
- **Clues That Should Alert Family, Friends, and Parents to Inhalant Abuse:** Breath or clothing that smells like chemicals; paint or glue on face, fingers, or clothing; rashes around the mouth.

Psychiatric Symptoms From Substance Abuse

- *Drug withdrawal and drug intoxication can mimic medical and psychiatric disorders.*
- **Anxiety:** Sometimes anxiety symptoms may represent withdrawal symptoms from depressant medications such as opiates (e.g., heroin) or sedative-hypnotics (e.g., alcohol, benzodiazepines). Anxiety attacks can occur during intoxication with stimulants (e.g., cocaine) and hallucinogens (e.g., LSD).
- **Depression:** Many individuals with drug abuse have symptoms of depression. Cocaine addicts experience a profound period of depression ("crash") after a cocaine binge.
- **Polydrug Abuse:** Many individuals abuse more than one drug at a time. For example, as many as 75% of individuals with cocaine abuse will also have alcohol dependence.
- **Suicidal Ideation:** It is appropriate to directly ask a patient about intent to harm himself/herself or end his/her own life. Such questions will not provoke a suicide attempt and may instead give the patient a chance to unburden himself/herself.

Narcan Nasal Spray: Emergency Treatment for Narcotic Overdose

Deaths from drug overdose have risen greatly in the United States since 2000. In 2014, about 2 out of every 3 overdose deaths involved an opioid such as heroin or narcotic prescription pain medicine (Rudd et al). Narcan (naloxone) nasal spray is an emergency treatment that can help prevent deaths from narcotic overdose.

- **How does it work?** The medicine counteracts the life-threatening effects of a narcotic overdose. It is absorbed quickly across the nasal membranes into the bloodstream.
- **Who can give it?** It can be given by family members and friends.
- **When should someone give it?** It should be given right away if a narcotic overdose is suspected and the person is hard to arouse or wake up or has slow or shallow breathing.
- **What are symptoms of a narcotic overdose?** The main symptoms are severe sleepiness (or even coma) and slow or shallow breathing. The pupils are small (constricted).
- **What are the side effects?** People who use narcotics for a long time will likely develop sudden narcotic withdrawal symptoms after receiving Narcan. The symptoms may include nausea, vomiting, feeling anxious, shakes, and chills. If the person is using a narcotic to treat pain, after Narcan the pain will return until the Narcan wears off.
- **Should the caller call 911?** Yes. Narcan nasal spray is not a replacement for emergency care. Instruct callers to call 911 even if the patient's symptoms improve after Narcan is given. The medicine may wear off quickly and life-threatening symptoms may return.

SUICIDE CONCERNS

Definition
- Patient or caller has questions or concerns about suicide thoughts, threats, or attempts.

TRIAGE ASSESSMENT QUESTIONS

Call EMS 911 Now
- Patient attempted suicide
  R/O: physical injury or overdosage
  Note: If patient is alone, another triage nurse should call emergency medical services (EMS) 911.
- Patient is threatening suicide now
  Reason: triager considers risk of harm to be moderate to severe; patient has suicidal ideation with intent
  Note: If patient is alone, another triage nurse should call EMS 911.
- Patient is threatening to kill a specific person
  Reason: triager considers risk of harm to be moderate to severe; patient has homicidal ideation
  Note: Triager should contact police.
- Patient is very confused (disoriented, slurred speech) and NO other adult (e.g., friend or family member) available
  Reason: dispatch EMS to assess caller
  Note: Under normal circumstances, most patients are oriented times 3 and can answer questions about person, place, and day or date. Triage nurse should contact EMS.
- Difficult to awaken or acting very confused (disoriented, slurred speech) and of new onset
  R/O: drug overdose, subarachnoid hemorrhage, encephalitis, stroke
- Sounds like a life-threatening emergency to the triager

See More Appropriate Protocol
- Depression is the main symptom and is not threatening suicide
  Go to Protocol: Depression on page 103

Go to ED/UCC Now
(or to Office With PCP Approval)
- Patient sounds very sick or weak to the triager

Go to Office Now
- Patient is not threatening suicide now BUT has shared a suicide plan (e.g., overdose, gunshot) and access (e.g., hoarding pills, firearm in house)

See Today in Office
- Sometimes has thoughts of suicide
  Reason: triager considers risk of harm to be low; no current intent or plan
- Patient wants to be seen

Call Local Agency Today
- Requesting to talk with a counselor (mental health worker, psychiatrist, etc.)
- Patient is evasive or refuses to answer questions regarding intent to harm himself/herself

See Within 3 Days in Office
- Depression symptoms (sadness, hopelessness, decreased energy) interfere with work or school
  Reason: triager considers functional impairment to be moderate
  Note: Symptoms of depression include: decreased energy; increased sleeping or difficulty sleeping; difficulty concentrating; feelings of sadness, guilt, hopelessness, or worthlessness.
- Known or suspected alcohol or drug abuse
  R/O: substance abuse as cause or contributing factor for depression

Home Care
- Recent death of a loved one
  Reason: triager considers risk of harm to be low; no current suicidal intent or plan; normal grief reaction
- Referral phone numbers for crisis intervention and depression, questions about

HOME CARE ADVICE

General Information

❶ Reassurance:
- It sounds like you are feeling sad and depressed. Maybe even helpless. I am glad you had the courage to call.
- Let me help you with the next step.
- Encourage the caller to talk about his/her problems and feelings. Offer hope.

❷ Note to Triager—Suicide Attempt: All patients with a suicide attempt should be seen immediately for an evaluation even if they have no medical symptoms. Obtain the following caller information: WHO (patient name), WHERE (patient address or location), and PHONE (phone number; capture it from caller ID if needed).
- **Patient Is Alone:** Triager should stay on the phone with the patient until EMS or the police arrive and take over. Have a coworker call EMS 911 NOW. Give the police the patient's name, location (address), and phone number. In some situations, police might be able to locate caller with phone number.
- **Patient Is With a Responsible Adult:** If patient is with a responsible adult friend or family member, ask this person to call EMS 911 NOW. Ask the responsible adult to make sure patient doesn't have access to medications or firearms. Ask the responsible adult to not leave the patient alone.

❸ Note to Triager—Suicidal Ideation: All patients who are threatening suicide now (intent) should be seen immediately for an evaluation. If the patient also has a credible and lethal plan, the risk of harm increases from moderate to severe. Obtain the following caller information: WHO (patient name), WHERE (patient address or location), and PHONE (phone number; capture it from caller ID if needed).
- **Patient Is Alone:** Triager should stay on the phone with the patient until EMS or the police arrive and take over. Have a coworker call EMS 911 NOW. Give the police the patient's name, location (address), and phone number. In some situations, police might be able to locate caller with phone number.

- **Patient Is With a Responsible Adult:** If patient is with a responsible adult friend or family member, ask this person to call EMS 911 NOW. Ask the responsible adult to make sure patient doesn't have access to poisons, medications, knives, or guns. Ask the responsible adult to not leave the patient alone.
- **Patient Is With a Responsible Adult and Patient Is Cooperative:** If the patient is cooperative and with a responsible adult, an alternative disposition is to have the responsible adult drive the patient to the nearest emergency department (**Go to ED NOW**).

❹ Note to Triager—Homicidal Ideation: All patients who are threatening to kill someone should be seen immediately for an evaluation. If the patient also has a credible and lethal plan, the risk of harm increases from moderate to severe. The police should be notified. Obtain the following caller information: WHO (patient name), WHERE (patient address or location), and PHONE (phone number; capture it from caller ID if needed).
- **Patient Is Alone:** Triager should stay on the phone with the patient until EMS or the police arrive and take over. Have a coworker call EMS 911 NOW. Give the police the patient's name, location (address), and phone number. In some situations, police might be able to locate caller with phone number.
- **Patient Is With a Responsible Adult:** If patient is with a responsible adult friend or family member, ask this person to call EMS 911 NOW. The triager should also call the police immediately.

❺ Local Agency or Suicide Hotline Phone Numbers:
- If available, local suicide hotline or crisis phone number:

  __ __ __ - __ __ __ - __ __ __ __

- If available, local psychiatric crisis service at _____ hospital:

  __ __ __ - __ __ __ - __ __ __ __

❻ Call Back If:
- You feel like harming yourself or feel more depressed.
- Situation becomes worse.

Recent Death of a Loved One

❶ Reassurance:
- Sadness and depression symptoms are common and normal after the death of a loved one.
- Encourage the caller to talk about his/her troubles.
- Let the caller know that taking time to grieve is important, and it is part of the healing process. Suggest reviewing a photo album or sharing your favorite memories with a friend or family member.
- Support of family and friends is important.

❷ Note to Triager—Phrases to Use or Avoid:
- **Use:** Tell me more about how you are doing; I'm sorry; what is the hardest part of your day?
- **Avoid:** I understand how you feel; he is in the Lord's hands; it is for the best.

❸ Suggestions for Healthy Living: Healthy living habits can improve one's sense of well-being.
- **Eat Healthy:** Eat a well-balanced diet.
- **Get More Sleep:** Most people need 7-8 hours of sleep each night. Being well rested improves your attitude and your sense of physical well-being.
- **Communicate:** Share how you are feeling with someone in your life who is a good listener. Make certain that your spouse, family, or friends know how you are feeling.
- **Exercise Regularly:** Take a daily walk or try swimming, biking, or yoga. Perhaps arrange to do this with a friend or family member.
- **Avoid Alcohol.**

❹ Call Back If:
- Sadness or depression symptoms last > 2 weeks.
- You want to talk with a counselor.
- You feel like harming yourself.
- You become worse.

Additional Resources

❶ United States—Crisis and Suicide Hotline:
- Kristin Brooks Hope Center IMALIVE: https://www.imalive.org
- National Suicide Prevention Lifeline in the United States: 800/273-8255

❷ United States—Veterans Crisis Line
- https://www.veteranscrisisline.net
- 800/273-8255
- *"…connects Veterans in crisis and their families and friends with qualified, caring VA responders through a confidential, toll-free hotline, online chat, and text-messaging service."*

❸ United States—Substance Abuse and Mental Health Services Administration (SAMHSA) National Helpline:
- The SAMHSA National Helpline (http://samhsa.gov/treatment) is a *"confidential, free, 24-hour-a-day, 365-day-a-year, information service, in English and Spanish, for individuals and family members facing substance abuse and mental health issues. This service provides referrals to local treatment facilities, support groups, and community-based organizations. Callers can also order free publications and other information in print on substance abuse and mental health issues."*
- The phone number is 800/662-HELP (4357).

❹ United States—NAMI HelpLine:
- National Alliance on Mental Illness.
- The NAMI HelpLine is an information and referral source for locating community mental health programs. *"Our toll-free NAMI HelpLine allows us to respond personally to hundreds of thousands of requests each year, providing free referral, information and support—a much-needed lifeline for many."*
- Toll-free phone number: 800/950-NAMI (6264), Monday through Friday, 10:00 am–6:00 pm, Eastern time.
- E-mail: info@nami.org.
- Web site: www.nami.org.

❺ United States—Mood Disorders Organizations:
- Anxiety and Depression Association of America (ADAA).
- There is a "Find a Therapist" link on the home page.
- Web site: www.adaa.org.
- Telephone: 240/485-1001.

❻ Canada—Hotlines and Helplines:
- **Alberta:** Quick links to addiction and substance abuse services are available at: www.albertahealthservices.ca/amh/Page3338.aspx.
- **Canadian Harm Reduction Network:** This Web site provides an extensive listing of Internet resources: www.canadianharmreduction.com.
- **New Brunswick:** Department of Health and Wellness Addiction Services: www2.gnb.ca/content/gnb/en/departments/health/Addiction.html. Services offered by region.
- **Newfoundland and Labrador:** Newfoundland and Labrador Addictions Services: www.health.gov.nl.ca/health/addictions/services.html. Services offered by region.
- **Northwest Territories:** Nats'ejée K'éh Treatment Centre crisis line—800/661-0846.
- **Ontario:** ConnexOntario: Provides access to addiction, mental health, and problem gambling services. Available at: www.connexontario.ca. The phone number for the helpline is 866/531-2600.

❼ Canada—Mood Disorder Organizations:
- **Ontario:** Mood Disorders Association of Ontario (MDAO)—866/363-MOOD (6663)
- Web site: www.mooddisorders.ca

❽ Call Back If:
- You have more questions.

FIRST AID

First Aid Advice for Breathing Stopped or Cardiac Arrest

Hands-Only CPR
- Call 911.
- Push hard and fast on the center of the chest.

Special Notes:
- **High-quality CPR:** Rescuers should push hard to a depth of at least 2" (5 cm), at a rate of at least 100 compressions per minute; allow full chest recoil; and minimize interruptions in chest compressions. The disco song "Stayin' Alive" has the right beat for CPR.
- The American Heart Association (AHA) provides a 1-minute instructional video on Hands-Only CPR at: http://handsonlycpr.org. Be prepared. Watch it now, before you need it!
- Answers to frequently asked questions about Hands-Only CPR are available at: http://cpr.heart.org/AHAECC/CPRAndECC/Programs/HandsOnlyCPR/UCM_475604_Learn-More-about-How-to-Save-a-Life-with-Hands-Only-CPR.jsp.
- You are strongly encouraged to get training in CPR from the American Red Cross or the AHA.
- Hands-Only CPR is a trademark of the AHA.

"All rescuers, regardless of training, should provide chest compressions to all cardiac arrest victims. Because of their importance, chest compressions should be the initial CPR action for all victims regardless of age. Rescuers who are able should add ventilations to chest compressions. Highly trained rescuers working together should coordinate their care and perform chest compressions as well as ventilations in a team-based approach." Source: 2010 AHA Guidelines for Cardiopulmonary Resuscitation and Emergency Cardiovascular Care

CPR by Trained Rescuers
Trained (confident) rescuers should add ventilations to chest compressions while waiting for paramedics to arrive:
- Call 911.
- Perform chest compressions and mouth-to-mouth breathing in cycles of 30 compressions and then 2 breaths.

Special Notes:
- Rescuers should push hard to a depth of at least 2" (5 cm), at a rate of at least 100 compressions per minute; allow full chest recoil; and minimize interruptions in chest compressions.

BACKGROUND

Key Points

- **Alternatives:** Suicidal patients often feel they have no alternatives. It is important for the triager to offer hope and to show such patients how they can get help.
- **Intent:** It is appropriate to directly ask patients about their intent to harm themselves or end their own life. Such questions will not provoke a suicide attempt and may instead give patients a chance to unburden themselves. *Any patient who is threatening self-harm NOW needs to be seen immediately for evaluation.*
- **Plan:** This refers to the extent to which the patient has prepared for a suicide attempt. Does the patient have a specific method in mind (e.g., gun, knife, overdose)? Does the patient have access to the verbalized method (e.g., hoarded pills, firearm in house)? Access to lethal methods increases the risk of suicide attempt and death. Generally, a patient with a specific plan is considered at higher suicide risk than a patient who is threatening suicide but has no plan.

Risks for Suicide Attempt

- Prior treatment for or diagnosis of mental health or chemical dependence problem
- **Addiction:** Alcohol, drug, gambling
- Serious or chronic medical illness
- **Lack of Social Support:** Living alone, divorced, widowed
- **Recent Losses:** Recent bereavement, separation, divorce, unemployment
- Prior suicide attempt
- Family history of completed suicide
- Age > 60 or < 25 years old

Risks for Suicide Completion (Death)

- Older
- Male
- Living alone
- Physical illness
- Access to lethal methods, such as a gun

Dos for the Triager

- Do ask about suicidal thoughts; be direct in questioning.
- Do assess for access to lethal methods (eg, pills, gun).
- Do listen and show interest.
- Do utilize friends and family.
- Do show support for courage to call.
- Do offer hope.
- Do show you care.

Don'ts for the Triager

- Don't try to cheer the patient up (e.g., jokes).
- Don't be judgmental.

SUNBURN

Definition
- Red, painful skin following sun exposure.
- The pain and swelling starts at 4 hours, peaks at 24 hours, and improves after 48 hours.
- Sunburn to the cornea (ultraviolet keratitis) is included in this protocol.

Sunburn Pain Severity Scale
- **Mild (1-3):** Doesn't interfere with normal activities.
- **Moderate (4-7):** Interferes with normal activities or awakens from sleep.
- **Severe (8-10):** Excruciating pain, unable to do any normal activities.

TRIAGE ASSESSMENT QUESTIONS

Call EMS 911 Now
- ● Difficult to awaken or acting confused (e.g., disoriented, slurred speech)
  R/O: heatstroke, shock
- ● Passed out (i.e., fainted, collapsed and was not responding)
  R/O: heat exhaustion or dehydration
- ● Sounds like a life-threatening emergency to the triager

See More Appropriate Protocol
- ● Sunburn-like rash BUT minimal or no sun exposure
  Go to Protocol: Rash or Redness, Widespread on page 330
- ● Heatstroke, sunstroke, or heat exhaustion suspected
  Go to Protocol: Heat Exposure (Heat Exhaustion and Heatstroke) on page 214

Go to ED/UCC Now
(or to Office With PCP Approval)
- ● Too weak to stand
  R/O: heat exhaustion
- ● Fever > 103° F (39.4° C)
  R/O: impending heatstroke
- ● Blisters (second-degree burn) covering > 10% BSA
- ● Patient sounds very sick or weak to the triager
  Reason: severe acute illness or serious complication suspected

See Today in Office
- ◐ SEVERE sunburn pain (e.g., excruciating)
  Reason: may need narcotic analgesic
- ◐ SEVERE eye pain or blurred vision that follows sun exposure (welding or other significant light exposure)
  R/O: ultraviolet photokeratitis needing patching
  Note: Photokeratitis can occur after exposure to the sun, tanning lamps, and broken mercury vapor lamps.
- ◐ Looks infected (e.g., spreading redness, pus, red streak)
  Reason: may need antibiotics

See Today or Tomorrow in Office
- ◐ Patient wants to be seen

Discuss With PCP and Callback by Nurse Today
- ◐ Sunburn following brief sun exposure and taking photosensitizing drug (e.g., tetracycline, doxycycline, Elidel, Protopic, griseofulvin, sulfa drugs)

See Within 3 Days in Office
- ◐ Blisters on the face
  Reason: cosmetic concerns
- ◐ Blisters (second-degree burn) covering > 2% BSA (i.e., > 2 palms)
- ◐ Blister > 1" (2.5 cm)

Home Care
- ○ Mild sunburn
- ○ Mild eye symptoms that follows sun exposure (or other significant light exposure)
  Reason: probably mild ultraviolet photokeratitis
  Note: Photokeratitis can occur after exposure to the sun, tanning lamps, and broken mercury vapor lamps.
- ○ Sunscreen and protection from the sun, questions about

HOME CARE ADVICE

Mild Sunburn

❶ **Ibuprofen for Pain:** For pain relief, begin taking ibuprofen (e.g., Advil, Motrin) as soon as possible. Adult dosage is 400 mg every 6 hours. If anti-inflammatory agents such as ibuprofen are begun within 6 hours of sun exposure and continued for 2 days, they can greatly reduce your discomfort.
  - Do not take ibuprofen if you have stomach problems, have kidney disease, are pregnant, or have been told by your doctor to avoid this type of anti-inflammatory drug. Do not take ibuprofen for > 7 days without consulting your doctor.
  - If you can't take ibuprofen, use acetaminophen (e.g., Tylenol) instead.
  - Do not take acetaminophen if you have liver disease.
  - *Before taking any medicine, read all the instructions on the package.*

❷ **Hydrocortisone Cream:**
  - Hydrocortisone may help reduce the redness and may be used for small areas of sunburn.
  - Put 1% hydrocortisone cream on the red area 3 times a day. Use it for 3 days.
  - This is an over-the-counter (OTC) drug. You can buy it at the drugstore.
  - Some people like to keep the cream in the refrigerator. It feels even better if the cream is used when it is cold.
  - CAUTION: Do not use hydrocortisone cream for > 1 week without talking to your doctor.
  - *Before taking any medicine, read all the instructions on the package.*

❸ **Cool Baths:** Apply cool compresses to the burned area several times a day to reduce pain and burning. For larger sunburns, give cool baths for 10 minutes. *(Caution: Avoid any chill.)* Add 2 oz (60 g) baking soda per tub. Avoid soap on the sunburn.

❹ **Extra Fluids:** Drink extra water on the first day to replace the fluids lost into the sunburn and to prevent dehydration and dizziness.

❺ **Broken Blisters:**
  - For broken blisters, trim off the dead skin with fine scissors.
    (Reason: These hidden pockets can become a breeding ground for infection.)
  - Apply antibiotic ointment (e.g., bacitracin) to the raw skin under broken blisters. Reapply twice daily for 3 days.
  - CAUTION: Leave intact blisters alone.
    (Reason: The intact blister protects the skin and allows it to heal.)

❻ **Expected Course:** Pain usually stops after 2 or 3 days. Skin flaking and peeling usually occur 5-7 days after the sunburn.

❼ **Call Back If:**
  - Pain becomes severe and not improved after taking pain medication.
  - Pain does not improve after 3 days.
  - Sunburn looks infected.
  - You become worse.

Mild Photokeratitis

❶ **Photokeratitis** (sunburn of cornea):
  - **Definition:** Photokeratitis can be thought of as a sunburn of the cornea. Exposure to intense light can cause corneal irritation (keratitis), especially if a person uses inadequate eye protection.
  - **Causes:** This is most commonly seen in individuals with inadequate eye protection while outside on a bright sunny day (e.g., water sports, snow skiing). It can also occur in individuals who do not use eye protection while using a tanning booth. This can occur in welders, as well.

❷ **Eye Treatment:**
  - Apply cool, wet compresses to the eyes.
  - Try to rest with your eyes closed.
  - Do not wear contacts until your eyes are completely better.
  - Avoid rubbing your eyes.

❸ **Expected Course:**
  - Symptoms should disappear completely over the next 24 hours. There should be no permanent damage to the cornea.
  - You can prevent future eye symptoms from sun exposure by wearing sunglasses.

❹ **Call Back If:**
  - Severe pain occurs.
  - Pain lasts > 24 hours.
  - Pus or yellow/green discharge occurs.
  - Blurred vision occurs.
  - You become worse.

How to Prevent Sunburn

❶ Prevention—Reduce Sun Exposure:

- Try to avoid all sun exposure between 10:00 am and 3:00 pm.
- You can get a sunburn while swimming. Water only blocks the ultraviolet radiation a little.

❷ Prevention—Clothing:

- Wear a wide-brimmed hat; it protects your face and neck from the sun.
- Wear shirts with long sleeves when outdoors and pants that go down to at least your knees.

❸ Prevention—Use Sunscreen:

- Apply sunscreen to areas that can't be protected by clothing. Generally, an adult needs about 1 oz (30 g) of sunscreen to cover the entire body.
- You should reapply the sunscreen every 2-4 hours. You should also reapply after swimming, exercising, or sweating.
- A sunscreen with a rating of sun protection factor (SPF) 15-30 should be used. Sunscreens with ratings > 30 provide minimal additional protection.
- Sunscreens help prevent sunburn but do not completely prevent skin damage. Thus, sun exposure can still increase your risk of skin aging and skin cancer.

❹ Vitamins C and E: Vitamins C and E have antioxidant properties, which means they help prevent sun damage to cells in your skin. Taking vitamins C and E by mouth may partially reduce the sunburn reaction.

- **Adult Dosage of Vitamin C** (ascorbic acid): 2 g by mouth once a day.
- **Adult Dosage of Vitamin E** (d-alpha-tocopherol): 1,000 IU by mouth once a day.
- CAUTION: Prevention is the key. Remember to reduce sun exposure and use sunscreens.
- *Before taking any medicine, read all the instructions on the package.*

Questions About Sunglasses

❶ The Sun and Your Eyes:

- The cornea can also get sunburned. This can cause eye pain, watery eyes, difficulty looking at lights, and blurred vision.
- Long-term sun exposure can also cause eye cataracts.

❷ Sunglasses:

- You can protect your eyes from the sun by wearing sunglasses.
- When you buy sunglasses, look for glasses that block 99%-100% of the full ultraviolet (UV) spectrum.

FIRST AID

First Aid Advice for Heatstroke or Sunstroke:

- Call EMS 911 immediately
- Move to a cool shady area. If possible, move into an air-conditioned place.
- Remove excess clothing or equipment (e.g., sports gear, protective work uniforms).
- Sponge the entire body surface with cool water (as cool as tolerated without shivering). If available, place ice packs on the neck, armpits, and groin. Fan the patient to increase evaporation.
- Keep the feet elevated to counteract shock.
- If the patient is awake, give as much cold water or sports drink (e.g., Gatorade, Powerade) as he or she can tolerate.
- Fever medicines are of no value for heatstroke.

First Aid Advice for Heat Exhaustion:

- Put the patient in a cool place. Lie down with the feet elevated.
- Undress patient (except for underwear) so the body surface can give off heat.
- Sponge the entire body surface continuously with cool water (as cool as tolerated without shivering). Fan the patient to increase evaporation.
- After 2 or 3 glasses of water, drive the patient in to be seen. During the drive, provide unlimited amounts of water.

BACKGROUND

Key Points

- Sunburn may cause a first-degree (redness and pain) or a second-degree (blistering) burn to the sun-exposed areas of the body.
- The triager should document the percentage of body surface area (BSA) involvement of blistering.
- Long-term sun exposure increases the risk for skin cancer and causes aging of the skin. Long-term sun exposure can also cause eye cataracts.
- Vitamins C and E are antioxidants. Taking vitamins C and E by mouth may partially reduce the sunburn reaction (Eberlein-Konig). More research is needed to prove whether there is any true benefit.

Degrees of Sunburn

- **First Degree:** Most sunburn is a first-degree burn which turns the skin pink or red. The pain and swelling starts at 4 hours, peaks at 24 hours, and improves after 48 hours.
- **Second Degree:** Prolonged sun exposure can cause blistering and a second-degree burn.
- **Third Degree:** Sunburn never causes a third-degree burn or scarring.

Causes of Sunburn

- **Broken Mercury-vapor Lamps** (overhead lighting): Damaged mercury-vapor (metal halide) lamps are known to cause outbreaks of UV-radiation "sunburns" and photokeratitis (corneal irritation).
- **Tanning lamps.**
- **The Sun.**

Photokeratitis (sunburn of cornea)

- **Definition:** Photokeratitis can be thought of as a sunburn of the cornea. Exposure to intense light can cause corneal irritation (keratitis), especially if a person uses inadequate eye protection.
- **Pain:** Usually bilateral eye pain; tearing; light bothers eyes.

- **Vision Loss:** Usually minimal vision change (haziness) to none. More severe photokeratitis can cause blurred vision; all patients with blurred vision require medical evaluation; in skiers this is referred to as snow blindness.
- **Causes:** This is most commonly seen in individuals with inadequate eye protection while outside on a bright sunny day (e.g., water sports, snow skiing). It can also occur in individuals who do not use eye protection while using a tanning booth. This can occur in welders, as well.

Polymorphous Light Eruption ("sun poisoning")

- **Definition:** Polymorphous light eruption (PMLE) is a type of itchy skin rash that appears on sun-exposed areas of the skin hours to sometimes days after prolonged sun exposure. PMLE is also sometimes called "sun poisoning."
- **Epidemiology:** More common during the first 3 decades of life. Perhaps 10% of the white population are susceptible to getting this; most are female and typically with a fair complexion.
- **Cause:** Unknown. It is probably some type of hypersensitivity (allergic) reaction; there is a genetic component, as family members commonly share this susceptibility.
- **Symptoms:** Itchy rash that can be skin-colored or erythematous (red), appearing as papules (small spots) or plaques (broader areas). Occasionally there may be vesicles (small blisters).
- **Expected Course:** The rash resolves over 7-10 days, if further sun exposure is avoided.
- **Treatment:** The main treatment is to avoid sun exposure by wearing a hat and a long-sleeved shirt and by using sunscreen. More serious cases may benefit from prescription topic corticosteroid creams.

Rule of 9s for Estimating Burn Size: Each part of the body contributes a predictable portion of the total body surface area (BSA):

- **Head and Neck:** 9%
- **Each Arm:** 9%
- **Anterior Chest and Abdomen:** 18%
- **Entire Back:** 18%
- **Each Leg:** 18%
- **Genital Region:** 1%

Rule of Palms for Estimating Burn Size

- A person's palm (not including the fingers) represents 1% of the total BSA.
- For example, if a person had blistering of the left shoulder the size of 2 palms, the total area of blistering would be 2% of the BSA.

Caution: Toxic Shock Syndrome

- The rash is a widespread erythroderma (painless "sunburn") that usually fades in 72 hours. It is followed by skin desquamation (peeling), especially of the palms and soles.
- Other signs and symptoms of the syndrome include fever, muscle aches, vomiting or diarrhea, multi-organ dysfunction (liver, kidney), confusion, shock, and death.
- Those at risk include menstruating women using tampons, postsurgical patients, and patients with nasal packings.
- Patients suspected of having this condition should be seen immediately.

SUTURE OR STAPLE QUESTIONS

Definition
- Questions about sutured or stapled wounds

TRIAGE ASSESSMENT QUESTIONS

Call EMS 911 Now
- ● Major abdominal surgical wound and visible internal organs
- ● Sounds like a life-threatening emergency to the triager

See More Appropriate Protocol
- ● Wound looks infected
  Go to Protocol: Wound Infection on page 443
- ● New cut and caller wonders if it needs stitches
  Go to Protocol: Skin Injury on page 361

Go to ED/UCC Now
(or to Office With PCP Approval)
- ● Bleeding won't stop after 10 minutes of direct pressure (using correct technique)
- ● Wound gaping open and < 48 hours since sutures placed
  R/O: dehiscence
  Reason: evaluate for infection; may re-suture, glue, or Steri-Strip
- ● Patient sounds very sick or weak to the triager
  Reason: severe acute illness or serious complication suspected

Go to Office Now
- ● Major surgical wound that is starting to open up
  R/O: dehiscence (site: if possible, refer to surgeon who performed surgery)

See Today in Office
- ◐ Wound gaping open and length of opening > ½" (6 mm)
- ◐ Wound gaping open and on face
  R/O: cosmetic concerns
- ◐ Suture or staple removal is overdue
- ◐ Suture (or staple) came out early and > 48 hours since sutures placed, and caller wants wound checked

See Today or Tomorrow in Office
- ◐ Patient wants to be seen

See Within 3 Days in Office
- ◐ Numbness extends beyond the wound edges and lasts > 8 hours

Home Care
- ○ Suture (or staple) came out early and > 48 hours since sutures placed
- ○ Care of sutured (or stapled) wound, questions about
- ○ Suture (or staple) removal date, questions about

HOME CARE ADVICE

General Care Advice for the Sutured or Stapled Wound

❶ **Suture Care for a Normal Sutured Wound:**
- Can get wound wet (e.g., bathing or swimming) after 24 hours.
- Apply antibiotic ointment 3 times a day.
  (Reason: to prevent infection and a thick scab)
- Cleanse with warm water once daily or if it becomes soiled.
- Change wound dressing when wet or soiled.
- Dressing no longer needed when edge of wound closed (usually 48 hours).
  (Exception: Dressing needed to prevent sutures from catching on clothing.)

❷ **Removal Date:** Guidelines for when particular sutures (stitches) or staples should be removed:
- **Face:** 4-5 days
- **Neck:** 7 days
- **Scalp:** 7-10 days
- **Chest or Abdomen:** 7-10 days
- **Arms and Back of Hands:** 7-10 days
- **Legs and Top of Feet:** 10 days
- **Back:** 10 days
- **Palms and Soles:** 12-14 days
- **Overlying a Joint:** 12-14 days

❸ **Removal Delays:** Don't miss your appointment for removing stitches. Stitches removed late can leave unnecessary skin marks and occasionally cause scarring. Delays also make suture removal more difficult.

❹ **Suture Out Early:** If the sutures come out early, reinforce the wound with tape or butterfly Band-Aids until the office visit.

❺ **Wound Protection:** After removal of sutures:
- Protect the wound from injury during the following month.
- Avoid sports that could reinjure the wound. If a sport is essential, apply tape before playing.
- Allow the scab to fall off on its own. Do not try to remove it.

❻ **Pain Medicines:**
- For pain relief, you can take either acetaminophen, ibuprofen, or naproxen.
- They are over-the-counter (OTC) pain drugs. You can buy them at the drugstore.

Acetaminophen (e.g., Tylenol):
- **Regular Strength Tylenol:** Take 650 mg (two 325 mg pills) by mouth every 4-6 hours as needed. Each Regular Strength Tylenol pill has 325 mg of acetaminophen.
- **Extra Strength Tylenol:** Take 1,000 mg (two 500 mg pills) every 8 hours as needed. Each Extra Strength Tylenol pill has 500 mg of acetaminophen.
- The most you should take each day is 3,000 mg (10 Regular Strength or 6 Extra Strength pills a day).

Ibuprofen (e.g., Motrin, Advil):
- Take 400 mg (two 200 mg pills) by mouth every 6 hours.
- Another choice is to take 600 mg (three 200 mg pills) by mouth every 8 hours.
- The most you should take each day is 1,200 mg (six 200 mg pills), unless your doctor has told you to take more.

Naproxen (e.g., Aleve):
- Take 220 mg (one 220 mg pill) by mouth every 8 hours as needed. You may take 440 mg (two 220 mg pills) for your first dose.
- The most you should take each day is 660 mg (three 220 mg pills a day), unless your doctor has told you to take more.

❼ **Pain Medicines—Extra Notes:**
- Use the lowest amount of medicine that makes your pain better.
- Acetaminophen is thought to be safer than ibuprofen or naproxen in people > 65 years old. Acetaminophen is in many OTC and prescription medicines. It might be in more than one medicine that you are taking. You need to be careful and not take an overdose. An acetaminophen overdose can hurt the liver.
- McNeil, the company that makes Tylenol, has different dosage instructions for Tylenol in Canada and the United States. In Canada, the maximum recommended dose per day is 4,000 mg or 12 Regular Strength (325 mg) pills. In the United States, McNeil recommends a maximum dose of 10 Regular Strength (325 mg) pills.
- CAUTION: Do not take acetaminophen if you have liver disease.
- CAUTION: Do not take ibuprofen or naproxen if you have stomach problems, have kidney disease, are pregnant, or have been told by your doctor to avoid this type of anti-inflammatory drug. Do not take ibuprofen or naproxen for > 7 days without consulting your doctor.
- *Before taking any medicine, read all the instructions on the package.*

❽ **Call Back If:**
- Looks infected.
- Fever.
- Sutures come out early.
- You become worse.

Preventing Scars—Questions About

❶ **Scarring:**
- Scarring is unfortunately a natural part of the healing process after a cut or wound from surgery or trauma.
- The more serious the injury and the larger the wound/cut, the greater the likelihood of scarring.
- Almost all cuts that require closure with sutures, staples, or skin glue will heal with some scarring.
- Some people are more prone to scarring than others.

❷ **Preventing Scarring:**
- Be certain to get the sutures removed during the time frame that your doctor recommended. *(Reason: If you leave them in too long they can leave "railroad tracks.")*
- Avoid getting a sunburn in this area for 2 months.
- Avoid reinjuring this area.
- Some people apply vitamin E lotion (or cream) to a healing wound to prevent scarring. Research has not shown that this helps.

FIRST AID

First Aid Advice for Bleeding:

Apply direct pressure to the entire wound with a clean cloth.

First Aid Advice for Surgical Wound That Is Opening:

Cover wound with a clean gauze or dressing.

BACKGROUND

Sutures or Staples That Fall Out

Sutures that pull out early are one of patients' main reasons for calling. The following rules generally apply:
- **Face:** If the wound is on the face and it has reopened, the patient should be seen regardless of how long it's been since the sutures were placed.
- **Body:** If the wound is elsewhere on the body, the patient should be seen if the wound is gaping and the sutures were placed < 48 hours ago. After 48 hours, re-suturing is rarely done (except on the face). After 48 hours, have the caller reinforce the wound with tape.

Suture and Staple Removal Dates

Here are some guidelines for when sutures (or staples) should be removed:
- **Face:** 4-5 days.
- **Neck:** 7 days.
- **Scalp:** 7-10 days.
- **Chest, Abdomen, and Back:** 7-10 days.
- **Arms and Back of Hands:** 7 days.
- **Legs and Top of Feet:** 10 days.
- **Fingers and Toes:** 10-14 days.
- **Palms and Soles:** 12-14 days.
- **Overlying a Joint:** 12-14 days.
- **Note:** If patient recalls that the doctor told him/her a different time frame, have patient call PCP or surgeon during normal office hours to confirm.

Numbness of Skin Near a Laceration

- **Local Anesthesia—Duration of Action:** Duration of numbness from local anesthesia depends on what type of local anesthesia was used. Numbness can last from 1-8 hours.
- **Numbness From the Laceration Itself:** Some people report a small area of numbness right along the edges of the sutured wound. This can last 1-3 weeks.
- **Nerve Injury:** Sometimes a cut can be deep enough that it cuts an important nerve. This should be suspected if the area of numbness extends beyond just the edges of the wound and lasts > 8 hours. An example of this would be a digital nerve injury of the finger; the patient might report persisting numbness of one side of the finger. A patient with a suspected nerve injury should be referred to the doctor within 3 days.

TICK BITE

Definition
- A tick (small brown bug) is attached to the skin.
- A tick recently was removed from the skin.

TRIAGE ASSESSMENT QUESTIONS

See More Appropriate Protocol
- Not a tick bite
  Go to Protocol: Insect Bite on page 257

Go to ED/UCC Now
(or to Office With PCP Approval)
- Patient sounds very sick or weak to the triager
  Reason: severe acute illness or serious complication suspected

Go to Office Now
- Fever or severe headache occurs, 2-14 days following the bite
  R/O: Rocky Mountain spotted fever
- Widespread rash occurs, 2-14 days following the bite
- Can't remove live tick (after using Home Care Advice)
  Reason: needs removal to prevent disease
- Can't remove tick's head that was broken off in the skin (after using Home Care Advice)
  Reason: tick's mouthparts need removal to prevent localized infection or granuloma
  Note: If the removed tick is moving, it was completely removed.
- Fever and area is red
  R/O: cellulitis, lymphangitis
  Reason: fever and looks infected
- Fever and area is very tender to touch
  R/O: cellulitis, lymphangitis
  Note: Skin infection is rare after a tick bite.
- Red streak or red line and length > 2" (5 cm)
  R/O: lymphangitis
  Note: Lymphangitis looks like a red streak or line originating at the wound and ascending the arm or leg toward the heart. Rare after a tick bite.

See Today in Office
- Red ring or bull's-eye rash occurs around a deer tick bite
  R/O: Lyme disease
- Probable deer tick that was attached > 36 hours (or tick appears swollen, not flat)
  Reason: consider antibiotic prophylaxis, especially if Lyme disease prevalent in the area
- Patient wants to be seen

Home Care
- Tick bite with no complications
- Prevention of tick bites and insect repellents (e.g., DEET), questions about
  R/O: cellulitis, lymphangitis
  Reason: fever and looks infected
  Note: Skin infection is rare after a tick bite.

HOME CARE ADVICE

Home Care Advice for Tick Bite
❶ Wood Tick Removal:
- Use a pair of tweezers and grasp the wood tick close to the skin (on its head). Pull the wood tick straight upward without twisting or crushing it. Maintain a steady pressure until it releases its grip.
- If tweezers aren't available, use fingers, a loop of thread around the jaws, or a needle between the jaws for traction.
- **Note:** Covering the tick with petroleum jelly, nail polish, or rubbing alcohol doesn't work. Neither does touching the tick with a hot or cold object.

❷ Tiny Deer Tick Removal:
- Deer ticks are very small and need to be scraped off with a credit card edge or the edge of a knife blade.
- Place tick in a sealed container (e.g., glass jar, resealable plastic bag), in case your doctor wants to see it.

❸ **Tick's Head Removal:**
- If the wood tick's head breaks off in the skin, it must be removed. Clean the skin. Then use a sterile needle to uncover the head and lift it out or scrape it off.
- If a very small piece of the head remains, the skin will eventually slough it off.

❹ **Antibiotic Ointment:** Wash the wound and your hands with soap and water after removal to prevent catching any tick disease. Apply an over-the-counter antibiotic ointment (e.g., bacitracin) to the bite once.

❺ **Expected Course:** Tick bites normally do not itch or hurt. That is why they often go unnoticed.

❻ **Call Back If:**
- You can't remove the tick or the tick's head.
- Fever or rash occur in the next 2 weeks.
- Bite begins to look infected.
- You become worse.

How to Prevent a Tick Bite

❶ **Prevention—General:**
- Prevention is important if you are hiking in tick-infested areas.
- Wear long pants and a long-sleeved shirt. Tuck your shirt into your pants. Tuck the cuffs of your pants into your socks or boots. Light-colored clothing is better because the ticks can be seen more easily.
- Inspect your entire body and your clothing every couple hours. Favorite places are in the hair, so be certain to check your scalp, neck, armpits, and groin.
- A shower at the end of a hike will help rinse off any tick that is not firmly attached.

❷ **Prevention With Insect Repellent—DEET:**
- DEET is a very effective tick repellent. It also repels mosquitoes and other bugs.
- Apply to exposed areas of skin. Do not apply to eyes, mouth, or irritated areas of skin. Remember to wash it off with soap and water when you return indoors.
- Pregnant and breastfeeding women may use DEET. No problems have been reported (Source: Insect Repellent Use and Safety, Centers for Disease Control and Prevention).
- *Be certain to read the package instructions on any product that you use.*

❸ **Permethrin—an Insect Repellent for Your Clothing and Gear:**
- Products that have permethrin (e.g., Duranon, Permanone, Congo Creek Tick Spray) are very effective mosquito repellents. Permethrin also repels ticks. You put permethrin on your clothing instead of your skin.
- Spray it on your clothes before you put them on. You can also put it on other outdoor items (shoes, mosquito screen, sleeping bags).
- It continues to work even after your clothes are washed several times.
- Do not put this type of repellent on your skin.
- *Read and follow the package directions carefully.*

BACKGROUND

Key Points
- The bite is painless and doesn't itch, so ticks may go unnoticed for a few days. Ticks eventually fall off on their own after sucking blood for 3-6 days.
- Ticks can transmit many diseases, including Lyme disease, Rocky Mountain spotted fever, Colorado tick fever, and relapsing fever.
- After feeding on blood, ticks become quite swollen and easier to see.

Types of Ticks
- The **deer tick** (black-legged tick) is between the size of a poppy seed (pinhead) and an apple seed and is the tick that usually transmits Lyme disease. A southern form of Lyme disease can be caused by contact with the lone star tick (this is a large tick).
- The **lone star tick** is the size of a watermelon seed. The lone star tick is the same size and the most common vector for ehrlichiosis (human monocytic ehrlichiosis [HME]). It also occasionally transmits Lyme disease.
- The **wood tick** (dog tick) is the size of a watermelon seed and can sometimes transmit Rocky Mountain spotted fever and Colorado tick fever.

Lyme Disease

- Lyme disease has become the most common tick-borne illness in the United States. The risk of Lyme disease following a recognized deer tick bite is approximately 1%.
- **Endemic Areas:** Lyme disease is common (i.e., endemic) in only certain areas of the United States. > 90% of Lyme disease occurs in the following 11 states: Connecticut, Rhode Island, New York, Pennsylvania, Delaware, New Jersey, Maryland, Massachusetts, Maine, Wisconsin, and Minnesota.
- **Erythema Migrans Rash:** The majority of cases of Lyme disease start with erythema migrans (bull's-eye rash) at the site of the tick bite. The rash can occur days to weeks (typically 7-10 days) after a tick bite. Treatment with antibiotics is indicated if this rash appears. Mild flu-like symptoms may accompany the erythema migrans rash, including: fever, chills, headaches, muscle aches, and fatigue.
- **Vaccine:** There is no Lyme disease vaccine currently available. The vaccine manufacturer discontinued production in 2002 because of insufficient consumer demand.

Antibiotic Prophylaxis After Deer Tick Bite

- Research has demonstrated that the risk of Lyme disease is zero for attachments of < 24-48 hours or if the tick appears flat (not swollen or engorged from feeding).
- Deer ticks go through 3 states in their life cycle: larval, nymphal, and adult. During the nymphal and adult states they may attach to humans, feed, and potentially transmit Lyme disease. Transmission occurs more often in the nymphal stage, presumably because the nymphal tick is smaller, more easily missed, and, thus, remains attached for a longer period.
- A recent article showed that a single 200 mg dose of doxycycline was effective at preventing Lyme disease if given within 72 hours of a deer tick bite (Nadelman et al).
- Thus, prophylactic antibiotic may sometimes be indicated in the following circumstances: (1) deer tick AND (2) has been attached for > 24 hours or appears swollen (engorged from feeding) AND (3) Lyme disease is relatively common in the region.

How to Remove a Wood Tick

- **Best Method—Tweezers:** Use a tweezers and grasp the wood tick close to the skin (on its head). Pull the wood tick straight upward without twisting or crushing it. Maintain a steady pressure until it releases its grip. If tweezers aren't available, use fingers, a loop of thread around the jaws, or a needle between the jaws for traction. Research (Needham) has demonstrated that this is the best method for tick removal.
- **Methods That Do Not Work:** Covering a tick with petroleum jelly, 70% rubbing alcohol, or fingernail polish does not work. Touching a tick with a red-hot match does not work (Source: Needham).

How to Remove a Tiny Deer Tick

Deer ticks are very small and need to be scraped off with a credit card edge or the edge of a knife blade.

How to Remove Lone Star Ticks (seed ticks, turkey ticks, turkey mites)

- "Seed ticks," "turkey ticks," and "turkey mites" are all layperson terms for the larval stage of the lone star tick. A female tick can lay several thousand eggs at a time. These eggs hatch at about the same time. If a potential host (animal, human) brushes past, hundreds of these tiny larvae can attach nearly simultaneously.
- **It is believed that lone star ticks do not spread any disease.** This makes sense because they are at the larval stage and have not yet eaten a blood meal from an animal.
- **Symptoms:** A person will note tens or hundreds of tiny poppy seed–sized moving black dots on his or her skin.
- **How to Remove Lone Star Ticks:** Various removal strategies have been described. Probably the best way to remove lone star ticks that are newly attached is to take a shower and use soap and a washcloth. Packaging tape or any adhesive tape will also work. You should be able to see the lone star ticks on the tape after you pull the tape off the skin. Using tweezers is unnecessary and tedious.

TOE INJURY

Definition
- Injuries to toe(s).
- Toe injuries include cuts, abrasions, stubbed toe, smashed toe, toenail injuries, subungual hematoma, dislocations, and fractures.

TRIAGE ASSESSMENT QUESTIONS

Call EMS 911 Now
- Major bleeding (actively dripping or spurting) that can't be stopped
  First Aid: Apply direct pressure to the entire wound with a clean cloth.
- Amputation of toe
  First Aid: Apply direct pressure to the entire wound with a clean cloth.
- Sounds like a life-threatening emergency to the triager

See More Appropriate Protocol
- Looks infected (e.g., spreading redness, pus, red streak)
  Go to Protocol: Wound Infection on page 443

Go to ED Now
- High-pressure injection injury (e.g., from paint gun, usually work related)
  Reason: deep tissue damage may exceed superficial injury

Go to ED/UCC Now (or to Office With PCP Approval)
- Looks like a broken bone or dislocated joint (e.g., crooked or deformed)
  R/O: dislocation or angulated fracture
- Skin is split open or gaping (length > ½" or 12 mm)
  Reason: may need laceration repair (e.g., sutures)
- Bleeding won't stop after 10 minutes of direct pressure (using correct technique)
- Dirt in the wound and not removed after 15 minutes of scrubbing
  Reason: needs irrigation or debridement
- Sounds like a serious injury to the triager

Go to Office Now
- Looks infected (e.g., spreading redness, pus, red streak)
  R/O: cellulitis, lymphangitis
- Toenail is completely torn off
- Base of toenail has popped out from under skinfold
  Reason: needs to be reinserted

See Today in Office
- SEVERE pain (e.g., excruciating)
  R/O: dislocation or displaced fracture
- MODERATE-SEVERE pain and blood present under the nail (usually > 50% of nail bed)
  R/O: severe subungual hematoma needing drainage

See Today or Tomorrow in Office
- Wound and no tetanus booster in > 5 years (or > 10 years for clean cuts)
  Reason: may need a tetanus booster shot (vaccine)
- Bad limp or can't wear shoes/sandals
  R/O: toe fracture
- Patient wants to be seen

See Within 3 Days in Office
- Injury interferes with work or school
- Injury and pain has not improved after 3 days
- Injury is still painful or swollen after 2 weeks
- Small cut or scrape and has diabetes mellitus
  Reason: wounds heal slower in diabetics

Home Care
- Minor toe injury
  R/O: minor bruise or sprain, scrapes, small subungual hematoma

HOME CARE ADVICE

Treatment of a Minor Bruise of the Toenail or Toe

❶ Reassurance—Bruised Toenail (Subungual Hematoma):
- A direct blow to the end of your toe can cause bruising under the toenail. There is bleeding underneath the nail. The medical term for this is subungual hematoma.
- Symptoms are bruising under the toenail and mild-moderate pain. Usually, the larger the bruise under the nail, the greater the pain.
- *Here is some care advice that should help.*

❷ Reassurance—Bruised Toe (Contusion, Bruise):
- A direct blow to your toe can cause a contusion. Contusion is the medical term for bruise.
- Symptoms are mild pain, swelling, and/or bruising.
- *Here is some care advice that should help.*

❸ Apply a Cold Pack:
- Apply a cold pack or an ice bag (wrapped in a moist towel) to the area for 20 minutes. Repeat in 1 hour, then every 4 hours while awake.
- Continue this for the first 48 hours after an injury.
- This will help decrease pain and swelling.

❹ Elevate the Foot:
- When you are sitting down reading or watching TV, place your foot up on a pillow.
- This can also help decrease swelling and pain.

❺ Protect the Toe: Wear a comfortable pair of shoes that do not rub on the injured toe.

❻ Expected Course:
- Pain, swelling, and bruising usually start to get better 2-3 days after an injury.
- It may take 2 weeks for the pain and tenderness to go away.
- A toenail bruise can take 6-12 weeks to go away. That is the amount of time needed for a nail to grow back completely. Sometimes the toenail falls off.

❼ Call Back If:
- Pain becomes severe.
- Pain does not improve after 3 days.
- Pain or swelling lasts > 2 weeks.
- You become worse.

Treatment of a Minor Sprain (Stubbed or Jammed Toe)

❶ Reassurance—Sprained Toe (Stubbed or Jammed Toe):
- Sprain is the medical terms used to describe over-stretching of the ligaments of the toe. This can happen when the toe is twisted or bent in the wrong way. It can happen when the toe is "stubbed" while walking.
- The main symptom is pain that is worse with movement. Swelling can occur. There is usually no bruising; if bruising is present it can be a sign that there is a small fracture.
- *Here is some care advice that should help.*

❷ Apply a Cold Pack:
- Apply a cold pack or an ice bag (wrapped in a moist towel) to the area for 20 minutes. Repeat in 1 hour, then every 4 hours while awake.
- Continue this for the first 48 hours after an injury.
- This will help decrease pain and swelling.

❸ Apply Heat to the Area:
- Beginning 48 hours after an injury, apply a warm washcloth or heating pad for 10 minutes 3 times a day.
- This will help increase blood flow and improve healing.

❹ Buddy-Tape Splinting:
- Protect your injured toe by "buddy-taping" it to the next toe.
- Use 2 pieces of tape. Place one around the base of both toes. Place the other around the ends of both toes.
- Wear a comfortable pair of shoes that do not rub on the injured toe.

❺ Rest Versus Movement:
- Movement is generally more healing in the long term than rest.
- Continue normal activities as much as your pain permits.
- If it really hurts to use the toe at all, you will need to see the doctor.

❻ Expected Course:
- Pain and swelling usually start to get better 2-3 days after an injury.
- Swelling most often is gone after 1 week.
- It may take 2 weeks for the pain to go away.

❼ Call Back If:
- Pain becomes severe.
- Pain does not improve after 3 days.
- Pain or swelling lasts > 2 weeks.
- You become worse.

Treatment of a Small Cut or Scrape

❶ **Reassurance—Superficial Laceration (Cut or Scratch) or Abrasion (Scrape):**
  • This sounds like a small cut or scrape that we can treat at home.
  • *Here is some care advice that should help.*

❷ **Bleeding:** Apply direct pressure for 10 minutes with a sterile gauze to stop any bleeding.

❸ **Cleaning the Wound:**
  • Wash the wound with soap and water for 5 minutes.
  • For any dirt, scrub gently with a washcloth.
  • For any bleeding, apply direct pressure with a sterile gauze or clean cloth for 10 minutes.

❹ **Antibiotic Ointment:**
  • Apply an antibiotic ointment (e.g., OTC bacitracin), covered by a Band-Aid or dressing. Change daily or if it becomes wet.
  • Option: A Telfa dressing won't stick to the wound when it is removed.
  • Option: Another option is to use a liquid skin bandage that only needs to be applied once. Don't use antibiotic ointment if you use a liquid skin bandage.

❺ **Liquid Skin Bandage:**
  • You can use a liquid skin bandage instead of antibiotic ointment and a dressing or a Band-Aid.
  • **Benefits:** Liquid skin bandage has several benefits when compared with a regular bandage (e.g., a dressing or a Band-Aid). You only need to put a liquid bandage on once to minor cuts and scrapes. It helps stop minor bleeding. It seals the wound and may promote faster healing and lower infection rates. However, it also costs more.
  • **How to Use It:** First clean and dry the wound. You put on the liquid as spray or with a swab. It dries in < 1 minute and usually lasts a week. You can get it wet.
  • **Examples:** Liquid skin bandage is available over the counter. Examples are Band-Aid Liquid Bandage, New Skin, Curad Spray Bandage, and 3M No Sting Liquid Bandage Spray.

❻ **Call Back If:**
  • Looks infected (pus, redness, increasing tenderness).
  • Doesn't heal within 10 days.
  • You become worse.

Treatment of a Torn Toenail

❶ **Reassurance—Torn Toenail (From Catching It on Something):**
  • Symptoms are mild pain and a torn or cracked nail.
  • *Here is some care advice that should help.*

❷ **Trimming the Nail:**
  • For a cracked nail without rough edges, leave it alone.
  • For a large flap of nail that is almost torn through, use a sterile scissors to cut it off along the line of the tear. This will keep the nail from catching on clothes or other things and tearing further.
  • Apply an antibiotic ointment and cover with a Band-Aid. Change daily.

❸ **Expected Course:**
  • After about 7 days, the nail bed should be covered by new skin and no longer hurt.
  • It takes about 6-12 weeks for a toenail to grow back completely.

❹ **Call Back If:**
  • Looks infected (pus, redness, increasing tenderness).
  • You become worse.

Over-the-counter Pain Medicines

❶ **Pain Medicines:**
  • For pain relief, you can take either acetaminophen, ibuprofen, or naproxen.
  • They are over-the-counter (OTC) pain drugs. You can buy them at the drugstore.

  Acetaminophen (e.g., Tylenol):
  • **Regular Strength Tylenol:** Take 650 mg (two 325 mg pills) by mouth every 4-6 hours as needed. Each Regular Strength Tylenol pill has 325 mg of acetaminophen.
  • **Extra Strength Tylenol:** Take 1,000 mg (two 500 mg pills) every 8 hours as needed. Each Extra Strength Tylenol pill has 500 mg of acetaminophen.
  • The most you should take each day is 3,000 mg (10 Regular Strength or 6 Extra Strength pills a day).

  Ibuprofen (e.g., Motrin, Advil):
  • Take 400 mg (two 200 mg pills) by mouth every 6 hours.
  • Another choice is to take 600 mg (three 200 mg pills) by mouth every 8 hours.
  • The most you should take each day is 1,200 mg (six 200 mg pills), unless your doctor has told you to take more.

Naproxen (e.g., Aleve):
- Take 220 mg (one 220 mg pill) by mouth every 8 hours as needed. You may take 440 mg (two 220 mg pills) for your first dose.
- The most you should take each day is 660 mg (three 220 mg pills a day), unless your doctor has told you to take more.

❷ **Pain Medicines—Extra Notes:**
- Use the lowest amount of medicine that makes your pain better.
- Acetaminophen is thought to be safer than ibuprofen or naproxen in people > 65 years old. Acetaminophen is in many OTC and prescription medicines. It might be in more than one medicine that you are taking. You need to be careful and not take an overdose. An acetaminophen overdose can hurt the liver.
- McNeil, the company that makes Tylenol, has different dosage instructions for Tylenol in Canada and the United States. In Canada, the maximum recommended dose per day is 4,000 mg or 12 Regular Strength (325 mg) pills. In the United States, McNeil recommends a maximum dose of 10 Regular Strength (325 mg) pills.
- CAUTION: Do not take acetaminophen if you have liver disease.
- CAUTION: Do not take ibuprofen or naproxen if you have stomach problems, have kidney disease, are pregnant, or have been told by your doctor to avoid this type of anti-inflammatory drug. Do not take ibuprofen or naproxen for > 7 days without consulting your doctor.
- *Before taking any medicine, read all the instructions on the package.*

❸ **Call Back If:**
- You have more questions.
- You become worse.

FIRST AID

First Aid Advice for Bleeding:
Apply direct pressure to the entire wound with a clean cloth.

First Aid Advice for Penetrating Object:
If penetrating object is still in place, don't remove it. *Reason: Removal could increase bleeding.*

First Aid Advice for Shock:
Lie down with the feet elevated.

First Aid Advice for a Sprain of the Toe:
- Remove any rings or jewelry from the injured toe.
- Tape the injured toe to the toe next to it (this is called a buddy splint).
- Apply a cold pack or an ice bag (wrapped in a moist towel) to the area for 20 minutes.

First Aid Advice for Suspected Fracture or Dislocation of the Toe:
- Remove any rings or jewelry from the injured toe.
- Tape the injured toe to the toe next to it (this is called a buddy splint).
- Apply a cold pack or an ice bag (wrapped in a moist towel) to the area for 20 minutes.

First Aid Advice for Transport of an Amputated Toe:
- Briefly rinse amputated part with water (to remove any dirt).
- Place amputated part in plastic bag (to protect and keep clean).
- Place plastic bag containing part in a cup of ice water (to keep cool and preserve tissue).

BACKGROUND

Types of Toe Injuries

❶ **Cuts, Abrasions (Skinned Toes), and Bruises:** The most common injuries.

❷ **Jammed or Stubbed Toe:** The end of a straightened toe receives a blow (usually from stubbing the toe on a table leg or bed corner while barefoot). The energy is absorbed by the joints' surfaces and the injury occurs there (a traumatic arthritis or sprain). These injuries are usually mild, and the severe pain is transient.

❸ **Smashed Toe** (e.g., from dropping heavy object on it): Usually the toe receives a few cuts, a blood blister, or a bruise. Occasionally the nail is damaged. Associated fractures of the phalanx can sometimes occur; there is a minor risk of osteomyelitis if there is a wound overlying a fracture.

❹ **Nail Injury:** If the nail bed is lacerated, it needs sutures to prevent a permanently deformed nail. This is less important for toenails than for fingernails.

❺ **Subungual Hematoma:**
  - A blood clot forms under the nail.
  - Usually caused by a crush injury from a heavy object falling on the toe while it is on a firm surface.
  - Most are only mildly painful, and blood is typically under < 50% of nail bed.
  - Some are severely painful and throbbing. These may need the pressure released to prevent loss of the toenail and to relieve pain. This is best done by a doctor (or nurse practitioner or physician assistant) and involves making a small hole in the nail to release the blood.

❻ **Fractures or Dislocations:** Fractures of the great toe may require splinting and crutches. Fractures of the lesser toes usually need buddy-taping or no splinting at all. Delayed intervention within 24 hours is acceptable.

❼ **Turf Toe:** This is a sprain injury to the first metatarsophalangeal joint. It is seen in athletes (e.g., football players) and seems to be related to increasing use of artificial playing surfaces.

What Cuts Need to Be Sutured?
  - Any cut that is split open or gaping probably needs sutures (or staples or skin glue).
  - Cuts > ½" (1 cm) usually need sutures.
  - Any open wound that may need sutures should be evaluated by a physician regardless of the time that has passed since the initial injury.

When Does an Adult Need a Tetanus Booster (Tetanus Shot)?
  - **Clean Cuts and Scrapes—Tetanus Booster Needed Every 10 Years:** Patients with clean minor wounds AND who have previously had ≥ 3 tetanus shots (full series) need a booster every 10 years. Examples of minor wounds include a superficial abrasion or a shallow cut from a clean knife blade. Obtain booster within 72 hours.
  - **Dirty Wounds—Tetanus Booster Needed Every 5 Years:** Patients with dirty wounds need a booster if it has been > 5 years since the last booster. Examples of dirty wounds include those contaminated with soil, feces, and/or saliva and more serious wounds from deep punctures, crushing, and burns. Obtain booster within 72 hours.

TOOTH INJURY

Definition
- Injury to tooth or teeth.
- **Note:** Other mouth injuries are covered in the Mouth Injury protocol on page 286.

TRIAGE ASSESSMENT QUESTIONS

Call EMS 911 Now
- Knocked out (unconscious) > 1 minute
  R/O: concussion
- Difficult to awaken or acting confused (e.g., disoriented, slurred speech)
  R/O: concussion, intoxication
- SEVERE neck pain (e.g., excruciating)
  R/O: cervical spine injury
  First Aid: Protect the neck from movement.
- Sounds like a life-threatening emergency to the triager

See More Appropriate Protocol
- Wound looks infected
  Go to Protocol: Wound Infection on page 443

Go to ED or Dentist Now
- Tooth knocked out
  First Aid: See First Aid for knocked-out tooth.
- Tooth is almost falling out
- Bleeding won't stop after 10 minutes of direct pressure (using correct technique)
  R/O: need for sutures
- Sounds like a serious injury to the triager

Call Dentist Now
- SEVERE pain (e.g., excruciating)
- Chipped tooth (piece missing)
  R/O: possible fracture into pulp or dentine
- Tooth pushed out of its normal position
  Reason: displaced tooth needs repositioning and stabilizing
- Tooth sensitive to cold fluids
  R/O: dentin exposure
- Can see a crack in the tooth
  R/O: tooth fracture

See Today or Tomorrow in Office
- Suspicious history for the injury
  R/O: domestic violence or elder abuse

Call Dentist Today
- Caller tries to move the tooth and it feels very loose
- Tooth becomes darker
  R/O: pulp necrosis
- Patient wants to be seen

Home Care
- Minor tooth injury

HOME CARE ADVICE

❶ **Apply a Cold Pack:** For pain, apply a piece of ice or a Popsicle to the injured gum area for 20 minutes.

❷ **Pain Medicines:**
- For pain relief, you can take either acetaminophen, ibuprofen, or naproxen.
- They are over-the-counter (OTC) pain drugs. You can buy them at the drugstore.

Acetaminophen (e.g., Tylenol):
- **Regular Strength Tylenol:** Take 650 mg (two 325 mg pills) by mouth every 4-6 hours as needed. Each Regular Strength Tylenol pill has 325 mg of acetaminophen.
- **Extra Strength Tylenol:** Take 1,000 mg (two 500 mg pills) every 8 hours as needed. Each Extra Strength Tylenol pill has 500 mg of acetaminophen.
- The most you should take each day is 3,000 mg (10 Regular Strength or 6 Extra Strength pills a day).

Ibuprofen (e.g., Motrin, Advil):
- Take 400 mg (two 200 mg pills) by mouth every 6 hours.
- Another choice is to take 600 mg (three 200 mg pills) by mouth every 8 hours.
- The most you should take each day is 1,200 mg (six 200 mg pills), unless your doctor has told you to take more.

Naproxen (e.g., Aleve):
- Take 220 mg (one 220 mg pill) by mouth every 8 hours as needed. You may take 440 mg (two 220 mg pills) for your first dose.
- The most you should take each day is 660 mg (three 220 mg pills a day), unless your doctor has told you to take more.

❸ **Soft Diet:** If you have any loose teeth, eat a soft diet for 3 days. After 3 days, they should be tightening up.

❹ **Call Your Dentist If:**
- Pain becomes severe.
- Tooth becomes sensitive to hot or cold fluids.
- Tooth becomes a darker color.
- You become worse.

FIRST AID

First Aid Advice for Knocked-Out Tooth

To save the tooth, it must be put back in its socket as soon as possible (2 hours is the maximum limit for survival). Use the following technique:
- Rinse off the tooth with saliva or water. Do not scrub the tooth.
- Replace it in the socket facing the correct way.
- Press down on the tooth with your thumb until the crown is level with the adjacent tooth.
- Lastly, bite down on a wad of cloth to stabilize the tooth until you can be seen by a dentist.
- **Transporting a Knocked-Out Tooth:** Follow these instructions if you are not able to put the tooth back in its socket:
- It is very important to keep the tooth moist. Do not let it dry out.
- Transport the tooth in saliva or milk.

BACKGROUND

Types of Tooth Injuries

❶ **Avulsion of Tooth** (knocked-out tooth): This is a dental emergency. The avulsed permanent tooth needs to be placed back in its socket as soon as possible, ideally within minutes, and certainly within 2 hours.

❷ **Concussion of Tooth** (tooth was bumped but is not loose): An injury to a tooth without displacement, loosening, or fracture. This is the most common dental injury. No immediate dental care is needed. A soft diet should be recommended. Rarely, a concussed tooth can undergo pulpal necrosis (tooth death) days to weeks later; this can be recognized when the tooth becomes darker than the adjacent teeth.

❸ **Crown Fracture—Complicated** (enamel-dentin fracture with pulp exposure): A fracture that enters into the pulp of a tooth is referred to as complicated. Typically, it is quite painful and is very sensitive to air and cold liquids. The caller will usually describe that a large piece of the tooth is broken off. The caller may be also able to see a small red dot or pink blush (the pulp) in the fractured area. To reduce pain and prevent pulpal damage, fractures into the pulp need to be treated urgently. Treatment in an ED may consist of temporarily covering the fracture with a dental cement or calcium hydroxide. Subsequent dental care is mandatory; most of these fractures will require root canal therapy.

❹ **Crown Fracture—Uncomplicated** (enamel-dentin fracture; chipped tooth; no pulp exposure): A small, painless chipped tooth can wait 24-72 hours for evaluation by a dentist.

❺ **Cracked Tooth** (infraction): This is a small hairline crack of a tooth. The caller will report a thin fracture line without any missing piece of tooth. Generally, this should be evaluated by a dentist in 24-72 hours.

❻ **Intruded Tooth** (pushed into gum): The tooth is pushed deeper into the gum and tooth socket. Generally, this should be evaluated by a dentist in 24-72 hours.

❼ **Loosened Tooth** (subluxation): If there is only mild looseness, the tooth usually tightens up on its own (may bleed a little from the gums).

❽ **Loosened and Displaced Tooth** (luxation): Need to see a dentist to assess damage. Displaced teeth that interfere with biting, chewing, or closing the mouth need to be repositioned within 4 hours for reasons of comfort and function. Mild displacement deserves evaluation within 24 hours.

Causes

- Contact sports
- Falls
- **Fights:** Direct blow from punch, kick, or object
- Motor vehicle accidents

Caution: Associated Head and Neck Trauma

- Head trauma should be considered in all patients with a mouth and dental injury. Signs of significant head injury include loss of consciousness, amnesia, unsteady walking, confusion, and slurred speech.
- Neck trauma should also be considered in all patients with a facial injury. Concerning findings include numbness, weakness, and neck pain.
- After using the Tooth Injury protocol, if the triager or caller has remaining concerns about head or neck trauma, the patient also should be triaged using the Head Injury and/or Neck Injury protocol on pages 201 and 290, respectively.

TOOTHACHE

Definition
- Pain or discomfort in a tooth
- Not due to a traumatic injury

Pain Severity Scale
- **Mild (1-3):** Doesn't interfere with chewing.
- **Moderate (4-7):** Interferes with chewing, interferes with normal activities, awakens from sleep.
- **Severe (8-10):** Unable to eat, unable to do any normal activities, excruciating pain.

TRIAGE ASSESSMENT QUESTIONS

Call EMS 911 Now
- Pale cold skin and very weak (can't stand)
  R/O: shock
- Similar pain previously and it was from "heart attack"
  R/O: cardiac ischemia, myocardial infarction
- Similar pain previously and it was from "angina" and not relieved by nitroglycerin
  R/O: cardiac ischemia, myocardial infarction
- Sounds like a life-threatening emergency to the triager

See More Appropriate Protocol
- Chest pain
  Go to Protocol: Chest Pain on page 73
- Toothache followed tooth injury
  Go to Protocol: Tooth Injury on page 408

Go to ED/UCC Now
(or to Office With PCP Approval)
- Patient sounds very sick or weak to the triager
  Reason: severe acute illness or serious complication suspected

Go to Office Now
- Face is swollen
  R/O: dental abscess with secondary facial cellulitis
- Fever
  R/O: dental abscess

Call Dentist Now
- SEVERE toothache pain

Call Dentist Today
- Toothache present > 24 hours
  R/O: tooth decay, enamel fracture
- Brown cavity visible in the painful tooth
  R/O: tooth decay
- Red or yellow lump present at the gumline of the painful tooth
  R/O: periapical gum abscess
- Lost crown
  Reason: replace crown; see FIRST AID
- Lost filling
  Reason: replace filling; see FIRST AID
- Broken braces wire or end of braces wire is jabbing into gum, cheek, or tongue
  Reason: fix orthodontia wire; see FIRST AID
- Patient wants to be seen

Home Care
- ○ Mild toothache present < 24 hours

HOME CARE ADVICE

❶ **Reassurance:**
- Most toothaches are temporary and due to a sensitive tooth. If the pain becomes worse or does not resolve in 24 hours, it could be due to a small cavity.
- *Here is some care advice that should help.*

❷ **Floss:** Floss on either side of the painful tooth to remove any wedged food.

❸ **Pain Medicines:**
- For pain relief, you can take either acetaminophen, ibuprofen, or naproxen.
- They are over-the-counter (OTC) pain drugs. You can buy them at the drugstore.

Acetaminophen (e.g., Tylenol):
- **Regular Strength Tylenol:** Take 650 mg (two 325 mg pills) by mouth every 4-6 hours as needed. Each Regular Strength Tylenol pill has 325 mg of acetaminophen.
- **Extra Strength Tylenol:** Take 1,000 mg (two 500 mg pills) every 8 hours as needed. Each Extra Strength Tylenol pill has 500 mg of acetaminophen.
- The most you should take each day is 3,000 mg (10 Regular Strength or 6 Extra Strength pills a day).

Ibuprofen (e.g., Motrin, Advil):
- Take 400 mg (two 200 mg pills) by mouth every 6 hours.
- Another choice is to take 600 mg (three 200 mg pills) by mouth every 8 hours.
- The most you should take each day is 1,200 mg (six 200 mg pills), unless your doctor has told you to take more.

Naproxen (e.g., Aleve):
- Take 220 mg (one 220 mg pill) by mouth every 8 hours as needed. You may take 440 mg (two 220 mg pills) for your first dose.
- The most you should take each day is 660 mg (three 220 mg pills a day), unless your doctor has told you to take more.

❹ **Pain Medicines—Extra Notes:**
- Use the lowest amount of medicine that makes your pain better.
- Acetaminophen is thought to be safer than ibuprofen or naproxen in people > 65 years old. Acetaminophen is in many OTC and prescription medicines. It might be in more than one medicine that you are taking. You need to be careful and not take an overdose. An acetaminophen overdose can hurt the liver.
- McNeil, the company that makes Tylenol, has different dosage instructions for Tylenol in Canada and the United States. In Canada, the maximum recommended dose per day is 4,000 mg or 12 Regular Strength (325 mg) pills. In the United States, McNeil recommends a maximum dose of 10 Regular Strength (325 mg) pills.
- CAUTION: Do not take acetaminophen if you have liver disease.
- CAUTION: Do not take ibuprofen or naproxen if you have stomach problems, have kidney disease, are pregnant, or have been told by your doctor to avoid this type of anti-inflammatory drug. Do not take ibuprofen or naproxen for > 7 days without consulting your doctor.
- *Before taking any medicine, read all the instructions on the package.*

❺ **Apply Cold to the Area:** Apply an ice pack to the painful jaw for 20 minutes.

❻ **Expected Course:** Most minor causes of toothache resolve in < 1 day.

❼ **Call Your Dentist If:**
- Toothache lasts > 24 hours.
- The toothache becomes worse.

FIRST AID

First Aid Advice for Lost Crown:
- Obtain some over-the-counter dental cement from your local pharmacy.
- Coat the inside of the crown with the dental cement.
- Place the crown back over the tooth.

Notes:
- You can use dental adhesive if you cannot obtain dental cement.
- Remember to see your dentist as soon as possible.

First Aid Advice for Lost Filling:
Push a piece of sugarless chewing gum into the cavity hole.

Notes:
- You can use over-the-counter dental cement instead of chewing gum.
- Remember to see your dentist as soon as possible.

First Aid Advice for Pain From Braces Wire Poking Cheek, Gum, or Tongue:
Cover the end of the wire with orthodontic wax or a cotton ball.

BACKGROUND

The main cause of toothache is tooth decay (cavities). Complications of tooth decay can also cause pain. For example, a periapical abscess (pus pocket) can develop around the base of a tooth with a cavity.

Dental Causes of Toothache

- **Dental Caries** (tooth decay): Pulpitis, periapical abscess
- Food stuck between teeth
- Lost crown
- Lost filling
- **Periodontal Disease** (gum disease): Gingivitis, periodontal abscess, pericoronitis
- Tooth fracture (broken or cracked tooth)

Other Causes of Toothache

- Canker sore (aphthous ulcer)
- Cardiac ischemia
- Ludwig angina
- Sinusitis
- Temporomandibular disorder
- Trigeminal neuralgia

Complications of Tooth Decay

- Cellulitis of the cheek
- Periapical dental abscess
- **Ludwig Angina:** This serious infection is a rapidly progressive cellulitis of the floor of the mouth that usually is a complication of a dental abscess or tooth extraction. The presenting symptoms are fever, a swollen/tender tongue, and difficulty swallowing.
- Submandibular lymphadenitis

Caution—Cardiac Ischemia

- Rarely, patients may present with toothache or jaw pain as the sole symptom of a myocardial infarction. Usually there will be other associated symptoms of cardiac ischemia: chest pain, shortness of breath, nausea, and/or diaphoresis.
- Cardiac ischemia should be suspected in any patients with risk factors for cardiac disease. These include: hypertension, smoking, diabetes, hyperlipidemia, a strong family history of heart disease, and age > 50.

URINALYSIS RESULTS FOLLOW-UP CALL

Definition

- Urinalysis or urine dipstick done and results called to triage nurse by the laboratory, PCP, or adult caller.
- Patient has been previously triaged by triage nurse or examined by PCP.
- Patient has some symptom(s) of a urinary tract infection (e.g., dysuria, frequency, urgency, foul-smelling urine, or hematuria).
- In most cases, the triage nurse needs to call the patient.

TRIAGE ASSESSMENT QUESTIONS

See More Appropriate Protocol

- ● Female taking antibiotic for diagnosed urine infection
  Go to Protocol: Urination Pain (Female) on page 418
- ● Male taking antibiotic for diagnosed urine infection
  Go to Protocol: Urination Pain (Male) on page 421

Go to ED/UCC Now
(or to Office With PCP Approval)

- ● Patient sounds very sick or weak to the triager
  Reason: severe acute illness or serious complication suspected

Call Transferred to PCP Now

- ● Positive urine test (i.e., LE+ or WBC > 10) and any of the following:
  - Fever > 100.5° F (38.1° C)
  - Side (flank) or lower back pain present
    R/O: pyelonephritis

See Today or Tomorrow in Office

- ● Negative urine test (i.e., LE- and WBC < 10) and urine symptoms continue or are worsening
  Note: Triager judgment regarding need for further triage.
- ● Patient wants to be seen

Discuss With PCP and Callback by Nurse Today

- ● Positive urine test (i.e., LE+ or WBC > 10) and NO standing order to call in prescription for antibiotic
  Reason: antibiotic prescription needed

- ● Positive urine test and any of the following:
  - Antibiotic treatment in past month for urine infection
  - Has urinary catheter (e.g., Foley)
  - Bedridden (e.g., nursing home patient, CVA, chronic illness, recovering from surgery)
  - Chronic urinary incontinence
    Reason: possible antibiotic resistance
- ● Positive urine test and any of the following:
  - Diabetes mellitus
  - Weak immune system (e.g., HIV positive, cancer chemotherapy, transplant patient)
  - Pregnant
  - Male
    Reason: special circumstances
- ● Triager uncertain how to interpret urine test results

Home Care

- ○ Positive urine test (i.e., LE+ or WBC > 10) and standing order to call in prescription for antibiotic
  Reason: antibiotic prescription needed for nonpregnant female with cystitis
- ○ Negative urine test (i.e., LE- and WBC < 10)

HOME CARE ADVICE

General Care Advice for Urination Pain

❶ **Fluids:** Drink extra fluids. Drink 8-10 glasses of liquids a day.
   (Reason: to produce a dilute, nonirritating urine)

❷ **Cranberry Juice:**
- Some people think that drinking cranberry juice may help in fighting urinary tract infections. However, there is no good research that has ever proved this.
- **Dosage Cranberry Juice Cocktail:** 8 oz (240 mL) twice a day.
- **Dosage 100% Cranberry Juice:** 1 oz (30 mL) twice a day.
- CAUTION: Do not drink > 16 oz (480 mL).
  (Reason: Too much cranberry juice can also be irritating to the bladder.)

❸ **Pain Medicines:**
- For pain relief, you can take either acetaminophen, ibuprofen, or naproxen.
- They are over-the-counter (OTC) pain drugs. You can buy them at the drugstore.

Acetaminophen (e.g., Tylenol):
- **Regular Strength Tylenol:** Take 650 mg (two 325 mg pills) by mouth every 4-6 hours as needed. Each Regular Strength Tylenol pill has 325 mg of acetaminophen.
- **Extra Strength Tylenol:** Take 1,000 mg (two 500 mg pills) every 8 hours as needed. Each Extra Strength Tylenol pill has 500 mg of acetaminophen.
- The most you should take each day is 3,000 mg (10 Regular Strength or 6 Extra Strength pills a day).

Ibuprofen (e.g., Motrin, Advil):
- Take 400 mg (two 200 mg pills) by mouth every 6 hours.
- Another choice is to take 600 mg (three 200 mg pills) by mouth every 8 hours.
- The most you should take each day is 1,200 mg (six 200 mg pills), unless your doctor has told you to take more.

Naproxen (e.g., Aleve):
- Take 220 mg (one 220 mg pill) by mouth every 8 hours as needed. You may take 440 mg (two 220 mg pills) for your first dose.
- The most you should take each day is 660 mg (three 220 mg pills a day), unless your doctor has told you to take more.

❹ **Pain Medicines—Extra Notes:**
- Use the lowest amount of medicine that makes your pain better.
- Acetaminophen is thought to be safer than ibuprofen or naproxen in people > 65 years old. Acetaminophen is in many OTC and prescription medicines. It might be in more than one medicine that you are taking. You need to be careful and not take an overdose. An acetaminophen overdose can hurt the liver.
- McNeil, the company that makes Tylenol, has different dosage instructions for Tylenol in Canada and the United States. In Canada, the maximum recommended dose per day is 4,000 mg or 12 Regular Strength (325 mg) pills. In the United States, McNeil recommends a maximum dose of 10 Regular Strength (325 mg) pills.

- CAUTION: Do not take acetaminophen if you have liver disease.
- CAUTION: Do not take ibuprofen or naproxen if you have stomach problems, have kidney disease, are pregnant, or have been told by your doctor to avoid this type of anti-inflammatory drug. Do not take ibuprofen or naproxen for > 7 days without consulting your doctor.
- *Before taking any medicine, read all the instructions on the package.*

❺ **Call Back If:**
- You become worse.

Positive Urine Test—Antibiotic Treatment for Urine Infection

❶ **Urine Test Positive:** Your urine test showed that you have an infection of your urine (bladder infection).

❷ **Recommended Antibiotic:** Follow office policy and physician practice rules. Call in a prescription for one of the following:
- **Trimethoprim-Sulfamethoxazole (Bactrim DS or Septra DS):** Take 1 pill by mouth twice a day for 3 days.
- **Nitrofurantoin (Macrobid):** Take 1 pill twice a day for 5 days.

❸ **Caution—Antibiotics:**
- Ask patient about allergies.
- Bactrim and Septra are sulfa-type antibiotics.

❹ **Warm Saline Sitz Baths to Reduce Pain:** Sit in a warm saline bath for 20 minutes to cleanse the area and to reduce pain. Add 2 oz (60 g) of table salt or baking soda to a tub of water.

❺ **OTC Phenazopyridine for Severe Dysuria and Frequency:**
- Phenazopyridine (Uristat) is available OTC (in United States only). Dosage is 2 pills by mouth 3 times a day.
- It is also available as a prescription medicine (Pyridium, Urodine, Urogesic). It has a numbing effect on the lining of the bladder and urethra. It can help reduce burning during urination, urgency, and frequency until the antibiotics start working.
- It does not have any antibacterial effect.
- *Before taking any medicine, read all the instructions on the package.*

❻ **Caution—Phenazopyridine:**
  - It turns the urine bright orange. This can cause staining of underwear. It can also sometimes stain contact lenses.
  - Do not take this medicine if you have kidney disease.
  - Do not use if pregnant.
    (Reason: class B; should discuss with PCP first)
  - Do not use if breastfeeding.
    (Reason: safety unknown; should discuss with PCP first)
  - Do not use > 2 days.

❼ **Call Back If:**
  - Fever > 100.5° F (38.1° C).
  - Urine symptoms do not improve by day 3 on antibiotics.
  - You become worse.

BACKGROUND

Key Points

- This guideline assumes that (1) the patient has ≥ 1 urine symptoms, (2) the clinician who ordered the urine test has a moderate suspicion that the patient has a urine infection, and (3) that it is safer to err on the side of antibiotic treatment.
- The urinalysis ("urine test") has 2 components: dipstick (chemical testing) and microscopic (look for cells in the urine under the microscope). In some doctors' offices, just the dipstick is performed.
- Antibiotic therapy is recommended in this protocol if the patient has a positive urine test (defined as follows).

Negative Urine Test—Normal Dipstick Urinalysis

The normal results for the chemical tests on the urine dipstick are as follows:
- **pH:** 4.8-7.5
- **Protein:** None or trace
- **Glucose:** None or trace
- **Ketones:** None
- **Hemoglobin:** None
- **Bilirubin:** None
- **Urobilinogen:** None
- **Leukocyte Esterase (LE):** Negative (LE-)
- **Nitrite:** Negative

Negative Urine Test—Normal Microscopic Urinalysis

The normal results for the microscopic analysis are as follows:
- **Red Blood Cells (RBC) per High-power Field (HPF):** 0-3.
- **White Blood Cells (WBC) per HPF:** 0-5.
- **Epithelial Cells:** May be present.
- **Bacteria:** None.
- **Crystals:** Small numbers are normal.

Positive Urine Test—Abnormal Urinalysis With Findings Suggestive of Urinary Tract Infection (UTI)

For the purposes of this guideline, each of the following results supports the presence of a UTI:
- **Nitrite (NI):** Positive (NI+)
- **LE:** Positive (LE +)
- **WBCs per HPF:** > 10

Types of Urine Infections

A urinalysis test is used to diagnose 2 main types of UTIs:
- **Cystitis:** An infection of the bladder mucosa. Painful urination, urinary frequency, and urgency are typically present. Blood in the urine may also be seen. There may be an associated mild midline suprapubic discomfort in the area of the bladder. In the 20- to 50-year-old, cystitis is 30x more common in women than men. This gender difference may reflect the much shorter length of the female urethra, which facilitates migration of bacteria up into the bladder. Risk factors for female cystitis in younger women include sexual intercourse, spermicidal usage, and pregnancy. Risk factors for cystitis in older females include institutionalization (i.e., nursing home), urinary catheterization (i.e., Foley), and recent urologic surgery.
- **Pyelonephritis:** An infection of the kidney. An untreated cystitis may progress into pyelonephritis. Commonly associated symptoms include flank pain, fever, and chills. Symptoms of cystitis (dysuria, frequency) may or may not be present.

UTI: Symptoms

- **Dysuria:** Discomfort (pain, burning, or stinging) when passing urine; the most common symptom of UTI.
- **Frequency and Urgency:** Frequency means urinating frequently and passing small amounts. Urgency refers to the periodic sensation of needing to rush to the bathroom (can't wait). Both are common symptoms of UTI.
- **Hematuria:** Blood in the urine; sometimes seen in UTI.
- **Flank Pain:** Pain in the side between the lower ribs and the top of the pelvis (iliac crest). Flank pain is a symptom of pyelonephritis.

Cranberry Juice for UTI

- Cranberry juice has been used for decades to help treat or prevent UTIs.
- **How It Might Work:** In the past it was believed that cranberry-derived products helped fight urine infections by (1) urine acidification and (2) a direct bacteriostatic effect. More recent research suggests that cranberry consumption helps by decreasing bacterial adherence (stickiness) to the bladder cells.
- **Treatment of UTI:** There is no good quality research evidence proving that cranberry juice helps in the treatment of UTI.
- **Prevention of UTI:** There is some decent research evidence suggesting that cranberry juice may decrease the number of UTIs in women.
- **Dosage Cranberry Juice Cocktail:** 8 oz (240 mL) twice a day.
- **Dosage 100% Cranberry Juice:** 1 oz (30 mL) twice a day.

OTC Phenazopyridine:

- Phenazopyridine (Uristat) is available OTC. Dosage is 2 pills by mouth 3 times a day. It is also available as a prescription medicine (Pyridium, Urodine, Urogesic).
- It has a numbing effect on the lining of the bladder and urethra. It can help reduce burning during urination, urgency, and frequency until the antibiotics start working.
- It does not have any antibacterial effect.
- It turns the urine orange and because of this it interferes with urine dipstick testing.

URINATION PAIN (FEMALE)

Definition

- Discomfort (pain, burning, or stinging) when passing urine.
- Associated symptoms may include urgency (can't wait) and frequency (passing small amounts) of urination.

Pain Severity Scale

- **Mild (1-3):** Complains slightly about urination hurting.
- **Moderate (4-7):** Interferes with normal activities.
- **Severe (8-10):** Excruciating; unwilling or unable to urinate because of the pain.

TRIAGE ASSESSMENT QUESTIONS

Call EMS 911 Now

- ● Shock suspected (e.g., cold/pale/clammy skin, too weak to stand)
  R/O: urosepsis, shock
  First Aid: Lie down with the feet elevated.
- ● Sounds like a life-threatening emergency to the triager

Go to ED/UCC Now
(or to Office With PCP Approval)

- ● Unable to urinate (or only a few drops) and bladder feels very full
  R/O: urinary retention
- ● Vomiting
- ● Patient sounds very sick or weak to the triager
  Reason: severe acute illness or serious complication suspected

Go to Office Now

- ● Severe pain with urination
- ● Fever > 100.5° F (38.1° C)
  R/O: pyelonephritis
- ● Side (flank) or lower back pain present

See Today in Office

- ◐ Taking antibiotic > 24 hours for UTI and fever persists
  R/O: complication, resistant organism, or need for IV antibiotics
- ◐ Taking antibiotic > 3 days for UTI and painful urination not improved
  R/O: resistant organism
- ◐ Unusual vaginal discharge
  R/O: vaginitis, urethritis (STI)
- ◐ > 2 UTIs in last year
  R/O: recurrent UTI
- ◐ Patient is worried about STIs
  R/O: UTI, urethritis (STI)
- ◐ Age > 50 years
  R/O: UTI
- ◐ Possibility of pregnancy
  Reason: needs pregnancy test and urinary testing
- ◐ Painful urination AND EITHER frequency or urgency
  R/O: uncomplicated cystitis
  Note: See antibiotic treatment option in Home Care Advice.
- ◐ All other females with painful urination, or patient wants to be seen
  R/O: UTI, urethritis (STI)

Home Care

- ○ Taking antibiotic < 24 hours for UTI and fever persists
  Reason: taking antibiotic and no complications
- ○ Taking antibiotic < 3 days for UTI and painful urination not improved
  Reason: taking antibiotic and no complications

HOME CARE ADVICE

General Care Advice for Urination Pain (Pending PCP Evaluation)

❶ **Fluids:** Drink extra fluids. Drink 8-10 glasses of liquids a day.
(Reason: to produce a dilute, nonirritating urine)

❷ **Cranberry Juice:**
- Some people think that drinking cranberry juice may help in fighting urinary tract infections (UTIs). However, there is no good research that has ever proved this.
- **Dosage Cranberry Juice Cocktail:** 8 oz (240 mL) twice a day.
- **Dosage 100% Cranberry Juice:** 1 oz (30 mL) twice a day.
- CAUTION: Do not drink > 16 oz (480 mL).
  (Reason: Too much cranberry juice can also be irritating to the bladder.)

❸ **Warm Saline Sitz Baths to Reduce Pain:** Sit in a warm saline bath for 20 minutes to cleanse the area and to reduce pain. Add 2 oz (60 g) of table salt or baking soda to a tub of water.

❹ **Call Back If:**
• You become worse.

Antibiotic Treatment Option for Uncomplicated Cystitis

❶ **Follow Policy and Physician's Practice Rules:**
• Some physicians are willing to initiate antibiotic therapy for uncomplicated cystitis over the telephone.
• Follow policy and the physician's practice rules.

❷ **Must Be Present:** Dysuria AND EITHER frequency or urgency. Not essential, but helpful: caller states that it feels just like prior "bladder/urine infection."
• **Must Be Absent:** New/changed vaginal discharge, fever, flank pain, age > 50, pregnancy, diabetes, or any other significant health problem.

❸ **Recommended Antibiotic:** Call in a prescription for one of the following:
• **Trimethoprim-Sulfamethoxazole (Bactrim DS or Septra DS):** Take 1 pill by mouth twice a day for 3 days.
• **Nitrofurantoin (Macrobid):** Take 1 pill twice a day for 5 days.

❹ **Caution—Antibiotics:** Ask patient about allergies. Bactrim is a sulfa-type antibiotic.

❺ **Call Back If:**
• Fever occurs.
• Back or flank pain occurs.
• Urine symptoms do not improve by day 3 on antibiotics.
• You become worse.

Already Receiving Antibiotic Treatment for UTI

❶ **Fluids:** Drink extra fluids. Drink 8-10 glasses of liquids a day.
(Reason: to produce a dilute, nonirritating urine)

❷ **Cranberry Juice:**
• Some people think that drinking cranberry juice may help in fighting urinary tract infections. However, there is no good research that has ever proved this.
• **Dosage Cranberry Juice Cocktail:** 8 oz (240 mL) twice a day.

• **Dosage 100% Cranberry Juice:** 1 oz (30 mL) twice a day.
• Do not drink > 12 oz (360 mL).
(Reason: Too much cranberry juice can also be irritating to the bladder.)

❸ **OTC Phenazopyridine for Severe Dysuria and Frequency:**
• Phenazopyridine (Uristat) is available OTC (in United States only). Dosage is 2 pills by mouth 3 times a day.
• It is also available as a prescription medicine (Pyridium, Urodine, Urogesic). It has a numbing effect on the lining of the bladder and urethra. It can help reduce burning during urination, urgency, and frequency until the antibiotics start working.
• It does not have any antibacterial effect.
• *Before taking any medicine, read all the instructions on the package.*

❹ **Caution—Phenazopyridine:**
• It turns the urine bright orange. This can cause staining of underwear. It can also sometimes stain contact lenses.
• Do not take this medicine if you have kidney disease.
• Do not use if pregnant.
(Reason: class B; should discuss with PCP first)
• Do not use if breastfeeding.
(Reason: safety unknown; should discuss with PCP first)
• Do not use > 2 days.

❺ **Call Back If:**
• Fever lasts > 24 hours on antibiotics.
• Pain does not improve by day 3 on antibiotics.
• Urine symptoms do not improve by day 3 on antibiotics.
• You become worse.

FIRST AID

First Aid Advice for Shock:
Lie down with the feet elevated.

BACKGROUND

Key Points

- Dysuria is the medical term that describes burning or pain with urination.
- Anything that irritates the urethral mucosa can cause dysuria. Urinary tract infections (UTIs) are the number one cause of dysuria. The term UTI is nonspecific and encompasses a number of more specific diagnoses.
- Half of all women experience at least one UTI at some point in their lifetime.

UTI Causes of Dysuria

- **Cystitis:** An infection of the bladder mucosa. Urinary frequency and urgency are typically present. Blood in the urine may also be seen. There may be an associated mild midline suprapubic discomfort in the area of the bladder. In the 20- to 50-year-old, cystitis is 30x more common in women than men. This gender difference may reflect the much shorter length of the female urethra, which facilitates migration of bacteria up into the bladder. Risk factors for female cystitis in younger women include sexual intercourse, spermicidal usage, and pregnancy. Risk factors for cystitis in older females include institutionalization (i.e., nursing home), urinary catheterization (i.e., Foley), and recent urologic surgery.
- **Pyelonephritis:** An infection of the kidney. An untreated cystitis may develop into pyelonephritis. Commonly associated symptoms include flank pain, fever, and chills. Symptoms of cystitis (dysuria, frequency) may or may not be present.
- **Urethritis:** Urethritis is a sexually transmitted infection (STI). The 2 principal organisms responsible for urethritis are gonorrhea and chlamydia. Suprapubic pain and hematuria are absent.

Other Causes of Dysuria

- **Labial Sores:** If a woman has a scratch or any type of sore on the labia near the urethra, the exiting warm urine may cause some pain. Many women will note that it "hurts outside." And unlike a cystitis, there is no frequency or urgency.
- **Vaginitis:** Vaginitis is a general term that means "vaginal inflammation." Vaginitis can have chemical etiology (excessive douching or excessive use of OTC yeast medication). Vaginitis may have an infectious etiology: *Trichomonas* or yeast (*Candida*).

- **Vaginitis, Atrophic:** In postmenopausal women, the vaginal mucosa thins because of lack of estrogen. Some women complain of mild dysuria, others experience itching, and others describe dyspareunia (painful intercourse).

Antibiotic Treatment Option for Uncomplicated Cystitis

- Some physicians are willing to initiate antibiotic therapy for uncomplicated cystitis over the telephone. Follow policy and the physician's practice rules.
- **Must Be Present:** Dysuria AND EITHER frequency or urgency. Not essential, but helpful: caller states that it feels just like prior "bladder/urine infection."
- **Must Be Absent:** New/changed vaginal discharge, fever, flank pain, age > 50, pregnancy, diabetes, or any other significant health problem.
- **Recommended Antibiotic:** Trimethoprim-sulfamethoxazole (Bactrim DS or Septra DS; 1 by mouth twice a day for 3 days), nitrofurantoin (Macrobid; 1 by mouth twice a day for 3 days), or ciprofloxacin (Cipro; 250 mg by mouth twice a day for 3 days).

Cranberry Juice for UTI

- Cranberry juice has been used for decades to help treat or prevent UTIs.
- **How It Might Work:** In the past it was believed that cranberry-derived products helped fight urine infections by (1) urine acidification and (2) a direct bacteriostatic effect. More recent research suggests that cranberry consumption helps by decreasing bacterial adherence (stickiness) to the bladder cells.
- **Treatment of UTI:** There is no good quality research evidence proving that cranberry juice helps in the treatment of UTI.
- **Prevention of UTI:** There is some decent research evidence suggesting that cranberry juice may decrease the number of UTIs in women.
- **Dosage Cranberry Juice Cocktail:** 8 oz (240 mL) twice a day.
- **Dosage 100% Cranberry Juice:** 1 oz (30 mL) twice a day.

URINATION PAIN (MALE)

Definition
- Discomfort (pain, burning, or stinging) when passing urine.
- Associated symptoms may include urgency (can't wait) and frequency (passing small amounts) of urination.

Pain Severity Scale
- **Mild (1-3):** Complains slightly about urination hurting.
- **Moderate (4-7):** Interferes with normal activities.
- **Severe (8-10):** Excruciating; unwilling or unable to urinate because of the pain.

TRIAGE ASSESSMENT QUESTIONS

Call EMS 911 Now
- Shock suspected (e.g., cold/pale/clammy skin, too weak to stand)
  R/O: urosepsis, shock
  First Aid: Lie down with the feet elevated.
- Sounds like a life-threatening emergency to the triager

Go to ED/UCC Now
(or to Office With PCP Approval)
- Unable to urinate (or only a few drops) and bladder feels very full
  R/O: urinary retention
- Pain in scrotum or testicle that persists > 1 hour
  R/O: torsion of testis or appendix testis, epididymitis
- Swollen scrotum
  R/O: torsion of testis, strangulated hernia, orchitis, epididymitis
- Fever > 100.5° F (38.1° C)
  R/O: pyelonephritis
- Vomiting
- Patient sounds very sick or weak to the triager
  Reason: severe acute illness or serious complication suspected

Go to Office Now
- Severe pain with urination
  R/O: severe urethritis or cystitis
- Side (flank) or lower back pain present
  R/O: pyelonephritis

See Today in Office
- Taking antibiotic > 24 hours for UTI and fever persists
  R/O: complication, resistant organism, or need for IV antibiotics
- Taking antibiotic > 3 days for UTI and painful urination not improved
  R/O: resistant organism
- Taking treatment > 3 days for STI (e.g., penile discharge from gonorrhea, chlamydia) and painful urination not improved
  R/O: resistant organism
- All other males with painful urination, or patient wants to be seen
  R/O: UTI, urethritis (STI)

Home Care
- Taking antibiotic < 24 hours for UTI and fever persists
  Reason: taking antibiotic and no complications
- Taking antibiotic < 3 days for UTI and painful urination not improved
  Reason: taking antibiotic and no complications
- Taking antibiotic < 3 days for STI and painful urination not improved
  Reason: taking antibiotic and no complications

HOME CARE ADVICE

General Care Advice for Urination Pain (Pending PCP Evaluation)
1. **Fluids:** Drink extra fluids.
   (Reason: to produce a dilute, nonirritating urine)
2. **Call Back If:**
   - You become worse.

Already Receiving Antibiotic Treatment for Urinary Tract Infection (UTI)
1. **Fluids:** Drink extra fluids.
   (Reason: to produce a dilute, nonirritating urine)
2. **Call Back If:**
   - Fever lasts > 24 hours on antibiotics.
   - Pain does not improve by day 3 on antibiotics.
   - Urine symptoms do not improve by day 3 on antibiotics.
   - You become worse.

FIRST AID

First Aid Advice for Shock:

Lie down with the feet elevated.

BACKGROUND

Key Points

- Dysuria is the medical term that describes burning or pain with urination. Adult males with dysuria require examination and laboratory evaluation to determine if an infection is present.
- Anything that irritates the urethral mucosa can cause dysuria. Urinary tract infections (UTIs) are the most common cause of dysuria. The term UTI is nonspecific and encompasses a number of more specific diagnoses: cystitis, urethritis, prostatitis.
- In younger men, it is more likely that the dysuria is the result of urethritis from a sexually transmitted infection (STI).
- In older men, cystitis becomes the more likely culprit and the infection is caused by coliform bacteria like *Escherichia coli.*

UTI Causes of Dysuria

- **Cystitis:** An infection of the bladder mucosa. Urinary frequency and urgency may be present. There may be an associated mild midline suprapubic discomfort in the area of the bladder. Cystitis is much less common in men than women. Cystitis is rare in healthy young to middle-aged men. Risk factors for male cystitis include age > 60, urinary catheterization (i.e., Foley), and recent urologic surgery.
- **Pyelonephritis:** An infection of the kidney. Untreated cystitis may develop into pyelonephritis. Commonly associated symptoms include flank pain, fever, and chills. Symptoms of cystitis (dysuria, frequency) may or may not be present.
- **Prostatitis:** An infection of the prostate. Dysuria and other urine symptoms may be mild or absent. Sometimes there is fever and a vague poorly localized lower abdominal or lower back pain.
- **Orchitis/Epididymitis:** An infection of the testicle or epididymis. The presenting complaint is usually pain and swelling in and around the testicle.
- **Urethritis:** Urethritis is an STI. The 2 principal organisms responsible for urethritis are gonorrhea and chlamydia. Most men with urethritis will describe a clear-white to light-yellow discharge from the penis.

Other Causes of Dysuria

- **Trauma:** Injuries to the penis with urethral damage can cause dysuria; the urine irritates the injured section of the male urethra.
- **Urethral Lithiasis:** Secondary to passing a kidney stone. As the stone passes through the male urethra, transient discomfort occurs.
- **Urinary Retention:** Prostate enlargement or a urethral stricture can cause obstructive symptoms and discomfort. True dysuria is usually absent, unless there is a concomitant UTI.

URINE, BLOOD IN

Definition

- Blood in the urine can make it red, pink, brown, or tea colored.

TRIAGE ASSESSMENT QUESTIONS

Call EMS 911 Now

- Shock suspected (e.g., cold/pale/clammy skin, too weak to stand, low BP, rapid pulse)
  R/O: urosepsis, shock
  First Aid: Lie down with the feet elevated.
- Sounds like a life-threatening emergency to the triager

Go to ED Now

- Recent back or abdominal injury
  R/O: kidney or bladder injury
- Recent genital injury
  R/O: urethral injury
- Unable to urinate (or only a few drops) > 4 hours and bladder feels very full (e.g., palpable bladder or strong urge to urinate)
  R/O: acute urinary retention
- Passing pure blood or large blood clots (i.e., larger than a dime or grape)

Go to ED/UCC Now
(or to Office With PCP Approval)

- Fever > 100.5° F (38.1° C)
  R/O: pyelonephritis
- Patient sounds very sick or weak to the triager
  Reason: severe acute illness or serious complication suspected

Go to Office Now

- Known sickle cell disease
  R/O: papillary necrosis
- Taking Coumadin (warfarin) or other strong blood thinner, or known bleeding disorder (e.g., thrombocytopenia)
  Reason: higher risk of serious bleeding; may need testing of INR, prothrombin time, or platelet count
  Note: Besides Coumadin, other strong blood thinners include Arixtra (fondaparinux), Eliquis (apixaban), Pradaxa (dabigatran), and Xarelto (rivaroxaban). Plavix (clopidogrel; antiplatelet drug) also increases risk in head injury.

See Today in Office

- Side (flank) or back pain present
  R/O: kidney stone (ureteral colic)
- Pain or burning with passing urine
  R/O: cystitis
- Patient wants to be seen

See Today or Tomorrow in Office

- Pink or red-colored urine and likely from food (beets, rhubarb, red food dye) and lasts > 24 hours after stopping food
  Reason: sometimes eating a large amount of red-colored food like beets can give a pink or red color to the urine; however, this should go away soon after stopping the suspected food
- All other patients with blood in urine
  (Exception: could be normal menstrual bleeding)
  Reason: evaluation for hematuria

Home Care

- ○ Female and before menopause and could be normal menstrual bleeding
- ○ Pink or red-colored urine and likely from food (beets, rhubarb, red food dye)

HOME CARE ADVICE

General Care Advice for Blood in Urine

❶ **Fluids:** Drink extra fluids.
  (Reason: to produce a dilute, nonirritating urine)
❷ **Call Back If:**
  • You become worse.

Blood in Urine From Menstrual Bleeding

❶ **Call Back If:**
  • You decide the blood in the urine is not from normal menstrual bleeding.
  • You become worse.

Pink or Red-Colored Urine From Food

❶ **Reassurance:**
  • From what you told me, you have eaten something that can change your urine color.
  • You have also told me that you have no other symptoms or injury.
  • Certain foods, such as beets, rhubarb, or red food dye, can make your urine pink or red colored.
  • Your urine will likely turn back to normal color when you stop this food.
❷ **Stop** eating the red-colored food.
❸ **Call Back If:**
  • You stop eating the red-colored food and the pink or red color of your urine lasts > 24 hours.
  • You develop any new symptoms (e.g., fever, pain with urination, blood clots seen in urine).
  • You become worse.

BACKGROUND

Key Points

• **Gross Hematuria:** Medical term for visible blood in the urine. Even a small amount of blood can make the urine appear quite red.
• **Foods:** Certain foods can temporarily give a red tint to the urine. Examples include beets, rhubarb, and red food coloring.
• **Drugs:** Certain drugs can also temporarily give an orange or red tint to the urine. Pyridium (phenazopyridine) is a bladder anesthetic that is used in treating patients with cystitis; it turns the urine bright orange. Rifampin is an antibiotic; it turns the urine red-orange.

Common Causes of Gross Hematuria

• Benign prostatic hypertrophy (men)
• Bladder surgery
• Cancer (kidney, bladder, or prostate)
• Coagulopathy (excessive Coumadin, bleeding disorders)
• Infection (cystitis, pyelonephritis)
• Kidney or ureteral stone
• Nephritis
• Procedures (urinary tract stenting, biopsy of prostate)
• Prostate surgery (transurethral resection of the prostate [TURP])
• Trauma (injury to urethra, bladder, ureter, kidney)

VAGINAL BLEEDING, ABNORMAL

Definition

Menstrual bleeding is abnormal or excessive when any of the following occur:

- > 7 days (1 week) of bleeding.
- > 6 well-soaked pads or tampons per day.
- > 21 pads or tampons per menstrual period.
- Large blood clots (e.g., large coin, golf ball).
- Periods occur more frequently than every 21 days.
- Periods occur less frequently than every 35 days.
- Any bleeding or spotting between regular periods.
- Has been diagnosed with anemia.

Note: On a practical level, if the woman feels that the amount of bleeding is excessive or heavier than normal periods, she should probably be seen and evaluated.

Includes: Health information for abnormal vaginal bleeding associated with Depo-Provera, Norplant, birth control patches, missed birth control pills, contraceptive ring (i.e., NuvaRing), and Mirena IUD.

Vaginal Bleeding Severity:

- **Spotting:** Pinkish/brownish mucus discharge; does not fill panty liner or pad.
- **Mild:** < 1 pad/hour; < patient's usual menstrual bleeding.
- **Moderate:** 1-2 pads/hour; small-medium blood clots (e.g., pea, grape, small coin).
- **Severe:** Soaking ≥ 2 pads/hour for ≥ 2 hours; bleeding not contained by pads or continuous red blood from vagina; large blood clots (e.g., golf ball, large coin).

TRIAGE ASSESSMENT QUESTIONS

Call EMS 911 Now

- SEVERE vaginal bleeding (e.g., continuous red blood from vagina or large blood clots) and very weak (can't stand)
  R/O: shock
  First Aid: Lie down with the feet elevated.
- Passed out (i.e., fainted, collapsed and was not responding)
  R/O: shock
  First Aid: Lie down with the feet elevated.
- Difficult to awaken or acting confused (e.g., disoriented, slurred speech)
  R/O: shock
  First Aid: Lie down with the feet elevated.
- Shock suspected (e.g., cold/pale/clammy skin, too weak to stand)
  R/O: shock
  First Aid: Lie down with the feet elevated.
- Sounds like a life-threatening emergency to the triager

See More Appropriate Protocol

- Vaginal discharge is the main symptom and bleeding is slight
  Go to Protocol: Vaginal Discharge on page 431

Go to ED Now

- SEVERE abdominal pain (e.g., excruciating)
  R/O: ectopic pregnancy
- SEVERE dizziness (e.g., unable to stand, requires support to walk, feels like passing out now)
  R/O: anemia

Go to ED/UCC Now
(or to Office With PCP Approval)

- SEVERE vaginal bleeding (i.e., soaking 2 pads or tampons per hour and present ≥ 2 hours)
  Reason: severe bleeding
- MODERATE vaginal bleeding (i.e., soaking pad or tampon per hour and present > 6 hours)
  Reason: prolonged moderate bleeding
- Pale skin (pallor) of new onset or worsening
- Constant abdominal pain lasting > 2 hours
  R/O: endometritis, ectopic pregnancy
- Patient sounds very sick or weak to the triager
  Reason: severe acute illness or serious complication suspected

See Today in Office

● Taking Coumadin (warfarin) or other strong blood thinner, or known bleeding disorder (e.g., thrombocytopenia)
Reason: higher risk of serious bleeding; may need testing of INR, prothrombin time, or platelet count
Note: Besides Coumadin, other strong blood thinners include Arixtra (fondaparinux), Eliquis (apixaban), Pradaxa (dabigatran), and Xarelto (rivaroxaban). Plavix (clopidogrel; antiplatelet drug) also increases risk in head injury.

● Skin bruises or nosebleed and not caused by an injury
R/O: bleeding disorder

● Bleeding/spotting after procedure (e.g., biopsy) or pelvic examination (e.g., Papanicolaou [Pap] smear) that persists > 3 days

● Patient wants to be seen

Discuss With PCP and Callback by Nurse Today

● Passed tissue (e.g., gray-white)
Reason: patient reports that she is not pregnant, so probably not a miscarriage; still, a home pregnancy test should be performed to be certain

See Within 3 Days in Office

● Periods with > 6 soaked pads or tampons per day
Reason: excessive vaginal bleeding, check for anemia

See Within 2 Weeks in Office

● Periods last > 7 days
Reason: excessive vaginal bleeding, check for anemia

● Missed period has occurred ≥ 2 times in the last year and the cause is not known
Reason: may need further evaluation and testing

● Menstrual cycle < 21 days OR > 35 days, and occurs > 2 cycles (2 months) this past year
Reason: may need further evaluation and testing

● Bleeding or spotting between regular periods occurs > 2 cycles (2 months)
R/O: dysfunctional uterine bleeding, fibroids, secondary anemia

● Bleeding or spotting between regular periods occurs > 2 cycles (2 months), and using birth control medicine (e.g., pills, patch, Depo-Provera, Implanon, vaginal ring, Mirena IUD)
Reason: evaluation and counseling; change in management may be needed

● Bleeding or spotting occurs after hysterectomy
Reason: no menses should occur after hysterectomy

● Age > 39 years with irregular or excessive bleeding
R/O: anovulatory bleeding from endometrial carcinoma
Reason: endometrial assessment may be needed

● Bleeding or spotting occurs after sex (Exception: first intercourse)
Reason: no bleeding should occur after sex, unless it is related to menses

Home Care

○ Normal menstrual flow

○ MILD bleeding or SPOTTING and could be pregnant (e.g., missed last period)
Reason: check home pregnancy test and call back if positive; all triage questions negative

○ MILD bleeding or SPOTTING after procedure (e.g., biopsy) or pelvic examination (e.g., Pap smear) persisting < 4 days

○ MILD bleeding or SPOTTING and immediately follows first intercourse

○ Taking birth control pills and hasn't missed taking any pills
R/O: breakthrough bleeding

○ Taking birth control pills and has missed ≥ 1 pills; or took a progestin-only pill late
R/O: expected breakthrough bleeding or spotting

○ Using Depo-Provera subdermal implant
R/O: hormone side effect

○ Has Implanon subdermal implant
Reason: bleeding is probably a common side effect of birth control hormone

○ Using birth control patch (i.e., transdermal contraceptive system)
R/O: breakthrough bleeding

○ Using vaginal contraceptive ring (i.e., NuvaRing)
R/O: breakthrough bleeding

○ Using Mirena IUD (a special IUD that releases the hormone progestin)
R/O: irregular bleeding or spotting from this hormonal IUD

HOME CARE ADVICE

Mild Vaginal Bleeding

❶ **Pregnancy Test, When in Doubt:**
- If there is a chance that you might be pregnant, use a urine pregnancy test.
- You can buy a pregnancy test at the drugstore.
- It works best if you test your first urine in the morning.
- Call back if you are pregnant.
- *Follow the instructions included in the package.*

❷ **Spotting After a Procedure or Pelvic Examination:** The cervix bleeds easily and even an internal exam, Pap smear, or biopsy of the cervix can cause some spotting. This spotting should subside within 24-72 hours.

❸ **Spotting After First Intercourse:** Mild bleeding or spotting with first intercourse is common. It should stop within 48 hours and not recur.

❹ **Iron and Anemia:** Heavy periods are the most common cause of iron deficiency anemia in women of childbearing age. Women with heavy periods should eat a diet rich in iron or take a daily multivitamin pill with iron.

❺ **Call Back If:**
- Pregnancy test is positive.
- You have difficulties with the home pregnancy test.
- Bleeding becomes worse.
- You become worse.

Irregular Vaginal Bleeding While Using Birth Control Medicine

❶ **Spotting Between Periods and Taking Birth Control Pills:** Breakthrough bleeding or spotting is common with most current birth control pills, especially during the first 3 pill pack cycles.

❷ **Irregular Bleeding and You Are Using Implanon or Depo-Provera:** Irregular bleeding is a common side effect. It may include heavier, lighter, more frequent, or less frequent bleeding than your normal periods.

❸ **Irregular Bleeding and You Are Using the Birth Control Patch:** Breakthrough bleeding or spotting is common with current birth control patches, especially during the first 3 cycles (months).

❹ **Irregular Bleeding and You Are Using the Vaginal Contraceptive Ring (i.e., NuvaRing):** Breakthrough bleeding or spotting is not common with the vaginal contraceptive ring (i.e., NuvaRing). However, it can occur, especially during the first 1 or 2 months of use (first 2 cycles).

❺ **Irregular Bleeding and You Are Using the Mirena IUD:**
- Bleeding and spotting may increase during the first several months after you get a Mirena IUD and your periods may be irregular.
- Over time your menstrual periods may become shorter or lighter.
- At some point your menstrual periods may stop completely. Your period will return after the IUD is removed by your health care professional.

❻ **Diary:** Keep a record of the days you have any bleeding or spotting.

❼ **Call Back If:**
- Irregular bleeding occurs > 2 cycles (2 months).
- Bleeding becomes worse.
- You become worse.

Missed Combined Hormone Birth Control Pill— Placebo or Reminder Pill

❶ **Directions for Missed Placebo Pills:**
- *Follow these directions if you missed ≥ 1 placebo pills (reminder pills).*
- Throw away the missed pill or pills.
- Continue taking the rest of the pills on the usual day.
- You are not at increased risk for pregnancy.
- You do not need to use a backup form of birth control.
- **Example:** Missed pill(s) during days 22-28 of a 28-day pack.

❷ **Tips for Remembering to Take Pills on Time:**
- Set an alarm on your watch or phone.
- Combine taking the pill with a daily routine.
- For example, take it after brushing your teeth in the morning.
- When traveling, keep your pill pack with you in your purse or carry-on bag.

❸ **Call Back If:**
- You have other questions or concerns.
- You become worse.

Missed or Late Taking Combined Hormone Birth Control Pill—Active Hormone Pill

❶ Late Taking 1 Active Pill (< 24 Hours Since a Pill Should Have Been Taken):
- *Follow these directions if you are late taking an active hormone pill (not placebo pills).*
- Take the late pill as soon as possible.
- Take the next pill at the usual time. This means you may need to take 2 pills at one time or 2 pills on the same day.
- There is little or no risk of becoming pregnant with one late pill.
- You do not need to use a backup method of birth control.

❷ Missed 1 Active Pill (24-48 Hours Since a Pill Should Have Been Taken):
- *Follow these directions if you missed one active hormone pill (not placebo pill).*
- Take the missed pill as soon as possible.
- Take your next pill at the usual time. This means you may need to take 2 pills at one time or 2 pills on the same day.
- There is little or no risk of becoming pregnant with one missed pill.
- You do not need to use a backup method of birth control.

❸ Missed ≥ 2 Pills on Days 1-14— 21-Day or 28-Day Pack Users:
- *Follow these directions if you missed ≥ 2 active hormone pills (not placebo pills).*
- Take one of the missed pills (most recently missed) as soon as possible.
- Throw away other missed pills.
- Continue taking the rest of your pills in your pack on the usual time, even if this means you take 2 pills on the same day.
- Use a backup contraception method (e.g., condom) or avoid having sex until you have taken the pills for 7 days in a row without missing any.
- Consider emergency contraception if unprotected sex in the past 5 days.

❹ Missed ≥ 2 Pills on Days 15-21— 21-Day or 28-Day Pack Users:
- *Follow these directions if you missed ≥ 2 active hormone pills (not placebo pills).*
- Take one of the missed pills (most recently missed) as soon as possible. Throw away other missed pills.
- Continue taking the rest of your pills in your pack on the usual time, even if this means you take 2 pills on the same day.
- Skip the placebo (reminder) pills (or hormone-free week if using a 21-day pack). Start a new pack the very next day.
- Use a backup contraception method (e.g., condom) or avoid having sex until you have taken the pills for 7 days in a row without missing any.
- Consider emergency contraception if unprotected sex in the past 5 days.

❺ Pregnancy Test, When in Doubt:
- If there is a chance that you might be pregnant, use a urine pregnancy test.
- You can buy a pregnancy test at the drugstore.
- It works best if you test your first urine in the morning.
- Call back if you are pregnant.
- *Follow the instructions included in the package.*

❻ Emergency Contraceptive Pills (ECPs)— When to Consider:
- Emergency contraception pills (ECPs) can be used by any woman who is worried she might become pregnant.
- ECPs should be taken as soon as possible within 5 days after unprotected sex.
- The sooner ECPs are taken, the more effective they are.

❼ Call Back If:
- You have other questions or concerns.
- You become worse.

Missed or Late Taking Progestin-Only Pill (POP)

❶ Progestin-Only Pill (POP):

- The progestin-only pill (POP), also called the "mini-pill," is different from combined birth control pills.
- POPs contain only one hormone (progestin) instead of 2 (progestin and estrogen).

❷ POP—Directions for Missed or Late Pills:

- *Follow these directions if you miss a pill or take a pill > 3 hours late.*
- Take the missed or late pill as soon as possible.
- Keep taking the rest of your pills at your usual time every day.
- This means you may need to take 2 at one time or 2 pills on the same day.

❸ Backup Form of Birth Control Is Needed:

- *Follow these directions if you miss a pill or take a pill > 3 hours late.*
- Avoid having sex, or use a backup method of birth control.
- You will need to do this until you have taken pills on time for 2 days in a row.
- Examples of backup birth control include condoms, spermicide, diaphragm, or sponge.

❹ Emergency Contraceptive Pills (ECPs)— When to Consider:

- Emergency contraception pills (ECPs) can be used by any woman who is worried she might become pregnant.
- Emergency contraception should be considered if the woman has had unprotected sexual intercourse.
- ECPs should be started as soon as possible within 5 days after unprotected sex.
- The sooner ECPs are taken, the more effective they are.

❺ Pregnancy Test, When in Doubt:

- If there is a chance that you might be pregnant, use a urine pregnancy test.
- You can buy a pregnancy test at the drugstore.
- It works best if you test your first urine in the morning.
- Call back if you are pregnant.
- *Follow the instructions included in the package.*

❻ Tips for Remembering to Take Pills on Time:

- Set an alarm on your watch or phone.
- Combine taking the pill with a daily routine.
- For example, take it after brushing your teeth in the morning.
- When traveling, keep your pill pack with you in your purse or carry-on bag.

❼ Call Back If:

- You have other questions or concerns.
- You become worse.

FIRST AID

First Aid Advice for Shock:

Lie down with the feet elevated.

BACKGROUND

Key Points

- The first day of menstrual bleeding is considered the first day of a new menstrual cycle.
- Menstrual bleeding typically lasts 3-7 days. The heaviest flow usually occurs during the first 1-3 days.
- Ovulation generally occurs around day 14 of the cycle.
- The length of the menstrual cycle varies from woman to woman. The range is from 24-35 days. The average is 28 days.
- Excessive vaginal bleeding is the most common cause of iron deficiency anemia in women of childbearing age.

Causes of Abnormal Vaginal Bleeding, Age 12-18 Years

Menarche is the first menstrual cycle. Worldwide the average age of menarche is 13 years old. Teens (age 12-18 years) may have abnormal vaginal bleeding during the year after menarche. This is normal. It does not require immediate evaluation unless the bleeding is unusually prolonged, quite severe, or associated with signs and symptoms of severe anemia (e.g., pale skin, weakness).

Coagulopathy is a rare cause of excessive vaginal bleeding. Von Willebrand disease is a type of inherited coagulopathy in which there is a problem with platelet function. It may be first diagnosed in the teenage years because of excessive vaginal bleeding.

Causes of Abnormal Vaginal Bleeding, Age 18 Years to Menopause

Women from age 18 years to menopause may have abnormal bleeding from a number of common causes, including anovulation, uterine leiomyomas, or as a side effect of hormonal contraceptive use.

Obtaining a prior history of vaginal bleeding problems can sometimes be helpful with triage. For example, a known history of polycystic ovarian disease with no recent increase in symptoms might reduce the urgency of the disposition. Pregnancy must be considered as a cause of abnormal uterine bleeding in all women of reproductive age.

Unfortunately, endometrial cancer can occur at any age. However, it becomes a more common cause and real concern in women > 35-40 years of age. Abnormal vaginal bleeding in women > 40 should be evaluated by the primary care physician for the possibility of endometrial cancer.

Here is a list of causes of abnormal vaginal bleeding:
- **Adenomyosis:** Endometriosis of the muscular wall of the uterus
- Anovulatory uterine bleeding (e.g., from hyperprolactinemia, hypothyroidism, polycystic ovarian disease)
- Cervical cancer
- Coagulopathy (e.g., Von Willebrand)
- Dysfunctional uterine bleeding
- Endometritis
- Medication effect (e.g., birth control medications)
- Recent dilation and curettage
- Recent gynecologic biopsy
- Recent treatment for abnormal Pap smear
- Uterine cancer
- Uterine (endometrial) hyperplasia
- Uterine polyps
- Uterine leiomyoma (fibroids of the uterus)

Caution: Pregnancy

- The possibility of pregnancy must be considered in all women in their childbearing years who have vaginal bleeding.
- In early pregnancy, vaginal bleeding can be a sign of serious problems like miscarriage (spontaneous abortion) or ectopic pregnancy.
- In late pregnancy, vaginal bleeding can be a sign of serious problems like placenta previa or abruptio placentae.

VAGINAL DISCHARGE

Definition
- Vaginal discharge

TRIAGE ASSESSMENT QUESTIONS

See More Appropriate Protocol
- Pain or burning with passing urine is the main symptom
  Go to Protocol: Urination Pain (Female) on page 418

Go to ED/UCC Now
(or to Office With PCP Approval)
- SEVERE abdominal pain (e.g., excruciating)
  R/O: acute salpingitis, ectopic pregnancy, appendicitis
- Patient sounds very sick or weak to the triager
  Reason: severe acute illness or serious complication suspected

Go to Office Now
- Yellow or green vaginal discharge and has a fever
  R/O: acute salpingitis
- Constant abdominal pain lasting > 2 hours
  R/O: acute salpingitis, ectopic pregnancy, appendicitis

See Today in Office
- Mild lower abdominal pain comes and goes (cramps) that lasts > 24 hours
  R/O: salpingitis
- Genital area looks infected (e.g., draining sore, spreading redness)
  R/O: STI, cellulitis, Bartholin cyst
- Rash is tiny water blisters (≥ 3)
  R/O: herpes simplex, pustules
- Patient wants to be seen

See Today or Tomorrow in Office
- Rash (e.g., redness, tiny bumps, sore) of genital area present > 24 hours
  R/O: herpes, pubic lice, genital warts, or other STI

See Within 3 Days in Office
- Bad smelling vaginal discharge
  R/O: vulvovaginitis from trichomonas or bacterial vaginosis
- Abnormal color vaginal discharge (i.e., yellow, green, gray)
  R/O: vulvovaginitis from trichomonas or bacterial vaginosis
- Symptoms of a yeast infection (i.e., itchy, white discharge, not bad smelling) and not improved > 3 days following Home Care Advice
- ≥ 4 episodes of vaginal infection in past year
  Reason: recurrent vulvovaginitis; consider diabetes or other medical disorder
- Diabetes mellitus or weak immune system (e.g., HIV positive, cancer chemotherapy, splenectomy, organ transplant, chronic steroids)
  R/O: complicated vulvovaginitis
- Patient is worried about an STI
  Reason: to relieve fear or prevent spread of STI
- Pain with sexual intercourse (dyspareunia)
  (Exception: vaginal yeast infection suspected)
  R/O: salpingitis, STI

Home Care
- Normal vaginal discharge
  R/O: physiologic discharge
- Symptoms of a vaginal yeast infection (i.e., white, thick, cottage-cheese–like, itchy, not bad-smelling discharge)
  Reason: probable vaginal yeast infection

HOME CARE ADVICE

❶ **Pregnancy Test, When in Doubt:**
  - If there is a chance that you might be pregnant, use a urine pregnancy test.
  - You can buy a pregnancy test at the drugstore.
  - It works best if you test your first urine in the morning.
  - Call back if you are pregnant.
  - *Follow the instructions included in the package.*

❷ Antifungal Medicine for Vaginal Yeast Infection:
There are a number of over-the-counter medications for the treatment of vaginal yeast infections.
- **Available in the United States:** Femstat-3, miconazole (Monistat-3), clotrimazole (Gyne-Lotrimin-3, Mycelex-7), butoconazole (Femstat-3).
- **Available in Canada:** Miconazole (Monistat-3) and clotrimazole (Canesten-3, Myclo-Gyne).
- Do not use yeast medication during the 24 hours prior to a physician appointment.
  (*Reason: interferes with examination*)
- CAUTION: If you are pregnant, speak with your doctor before using.
- *Before taking any medicine, read all the instructions on the package.*

❸ Genital Hygiene:
- Keep your genital area clean. Wash daily.
- Keep your genital area dry. Wear cotton underwear or underwear with a cotton crotch.
- Do not douche.
- Do not use feminine hygiene products.

❹ Call Back If:
- Pregnancy test is positive.
- You have difficulties with the home pregnancy test.
- There is no improvement after treating yourself for a vaginal yeast infection.
- You become worse.

BACKGROUND

Normal Vaginal Discharge
- Normal vaginal discharge may be clear or white, thin or thick.
- It is not odorous and there is no itching.

Abnormal Vaginal Discharge
- **Color:** Yellow, green, or gray-colored vaginal discharge is usually abnormal. Vulvovaginitis from *Trichomonas* or bacterial vaginosis should be suspected.
- **Smell:** Bad or foul-smelling discharge is usually abnormal. Vulvovaginitis from *Trichomonas* or bacterial vaginosis should be suspected.
- **Consistency:** A thick, white, cottage-cheese–like, non-odorous, itchy discharge is usually abnormal. A yeast infection (vulvovaginitis from *Candida*) should be suspected.

Causes of Vaginal Discharge
- **Atrophic Vaginitis:** Perimenopausal and post-menopausal women will often describe itching and dryness of the vulvovaginal area. This is the result of atrophic changes in this area from the lack of estrogen stimulation.
- **Cervicitis:** Gonorrhea and chlamydia are sexually transmitted infections (STIs) that can cause cervicitis. Symptoms can include vaginal discharge, dysuria, pelvic pain, and bleeding.
- **Contact Dermatitis and Irritation:** Douching, soaps, and other chemical products can sometimes cause symptoms of itching and irritation.
- **Pelvic Inflammatory Disease (PID):** PID is an infection of the tubes connecting the ovaries to the uterus. PID is a serious illness which, in some cases, requires hospitalization and IV antibiotics. The clinical presentation of PID is variable, but symptoms classically include lower abdominal/pelvic pain, fever, and vaginal discharge.
- **Vaginal Foreign Bodies (FBs):** Vaginal FBs must be removed to prevent a vaginal infection. Sometimes FBs are not discovered until after the patient comes in for a bad-smelling yellow vaginal discharge. Most vaginal FBs can be easily removed in the doctor's office.
- **Vulvovaginitis:** Vaginal discharge and vulvovaginal itching are the symptoms of vulvovaginitis. The 3 main types of vulvovaginitis are candidiasis ("yeast infection"; symptoms of thick, white, cottage-cheese–like, non-odorous discharge), *Trichomonas* (foamy, yellow-green, foul-smelling discharge), and bacterial vaginosis (white-gray discharge, fishy odor).

Caution: Pregnancy
- The possibility of pregnancy must be considered in all women in their childbearing years.
- In the second half of pregnancy, increasing vaginal discharge can be a subtle sign of preterm labor.

VOMITING

Definition
- Vomiting ("throwing up") is the forceful emptying of a portion of the stomach's contents through the mouth.

Severity:
- **Mild:** 1-2 times/day.
- **Moderate:** 3-5 times/day, decreased oral intake without significant weight loss or symptoms of dehydration.
- **Severe:** ≥ 6 times/day, with significant weight loss, symptoms of dehydration.

Notes:
- Retching ("dry heaves") describes rhythmic contractions of the abdominal and intercostal muscles against a closed glottis (no vomit).
- Multiple episodes of retching (heaves, stomach contractions) do not count as separate episodes of vomiting. At least 5-10 minutes need to pass before one considers it another episode of vomiting.

TRIAGE ASSESSMENT QUESTIONS

Call EMS 911 Now
- Shock suspected (e.g., cold/pale/clammy skin, too weak to stand)
  R/O: shock
  First Aid: Lie down with the feet elevated.
- Difficult to awaken or acting confused (e.g., disoriented, slurred speech)
  R/O: shock
  First Aid: Lie down with the feet elevated.
- Sounds like a life-threatening emergency to the triager

See More Appropriate Protocol
- Vomiting occurs only while coughing
  Go to Protocol: Cough on page 95
- Chest pain
  Go to Protocol: Chest Pain on page 73
- Headache is main symptom
  Go to Protocol: Headache on page 207

Go to ED Now
- SEVERE vomiting (e.g., ≥ 6 times/day)
  Reason: greater risk for dehydration
- MODERATE vomiting (e.g., 3-5 times/day) and age > 60
- Vomiting contains bile (green color)
  R/O: intestinal obstruction
- Vomiting red blood or black (coffee-ground) material
  R/O: gastritis, peptic ulcer
- Insulin-dependent diabetes and glucose > 240 mg/dL (13 mmol/L)
  R/O: DKA
- Recent head injury (within 3 days)
  R/O: subdural hematoma
- Recent abdominal injury (within 7 days)
  R/O: traumatic pancreatitis

Go to ED/UCC Now
(or to Office With PCP Approval)
- Drinking very little and has signs of dehydration (e.g., no urine > 12 hours, very dry mouth, very light-headed)
  Reason: IV therapy needed
- Constant abdominal pain lasting > 2 hours
  R/O: GI obstruction
- HIGH-RISK adult (e.g., brain tumor, ventriculoperitoneal shunt, hernia)
- Severe pain in one eye
  R/O: acute glaucoma
- Patient sounds very sick or weak to the triager
  Reason: severe acute illness or serious complication suspected

Go to Office Now
- MILD-MODERATE vomiting (e.g., 1-5 times/day) and abdomen looks much more swollen than usual
  R/O: intestinal obstruction
- Fever > 103° F (39.4° C)
- Fever > 100.5° F (38.1° C) and > 60 years of age
- Fever > 100.0° F (37.8° C) and has a weak immune system (e.g., HIV positive, cancer chemotherapy, organ transplant, splenectomy, chronic steroids)

● Fever > 100.0° F (37.8° C) and bedridden (e.g., nursing home patient, stroke, chronic illness, recovering from surgery)
Reason: higher risk of bacterial infection
Note: May need ambulance transport to ED.

● Taking any of the following medications: digoxin (Lanoxin), lithium, theophylline, phenytoin (Dilantin)
R/O: drug toxicity

Callback by PCP Within 1 Hour

● Severe headache and vomiting
R/O: migraine, increased ICP

See Today in Office

● MILD-MODERATE vomiting (e.g., 1-5 times/day) and lasts > 48 hours (2 days)
● Fever present > 3 days (72 hours)
● Patient wants to be seen

Callback by PCP Today

● Vomiting a prescription medication
Reason: the medication may be important for health; a new medication may be causing vomiting

See Within 3 Days in Office

● Alcohol abuse, known or suspected

See Within 2 Weeks in Office

● Vomiting is a chronic symptom (recurrent or ongoing AND lasting > 4 weeks)

Home Care

○ Vomiting
○ Vomiting with diarrhea

HOME CARE ADVICE

Vomiting

❶ Reassurance—Severe Vomiting:
• Sometimes patients vomit everything for 3 or 4 hours, even if drinking small amounts. From what you've told me, you are well hydrated.
• Vomiting can be caused by many types of illnesses. It can be caused by a stomach flu virus. It can be caused by eating or drinking something that disagreed with your stomach.
• Adults with vomiting need to stay hydrated. This is the most important thing. If you don't drink and replace lost fluids, you may get dehydrated.

• You can treat vomiting, even if there is mild dehydration, at home.
• *Here is some care advice that should help.*

❷ Reassurance—Mild-Moderate Vomiting:
• Vomiting can be caused by many types of illnesses. It can be caused by a stomach flu virus. It can be caused by eating or drinking something that disagreed with your stomach.
• Adults with vomiting need to stay hydrated. This is the most important thing. If you don't drink and replace lost fluids, you may get dehydrated.
• You can treat vomiting, even if there is mild dehydration, at home.
• *Here is some care advice that should help.*

❸ For Nonstop Vomiting, Try Sleeping:
• Try to go to sleep.
(Reason: Sleep often empties the stomach and relieves the need to vomit.)
• When you awaken, resume drinking liquids. Water works best initially.

❹ Clear Liquids: Try to sip small amounts (1 tablespoon or 15 mL) of liquid frequently (every 5 minutes) for 8 hours, rather than trying to drink a lot of liquid all at one time.
• Sip water or a ½-strength sports drink (e.g., Gatorade or Powerade).
• **Other Options:** ½-strength flat lemon-lime soda or ginger ale.
• After 4 hours without vomiting, increase the amount.

❺ Solid Food:
• You may begin eating bland foods after 8 hours without vomiting.
• Start with saltine crackers, white bread, rice, mashed potatoes, cereal, applesauce, etc.
• You can resume a normal diet in 24-48 hours.

❻ Avoid Nonprescription Medicines:
• Stop all nonprescription medicines for 24 hours.
(Reason: They may make vomiting worse.)
• Call if vomiting a prescription medicine.

❼ Contagiousness: You can return to work or school after vomiting and fever are gone.

❽ Expected Course:
- Vomiting from viral gastritis usually stops in 12-48 hours.
- If diarrhea is present, it usually lasts for several days.
- People with mild dehydration can usually treat themselves at home, by drinking more liquids.
- People with moderate-severe dehydration may need medical care. Signs of this include very dry mouth, dizziness, weakness, and decreased urination.

❾ Call Back If:
- Vomiting lasts for > 2 days (48 hours).
- Signs of dehydration occur.
- You become worse.

Vomiting With Diarrhea

❶ Reassurance:
- Vomiting and diarrhea are often caused by viral gastroenteritis (stomach flu) or mild food poisoning.
- Adults with vomiting need to stay hydrated. This is the most important thing. If you don't drink and replace lost fluids, you may get dehydrated.
- You can treat vomiting, even if there is mild dehydration, at home.
- *Here is some care advice that should help.*

❷ Clear Liquids: Try to sip small amounts (1 tablespoon or 15 mL) of liquid frequently (every 5 minutes) for 8 hours, rather than trying to drink a lot of liquid all at one time.
- Sip water or a ½-strength sports drink (e.g., Gatorade or Powerade).
- **Other Options:** ½-strength flat lemon-lime soda or ginger ale.
- After 4 hours without vomiting, increase the amount.

❸ Solid Food:
- You may begin eating bland foods after 8 hours without vomiting.
- Start with saltine crackers, white bread, rice, mashed potatoes, cereal, applesauce, etc.
- You can resume a normal diet in 24-48 hours.

❹ Avoid Nonprescription Medicines:
- Stop all nonprescription medicines for 24 hours. *(Reason: They may make vomiting worse.)*
- Call if vomiting a prescription medicine.

❺ Expected Course:
- Vomiting from viral gastroenteritis (stomach flu) or mild food poisoning usually stops in 12-48 hours.
- Diarrhea often lasts for several days. For mild diarrhea, follow the care advice for vomiting; you don't need to do anything special for mild diarrhea.
- People with mild dehydration can usually treat themselves at home, by drinking more liquids.
- People with moderate-severe dehydration may need medical care. Signs of this include very dry mouth, dizziness, weakness, and decreased urination.

❻ Call Back If:
- Vomiting lasts for > 2 days (48 hours).
- Diarrhea lasts > 7 days.
- Signs of dehydration occur.
- You become worse.

Vomiting a Prescription Medicine

❶ Did See Pill in Vomit (usually < 30 minutes after taking pill):
- If you see the pill in your vomit it is OK to take that pill again.
- You might want to wait a little while until your stomach is less upset. You might want to take it with a little bit of water and simple food, like a cracker.

❷ Did Not See Pill in Vomit: You should wait until the next time you are supposed to take this drug.

❸ Call Back If:
- Vomiting lasts for > 2 days (48 hours).
- Signs of dehydration occur.
- You have more questions.
- You become worse.

FIRST AID

First Aid Advice for Shock:
Lie down with the feet elevated.

BACKGROUND

Key Points

- Vomiting can occur in many type of illnesses.
- Nausea and abdominal discomfort usually precede each bout of vomiting.
- Vomiting occurring with diarrhea is suggestive of gastroenteritis (stomach flu) or some type of food poisoning. Most such patients can be managed at home.
- Maintaining hydration is the cornerstone of treatment of adults with acute vomiting. Patients with moderate-severe dehydration will require medical evaluaion, usually in an ED or UCC.
- In general, an adult who is alert, feels well, and who is not thirsty or dizzy is NOT dehydrated.

Causes of Vomiting

- **Appendicitis.**
- **Bowel obstruction.**
- **Central Nervous System:** Increased intracranial pressure may lead to vomiting.
- **Diabetic Ketoacidosis (DKA):** This is seen in people with diabetes who are taking insulin. Vomiting in people with insulin-dependent diabetes should be taken seriously and usually requires an ED disposition.
- **Emotional response to certain smells.**
- **Food allergy.**
- **Food-borne Illness** ("food poisoning"): Food poisoning is caused by toxins produced by bacteria growing in poorly refrigerated foods (e.g., *Staphylococcus* toxin in egg salad or *Bacillus cereus* toxin in rice dishes). Food-borne illnesses usually present with gastrointestinal symptoms of vomiting, diarrhea, and/or abdominal pain. The symptoms and their duration depend on the type of infection.
- **Gastritis and Gastroenteritis** ("stomach flu"): There are many viral and bacterial causes. This is a common cause.
- **Hepatitis.**
- **Labyrinthine Disorders:** This grouping includes labyrinthitis and motion sickness. Typical symptoms are episodes of vertigo with nausea and vomiting.
- **Medications:** This may be the most common cause in adults and certainly should be considered in elderly adults. Some examples include digoxin, narcotics, erythromycin, NSAIDs, and anticancer drugs.
- **Migraine Headaches:** Vomiting occurs commonly in some patients with migraine or cluster headaches.

- **Neurologic Disease:** Meningitis, encephalitis, Reye syndrome, blocked ventriculoperitoneal shunt, head trauma, and other causes of increased intracranial pressure.
- **Postoperative vomiting.**
- **Renal Colic** (kidney stone attack): Nausea and vomiting commonly accompany the flank pain of a kidney stone attack.
- **Vomiting in first trimester of pregnancy** (i.e., morning sickness).

Dehydration: Estimation by Telephone

Mild Dehydration

❶ **Urine Production:** Slightly decreased

❷ **Mucous Membranes:** Normal

❸ Heart rate < 100 beats/minute

❹ Slightly thirsty

❺ **Capillary Refill:** < 2 seconds

❻ **Treatment:** Can usually treat at home.

Moderate Dehydration

❶ **Urine Production:** Minimal or absent.

❷ **Mucous Membranes:** Dry inside of mouth.

❸ Heart rate 100-130 beats/minute.

❹ Thirsty, light-headed when standing.

❺ **Capillary Refill:** > 2 seconds.

❻ **Treatment:** Must be seen; go to ED NOW (or PCP triage).

Severe Dehydration

❶ **Urine Production:** None > 12 hours.

❷ **Mucous Membranes:** Very dry inside of mouth.

❸ Heart rate > 130 beats/minute.

❹ Very thirsty, very weak, and light-headed; fainting may occur.

❺ **Capillary Refill:** > 2-4 seconds.

❻ **Treatment:** Must be seen immediately; go to ED NOW or call EMS 911 NOW.

Signs of Shock

❶ Confused, difficult to awaken, or unresponsive.

❷ Heart rate (pulse) is rapid and weak.

❸ Extremities (especially hands and feet) are bluish or gray, and cold.

❹ Too weak to stand or very dizzy when tries to stand.

❺ **Capillary Refill:** > 4 seconds.

❻ **Treatment:** Lie down with the feet elevated; call EMS 911 NOW.

VULVAR SYMPTOMS

Definition
- Itching or dryness of external female genital area (vulva)
- Rashes of external female genital area including: sores, redness, blisters, lumps

Note:
- If vaginal discharge is the main symptom, see Vaginal Discharge protocol on page 431.

TRIAGE ASSESSMENT QUESTIONS

See More Appropriate Protocol
- Pain or burning with passing urine is the main symptom
  Go to Protocol: Urination Pain (Female) on page 418
- Vaginal discharge is the main symptom
  Go to Protocol: Vaginal Discharge on page 431
- Pubic lice suspected
  Go to Protocol: Pubic Lice on page 317
- STI exposure and prevention, question about
  Go to Protocol: STI Exposure and Prevention on page 377

Go to ED/UCC Now
(or to Office With PCP Approval)
- Patient sounds very sick or weak to the triager
  Reason: severe acute illness or serious complication suspected

Go to Office Now
- SEVERE pain (e.g., excruciating)
  R/O: Bartholin cyst, herpes simplex

See Today in Office
- Genital area looks infected (e.g., draining sore, spreading redness)
  R/O: STI, cellulitis, Bartholin cyst
- Rash with painful tiny water blisters
  R/O: herpes simplex
- Patient wants to be seen

See Today or Tomorrow in Office
- MODERATE-SEVERE itching
  (i.e., interferes with school, work, or sleep)
  R/O: contact dermatitis, poison ivy, pubic lice
- Rash (e.g., redness, tiny bumps, sore) of genital area present > 24 hours
  R/O: herpes, pubic lice, genital warts
- Tender lump (swelling or "ball") at vaginal opening
  R/O: Bartholin cyst
  Note: The cyst is in the left or right labia.
- Vulvar itching and not improved > 3 days following Home Care Advice
  R/O: contact dermatitis, lichen sclerosis, STI
- Symptoms of a "yeast infection" (i.e., itchy, white discharge, not bad smelling) and not improved > 3 days following Home Care Advice

See Within 3 Days in Office
- Patient is worried about an STI
  Reason: to relieve fear or prevent spread of STI

See Within 2 Weeks in Office
- Itching or dryness of genital area and nearing menopause or after menopause
  R/O: atrophic vaginitis, dermatoses
- Pain in genital area is a chronic symptom (recurrent or ongoing AND lasting > 4 weeks)
  R/O: vulvodynia
- ALL other vulvar symptoms
  (Exception: feels like prior yeast infection, or rash < 24-hour duration)
  R/O: skin dermatoses or cancer, atrophic changes, psoriasis

Home Care
- Symptoms of a "yeast infection" (i.e., itchy, white discharge, not bad smelling), which feels like prior vaginal yeast infections
  R/O: yeast vulvovaginitis
- Rash (e.g., redness, tiny bumps, sore) of genital area present < 24 hours
  R/O: minor abrasion, mild irritation, or contact dermatitis
- Mild vulvar itching
  R/O: contact dermatitis, excess moisture

HOME CARE ADVICE

General

❶ Pregnancy Test, When in Doubt:
- If there is a chance that you might be pregnant, use a urine pregnancy test.
- You can buy a pregnancy test at the drugstore.
- It works best if you test your first urine in the morning.
- Call back if you are pregnant.
- *Follow the instructions included in the package.*

❷ Call Back If:
- Pregnancy test is positive or if you have difficulties with the home pregnancy test.
- Rash lasts > 24 hours.
- Rash spreads or becomes worse.
- Fever occurs.
- No improvement after 3 days.
- You become worse.

Symptoms of a Vaginal Yeast Infection

❶ Genital Hygiene:
- Keep your genital area clean. Wash daily.
- Keep your genital area dry. Wear cotton underwear or underwear with a cotton crotch.
- Do not douche.
- Do not use feminine hygiene products.

❷ Antifungal Medicine for Yeast Infection: There are a number of over-the-counter medications for the treatment of yeast infections.
- **Available in the United States:** Femstat-3, miconazole (Monistat-3), clotrimazole (Gyne-Lotrimin-3, Mycelex-7), butoconazole (Femstat-3).
- **Available in Canada:** Miconazole (Monistat-3) and clotrimazole (Canesten-3, Myclo-Gyne).
- Do not use yeast medication during the 24 hours prior to a physician appointment. *(Reason: interferes with examination)*
- CAUTION: If you are pregnant, speak with your doctor before using.
- *Before taking any medicine, read all the instructions on the package.*

❸ Expected Course: If there is no improvement within 3 days, then you will need to be examined.

❹ Call Back If:
- Any rash lasts > 24 hours.
- Fever occurs.
- Yellow or green vaginal discharge occurs.
- No improvement in "yeast infection" within 3 days.
- You become worse.

Mild Vulvar Itching

❶ Reassurance:
- Common causes of mild vaginal itching are new soaps/detergent, perfumed toilet products, hormone changes, and excessive perspiration. Sometimes itching can be caused by a yeast infection.
- *Here is some care advice that should help.*

❷ Genital Hygiene:
- Keep your genital area clean. Wash daily.
- Keep your genital area dry. Wear cotton underwear or underwear with a cotton crotch.
- Do not douche.
- Do not use feminine hygiene products.

❸ Cleaning: Wash the area once thoroughly with unscented soap and water to remove any irritants.

❹ Take a Sitz Bath:
- Take a 10- to 15-minute sitz bath once or twice a day. Sitting in the warm water will help soothe the irritated skin. You can make a sitz bath by adding 2 oz (60 g) of baking soda to a bathtub containing warm water.
- Afterward, dry the area by gently patting it with a towel.
- Lastly, apply a small amount of ointment or cream to help seal in the moisture. Good choices for this are Vaseline ointment or Eucerin.

❺ Call Back If:
- Any rash lasts > 24 hours.
- Fever occurs.
- Yellow or green vaginal discharge occurs.
- No improvement in "yeast infection" within 3 days.
- You become worse.

BACKGROUND

Causes

- Any preexisting skin disorders/rashes can also occur on the vulva (e.g., psoriasis, eczema, drug rashes).
- Bartholin cyst.
- Candidal vulvovaginitis (aka, "yeast infection").
- Contact dermatitis (e.g., soaps, feminine hygiene products).
- Irritation after sexual intercourse (e.g., inadequate lubrication, latex-condom allergy).
- Poison ivy.
- Skin cancer.
- Skin dermatoses (e.g., lichen sclerosis, squamous hyperplasia).
- STIs (e.g., herpes simplex, syphilis, pubic lice, genital warts).

Common Causes of Vulvar Itching

- **Contact Dermatitis—Irritant:** There are 2 different types of vulvar contact dermatitis: irritant and allergic. Products like soaps, detergents, and douches can cause local irritation. Urinary incontinence can result in the vulva being irritated by constant moisture. The treatment for irritant contact dermatitis is to avoid irritating products and to keep the vulvar area clean and dry (maintain good genital hygiene).
- **Contact Dermatitis—Allergic:** Women can develop an allergic skin reaction to a number of different OTC products. These products include: benzocaine (in Vagisil anti-itch cream), neomycin (antibiotic ointment), latex condoms, nail polish, and perfumes. The treatment for allergic contact dermatitis is to avoid allergic products and to keep the vulvar area clean and dry (maintain good genital hygiene).
- **Menopause:** At menopause the ovaries stop functioning, and as result the body produces less estrogen. Without estrogen, the skin in the genital area can become thin and women notice increased dryness. There are estrogen-based vaginal crèmes or lubricants that the physician can prescribe to reduce this itching and dryness.
- **Yeast Vulvovaginitis (Yeast Infection):** Sometimes itching can be caused by a yeast infection (*Candida*). Often there is a new or an increased vaginal discharge (thick, white, cottage-cheese–like, non-odorous discharge). There are a number of over-the-counter medications for the treatment of vaginal yeast infections.

WEAKNESS (GENERALIZED) AND FATIGUE

Definition
- Patient complains of generalized body weakness.
- Patient complains of fatigue (tiredness, lack of energy).

Severity:
- **Mild:** Feels weak or tired but does not interfere with work, school, or normal activities.
- **Moderate:** Able to stand and walk; weakness interferes with work, school, or normal activities.
- **Severe:** Unable to stand or walk.

TRIAGE ASSESSMENT QUESTIONS

Call EMS 911 Now
- SEVERE difficulty breathing (e.g., struggling for each breath, speaks in single words)
  R/O: respiratory failure, hypoxia
- Shock suspected (e.g., cold/pale/clammy skin, too weak to stand)
  R/O: shock
  First Aid: Lie down with the feet elevated.
- Difficult to awaken or acting confused (e.g., disoriented, slurred speech)
  R/O: shock
  First Aid: Lie down with the feet elevated.
- Fainted > 15 minutes ago and still feels too weak or dizzy to stand
  R/O: hypovolemia, arrhythmia
- SEVERE weakness (i.e., unable to walk or barely able to walk, requires support) and new onset or worsening
  Reason: severe weakness, acute
  R/O: anemia, cardiac problem, serious infection, volume depletion, metabolic abnormality
- Sounds like a life-threatening emergency to the triager

See More Appropriate Protocol
- Weakness of the face, arm, or leg on one side of the body
  Go to Protocol: Neurologic Deficit on page 298
- Has diabetes and weakness from low blood sugar (i.e., < 60 mg/dL or 3.5 mmol/L)
  Go to Protocol: Diabetes (Low Blood Sugar) on page 116

- Recent heat exposure, suspected cause of weakness
  Go to Protocol: Heat Exposure (Heat Exhaustion and Heatstroke) on page 214
- Vomiting is the main symptom
  Go to Protocol: Vomiting on page 433
- Diarrhea is the main symptom
  Go to Protocol: Diarrhea on page 123

Go to ED Now
- Difficulty breathing
  R/O: hypoxia with need for oxygen, acidosis
- Heart beating < 50 beats per minute OR > 140 beats per minute
  Reason: symptomatic bradycardia or tachycardia
- Extra heartbeats OR irregular heart beating (i.e., "palpitations")
  R/O: dysrhythmia
- Follows bleeding (e.g., from vomiting, rectum, vagina)
  R/O: hypovolemic shock from major blood loss
  (Exception: small transient weakness from sight of a small amount blood)
- Bloody, black, or tarry bowel movements
  R/O: GI bleed
  (Exception: chronic, unchanged black-gray bowel movements and is taking iron pills or Pepto-Bismol)

Go to ED/UCC Now
(or to Office With PCP Approval)
- MODERATE weakness from poor fluid intake with no improvement after 2 hours of rest and fluids
  Reason: may need IV hydration
- Drinking very little and dehydration suspected (e.g., no urine > 12 hours, very dry mouth, very light-headed)
  Reason: may need IV hydration
- Patient sounds very sick or weak to the triager
  Reason: severe acute illness or serious complication suspected

Go to Office Now
- MODERATE weakness (i.e., interferes with work, school, normal activities) and cause unknown *(Exceptions: weakness with acute minor illness, or weakness from poor fluid intake)*
- Fever > 103° F (39.4° C) and not able to get the fever down using Home Care Advice
- Fever > 100.0° F (37.8° C) and bedridden (e.g., nursing home patient, stroke, chronic illness, recovering from surgery)
  Reason: higher risk of bacterial infection
  Note: May need ambulance transport to ED.
- Fever > 100.5° F (38.1° C) and > 60 years of age
- Fever > 100.0° F (37.8° C) and diabetes mellitus or weak immune system (e.g., HIV positive, cancer chemotherapy, splenectomy, organ transplant, chronic steroids)
- Pale skin (pallor)

See Today in Office
- MODERATE weakness (i.e., interferes with work, school, normal activities) and persists > 3 days
- Taking a medicine that could cause weakness (e.g., blood pressure medications, diuretics)
- Patient wants to be seen

See Within 3 Days in Office
- MILD weakness (i.e., does not interfere with ability to work, go to school, normal activities) and persists > 1 week
  R/O: depression, stress, anemia, viral syndrome, broad range of other medical conditions
- Fatigue (i.e., tires easily, decreased energy) and persists > 1 week
  R/O: depression, stress, chronic fatigue syndrome, insufficient sleep, broad range of other medical conditions

See Within 2 Weeks in Office
- Weakness is a chronic symptom (recurrent or ongoing AND lasting > 4 weeks)
  Reason: reevaluation of chronic unchanged symptom.

Home Care
- MILD weakness or fatigue with acute minor illness (e.g., colds)
- Weakness from poor fluid intake

HOME CARE ADVICE

Weakness or Fatigue From Acute Minor Illness
(e.g., colds, viral syndrome)
❶ **Reassurance:**
- Weakness often accompanies viral illnesses (e.g., colds and flu).
- The weakness is usually worse the first 3 days of the illness, then gets better.
- A fever can make you feel weak.
- *Here is some care advice that should help.*
❷ **Fever Medicines:**
- For fevers > 101° F (38.3° C) take either acetaminophen or ibuprofen.
- They are over-the-counter (OTC) drugs that help treat both fever and pain. You can buy them at the drugstore.
- The goal of fever therapy is to bring the fever down to a comfortable level. Remember that fever medicine usually lowers fever 2° F (1-1½° C).

Acetaminophen (e.g., Tylenol):
- **Regular Strength Tylenol:** Take 650 mg (two 325 mg pills) by mouth every 4-6 hours as needed. Each Regular Strength Tylenol pill has 325 mg of acetaminophen.
- **Extra Strength Tylenol:** Take 1,000 mg (two 500 mg pills) every 8 hours as needed. Each Extra Strength Tylenol pill has 500 mg of acetaminophen.
- The most you should take each day is 3,000 mg (10 Regular Strength or 6 Extra Strength pills a day).

Ibuprofen (e.g., Motrin, Advil):
- Take 400 mg (two 200 mg pills) by mouth every 6 hours.
- Another choice is to take 600 mg (three 200 mg pills) by mouth every 8 hours.
- The most you should take each day is 1,200 mg (six 200 mg pills), unless your doctor has told you to take more.

❸ **Fever Medicines—Extra Notes:**
- Use the lowest amount of medicine that makes your fever better.
- Acetaminophen is thought to be safer than ibuprofen or naproxen in people > 65 years old. Acetaminophen is in many OTC and prescription medicines. It might be in more than one medicine that you are taking. You need to be careful and not take an overdose. An acetaminophen overdose can hurt the liver.

- McNeil, the company that makes Tylenol, has different dosage instructions for Tylenol in Canada and the United States. In Canada, the maximum recommended dose per day is 4,000 mg or 12 Regular Strength (325 mg) pills. In the United States, McNeil recommends a maximum dose of 10 Regular Strength (325 mg) pills.
- CAUTION: Do not take acetaminophen if you have liver disease.
- CAUTION: Do not take ibuprofen if you have stomach problems, have kidney disease, are pregnant, or have been told by your doctor to avoid this type of anti-inflammatory drug. Do not take ibuprofen for > 7 days without consulting your doctor.
- *Before taking any medicine, read all the instructions on the package.*

❹ **For All Fevers:**
- Drink cold fluids to prevent dehydration. *(Reason: Good hydration replaces sweat and improves heat loss via skin.)* Adults should drink 6-8 glasses of water daily.
- Dress in one layer of lightweight clothing and sleep with one light blanket.
- For fevers 100° F-101° F (37.8° C-38.3° C) this is the only treatment and fever medicine is not needed.

❺ **Call Back If:**
- Unable to stand or walk.
- Passes out.
- Breathing difficulty occurs.
- You become worse.

Weakness From Poor Fluid Intake

❶ **Reassurance:**
- Not drinking enough fluids and being a little dehydrated is a common cause of mild weakness.
- Vomiting and diarrhea can lead to dehydration.
- During hot weather you sweat more and can become dehydrated more easily.
- *Here is some care advice that should help.*

❷ **Fluids:** Drink several glasses of fruit juice, other clear fluids, or water. This will improve hydration and blood glucose.

❸ **Rest:** Lie down with the feet elevated for 1 hour. This will improve blood flow and increase blood flow to the brain.

❹ **Cool Off:** If the weather is hot, apply a cold compress to the forehead or take a cool shower or bath.

❺ **Call Back If:**
- Still feeling weak after 2 hours of rest and fluids.
- Passes out (faints).
- You become worse.

FIRST AID

First Aid Advice for Shock:
Lie down with the feet elevated.

BACKGROUND

Key Points
- **Weakness:** Weakness is a very nonspecific symptom. It can be caused by a wide range of medical conditions. It can accompany minor viral illness (e.g., colds, flu) but can also accompany major illness (e.g., GI bleeding, myocardial infarction, pneumonia). Weakness may also be a symptom of depression. Real weakness means that there is a decrease in muscle strength; this is a more concerning finding.
- **Fatigue:** Fatigue is somewhat different from weakness. It's a feeling of being tired and having decreased energy. Endurance is decreased. On testing, however, muscle strength is normal (i.e., no true weakness). Fatigue is often caused by insufficient sleep, inadequate caloric intake, stress, and viral infections.

Causes of Generalized Weakness and Fatigue
- Acute blood loss (e.g., gastrointestinal bleeding, vaginal bleeding).
- Cardiac disorders with decreased cardiac output (e.g., MI, arrhythmias, valvular heart disease, cardiomyopathies).
- Depression.
- Fever.
- Heat exhaustion.
- Hypoglycemia.
- Inadequate caloric intake.
- Infections (e.g., pneumonia, UTI).
- Insufficient sleep.
- Medication side effect.
- Metabolic (e.g., hypoglycemia, hyponatremia, hypokalemia).
- Stress.
- **Viral Syndrome:** Patients with viral illnesses (e.g., colds, flu) often report some generalized weakness along with all the other symptoms that they are experiencing.
- **Volume Depletion and Dehydration:** From vomiting, diarrhea, sweating.

WOUND INFECTION

Definition
- Traumatic wound (break in the skin) shows signs of infection. This includes sutured wounds, puncture wounds, and scrapes.
- *Use this protocol only if the patient has symptoms that match Wound Infection.*

Symptoms:
- Pus or cloudy fluid is draining from the wound.
- Pimple or yellow crust has formed on the wound.
  R/O: impetigo
- Increasing redness occurs around the wound.
  R/O: cellulitis
- Red streak is spreading from the wound toward the heart.
  R/O: lymphangitis
- Wound has become extremely tender.
  R/O: abscess, cellulitis, necrotizing fasciitis
- Wound has developed blebs, crepitus, severe pain, or black necrotic tissue.
  R/O: gangrene and myonecrosis
- Pain or swelling is increasing 48 hours after the wound occurred.
  R/O: abscess, cellulitis
- Lymph node draining that area of skin may become large and tender.
  R/O: lymphadenitis
- Onset of widespread bright-red rash.
  R/O: exotoxin from staph or strep wound infection
- Onset of fever.
- Wound hasn't healed within 10 days after the injury.

TRIAGE ASSESSMENT QUESTIONS

See More Appropriate Protocol
- Stitches and not infected
  Go to Protocol: Suture or Staple Questions on page 397

Go to ED/UCC Now
(or to Office With PCP Approval)
- Bright-red, widespread, sunburn-like rash
  R/O: staph or strep exotoxin
- Black (necrotic) or blisters develop in wound
- Looks infected (spreading redness, red streak, pus) and fever
  R/O: cellulitis
- Patient sounds very sick or weak to the triager
  Reason: severe acute illness or serious complication suspected

Go to Office Now
- Severe pain in the wound
  R/O: abscess or invasive strep
- Red streak runs from the wound
  R/O: lymphangitis
- Facial wound looks infected (spreading redness)
  Reason: cosmetic concerns
  Note: It may be difficult to determine the rash color in people with darker-colored skin.
- Finger wound and entire finger swollen
  R/O: tenosynovitis

See Today in Office
- Skin redness around the wound > 2" (5 cm)
  R/O: cellulitis
  Note: It may be difficult to determine the rash color in people with darker-colored skin.
- Pus or cloudy fluid draining from wound
  R/O: wound infection
- Taking antibiotic > 48 hours and fever persists
  R/O: complication, abscess, resistant organism, MRSA
- Taking antibiotic > 72 hours (3 days) and infected wound not improved (pain, pus, redness)
  R/O: complication, abscess, resistant organism, MRSA
- Patient wants to be seen

See Today or Tomorrow in Office

● Pimple where a stitch comes through the skin
R/O: stitch abscess

● Wound becomes more painful or swollen,
≥ 3 days after injury
R/O: wound infection

● Wound and no tetanus booster in > 5 years
(or > 10 years for clean cuts)
Reason: may need a tetanus booster shot (vaccine)

See Within 3 Days in Office

● Wound hasn't healed within 10 days after the injury
R/O: low-grade wound infection

Home Care

○ Taking antibiotic < 48 hours for wound infection
and fever persists
Reason: taking antibiotic and no complications

○ Taking antibiotic < 72 hours (3 days) and infected
wound doesn't look better
Reason: taking antibiotic and no complications

○ Wound doesn't sound infected, or only mild redness
Reason: all triage questions negative

HOME CARE ADVICE

❶ **Warm Soaks or Local Heat:** If the wound is open,
soak it in warm water or put a warm, wet cloth on
the wound for 20 minutes 3 times per day. Use a
warm saltwater solution containing 2 teaspoons of
table salt per quart of water. If the wound is closed,
apply a heating pad or warm, moist washcloth to
the reddened area for 20 minutes 3 times per day.

❷ **Antibiotic Ointment:** Apply an antibiotic ointment
3 times a day. If the area could become dirty, cover
with a Band-Aid or a clean gauze dressing.

❸ **Pain Medicines:**

• For pain relief, you can take either acetaminophen,
ibuprofen, or naproxen.

• They are over-the-counter (OTC) pain drugs.
You can buy them at the drugstore.

Acetaminophen (e.g., Tylenol):

• **Regular Strength Tylenol:** Take 650 mg
(two 325 mg pills) by mouth every 4-6 hours
as needed. Each Regular Strength Tylenol pill
has 325 mg of acetaminophen.

• **Extra Strength Tylenol:** Take 1,000 mg
(two 500 mg pills) every 8 hours as needed.
Each Extra Strength Tylenol pill has 500 mg
of acetaminophen.

• The most you should take each day is 3,000 mg
(10 Regular Strength or 6 Extra Strength pills
a day).

Ibuprofen (e.g., Motrin, Advil):

• Take 400 mg (two 200 mg pills) by mouth every
6 hours.

• Another choice is to take 600 mg (three 200 mg
pills) by mouth every 8 hours.

• The most you should take each day is 1,200 mg
(six 200 mg pills), unless your doctor has told
you to take more.

Naproxen (e.g., Aleve):

• Take 220 mg (one 220 mg pill) by mouth every
8 hours as needed. You may take 440 mg
(two 220 mg pills) for your first dose.

• The most you should take each day is 660 mg
(three 220 mg pills a day), unless your doctor
has told you to take more.

❹ **Pain Medicines—Extra Notes:**

• Use the lowest amount of medicine that makes
your pain better.

• Acetaminophen is thought to be safer than
ibuprofen or naproxen in people > 65 years old.
Acetaminophen is in many OTC and prescription
medicines. It might be in more than one medicine
that you are taking. You need to be careful and
not take an overdose. An acetaminophen overdose can hurt the liver.

• McNeil, the company that makes Tylenol, has
different dosage instructions for Tylenol in Canada
and the United States. In Canada, the maximum
recommended dose per day is 4,000 mg or
12 Regular Strength (325 mg) pills. In the United
States, McNeil recommends a maximum dose
of 10 Regular Strength (325 mg) pills.

• CAUTION: Do not take acetaminophen if you
have liver disease.

• CAUTION: Do not take ibuprofen or naproxen if
you have stomach problems, have kidney disease,
are pregnant, or have been told by your doctor to
avoid this type of anti-inflammatory drug. Do not
take ibuprofen or naproxen for > 7 days without
consulting your doctor.

• *Before taking any medicine, read all the instructions
on the package.*

❺ **Expected Course:** Pain and swelling normally peak on day 2. Any redness should go away by day 3 or 4. Complete healing should occur by day 10.

❻ **Contagiousness:** For true wound infections, you can return to work or school after any fever is gone and you have received antibiotics for 24 hours.

❼ **Call Back If:**
- Wound becomes more tender.
- Redness starts to spread.
- Pus, drainage, or fever occurs.
- You become worse.

BACKGROUND

Key Points

- When wounds become infected, the infection usually develops 24-72 hours after the initial break in the skin.
- CA-MRSA must be considered as a possible cause in newly infected wounds and in wounds that are not improving despite antibiotic therapy.

Community-Acquired Methicillin-Resistant *Staphylococcus aureus* (CA-MRSA)

- *Staphylococcus aureus* is bacteria that can cause a variety of skin infections, including pimples, boils, abscesses, cellulitis, wound infections, and impetigo. It can also cause more serious infections like staphylococcal pneumonia, sepsis, and toxic shock syndrome.
- In the 1960s strains of *S aureus* that were resistant to penicillin-type antibiotics started appearing in hospitals and health care settings. These were referred to as methicillin-resistant *S aureus* (MRSA) infections.
- More recently, strains of penicillin-resistant *S aureus* have increasingly become the cause of skin infections in healthy individuals in the community. These are now being referred to as community-acquired methicillin-resistant *S aureus* (CA-MRSA) infections. There have been outbreaks in athletes (e.g., wrestling teams) and in prison populations.
- CA-MRSA requires treatment with specific types of antibiotics.
- More information about CA-MRSA is available at: www.cdc.gov/mrsa/index.html.

What Is Tetanus?

- **Definition:** Tetanus is a rare infection caused by bacteria that are found in many places, especially in dirt and soil. The tetanus bacteria enter through a break in the skin and then spread through the body.
- **Symptoms:** Tetanus is commonly called "lockjaw" because the first symptom is a tightening of the muscles of the face. However, the final stage of the infection is much more serious. All of the muscles of the body go into severe spasm, including the muscles that control breathing. Eventually a person with a tetanus infection loses the ability to breath and may die in spite of intensive treatment in the hospital.
- **Prevention:** A tetanus booster protects you from getting a tetanus infection. It does not prevent other kinds of wound infection.

Tetanus Booster—When Does an Adult Need a Tetanus Shot?

- **Clean Cuts and Scrapes—Tetanus Booster Needed Every 10 Years:** Patients with clean minor wounds AND who have previously had ≥ 3 tetanus shots (full series) need a booster every 10 years. Examples of minor wounds include a superficial knee abrasion, a small cut from a clean knife blade, or a glass cut sustained while washing dishes. All wounds need wound care and cleaning right away. Obtain tetanus booster within 72 hours.
- **Dirty Wounds—Tetanus Booster Needed Every 5 Years:** Patients with dirty wounds need a booster every 5 years. Examples of dirty wounds include any cut contaminated with soil, feces, and/or saliva and more serious wounds from deep punctures, crushing, and burns. All wounds need to be cleaned right away. Dirty wounds usually need immediate care in a doctor's office, urgent care, or ED. A tetanus booster should be given as soon as possible, preferably at the time of wound care, and definitely within 72 hours.
- Contaminated major wounds (e.g., crush injuries, amputations, avulsions, gaping cuts, larger burns, or any other wound that needs debridement or irrigation) are all referred in immediately for wound care. For these patients, if a tetanus booster is required, it will be given on the day of the injury.

ZIKA VIRUS EXPOSURE

Definition
- Travel to or living in an area with recent local transmission of Zika virus
- Exposure to a person with Zika virus
- Questions about Zika virus

Exposure:
- Travel in the past 14 days to a Zika outbreak area
- Live in a Zika outbreak area
- Had unprotected sex (no condom) in the past 14 days with a person who lives in or has recently traveled to a Zika outbreak area

Refer to the Centers for Disease Control and Prevention for the most recent updates on Zika outbreak areas (areas where local transmission of Zika is occurring): www.cdc.gov/zika/geo/index.html. Or review information available on the World Health Organization Web site: www.who.int/mediacentre/factsheets/zika/en.

TRIAGE ASSESSMENT QUESTIONS

Call EMS 911 Now
- Sounds like a life-threatening emergency to the triager
- Difficult to awaken or acting confused (e.g., disoriented, slurred speech)
  R/O: sepsis, shock

See More Appropriate Protocol
- Has symptoms but has not had any exposure to Zika
  Go to a more appropriate symptom protocol (e.g., fever, rash, red eyes)

Go to ED/UCC Now
(or to Office With PCP Approval)
- Fever > 104° F (40° C)
  R/O: serious bacterial infection
- Patient sounds very sick or weak to the triager
  Reason: severe acute illness or serious complication suspected

Go to Office Now
- Fever > 101° F (38.3° C) and age > 60
- Fever > 100.0° F (37.8° C) and weak immune system (e.g., HIV positive, cancer chemotherapy, splenectomy, organ transplant, chronic oral steroids)

See Today in Office
- Pregnant and Zika EXPOSURE in past 14 days and new onset of fever, rash, red eyes, or joint aches
  R/O: Zika or other mosquito-borne illness

Discuss With PCP and Callback by Nurse Today
- Not pregnant and Zika EXPOSURE in past 14 days and new onset of fever, rash, red eyes, or joint aches
  R/O: Zika or other mosquito-borne illness

See Within 3 Days in Office
- Pregnant and recent travel to a Zika outbreak area
  Reason: CDC recommends that pregnant women who have traveled to a Zika outbreak area talk with their doctor or health care professional
- Pregnant and had unprotected sex (no condom) with a person who lives in or recently traveled to a Zika area
  Reason: CDC recommends that women discuss this with their doctor or health care professional
- Patient wants to be seen

See Within 2 Weeks in Office
- Pregnant or planning to become pregnant and has other concerns about Zika exposure (e.g., exposure earlier in pregnancy, travel plans)
  Reason: no recent exposure; need for prenatal counseling

Home Care
- Zika EXPOSURE and all other triage questions negative (e.g., no symptoms, not pregnant)
- Zika virus, questions about
- Preventing mosquito bites and insect repellents (e.g., DEET), questions about

HOME CARE ADVICE

Zika Virus

❶ Key Points:
- Zika is spread mainly by a bite of an infected *Aedes* species mosquito. It can also spread from person to person during sex.
- Most people who are infected do not get sick or have only mild symptoms.
- The main symptoms are fever, eye redness, rash, and joint pain.
- Zika may cause microcephaly (small head and brain) and other brain defects in babies born to women infected while pregnant.

❷ Symptoms:
- Most people do not even know they have it.
- Only 1 out of 5 people have symptoms.
- Common symptoms are mild fever, allover rash, red eyes, and joint pain.
- Symptoms last about 2-7 days.

❸ Risk Factors:
- Live in or recently traveled to a Zika outbreak area and bit by mosquitoes there.
- Have unprotected sex (no condom) with a person who lives in or recently traveled to a Zika outbreak area.

❹ How It Is Spread:
- Zika is spread mainly by a bite of an infected *Aedes* species mosquito.
- A mosquito bites a person who already has Zika. The mosquito then bites other people and infects them.
- It can also spread from a pregnant mother to her unborn baby or to the baby during birth.
- A man or women who has Zika can spread the virus to his/her partner through sex (vaginal, oral, or anal).
- There have been no known cases of infants getting Zika through breastfeeding.

❺ Treatment:
- Currently, there are no special medicines to treat Zika.
- Most people can treat their symptoms at home.
- Acetaminophen (Tylenol) can be used to treat fever and pain.

❻ Complications:
- Almost all people with Zika get better without any special treatment.
- Most people do not get sick and do not need to go to the hospital.
- **Pregnancy:** However, if a woman gets infected with the Zika virus while pregnant, it may harm the baby. A pregnant woman who has Zika can pass the virus to her unborn child. The virus may cause serious birth defects that affect the brain, including microcephaly (small brain and head). More studies are being done to learn how Zika harms unborn babies.

❼ Prevention:
- There is no vaccine to prevent Zika.
- The best way to not get Zika is to avoid mosquito bites.
- If a woman is planning to become pregnant, she and her partner should avoid travel to a Zika outbreak area if at all possible.
- Always use a condom (or avoid sex) if you have sex with a person who lives in or recently traveled to a Zika outbreak area.

❽ Note to Triager—Do Not Take Aspirin:
- Patient should not take aspirin or other NSAIDs (e.g., ibuprofen, naproxen) until dengue has been ruled out.
  (Reason: NSAIDs may increase the risk of bleeding with dengue.)

❿ Call Back If:
- You have more questions.

Zika Virus Exposure

❶ Reassurance—Exposure:
- It sounds like you may have been exposed to Zika.
- Many people who have Zika do not have any symptoms.
- If you do get sick, the symptoms are usually mild.
- The symptoms are mild fever, rash, red eyes, and achy joints.

❷ Precautions During Sex:
- A person with Zika can spread the virus to his/her partner during sex.
- This includes all kinds of sex (vaginal, oral, or anal).
- The virus has been found in vaginal secretions and semen.
- Because you might have Zika, it is important to avoid sex or use a condom every time you have sex. This is especially important if your partner is pregnant or planning to become pregnant.
- Talk to your doctor about these precautions and how long you need to follow them.

❸ Call Back If:
- You develop fever, rash, red eyes, or joint pain.
- You have other questions or concerns.

Preventing Mosquito Bites

❶ Preventing Mosquito Bites:
- If you live in or travel to a Zika outbreak area, protect yourself from mosquitoes.
- **Stay indoors** at sunrise, during early evening, and at sunset. These are times of the day mosquitoes bite the most.
- When outdoors, cover yourself well with clothing and use insect repellents.

❷ What to Wear When Outdoors:
- Wear long pants and long-sleeved shirts. Loose clothing is best.
- Tuck your pants into your socks.
- Wear shoes and socks (mosquitoes like to bite feet).
- Wear a hat (even better, a hat with a mosquito net).

❸ Insect Repellents:
- Use insect repellents on your uncovered skin when you are outdoors.
- Repellents that work very well and are safe are those made with DEET and picaridin. Look for these names in the active ingredients. You can use these types if you are pregnant or breast-feeding. No problems have been found.
- *Follow the package directions carefully.* The directions should tell you how to use it and how long it lasts.
- Do not put it on skin covered by clothes. Do not spray it near your eyes, nose, or mouth.
- DEET is a strong insect repellent that comes in different strengths. The higher the strength, the longer it lasts. The American Academy of Pediatrics recommends using 10%-30% DEET for children.
- Insect repellents should not be used on newborns and infants < 2 months old.

❹ Permethrin—an Insect Repellent for Your Clothing and Gear:
- Products that have permethrin (e.g., Duranon, Permanone, Congo Creek Tick Spray) are very effective mosquito repellents. They also repel ticks. You put permethrin on your clothing instead of your skin.
- Spray it on your clothes before you put them on. You can also put it on other outdoor items (shoes, mosquito screen, sleeping bags).
- It continues to work even after your clothes are washed several times.
- Do not put this type of repellent on your skin.
- *Read and follow the package directions carefully.*

❺ Internet Resources:
- You can find more information at the CDC Web site.
- **Mosquito Bite Prevention for Travelers:** www.cdc.gov/chikungunya/pdfs/fs_mosquito_bite_prevention_travelers.pdf.

❻ Call Back If:
- You have more questions.

BACKGROUND

Key Points

- Zika is a virus that spreads mainly through the bite of an *Aedes* species mosquito. It is the cause of the Zika virus infection, also called Zika fever.
- Zika can also be passed through having sex with a person who has Zika. Zika can be passed from a pregnant woman to her fetus.
- There have been outbreaks in Africa, Asia, the Pacific Islands, and Latin and South America. In 2016 there were some cases reported of Zika being spread by mosquitoes in parts of Florida (Miami-Dade County).
- Zika may cause microcephaly (small head and brain) and other brain defects in babies born to women infected while pregnant.

Symptoms

Most people do not even know they have the virus. Only 1 out of 5 people have symptoms. Symptoms usually last about 2-7 days. Common symptoms of the Zika infection are:

- **Eye Redness:** The whites of the eyes may become pink or red. There is no pus or discharge.
- **Fever:** Fever is usually low grade (< 101.5° F or 38.6° C).
- **Joint pain** or aching.
- Widespread pink-red **rash** (small flat spots or bumps).

Risk Factors

- Live in or recently traveled to a Zika outbreak area (where local transmission of Zika is occurring) and are bit by mosquitoes there.
- Unprotected sex (no condom) with a person who lives in or recently traveled to a Zika outbreak area.
- Unborn baby may be at risk if mother gets infected while pregnant.

Diagnosis

- It is hard to diagnose Zika. There are many other illnesses that have the same symptoms.
- There are blood tests that can help diagnose Zika. However, these tests are only available at the Centers for Disease Control and Prevention (CDC) and in some state health departments. Doctor's offices and EDs do not have this test. CDC testing information is available at: https://www.cdc.gov/zika/hc-providers/testing-for-zikavirus.html.

How It Is Spread

- The main way the virus is spread to others is through a bite from an *Aedes* species mosquito.
- A mosquito bites a person who already has Zika. The mosquito then bites other people and infects them.
- It can also spread from a pregnant mother to her unborn baby or to the baby during birth.
- A person who has Zika can spread the virus to his/her partner during sex. This includes vaginal, anal, or oral sex.
- There have been no known cases of infants getting Zika from breastfeeding. Because of the many benefits of breastfeeding, mothers are encouraged to continue breastfeeding even if they live in a Zika outbreak area (CDC).

Incubation Period

Health experts think this is likely a few days (range 2-12 days).

How Long Can a Person With Zika Spread the Virus Through Sex?

A person with Zika can spread the virus to his/her partner during sex (anal, oral, or vaginal).

- This can happen before the infected person starts to have symptoms, while they have symptoms, and after the symptoms end.
- The virus can remain in the semen longer than other body fluids such as vaginal secretions and blood.
- People with Zika should avoid sex or always use a condom correctly every time they have sex to prevent the spread of the virus to others.

The CDC recommends the following:

- Men with Zika should follow these precautions for 6 months after the start of their Zika symptoms.
- Men who have been exposed to Zika but do not have symptoms should also follow these precautions for 6 months after the date of their last exposure.
- If the partner is pregnant, these precautions should be followed for the rest of the pregnancy.
- Women with Zika should follow these precautions for 8 weeks after the start of their Zika symptoms.
- Women who are exposed to Zika but do not have symptoms should also follow these precautions for 8 weeks after the date of their last exposure.

Prevention

- There is no vaccine to prevent Zika.
- The best way to not get Zika is to avoid mosquito bites.
- If a woman is planning to become pregnant, she and her partner should avoid travel to a Zika outbreak area if at all possible.
- Always use a condom (or avoid sex) if you have sex with a person who lives in or recently traveled to a Zika outbreak area.

Complications

Almost all people with Zika get better without any special treatment. Most people do not get very sick and do not need to go to the hospital.

- However, if a woman gets infected with the Zika virus while pregnant, it may harm the baby.
- A pregnant woman who has Zika can pass the virus to her unborn child. The virus may cause serious birth defects that affect the brain, including microcephaly (small brain and head), More studies are being done to learn how Zika harms unborn babies.

There have been some reported cases of Guillain-Barré syndrome that occur with Zika.

- This is a rare problem that sometimes happens when the body's natural defense against infection attacks the nerves.
- Experts do not know for sure if or how this health problem is related to Zika infection.
- The main symptom is bilateral muscle weakness and paralysis. Most of the time this is short-lived and goes away in several weeks to months. However, it can be very serious and sometimes cause death.

Treatment

- Currently, there is no specific medical treatment for Zika.
- There are no antiviral medicines available to treat Zika.
- Most people can treat this at home. They can take acetaminophen (Tylenol) if needed to treat fever and muscle aches.
- The CDC advises against using aspirin and NSAIDs (ibuprofen, naproxen) if a Zika infection is suspected. The reason for this is because there is a small risk that the patient may have another type of mosquito-borne illness (e.g., dengue) instead of or in addition to Zika. NSAIDs may worsen a rare complication that can occur with some of these other infections.

Internet Resources

You should check with your state and national health authorities for the most up-to-date information and recommendations. Also, follow any related policies for screening and referrals set up by your call center or health organization.

- **Centers for Disease Control and Prevention (CDC):** www.cdc.gov/zika
- **World Health Organization (WHO):** www.who.int/mediacentre/factsheets/zika/en
- **European Centre for Disease Prevention and Control (ECDC):** http://ecdc.europa.eu/en/healthtopics/zika_virus_infection/Pages/index.aspx

Appendix A: User's Guide: How to Use *Adult Telephone Protocols: Office Version*

<u>Contents</u>

Introduction

This User's Guide is primarily written for those office personnel who perform telephone triage and provide health information over the phone.

The goals of this book are:

- To provide telephone triage protocols for use by the triage personnel in adult primary care offices.
- To provide adult health information and care advice for use by office telephone triage personnel.
- To serve as a training tool for office staff who are responsible for performing triage and communicating health care information to patients.

This book contains 115 protocols that cover more than 90% of adult telephone chief complaints. They are arranged alphabetically.

Using protocols is a key element in delivering safe and effective telephone triage in a primary care office. There are several reasons why they are important. Protocols make it possible for a primary care office to:

- Deliver consistent health information to callers, independent of which staff person is handling the call.
- Provide a structured decision-support tool to guide the triager through a standardized telephone interview.
- Develop a consensus among several different physicians within an office practice by giving them a document to review, amend as needed, and approve.
- Reduce risk-management challenges by including screening questions that the triager might not have otherwised considered.
- Reconstruct the interview of a past telephone triage call.

Medical Review – These protocols should not be used unless they have been reviewed, amended as necessary, and approved by a supervising physician or medical director responsible for overseeing their use.

Decision Support – These protocols are clinical guidelines that must be used in conjunction with critical thinking and clinical judgment. These protocols provide decision support but do not make the decision; the clinical decision of whether and when a patient needs to be seen must be made by the staff person performing the triage.

Therefore, these protocols are most suitable for use by physicians and clinically experienced nurses, nurse practitioners, and physician assistants. All licensed health professionals should receive special training before using these protocols. Non-licensed and non-health professionals (e.g., secretaries) should not use these protocols.

Principles of Triage Decision-making

Triage is the decision process of sorting patients to the level of care that best meets their medical needs. This decision process must take into consideration the seriousness (medical acuity) of the patient's medical complaint, the types of resources required to provide effective care, the patient's expectations, and several other factors. See Figure 1.

Medical Acuity – Medical acuity refers to the severity of the patient's problem or symptom. Medical acuity is the foundation; it is the fundamental deciding factor you will use to decide whether, when, and where a patient needs to be seen. A patient who is having an anaphylactic reaction (life-threatening allergic reaction) with shortness of breath and wheezing after a bee sting has a problem of high acuity. Based solely on the high acuity of this problem, you would recommend that the caller immediately contact an emergency ambulance service (Call EMS 911 NOW). In contrast, a patient who states they feel completely well except for a low-grade fever and a constant moderate sore throat of 2 days' duration has a problem of low acuity. You would likely recommend an appointment in the office today or tomorrow for evaluation (See Today or Tomorrow in Office). A patient with mild sunburn who calls for care advice has a problem of very low acuity. For such a patient, no appointment would be needed and instead you would provide brief health information on how to reduce the sunburn pain (Home Care Advice).

During your triage decision-making process you will always need to consider…

- **Is there an immediate threat to life or limb?** You should recommend an emergency medical services (EMS) transport team for patient problems for which there is a clear or high likelihood of life, limb, or organ threat. Such patients may require resuscitative efforts; treatment often can be initiated within minutes by EMS providers. Examples of symptoms that require you to call EMS 911 services include:

- Amputation
- Chest pain lasting longer than 10 minutes, not relieved by nitroglycerin
- Stopped breathing or severe difficulty breathing
- Unconscious, comatose, or confused

You may wish to review Appendix C. It contains a table listing further examples of patient symptoms and problems that generally require activation of the EMS system.

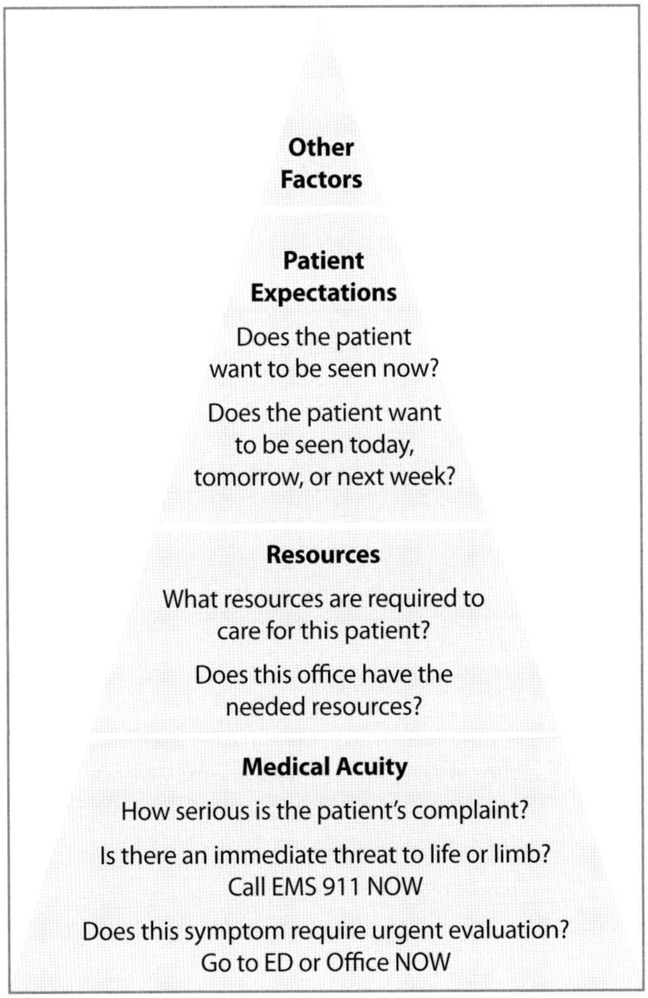

Other Factors

Patient Expectations

Does the patient want to be seen now?

Does the patient want to be seen today, tomorrow, or next week?

Resources

What resources are required to care for this patient?

Does this office have the needed resources?

Medical Acuity

How serious is the patient's complaint?

Is there an immediate threat to life or limb?
Call EMS 911 NOW

Does this symptom require urgent evaluation?
Go to ED or Office NOW

Figure 1. Factors Involved in the Telephone Triage Decision Process

- **Does the symptom require urgent evaluation?** Many symptoms are of such potentially high acuity that only through a complete medical evaluation can the diagnosis and necessary treatment be determined. Thus, you should recommend an immediate evaluation in the emergency department (ED) or office for patient problems for which there is an unclear or low to moderate likelihood of life, limb, or organ threat.

Examples of symptoms that often require urgent evaluation include:

- Chest pain
  R/O: heart attack, etc.
- Difficulty breathing
  R/O: pneumonia, etc.
- Abdominal pain persisting > 2 hours
  R/O: appendicitis, etc.
- Headache, fever, and stiff neck
  R/O: meningitis, etc.

You may wish to review Appendix D. It contains a table listing further examples of patient symptoms and problems that generally require an immediate visit to the office or emergency department for medical evaluation.

Resources – The resource needs of the patient's problem also impact your triage decision-making. "Resources" is a broad term describing the equipment, medications, supplies, and personnel skills needed for a specific patient problem.

During your triage decision-making process you will often need to consider...

- **What resources are required to care for this patient?** For example, a patient with a gaping 2-inch laceration on the hand needs treatment at a health care site that has the resources of suture material, a laceration repair tray, tetanus vaccine, and a provider skilled in performing laceration repair.

- **Does this office have the needed resources?**
  It is very helpful and improves your call efficiency if you know what resources your office has for provision of patient care. Try to avoid being in the situation of having to lean away from the phone and whisper, "Do we do _____ in this office? Do we have any tetanus shots left? Does Dr Smith remove insects from inside an ear?"

  You can tabulate the resources you have available in your office by using the forms in Appendix E. There are 3 basic categories of resources:

  - **Procedures** – e.g., foreign body removal, laceration repair, fracture reduction and casting, pelvic examination, intravenous fluid administration
  - **Tests** – e.g., electrocardiogram, chest radiograph, urine pregnancy, fingerstick glucose
  - **Medications** – e.g., tetanus vaccination, albuterol (metaproterenol) nebulizer treatment, acetaminophen (Tylenol)

Patient Expectations – A patient begins the telephone triage encounter with expectations about whether he or she needs to be seen in the office, and when an appointment would be convenient. From a customer service standpoint, the way to achieve patient satisfaction is to meet or exceed these expectations. If you are unable to meet the patient's expectations, to achieve patient satisfaction you will need to "manage" this expectation by successfully convincing the patient that an office visit is not needed or that it can be postponed.

- **Does the patient want to be seen in the office?**
  You should determine if the patient wants to be seen. Sometimes a patient calls with expectations to be seen in the office and other times the patient is just seeking health information for home care.
- **Does the patient want to be seen today, tomorrow, or next week?**
  What do you do if there are no office appointments available right now, today, tomorrow, or later this week? All too frequently office schedules are booked up with 2- to 8-week waits. If you have no appropriate open appointments, you may need to overbook the patient into the office schedule

according to your scheduling policy or after discussion with the physician. Alternatively, sometimes you may have to recommend that the patient be seen in the local emergency department.

Some primary care offices have successfully implemented a new paradigm, called "open access" or "advanced access." Open access means that if a patient requests an appointment, you give an appointment today. The patient decides whether to come in today, tomorrow, or next week. The theme of open access scheduling is, do today's work—today!

Another office model is to dedicate a block of time for urgent care in the daily office schedule, and staff this clinic with an advanced practice nurse or physician assistant.

Other Factors – There are a number of other factors that you will need to take into consideration during the triage process.

- **What social factors affect the triage disposition?**
  There are a number of social factors that may affect the disposition you recommend to a patient. For example, a healthy ambulatory elderly patient with a cough and a fever of 102.5° F probably needs an urgent office visit; whereas a similar bedridden patient would likely need to be directed to the emergency department via ambulance solely because of the bedridden status. See Table 1 for a list of other important social factors.
- **Does the patient have any chronic medical problems?**
  You will need to be more cautious in your triage of patients with chronic illness. See Table 2 for a listing of important illnesses.
- **Is the patient pregnant?**
- **Is the patient taking any medications, especially new medications? Could the patient be experiencing an adverse reaction to the medications?**

Table 1. Social Factors: RATE the Patient

Reliability	• Barriers from language, intoxication, or limited education • Second-party callers • Truthfulness
Abuse	• Partner and elder abuse
Travel Distance and Access	• Distance from hospital and office • Access to car or other transportation • Ambulatory or bedridden
Emotional	• Anxiety, fear, hysteria

Table 2. Chronic Illness

Important Medical Conditions	Relevance to Triage Decision-Making
Common	
• AIDS and HIV positive, cancer chemotherapy, chronic steroids, transplant patients	Weakened immune system; more prone to infection.
• Asthma, emphysema	Increased risk of pneumonia, pneumothorax.
• Cardiac disease	Higher risk for further cardiac events (e.g., heart attack, congestive heart failure); cardiac medications can cause weakness, dizziness, and electrolyte problems.
• Central venous line (e.g. Port-a-Cath)	Increased risk of catheter-related infections.
• Diabetes	Weakened immune system, thus more prone to infection. Hyperglycemia and hypoglycemia may present with frequent urination, weakness, dizziness, altered mental status, or coma.
• Coagulopathy, Coumadin therapy	Increased tendency for bleeding; must be more cautious in these patients whenever they bleed or have a traumatic injury.
• Feeding tube	Increased risk of aspiration pneumonia, bowel obstruction, osmotic diarrhea.
• Hypertension	Prone to stroke; hypertension medications can cause weakness, dizziness, and electrolyte problems.
• Liver disease	Prone to bleeding problems.
• Urinary catheter (e.g., Foley)	Increased risk of urinary retention, urinary tract infection.
Geriatric Concerns	
• Dementia	Problems with getting an accurate history, safety issues.
• Osteoporosis	Loss of bone density increases likelihood of fracture from minor falls.
• Polypharmacy	Elderly patients frequently are taking multiple drugs. There are risks of drug-drug and drug-disease interactions.
• Recent injury	Possible undiagnosed injury, wound infection.
• Recent surgery	Surgical complications including urinary infection, bleeding, wound infection; increased risk of pulmonary embolism after major surgery.
• Recent infection	Antibiotics can frequently cause rashes; some antibiotics can cause *Clostridium difficile* diarrhea.

Structure of a Telephone Triage Encounter

The typical triage call has a structure that can be organized in the following manner. The call begins with a greeting followed by a short period of active listening. Brief demographic information is obtained, a protocol is selected, triage is performed using the triage assessment questions in the protocol, then a disposition is recommended to the caller. The call concludes with the triager providing relevant care advice, answering any final questions, and instructing the caller to call back if symptoms worsen. See Table 3.

Let's look at each of the components of a telephone triage encounter in more detail.

Greeting – The call begins with a greeting, during which you introduce yourself and apologize for any delays. The greeting ends with an invitation to the caller to describe their problem or symptom. Many successful office practices have a specific scripted approach to this first part of the encounter. Your greeting might contain the following scripted elements:

- Greeting   *"Good morning."*
- Introduction   *"This is Donna,"*
- Title   *"the nurse working with Dr Smith."*
- Apology if   *"I am sorry that you had to wait on*
  indicated   *the phone."*
- Query   *"How can I help you this morning?"*

Remember to smile. The caller easily can hear the smile in your voice even when they cannot see it.

Active Listening, the Chief Complaint – During the second part of the triage call you listen to the caller describe the problem in an open-ended manner with minimal interruptions. During this part of the call the triager is actively listening to the caller with the primary goal of identifying the caller's main complaint. Ideally this part of the call should last 30 to 60 seconds. This part of the call is often the most challenging for new triagers because callers may often present their concerns in a disjointed and rambling manner. If more than 30 to 60 seconds elapse and you remain unclear about the caller's main question, it is productive at this point to become more directive in your call. For example, asking clarifying questions is often helpful:

- "So while you have a sore throat and runny nose, the main reason you are calling is the bad cough. Is this right?"
- "Besides the cough and runny nose for the last 3 days, do you have any other symptoms that you are really worried about?"
- "When you fell and injured your ankle, did you hurt any other part of your body?"
- "It sounds like a lot of things are bothering you right now. What's the worst thing?"

Demographic Information – During the third phase of the call, you should obtain brief identifying demographic information, if it was not provided previously. At the very least this usually consists of name, age,

Table 3. Structure of a Telephone Triage Encounter

Component	Description
Greeting	Greet caller. Introduce yourself as per approved office script. Apologize for any delays. Smile.
Active Listening, the Chief Complaint	Listen to the caller describe the problem or symptom. Try to avoid interrupting for the first 30 seconds. Determine the patient's main complaint or symptom. Select the correct protocol.
Demographic Information	Obtain or confirm patient identifying information: name, phone number, age, gender.
Chronic Illness, Social History, Pregnancy	Determine if there are chronic illnesses or social factors (RATE the patient) that may affect the disposition.
Triage Assessment Questions	Scan through the questions in the selected protocol. Ask questions in order provided. Assign a disposition level.
Home Care Advice	Provide care advice; give only First Aid advice to patients requiring immediate evaluation.
Closure	Confirm understanding and patient intent to follow recommendations. Provide Call Back If advice.

phone number, and gender. Obtaining several different phone numbers (e.g., home, mobile, pager) may save office time on callbacks. Some offices have a standard of obtaining demographic information before asking for any medical information. Some offices will only provide telephone advice to patients who have previously been seen in the office.

Chronic Illness, Social History, Pregnancy – During the fourth phase of the encounter it is important to inquire regarding the possibility of pregnancy, obtain any patient history of significant chronic illness, and identify any directly relevant social factors. See Tables 1 and 2.

Triage Assessment Questions – At this point in the telephone encounter, you will select the most relevant protocol and then systematically ask the triage assessment questions in the order presented in the protocol. You will be asking the highest acuity questions first. Be certain to ask the questions in the order presented until you obtain a positive response. The triage assessment questions in the protocol are organized under disposition categories.

Home Care Advice – You do not need to provide every piece of care advice listed for the protocol. Try to tailor the care advice to the patient's needs. Attempt to limit the care advice you provide to 2-3 instructions and keep your comments brief.

Closure – Closure is the end of the telephone triage encounter. The triager needs to confirm that the caller understands the care advice provided, has no further questions, and agrees with the recommended disposition. The triager and caller should be in agreement regarding the disposition before the call ends. The triager should conclude the conversation with a brief Call Back If statement. Suggested Call Back If statements are included at the bottom of the Home Care Advice section. Covering every worst-case scenario is impossible and will unduly alarm the caller. But at the least, the triager should instruct the patient to call back if *"you become worse."*

Structure of the Protocols in This Book

Each of the protocols in this book is organized identically and contain the following components.

- Title
- Definition
- Triage Assessment Questions
  - See More Appropriate Protocol
- Home Care Advice
- Background Information

Title – The title briefly describes the type of call for which the protocol is intended to be used. This is nearly always a symptom. For example, a patient might have "Sore Throat" or "Constipation." Some of the protocols have a diagnosis as a title; these are used in those limited clinical situations in which patients can reasonably diagnose themselves with a specific problem. For example, many patients will call up and state that they have "Poison Ivy/Oak/Sumac" or "Jock Itch."

Definition – From your review of the list of topics, you should find that most of the protocols are self-explanatory. The purpose of the symptom definition is to more specifically define the type of patient complaints for which a protocol is applicable. Read the symptom definition completely, especially the first time that you use a protocol. Make certain that your caller's complaint is specifically covered in this symptom definition. It is especially important to do this when using the protocols that have a diagnosis for a title (e.g. Jock Itch, Poison Ivy/Oak/Sumac, Pubic Lice).

Most of the protocols are symptom based. In general, symptoms mentioned by the patient can be accepted at face value (e.g., earache, headache, cough, head injury), but sometimes the definition requires clarification. For example, patients often diagnose themselves with hay fever; you should make certain that their symptoms match the Hay Fever (Nasal Allergies) definition.

As a general rule, neither the patient nor the triager should make diagnoses. However, there are exceptions such as adult illnesses that the average patient can easily recognize (e.g., Athlete's Foot, Pubic Lice, Asthma Attack). Patients may have had the illness previously or have friends or neighbors who suggest the diagnosis to them. For these patients, a diagnosis/disease-based protocol may be indicated. See Table 4.

The first safeguard in all of the disease-based protocols is that they start with a definition. The caller's description of the symptoms must match the definition before the protocol's triage assessment questions and care advice are used.

Table 4. Disease-Based Protocols

• Asthma Attack
• Athlete's Foot
• Cold Sores (Fever Blisters of Lip)
• Common Cold
• Ear, Swimmer's (Otitis Externa)
• Hay Fever (Nasal Allergies)
• Hives
• Influenza, Seasonal
• Jock Itch
• Poison Ivy/Oak/Sumac
• Pubic Lice
• Sunburn

A second safeguard is that the triager can use the See More Appropriate Protocol section; this keeps the triager from over-using the disease-based guideline. If the criteria in the definition are not met, the triager can be redirected to a more appropriate protocol. For example, the triager might be directed from Hives to Rash or Redness, Widespread.

There are several advantages to using a disease-based protocol over a symptom-based protocol. First, the triage questions and care advice are more specific and targeted to the patient's complaint. Secondly, the call is faster and more effective.

Triage Assessment Questions – The triage questions are arranged in descending order of acuity. Restated, the questions are arranged so that the most serious causes of a symptom are considered first.

- You should ask the caller these questions in the order listed, continuing on until you get a "yes" (positive response) to a question.
- Stop asking questions as soon as you get a positive response.
- The remaining questions and other information can be asked by the physician in the emergency department or the office when the patient comes in for evaluation.

Often you will find that the caller has provided the answer to many of these Triage Assessment Questions in the first portion of the call, when he or she was first describing their problem or symptom. You do not need to re-ask the Triage Assessment Question if you already have been given the answer.

Disposition Category – The Triage Assessment Questions are grouped within different disposition categories. The disposition categories, like the Triage Assessment Questions, are arranged in descending order of acuity. (See Figure 2.) The standard disposition categories are:

- **Call EMS 911 Now**
  Life-threatening emergencies.
- **Go to ED Now**
  Emergent patients who need an ED for management.
- **Go to ED/UCC Now (or to Office With PCP Approval)**
  Emergent patients. Discuss the best site with the primary care physician.

- **Go to Office Now**
  Less emergent patients who can be evaluated in most adult primary care offices.
- **See Today in Office**
  (by appointment)
  Urgent or uncomfortable patients.
  Also included here are "Patient wants to be seen."
- **See Today or Tomorrow in Office**
  (by appointment)
  Nonurgent patients.
- **See Within 3 Days in Office**
  (by appointment)
  Persisting symptoms or patients who are not getting better.
- **See Within 2 Weeks in Office**
  (by appointment)
  Chronic or recurrent symptoms that are not becoming worse.
- **Home Care**
  Do not see at all. All the triage questions are negative. Provide home treatment advice.

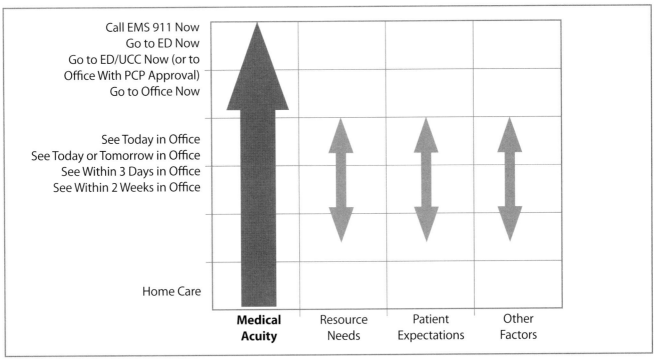

Figure 2. Disposition Categories

When it is seems medically safe, these protocols attempt to place the patient into the Home Care disposition category. Neither the patient nor the physician are interested in unnecessary visits. The triager can elect to move a patient to a higher disposition category (one of greater urgency and acuity). This is referred to as "upgrading" or overriding. Such upgrading of patients is medically harmless. Triagers should feel free to use their judgment and upgrade as they deem necessary.

The patient's desire to be seen should be respected. If the patient wants to be seen and the protocol recommends Home Care, the triager should make arrangements for the patient to be evaluated. In some cases this type of upgrade will turn out to be medically warranted, as the patient may have a medical illness that he or she was not able to communicate well or a medical illness with an atypical presentation. In other cases, this upgrade will turn out to be medically unwarranted, but the patient remains a customer of the office practice and meeting and exceeding the patient's expectations is important.

Downgrading is the term used to describe overriding the protocol disposition and giving the patient a home care or less urgent disposition. This should be done with great caution. Some office practices make it a policy to not downgrade; others allow downgrade only after discussing the patient with the physician. Of course, the patient may sometimes insist on a disposition lower than what the triager recommends. In such cases, the triager should document this. For example: *"Patient will not come into the office now as per my strong recommendation, instead the patient will come to the office at 5:00 pm."*

Home Care Advice – You do not need to provide every piece of care advice listed for the protocol. Try to tailor the care advice to the patient's needs. Attempt to limit the care advice you provide to 2-3 instructions and keep your comments brief. The reason for this is that the average caller cannot retain and act upon more than 2 or 3 key instructions.

Before giving advice, make sure that the caller has a paper and pen handy. This will serve as a memory aid for the caller, reduce callbacks, and ensure that medication dosages are correctly taken. It is often helpful to ask the caller, *"What treatment has the patient tried already?"* This keeps you from wasting the caller's and your time by going over familiar territory. A follow-up question to this is, *"How is this working?"*

Offer empathy, reassurance, and compliments. When a patient has injured himself or herself, it is appropriate to mirror the patient's own description of the pain. For example, the triager may wish to say: "That sounds like it hurts a lot." Callers are sometimes seeking reassurance that the symptoms they are experiencing are common (e.g., fever and muscle aches occur with a cold) and that the treatment they are using is correct (e.g., Tylenol dosing). A triager should provide reassurance whenever possible. Sometimes a sincere compliment is appreciated. Perhaps the patient has been following nearly all of the listed care advice already, in which case it may be appropriate for the triager to tell the caller that they are "doing everything just right." Such compliments provide the patient confidence to handle minor illness and injury on his or her own.

Background Information – Every protocol has some general background information that is provided for the patient's and your benefit. Some of this information is helpful when callers are simply seeking some health information. You should try to review all of the background information in this book as time permits.

Closure – Closure is the end of the telephone triage encounter. The triager will want to confirm that the caller understands the care advice provided, has no further questions, and is in agreement with the recommended disposition. The triager and the caller should be in alignment with the disposition before the call ends. The triager should conclude the conversation with a brief **Call Back If** statement. Suggested Call Back If statements are included at the bottom of the Home Care Advice section. Covering every worst-case scenario is impossible and will unduly alarm the caller. But at the least, the triager should instruct the patient to call back if *"you become worse."*

Selecting the Correct Protocol

Selecting the correct triage protocol is an important initial step in triaging calls.

What is the patient's main problem or symptom? Find the protocol that best matches that problem or symptom. In most circumstances the best protocol will be obvious. For example, a patient calling with a bad sore throat and minimal other symptoms would be triaged using the Sore Throat protocol.

Familiarize yourself with the alphabetic, anatomic, and category listings of protocols. By reviewing these lists you will be able quickly determine the best protocol.

If a caller has multiple symptoms, always select the most serious symptom. If none of the symptoms are serious, select the protocol that will result in the patient be seen the soonest. For most calls you should have to use only 1 protocol to triage a call. In approximately 5% of calls you will need to use 2 protocols.

Reason and Rule-Out Statements

Below many of the Triage Assessment Questions are rationale statements that provide useful information for the nurse triager.

"Rule-outs" (R/O) list the most likely conditions or diagnoses that could cause this symptom. "Reasons" provide the specific indications for a disposition. See Table 5.

Why Are These Reasons and Rule-Outs Provided?
The rationale statements allow physician reviewers to more easily critique the indications for seeing patients. Furthermore, the rationale statements allow the triager to:

- Understand the reasons behind each question.
- If unsure of patient's status, more easily create other questions to pursue relevant diagnoses.
- More easily memorize the questions (understanding increases recall).
- Increase triage nurse job satisfaction and improve nursing judgment.

Should the Caller Be Told the Listed Diagnosis?
Usually no. This should not be done for the following reasons:

- Generally, diagnoses should not be made without seeing the patient and performing a physical examination.

- Suggesting a diagnosis over the phone conveys to the patient that you know more than you actually do.
- A triager should not make a diagnosis over the phone.

If the caller asks you what he or she "might have," tell the caller, *"It's impossible to diagnose most conditions over the telephone, but from what you've told me, you need to be seen for a complete evaluation today."*

If the caller raises a diagnostic possibility, such as appendicitis, and you agree with it, tell the patient, *"It is a possibility and that's why you need to be evaluated today."*

Only as a last resort should you use "scare tactics" (i.e., telling potential diagnoses) to motivate a patient to comply with your recommendation to call an ambulance, go to the emergency department, or come to the office for an evaluation.

Table 5. Reason and Rule-Out Statements

Triage Assessment Question	Reasons and Rule-Outs
• Patient wants to be seen • Bleeding recurs 3 or more times in 24 hours despite direct pressure • Taking Coumadin or known bleeding disorder (e.g., thrombocytopenia) • Has skin bruises or bleeding gums, that are not caused by an injury • Health care provider inserted a nasal packing to control bleeding and now has fever > 100.5° F (38.1° C)	*Reason: need for testing of INR, prothrombin time* *R/O: bleeding disorder* *R/O: sinusitis*

Documentation

Every office should have a method for briefly documenting the telephone triage encounter. Often this takes the form of a telephone log with separate entries for each phone encounter. Some offices instead choose to use a memo pad, which they then tear off and place in the chart as a permanent record. Your office will need to decide on its own standard for documentation.

In Appendix F of this book you will find 3 sample telephone log sheets. Feel free to copy, modify, and use these samples. Simple, well-organized forms like these save you charting time and increase the number of calls you can take per hour.

Always record which protocol you used. If you used 2 protocols, write down the titles of both protocols.

If you decide to recommend EMS 911, direct the patient to the emergency department, or give the patient an appointment, then always list the reason for your decision. The reason is usually going to be the Triage Assessment Question to which you elicited a positive response. If you instead decide that the patient does not need to be seen and that home management is safe and appropriate, remember to document that "all triage questions are negative."

Be certain to document the name, dosage, and route of any medications that you instruct the patient to use. Callers commonly blame dosage errors on information that they received from the triager.

Because protocols are being used, documentation can be limited to pertinent positives.

You should write into the telephone log sheets while you are talking and listening to the caller. Do not try to write down the call afterward; such delayed documentation leads to errors and reduces your efficiency.

Prioritizing Calls

- Take **EMS 911 calls first.**
- Take or return **emergent/urgent** calls that may need to be **seen in the ED or office now next.**
- Take or return nonurgent calls last.

For busy signals or no answer: call back in 10 minutes and then again in 30 minutes.
If there is an answering machine, leave a message.
Document all of your attempts and any message that you leave in your telephone triage log.

May Need to Call EMS 911 Now

You should recommend an emergency medical services (EMS) transport team for patient problems for which there is a clear or high likelihood of life, limb, or organ threat. Such patients may require resuscitative efforts; treatment can often be initiated within minutes by EMS providers. You should immediately transfer the call to EMS. If your phone system cannot transfer a call in this manner, then you should instruct the patient to hang up and immediately call the local ambulance service. In most of the United States, emergency services are available by dialing 911.

Examples of symptoms that nearly always require EMS 911 services include:

- Stopped breathing or severe difficulty breathing
- Unconscious, comatose
- Chest pain lasting longer than 10 minutes, not relieved by nitroglycerin
- Amputation

You may wish to review Appendix C. It contains a table listing further examples of patient symptoms and problems that generally require activation of the EMS system.

In most circumstances the triager should provide no advice to the caller as this will delay the contacting of EMS 911. There are rare situations in which the triager might consider providing brief (10-15 seconds) lifesaving advice to the caller. Examples might include:

- **Choking:** Heimlich maneuver.
- **Fainting:** Lie down with feet elevated.
- **Active Bleeding:** Apply direct pressure to the wound.

What are the exceptions to transferring callers directly to EMS 911? The main exception is the suicidal caller. Such a patient is better served by continuing the conversation and having another staff person in the office call EMS 911 to dispatch a rescue squad. Continue to provide support and understanding until the police or paramedics arrive.

May Need to Be Seen in ED or Office Now

You should recommend an immediate evaluation in the emergency department (ED) or office for patient problems for which there is an low to moderate likelihood of life, limb, or organ threat or if the likelihood is unclear after telephone triage. Many symptoms are of such potentially high seriousness that only through a complete face-to-face medical evaluation can the diagnosis and necessary treatment be determined. Examples of symptoms that often require urgent/emergent evaluation include:

• Chest pain	*R/O: heart attack, etc.*
• Difficulty breathing	*R/O: pneumonia, etc.*
• Abdominal pain persisting > 2 hours	*R/O: appendicitis, etc.*
• Headache, fever, and stiff neck	*R/O: meningitis, etc.*
• Unexplained purple spots	*R/O: meningococcemia*
• Fever higher than 103° F	*R/O: bacterial infection, etc.*
• Severe pain	

You may wish to review Appendix D. It contains a table listing further examples of patient symptoms and problems that generally require an immediate visit to the office or emergency department for medical evaluation.

Nonurgent Calls

Return nonurgent calls last. Examples include cold and cough symptoms, most rashes, constipation, and minor injuries.

Training

1. The first step in training is to review this User's Guide. Ideally, you should read through it twice.
2. Make certain that you understand the structure of the typical telephone triage encounter.
3. Familiarize yourself with whatever documentation form your office uses for telephone triage calls.
4. Review your office's telephone care policies and procedures.
5. Study the Common Cold protocol. Read through and become acquainted with the different components o the protocol.
6. The next step is to review the following protocols. Knowledge of these protocols will prepare you for the most common telephone triage complaints.
7. After studying these protocols, observe an experienced nurse or physician manage phone calls for a minimum of 16 hours.
   - Learn how to select the correct protocol.
   - Learn how to recognize serious symptoms (e.g., choking, chest pain).
   - Learn how to use the Triage Assessment Questions and reach a disposition that is appropriate for your office.
8. Lastly, triage calls yourself for a minimum of 24 hours with an experienced nurse or physician observing.
9. Learning is an ongoing process. Never hesitate to ask the physician in your office or another mentor questions. Your goal is to provide safe and efficacious medical advice to the patients in your office practice.

Abdominal Pain (Female)	Headache
Abdominal Pain (Male)	Neurologic Deficit
Asthma Attack	Rash or Redness, Localized
Back Pain	Rash or Redness, Widespread
Bee Sting	Rectal Symptoms
Chest Pain	Sinus Pain and Congestion
Common Cold	Skin Injury
Constipation	Sore Throat
Cough	Urination Pain (Female)
Diarrhea	Vaginal Bleeding, Abnormal
Earache	Vomiting

Risk Management

- The patient's safety and well-being are always the highest priority.
- Telephone triage is a point of entry into the health care system. Do not use triage as a method of limiting access; instead use it as a method of improving access to primary care.
- Prevent delayed visits of seriously ill patients by taking a proactive and cautious triage stance. When in doubt, see the patient or make arrangements for the patient to be seen. If the problem could be serious, see the patient immediately.
- If the patient sounds very sick or weak to you as the triager, have the patient come in immediately even if none of the other triage assessment questions are positive.
- Any patient that has become confused or too weak to stand needs immediate evaluation. Usually this patient will require EMS activation.
- If the patient's condition sounds life-threatening or unstable, transfer the call to EMS 911 or call an ambulance yourself for the patient.
- A good exercise to improve your ability to recognize life-threatening or serious disease is to read the EMS 911 section of each protocol.
- After reviewing home care advice, ask the caller, "Do you feel comfortable with the plan?" Most will. If the caller does not, perform a callback in 1 hour or, even better, arrange for the patient to be seen. Always strive for "alignment" with the caller. If the caller insists that he or she needs to be seen, accommodate that request. From a risk management standpoint, it is challenging to defend a bad patient outcome when the patient insisted on being seen and the triager adamantly refused an appointment.
- The triager may override the protocol to suggest the patient goes to a higher level disposition. The triager should not override the protocol to a lower disposition, but instead should discuss with or refer such calls to the primary care physician.
- A nurse triager should not make a diagnosis over the phone. It may be appropriate in certain circumstances for a physician triager to provide a possible/probable diagnosis over the phone.
- Encourage all callers to call back if the condition worsens. Callers should be given specific reasons to call back. At the least, the triager should instruct the patient call back if "you become worse."
- Sometimes callers telephone seeking some brief health information and do not want to be triaged. When in doubt, perform a complete triage and document the call completely. For example, the 55-year-old male patient with "gas pressure" in his chest seeking information about the best antacid may actually be having a heart attack and should be triaged into the emergency department. The 22-year-old female who is calling with concerns about breastfeeding may actually have significant postpartum depression.
- Three calls equal a visit. If a patient calls seeking advice about the same problem 3 times, arrange an appointment. In fact, if the caller phones in 2 times in 12 hours, you usually should arrange an appointment. The reason you should see the patient is that either the caller was not reassured by the information provided over the phone or the patient is actually sicker than described. An exception to this rule is a patient calling in a second time to confirm a drug dosage.
- If a caller calls about a diagnosis (e.g., athlete's foot), do not accept the caller's diagnosis unless it meets the criteria listed in the definition at the beginning of the protocol.
- These protocols should be reviewed and amended as needed by the physicians in your medical practice.

References

Poole SR. *The Complete Guide: Providing Telephone Triage and Advice in a Family Practice.* Elk Grove Village, IL: American Academy of Pediatrics; 2011

Reisman AB, Stevens DL, eds. *Telephone Medicine: A Guide for the Practicing Physician.* Philadelphia, PA: American College of Physicians; 2002

Schmitt BD. *Pediatric Telephone Protocols: Office Version.* 16th ed. Itasca, IL: American Academy of Pediatrics; 2019

Wheeler S. *Telephone Triage: Theory, Practice and Protocol Development.* San Anselmo, CA: TeleTriage Systems Publishers; 1993

Appendix B

Red Flag Flowchart for Office Support Staff or Call Center Staff

Call Prioritization Index
Conceptual Flowchart

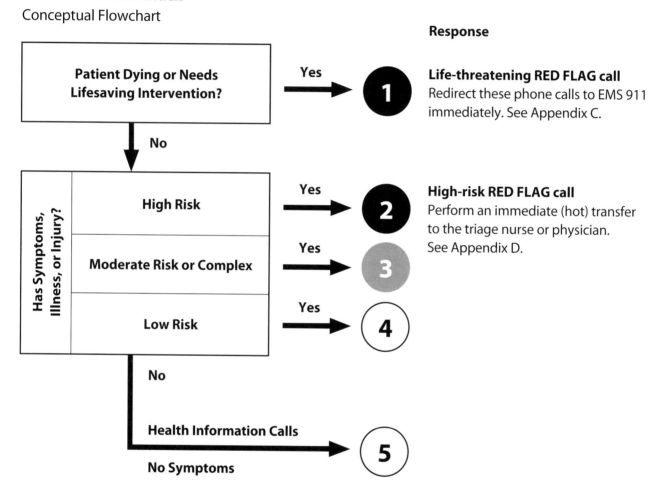

Response

Patient Dying or Needs Lifesaving Intervention? — Yes → **1** — **Life-threatening RED FLAG call** Redirect these phone calls to EMS 911 immediately. See Appendix C.

No

Has Symptoms, Illness, or Injury?

High Risk — Yes → **2** — **High-risk RED FLAG call** Perform an immediate (hot) transfer to the triage nurse or physician. See Appendix D.

Moderate Risk or Complex — Yes → **3**

Low Risk — Yes → **4**

No

Health Information Calls → **5**

No Symptoms

Appendix C

Prioritizing Calls

May Need to Call EMS 911 NOW

ABCs	Reason or Diagnosis
Airway ● Choking ● Stopped breathing	**Airway obstruction** **Respiratory arrest**
Breathing ● Severe difficulty breathing (e.g., struggling for each breath, unable to speak) ● Lips or face are bluish ● Rapid onset of cough, wheezing, or difficulty breathing after bee sting, insect bite, or other allergic exposure (e.g., medicine, food)	**Respiratory failure** **Hypoxia** **Anaphylaxis**
Circulation ● Signs of shock (e.g., cold/clammy, low blood pressure) ● Unconscious, coma ● Lethargic	**Shock from cardiac, hypovolemic, or septic cause**

Systems	Reason or Diagnosis
Allergic ● Rapid onset of cough, wheezing, or difficulty breathing after bee sting, insect bite, or other allergic exposure (e.g., medicine, food) ● Previous severe allergic reaction (anaphylaxis) to bees, yellow jackets, etc. (not just hives or swelling) and < 2 hours since sting	**Anaphylaxis**

Cardiovascular
● Fainted and still feels dizzy or light-headed
● Chest pain lasting longer than 5 minutes and any of the following:
  – Pain is crushing, pressure-like, or heavy
  – History of heart disease (e.g., angina, heart attack, bypass surgery, angioplasty)
  – Over 50 years old
  – Over 35 years old and one or more cardiac risk factors (i.e., high blood pressure, diabetes, high cholesterol, obesity, smoker, or strong family history of heart disease)
  – Took nitroglycerin and chest pain was not relieved
	Arrhythmia, shock
	Myocardial infarction or unstable angina

Infectious ● Too weak or sick to stand ● Fever and purple or blood-colored spots or dots ● Possible bioterrorism exposure	**Sepsis** **Meningococcemia** **Bioterrorism**
Neurologic ● Difficult to awaken or acting confused (disoriented, slurred speech) ● Weakness of the face, arm, or leg on one side of the body (new onset) ● Numbness of the face, arm, or leg on one side of the body (new onset) ● Loss of speech or garbled speech (new onset)	**Stroke (CVA)**
Psychiatric ● Intentional overdose or poisoning (suicide attempt) ● Suicide attempt ● Suicidal or homicidal ideation	
Traumatic ● Cut on the neck, chest, back, or abdomen that may go deep (e.g., stab wound) ● Major bleeding (actively dripping or spurting) that can't be stopped ● Amputation ● Head injury with loss of consciousness > 1 minute ● Second- or third-degree burn involving > 10% of body surface area	**Penetrating trauma** **Uncontrolled bleeding** **Epidural, subdural**

Appendix D

Prioritizing Calls   May Need to Be Seen in ED or Office NOW

General	Reason or Diagnosis

● Patient sounds very sick or weak to the triager
● Sounds like a serious injury to the triager
● Fever > 103° F (39.4° C)
● Fever > 100.4° F (38.0° C) and:
  – Over 60 years of age
  – Diabetes mellitus or a weakened immune system (e.g., HIV positive, chemotherapy, chronic steroid treatment, splenectomy)
  – Bedridden (e.g., nursing home patient, stroke, chronic illness, recovering from surgery)
  – Transplant patient (e.g., liver, heart, kidney)
● Drinking very little and signs of dehydration (e.g., no urine > 12 hours, very dry mouth, light-headed, etc.)
● Severe pain
	Bacterial infection
	Bacterial infection
	
	Dehydration
	Severe pain should be treated

Systems	Reason or Diagnosis

Cardiovascular
● Heart beating irregularly or very rapidly
● Chest pain with any of the following:
  – Pain also present in the shoulder(s), arm(s), or jaw
  – Difficulty breathing or unusual sweating
● Has known "angina" chest pain and pain has been increasing in severity or frequency
	Arrhythmia
	Acute myocardial infarction
	
	Unstable angina

Gastrointestinal ● Constant abdominal pain persisting > 2 hours ● Vomiting red blood or black ("coffee ground") material ● Blood in bowel movements ● Black or tarry bowel movements	Surgical cause of pain GI bleed
Infectious ● Fever and rash ● Purple or blood-colored spots or dots ● Looks infected (spreading redness, pus, red streak)	Rocky Mountain spotted fever Meningococcemia Cellulitis, lymphangitis
Neurologic ● Vision loss or change	

Respiratory
● Coughing up blood
● Difficulty breathing (new or worsening)
● Asthma and either:
  – Peak flow rate less than 50% of baseline level
  – Peak flow rate 50-80% of baseline level after nebulizer x 1 OR inhaler x 2 (2 puffs q 20 minutes)
● Wheezing, audible
	Pneumonia, CHF, pulmonary embolus
	Significant asthma attack

Traumatic ● Skin is split open or gaping ● Minor bleeding won't stop after 10 minutes of direct pressure ● Injury looks like a dislocated joint (crooked or deformed) ● Can't stand (bear weight) or walk ● Animal at risk for RABIES and any cut, puncture, or scratch ● Burn blisters (open or closed) over area larger than palm of hand (>1% BSA) ● Burn from acid or alkali (lye) burn	Laceration needing sutures or staples Fracture or dislocation Fracture or dislocation Rabies vaccination Large second-degree burn Chemical burn
Urologic ● Unable to urinate and bladder feels very full	Urinary retention

Appendix E

Office Resources

Procedures

If this procedure is needed, how often would it be performed in this office (rather than referred to the ED or a surgeon's office)?	Always or Nearly Always	Sometimes (Ask PCP)	Never (Refer to ED)	Referral Notes
IV fluid for dehydration				
IM or IV antibiotics				
Phlebotomy (blood draw from vein)				
Extremity laceration repair using sutures				
Facial laceration repair using sutures				
Facial laceration repair using Dermabond (skin glue)				
Mouth laceration repair using sutures				
Animal bite wound care (vigorous irrigation)				
Reduction of angulated forearm fracture				
Reduction of finger dislocation (PIP or DIP)				
Reduction of shoulder dislocation				
Reduction of a nursemaid elbow				
Sling/strapping non-displaced clavicle fracture				
Splinting non-displaced finger fracture				
Foreign body removal from cornea				
Foreign body removal from conjunctiva				
Foreign body removal from ear canal				
Foreign body removal from nasal canal				
Foreign body removal from subcutaneous skin				
Fishhook removal from skin				
Fluorescein examination for corneal abrasion				
Incision and drainage of an abscess				
Drainage of a subungual hematoma				
Nasal packing for epistaxis				
Nasal cautery for epistaxis				
Pelvic exam and Pap smear				
Pelvic exam and foreign body removal				
Minor facial burn treatment and follow-up				
Minor extremity burn treatment and follow-up				
Sigmoidoscopy				
Urinary catheter insertion (Foley or coudé)				
Lumbar puncture				
Arthrocentesis (joint aspiration) of knee				

Office Resources   Tests

If this test is needed, can it be performed in this office?	Yes	No	Notes
Plain radiograph (i.e., CXR, extremity film)			
Urine dipstick			
Urine pregnancy test			
Fingerstick hemoglobin			
Fingerstick blood glucose			
Rapid strep test			
Pulse oximetry			
Peak flow rate			
EKG			

Office Resources   Medications

If this medication is needed, is it available in this office?	Route	Yes	No	Notes
Albuterol inhaler (or other beta-agonist)	Inhaler			
Albuterol for nebulization (or other beta-agonist)	Nebulizer			
Epinephrine 1:1000 for SQ administration	SQ			
Nitroglycerine SL pills or nasal spray	SL or Nasal			
Diphenhydramine pills or liquid (e.g., Benadryl or other oral antihistamine)	Oral			
Aspirin pills	Oral			
Acetaminophen suppositories (e.g., Tylenol)	Rectal			
Acetaminophen pills or liquid (e.g., Tylenol)	Oral			
Ibuprofen pills or liquid (e.g., Motrin, Advil)	Oral			
Influenza vaccine	IM			
Tetanus immunization (e.g., Td, Tdap)	IM			

Appendix F

Sample Telephone Triage Logs

Date & Times – Call Received – Call Back – Call Finished	Patient's Name – Age, Sex – Phone Number Social Factors Chronic Illness	Brief History of Illness/Injury Document symptoms • Location, duration, severity List reason patient needs to be seen or mark "all triage questions negative"	Disposition	Comments – Special Advice – Drug Dosage – Follow-up Call Triager
		Protocol Reason to see _____ Or ☐ all triage questions negative	☐ EMS 911 ☐ ED Now ☐ Office Now ☐ See Today ☐ See Tomorrow ☐ See Later, protocol care advice given ☐ Home Care, protocol care advice given ☐ Patient agrees ☐ Refer call to PCP	
		Protocol Reason to see _____ Or ☐ all triage questions negative	☐ EMS 911 ☐ ED Now ☐ Office Now ☐ See Today ☐ See Tomorrow ☐ See Later, protocol care advice given ☐ Home Care, protocol care advice given ☐ Patient agrees ☐ Refer call to PCP	
		Protocol Reason to see _____ Or ☐ all triage questions negative	☐ EMS 911 ☐ ED Now ☐ Office Now ☐ See Today ☐ See Tomorrow ☐ See Later, protocol care advice given ☐ Home Care, protocol care advice given ☐ Patient agrees ☐ Refer call to PCP	

Time Phone Number	Patient Name Age/Sex	Problem/Symptom	Protocol Used	Disposition	Advice Per Protocol Drug Dosage

Date: _____   Triage Nurse: _____

Date	Time	Phone #	Patient
Age _____ Sex ☐ F ☐ M Symptoms Chronic Illness		Protocol Reason to See Or ☐ all triage questions negative	Disposition ☐ EMS 911 ☐ ED Now ☐ Office Now ☐ See Today ☐ See Tomorrow ☐ See Later, protocol care advice given ☐ Home Care, protocol care advice given ☐ Patient agrees ☐ Refer call to PCP
☐ Advice Per Protocol			Triager

Date	Time	Phone #	Patient
Age _____ Sex ☐ F ☐ M Symptoms Chronic Illness		Protocol Reason to See Or ☐ all triage questions negative	Disposition ☐ EMS 911 ☐ ED Now ☐ Office Now ☐ See Today ☐ See Tomorrow ☐ See Later, protocol care advice given ☐ Home Care, protocol care advice given ☐ Patient agrees ☐ Refer call to PCP
☐ Advice Per Protocol			Triager

Date	Time	Phone #	Patient
Age _____ Sex ☐ F ☐ M Symptoms Chronic Illness		Protocol Reason to See Or ☐ all triage questions negative	Disposition ☐ EMS 911 ☐ ED Now ☐ Office Now ☐ See Today ☐ See Tomorrow ☐ See Later, protocol care advice given ☐ Home Care, protocol care advice given ☐ Patient agrees ☐ Refer call to PCP
☐ Advice Per Protocol			Triager

Appendix G

Reviewers

The author is grateful to the following individuals for their time and expertise in reviewing the triage content that has been incorporated into these guidelines.

Call Center Medical Directors

Lee-Anne Facey-Crowther, MD, Medical Advisor, Sykes Assistance Services Corporation, Toronto, Ontario, Canada

Susan MacLean, MD, Medical Advisor, Sykes Assistance Services Corporation, Toronto, Ontario, Canada

Gary Marks, DO, CHWS, Medical Director Telemedicine & Telephone Nurse Triage, Asante, Medford, OR

Scott Pirkle, MD, Regional Director ECI Healthcare - Schumacher Clinical Partners, Chief Medical Officer Air Methods, Indianapolis, IN

Mark Rotty, MD, Medical Director, Medical Call Center, Children's Physician Network, Minneapolis, MN

Barton Schmitt, MD, Professor of Pediatrics, Medical Director, After-Hours Call Center, Children's Hospital Colorado, Aurora, CO

Gary Setnik, MD, Chair, Emergency Medicine, Mount Auburn Hospital, Cambridge, MA; Co-director, Division of Emergency Medicine, Harvard Medical School; Medical Director, SironaHealth, Portland, ME

Michael Wahl, MD, Medical Director, The Illinois Poison Center, Chicago, IL

Michael Weaver, MD, Medical Director, Fonemed; Medical Director, Clinical Forensic Care Program; VP Clinical Diversity, Saint Luke's Hospital, MO

Physicians

Charles Bareis, MD, General Internist, Chief Medical Officer, MacNeal Hospital and Health Network, Berwyn, IL

Gregor Blix, MD, Urologic Surgeon, Medical Director Healthcare Midwest Surgery Center, Bronson Methodist Hospital and Borgess Hospital, Kalamazoo, MI

Carolyn B. Bridges, MD, CDR, USPHS. Associate Director for Science (acting), Influenza Division, NCIRD (proposed), Centers for Disease Control and Prevention

John Brofman, MD, Pulmonologist, Medical Director of Critical Care, MacNeal Hospital and Health Network, Berwyn, IL

Dwayne Coad, MD, Emergency Physician and Hospice Physician, Yellowknife, Northwest Territories, Canada

Andrew Davis, MD, MPH, General Internist, Assistant Professor of Clinical Medicine, University of Chicago Hospitals, Chicago, IL

Robin Devan, MD, Palliative Care Program, Adult Sickle Cell Clinical Program, Assistant Professor, College of Medicine, University of Arkansas for Medical Sciences

Kellie Flood-Shaffer, MD, Assistant Professor, Division Director, Obstetrics and Gynecology, University of Cincinatti, Ohio

David Goldberg, MD, Director of Student Health, Assistant Professor of Medicine, Loyola University Medical Center, Maywood, IL

Mitchell Goldman, MD, Pediatric Emergency Medicine, Peyton Manning Children's Hospital at St Vincent, Indianapolis, IN

Michael Gottlieb, MD, Emergency Physician, John H. Stroger, Jr. of Cook County Hospital, Chicago, IL

Joseph Grubenhoff, MD, Assistant Professor, Section of Emergency Medicine, The Children's Hospital, Denver, CO

Jason Gutting, MD, Pediatrician, Pediatric Emergency Physician, Pediatric Telemedicine Specialist, Medical Director of Informatics SSM St. Joseph Hospital, Lake, St. Louis, MO

Kenneth Heinrich, MD, Emergency Physician; Regional Director, Emergency Consultants, Inc., Traverse City, MI

Inbar Kirson, MD, Attending, Obstetrics and Gynecology, Lutheran General Hospital, Park Ridge, IL

Tony Lang, MD, Intemist, Mercy Hospital and Medical Center, Chicago, IL

Matthew Levine, MD, Director of Trauma Services, Department of Emergency Medicine, Northwestern Memorial Hospital, Chicago, IL

Samantha Mckelvey, Obstetrics and Gynecology, University of Arkansas for Medical Sciences; ANGELS program (Antenatal and Neonatal Guidelines, Education and Learning System), Little Rock, AR

Katherine Nolan-Watson, MD, Assistant Professor in Obstetrics and Gynecology, Loyola University Medical Center, Maywood, IL

Roger Kaldawy, MD, Assistant Professor in Ophthalmology and Visual Sciences, Boston University School of Medicine, Boston, MA

Edward Otten, MD, Toxicologist, Professor of Emergency Medicine, University of Cincinnati Medical Center, OH

Greg Ozark, MD, Director, Med-Peds Residency, Loyola University Medical Center, Maywood, IL

Paula Podrazik, MD, Geriatrician, General Internist and ED Physician, University of Chicago Hospitals, Chicago, IL

Anna B. Reisman, MD, Assistant Professor, Department of Internal Medicine, Yale University School of Medicine, New Haven, CT

Theodora Rusinak, MD, Emergency Physician, Illinois Masonic Hospital, Chicago, IL

Daniel Stone, MD, MBA, Attending Physician and Clinical Instructor, Northwestern University Emergency Medicine Residency, Chicago, IL

Herb Sutherland, DO, Medical Director of Emergency Department and Medical Call Center, Central Dupage Hospital, Winfield, IL

Penny Tenzer, MD, Vice-Chair, Director of Family Medicine Residency, University of Miami Hospital and Medical School, FL

Diana Viravec, MD, Emergency Physician, Emergency Services, MacNeal Hospital and Health Network, Berwyn, IL

Gary Wainer, DO, Family Practice Attending, Chief Medical Officer, Chicago Health Systems, Chicago, IL

James Waymack, MD, Assistant Professor of Emergency Medicine at Southern Illinois University in Springfield, IL

Victoria Weston, MD, Emergency Physician, Northwestern Lake Forest Hospital; Past President, AAEM Resident and Student Association

James Wilkerson, MD, Attending Pathologist, Merced Pathology Laboratory, Merced, CA

David Zipes, MD, Pediatric Hospitalist, Peyton Manning Children's Hospital at St Vincent, Indianapolis, IN

Nurses

Mary Alexander, CRNI, Chief Executive Officer, Infusion Nurses Society (INS), Editor, *Journal of Infusion Nursing,* Norwood, MA

Charlene Brophy, Director of Client and Clinical Services, FONEMED, Newfoundland, Canada

Tina Butler, WHNP-BC, MNSc, University of Arkansas for Medical Sciences ANGELS program (Antenatal and Neonatal Guidelines, Education and Learning System), Little Rock, AR

Joanne Dedowicz, RN, Director of Resource and Referral, Behavioral Health, Edwards – Linden Hospital, Naperville, IL

Jenny DuFresne, RN, Manager for Valley Connection Call Center, Santa Clara Valley Hospital, Santa Clara, CA

Jeanine Feirer, RN, Clinical Coordinator, Proactive Health, Marshfield Clinic, Unity, WI

Lisbeth Gabrielski, RN, MSN, IBCLC, Clinical Manager, Lactation Services, The Children's Hospital, Denver, CO

Rebecca Gebhart, RN, MSN, Faculty, University of Phoenix AZ, Call Center Advisor, ExpertKnowledgeNetwork.com

Marlene Grasser, RN, LVM Systems, Phoenix, AZ

Deborah Gresham, RNC, MSN, Clinical Nurse Specialist, Center for Women's Health Care, Miami Valley Hospital, Dayton OH

Valerie Grossman, RN, BSN, CEN, Director of Medical-Surgical Services, Via Health Hospital, Rochester, NY

Teresa Hegarty, RN, Nurse Manager, Call Center Nurse, After-Hours Call Center Children's Hospital Colorado, Aurora, CO

Laura Mahlmeister, RN, PhD, Educational and Nurse Legal Consultant, L&D Nurse, Mahlmeister and Associates, San Francisco, CA

Kelli Massaro, RN, Telephone Triage Consultant, Call Center Nurse, After-Hours Call Center Children's Hospital Colorado, Aurora, CO

Melissa Masson, RN, BScN, MN(c), Clinical Practice Consultant, Sykes Assistance Services Corporation, Ontario, Canada

Donna Matthews, RN, Newfoundland, Canada

Nurses (*continued*)

Becky McGowan, RN, Call Center Nurse and Emergency Department Nurse, MacNeal Hospital and Health Network, Berwyn, IL

Kim McCormick, RN, Telephone Triage, Home Health and Hospice Nursing, MacNeal Home Health Care, Berwyn, IL

Cheryl Patterson, RNC, BSN, Educator Coordinator, Evergreen Healthline, Evergreen Hospital Medical Center, Kirkland, WA

Laurie Peachey, RN, Toronto, Ontario, Canada

Teresa Pounds, BSN, RN, Clinical Quality Coordinator for Citra Health Solutions, Portland, ME

Joan Rucker, RN, Perinatal and Maternal Educator, MacNeal Hospital and Health Network, Berwyn, IL

Susan Smith Dodson, MBA, BSN, RN, CCRC, Triage System Development Coordinator/Trainer, University of Arkansas for Medical Sciences ANGELS program (Antenatal and Neonatal Guidelines, Education and Learning System), Little Rock, AR

Beverley Tipsord-Klinkhammer, RN, MBA, Senior VP of Patient Services, Onslow Memorial Hospital, Jacksonville, NC

Michelle Violette, RN, BScN, MSc, Director of Chronic Disease Management, Sykes Assistance Services Corporation, Toronto, Ontario, Canada

Donna Williams, RN, Nurse Manager, University of Arkansas for Medical Sciences ANGELS program (Antenatal and Neonatal Guidelines, Education and Learning System), Little Rock, AR

Paramedics

Peter Dillman, EdD, EMT-P, St Vincent Health, Indianapolis, IN

Dentists

James Discipio, DDS, LaGrange, IL

Behavioral Health Counselors

Jennifer Vitagliano, MC, CPC, Helpline Coordinator, Behavioral Health Services, Banner Health System Call Center, Phoenix, AZ

Appendix H: References for All Protocols

Abdominal Pain (Female)

1. Barnhart KT. Clinical practice. Ectopic pregnancy. *N Engl J Med.* 2009;361(4):379–387
2. Bundy DG, Byerley JS, Liles EA, Perrin EM, Katznelson J, Rice HE. Does this child have appendicitis? *JAMA.* 2007;298(4):438–451
3. Cappell MS, Friedel D. Abdominal pain during pregnancy. *Gastroenterol Clin North Am.* 2003;32(1):1–58
4. Cardall T, Glasser J, Guss DA. Clinical value of the total white blood cell count and temperature in the evaluation of patients with suspected appendicitis. *Acad Emerg Med.* 2004;11(10):1021–1027
5. Cartwright SL, Knudson MP. Evaluation of acute abdominal pain in adults. *Am Fam Physician.* 2008;77(7):971–978
6. Condous G. Ectopic pregnancy—risk factors and diagnosis. *Aust Fam Physician.* 2006;35(11):854–857
7. Flasar MH, Cross R, Goldberg E. Acute abdominal pain. *Prim Care.* 2006;33(3):659–684, vi
8. Hendrickson M, Naparst TR. Abdominal surgical emergencies in the elderly. *Emerg Med Clin North Am.* 2003;21(4):937–969
9. Jacobs DO. Clinical practice. Diverticulitis. *N Engl J Med.* 2007;357(20):2057–2066
10. Kamin R, Nowicki TA, Courtney DS, Powers RD. Pearls and pitfalls in the emergency department evaluation of abdominal pain. *Emerg Med Clin North Am.* 2003;21(1):61–72, vi
11. Martinez JP, Hogan GJ. Mesenteric ischemia. *Emerg Med Clin North Am.* 2004;22(4):909–928
12. Martinez JP, Mattu A Abdominal pain in the elderly. *Emerg Med Clin North Am.* 2006;24(2):371–388, vii
13. North F, Odunukan O, Varkey P. The value of telephone triage for patients with appendicitis. *J Telemed Telecare.* 2011;17(8):417–420
14. Ranji SR, Goldman LE, Simel DL, Shojania KG. Do opiates affect the clinical evaluation of patients with acute abdominal pain? *JAMA.* 2006;296(14):1764–1774
15. Roy S, Weimersheimer P. Nonoperative cause of abdominal pain. *Surg Clin North Am.* 1997;77(6):1433–1454
16. Stewart C, Bosker G. Pelvic inflammatory disease. *Emerg Med Rep.* 1999;20(16):163–172
17. Wagner JM, McKinney WP, Carpenter JL. Does this patient have appendicitis? *JAMA.* 1996;276(19):1589–1594
18. Yamamoto W, Kono H, Maekawa M, Fukui T. The relationship between abdominal pain regions and specific diseases: an epidemiologic approach to clinical practice. *J Epidemiol.*1997;7(1):27–32

Abdominal Pain (Male)

1. Bundy DG, Byerley JS, Liles EA, Perrin EM, Katznelson J, Rice HE. Does this child have appendicitis? *JAMA.* 2007;298(4):438–451
2. Cardall T, Glasser J, Guss DA. Clinical value of the total white blood cell count and temperature in the evaluation of patients with suspected appendicitis. *Acad Emerg Med.* 2004;11(10):1021–1027
3. Cartwright SL, Knudson MP. Evaluation of acute abdominal pain in adults. *Am Fam Physician.* 2008;77(7):971–978
4. Flasar MH, Cross R, Goldberg E. Acute abdominal pain. *Prim Care.* 2006;33(3):659–684, vi
5. Hendrickson M, Naparst TR. Abdominal surgical emergencies in the elderly. *Emerg Med Clin North Am.* 2003;21(4):937–969
6. Jacobs DO. Clinical practice. Diverticulitis. *N Engl J Med.* 2007;357(20):2057–2066
7. Kamin R. Nowicki TA, Courtney DS, Powers RD. Pearls and pitfalls in the emergency department evaluation of abdominal pain. *Emerg Med Clin North Am.* 2003;21(1):61–72, vi
8. Martinez JP, Hogan GJ. Mesenteric ischemia. *Emerg Med Clin North Am.* 2004;22(4):909–928
9. Martinez JP, Mattu A Abdominal pain in the elderly. *Emerg Med Clin North Am.* 2006;24(2):371–388, vii

10. North F, Odunukan O, Varkey P. The value of telephone triage for patients with appendicitis. *J Telemed Telecare.* 2011;17(8):417–420
11. Pearigen PD. Unusual causes of abdominal pain. *Emerg Med Clin North Am.* 1996;14(3):593–613
12. Ranji SR, Goldman LE, Simel DL, Shojania KG. Do opiates affect the clinical evaluation of patients with acute abdominal pain? *JAMA.* 2006;296(14):1764–1774
13. Roy S, Weimersheimer P. Nonoperative cause of abdominal pain. *Surg Clin North Am.* 1997;77(6):1433–1454
14. Wagner JM, McKinney WP, Carpenter JL. Does this patient have appendicitis? *JAMA.* 1996;276(19):1589–1594
15. Yamamoto W, Kono H, Maekawa M, Fukui T. The relationship between abdominal pain regions and specific diseases: an epidemiologic approach to clinical practice. *J Epidemiol.* 1997;7(1):27–32

Abdominal Pain (Menstrual Cramps)

1. Apgar BS. Dysmenorrhea and dysfunctional uterine bleeding. *Prim Care.* 1997;24(1):161–178
2. Barnhart KT. Clinical practice. Ectopic pregnancy. *N Engl J Med.* 2009;361(4):379–387
3. Bundy DG, Byerley JS, Liles EA, Perrin EM, Katznelson J, Rice HE. Does this child have appendicitis? *JAMA.* 2007;298(4):438–451
4. Dawood MY. Primary dysmenorrhea: advances in pathogenesis and management. *Obstet Gynecol.* 2006;108(2):428–441
5. Duleba AJ. Diagnosis of endometriosis. *Obstet Gynecol Clin North Am.* 1997;24(2):331–346
6. Kamin R, Nowicki TA, Courtney DS, Powers RD. Pearls and pitfalls in the emergency department evaluation of abdominal pain. *Emerg Med Clin North Am.* 2003;21(1):61–72
7. Lethaby A, Augood C, Duckitt K, Farquhar C. Nonsteroidal anti-inflammatory drugs for heavy menstrual bleeding. *Cochrane Database Syst Rev.* 2007;(4):CD000400
8. Milsom I, Minic M, Dawood MY, et al. Comparison of the efficacy and safety of nonprescription doses of naproxen and naproxen sodium with ibuprofen, acetaminophen, and placebo in the treatment of dysmenorrhea. *Clin Ther.* 2002;24(9):1384–1400
9. Proctor ML, Hing W, Johnson TC, Murphy PA. Spinal manipulation for primary and secondary dysmenorrhoea. *Cochrane Database Syst Rev.* 2006;3:CD002119
10. Rainsford KD. Ibuprofen: pharmacology, efficacy and safety. *Inflammopharmacology.* 2009;17(6):275–342
11. Santer M, Wyke S, Warner P. What aspects of periods are most bothersome for women reporting heavy menstrual bleeding? Community survey and qualitative study. *C Womens Health.* 2007;7:8
12. Wagner JM, McKinney WP, Carpenter JL. Does this patient have appendicitis? *JAMA.* 1996;276(19):1589–1594
13. Warner PE, Critchley HO, Lumsden MA, Campbell-Brown M, Douglas A, Murray GD. Menorrhagia I: measured blood loss, clinical features, and outcome in women with heavy periods: a survey with follow-up data. *Am J Obstet Gynecol.* 2004;190(5):1216–1223
14. Warner PE, Critchley HO, Lumsden MA, Campbell-Brown M, Douglas A, Murray GD. Menorrhagia II: is the 80-mL blood loss criterion useful in management of complaint of menorrhagia? *Am J Obstet Gynecol.* 2004;190(5):1224–1229
15. Wilson ML, Murphy PA. Herbal and dietary therapies for primary and secondary dysmenorrhoea. *Cochrane Database Syst Rev.* 2001;(3):CD002124
16. Wong CL, Farquhar C, Roberts H, Proctor M. Oral contraceptive pill for primary dysmenorrhoea. *Cochrane Database Syst Rev.* 2009;(4):CD002120
17. Zhang WY, Li Wan Po A. Efficacy of minor analgesics in primary dysmenorrhoea: a systematic review. *Br J Obstet Gynaecol.* 1998;105(7):780–790

Abdominal Pain (Upper)

1. Bundy DG, Byerley JS, Liles EA, et al. Does this child have appendicitis? *JAMA.* 2007;298(4):438–451
2. Canto JG, Shlipak MG, Rogers WJ, et al. Prevalence, clinical characteristics, and mortality among patients with myocardial infarction presenting without chest pain. *JAMA.* 2000;283(24):3223–3229
3. Cartwright SL, Knudson MP. Evaluation of acute abdominal pain in adults. *Am Fam Physician.* 2008;77(7):971–980
4. Culic V, Eterovic D, Miric D, Silic N. Symptom presentation of acute myocardial infarction: influence of sex, age, and risk factors. *Am Heart J.* 2002;144(6):1012–1017
5. Edwards M, Chang AM, Matsuura AC, Green M, Robey JM, Hollander JE. Relationship between pain severity and outcomes in patients presenting with potential acute coronary syndromes. *Ann Emerg Med.* 2011;58(6):501–507
6. Flasar MH, Cross R, Goldberg E. Acute abdominal pain. *Prim Care.* 2006;33(3):659–684, vi
7. Lemire S. Assessment of clinical severity and investigation of uncomplicated gastroesophageal reflux disease and noncardiac angina-like chest pain. *Can J Gastroenterol.* 1997;11(suppl B):37B–40B
8. Martinez JP, Mattu A Abdominal pain in the elderly. *Emerg Med Clin North Am.* 2006;24(2):371–388, vii
9. North F, Odunukan O, Varkey P. The value of telephone triage for patients with appendicitis. *J Telemed Telecare.* 2011;17(8):417–420
10. Pearigen PD. Unusual causes of abdominal pain. *Emerg Med Clin North Am.* 1996;14(3):593–613
11. Ranji SR, Goldman LE, Simel DL, Shojania KG. Do opiates affect the clinical evaluation of patients with acute abdominal pain? *JAMA.* 2006;296(14):1764–1774
12. Roy S, Weimersheimer P. Nonoperative cause of abdominal pain. *Surg Clin North Am.* 1997;77(6):1433–1454
13. Sanson TG, O'Keefe KP. Evaluation of abdominal pain in the elderly. *Emerg Med Clin North Am.* 1996;14(3):615–627
14. Simrén M, Tack J. Functional dyspepsia: evaluation and treatment. *Gastroenterol Clin North Am.* 2003;32(2):577–599
15. Wagner JM, McKinney WP, Carpenter JL. Does this patient have appendicitis? *JAMA.* 1996;276(19):1589–1594
16. Yamamoto W, Kono H, Maekawa M, Fukui T. The relationship between abdominal pain regions and specific diseases: an epidemiologic approach to clinical practice. *J Epidemiol.* 1997;7(1):27–32

Alcohol Abuse and Dependence

1. Burge SK, Schneider FD. Alcohol-related problems: recognition and intervention. *Am Fam Physician.* 1999;59(2):361–372
2. Cherpitel CJ. Screening for alcohol problems in the emergency department. *Ann Emerg Med.* 1995;26(2):158–166
3. Dart RC, Kuffner EK, Rumack BH. Treatment of pain or fever with paracetamol (acetaminophen) in the alcoholic patient: a systematic review. *Am J Ther.* 2000;7(2):123–134
4. Fiellin DA, Reid MC, O'Connor PG. Outpatient management of patients with alcohol problems. *Ann Intern Med.* 2000;133(10):815–827
5. Mayo-Smith MF, Beecher LH, Fischer TL, et al; American Society of Addiction Medicine Working Group on the Management of Alcohol Withdrawal Delirium, Practice Guidelines Committee. Management of alcohol withdrawal delirium. An evidence-based practice guideline. *Arch Intern Med.* 2004;164(13):1405–1412
6. Stein MD. Medical consequences of substance abuse. *Psychiatr Clin North Am.* 1999;22(2):351–370
7. US Department of Health and Human Services, Public Health Service. *The Physicians' Guide to Helping Patients With Alcohol Problems.* Bethesda, MD: National Institutes of Health; 1995. NIH publication no. 95-3769
8. US Preventive Services Task Force. Screening for problem drinking. In: *Guide to Clinical Preventive Services.* 2nd ed. Alexandria, VA: International Medical Publishing, Inc; 1996:567–582

Anaphylaxis

1. American Academy of Allergy, Asthma and Immunology. The use of epinephrine in the treatment of anaphylaxis. Position statement #26. http://www.aaaai.org/Aaaai/media/MediaLibrary/PDF%20Documents/Practice%20and%20Parameters/Epinephrine-in-treating-anaphylaxis-2002.pdf. Accessed June 7, 2018
2. American Heart Association. 2005 Guidelines for Cardiopulmonary Resuscitation and Emergency Cardiovascular Care. Part 10: First Aid. *Circulation.* 2005;112:IV-196–IV-203
3. Anchor J, Settipane RA. Appropriate use of epinephrine in anaphylaxis. *Am J Emerg Med.* 2004;22(6):488–490
4. Braganza SC, Acworth JP, Mckinnon DR, Peake JE, Brown AF. Paediatric emergency department anaphylaxis: different patterns from adults. *Arch Dis Child.* 2006;91(2):159–163
5. Burks AW, Sampson HA. Anaphylaxis and food allergy. *Clin Rev Allergy Immunol.* 1999;17(3):339–360
6. Ellis AK, Day JH. Diagnosis and management of anaphylaxis. *CMAJ.* 2003;169(4):307–311
7. Fisher M. Treatment of acute anaphylaxis. *BMJ.* 1995;311(7007):731–733
8. Golden DB. Patterns of anaphylaxis: acute and late phase features of allergic reactions. *Novartis Found Symp.* 2004;257:101–110; discussion 110–150, 157–160, 276–285
9. Joint Task Force on Practice Parameters; American Academy of Allergy, Asthma and Immunology; American College of Allergy, Asthma and Immunology; Joint Council of Allergy, Asthma and Immunology. The diagnosis and management of anaphylaxis. *J Allergy Clin Immunol.* 1998;101(6 Pt 2):S465–S528
10. Joint Task Force on Practice Parameters; American Academy of Allergy, Asthma and Immunology; American College of Allergy, Asthma and Immunology; Joint Council of Allergy, Asthma and Immunology. The diagnosis and management of anaphylaxis: an updated practice parameter. *J Allergy Clin Immunol.* 2005;115(3 Suppl 2):S483–S523
11. Kennedy MS. Evaluation of chronic eczema and urticaria and angioedema. *Immunol Allergy Clin North Am.* 1998;18(4):759–772
12. Liew WK, Williamson E, Tang ML. Anaphylaxis fatalities and admissions in Australia. *J Allergy Clin Immunol.* 2009;123(2):434–442
13. Markenson D, Ferguson JD, Chameides L, et al. 2010 American Heart Association and American Red Cross Guidelines for First Aid. Part 17: First Aid. *Circulation.* 2010;122(18 suppl 3):S934–S946
14. Nowak-Wegrzyn A, Sampson HA. Adverse reactions to foods. *Med Clin North Am.* 2006;90(1):97–127
15. Sampson HA. Anaphylaxis and emergency treatment. *Pediatrics.* 2003;111(6 Pt 3):1601–1608
16. Sampson HA, Muñoz-Furlong A, Campbell RL, et al. Second symposium on the definition and management of anaphylaxis. *J Allergy Clin Immunol.* 2006;117(2):391–397
17. Sheikh A, Walker S. Food allergy. *BMJ.* 2002;325(7376):1337
18. Sicherer SH, Simons FE. Self-injectable epinephrine for first-aid management of anaphylaxis. *Pediatrics.* 2007;119(3):638–646
19. Simons FE, Ardusso LR, Bilò MB, et al; World Allergy Organization. 2012 update: World Allergy Organization guidelines for the assessment and management of anaphylaxis. *Curr Opin Allergy Clin Immunol.* 2012;12(4):389–399
20. Stark BJ, Sullivan TJ. Biphasic and protracted anaphylaxis. *J Allergy Clin Immunol.* 1986;78(1 Pt 1):76–83
21. Tang AW. A practical guide to anaphylaxis. *Am Fam Physician.* 2003;68(7):1325–1332

Animal Bite

1. Adams DA, Jajosky RA, Ajani U, et al. Summary of notifiable diseases—United States, 2012. *MMWR Morb Mortal Wkly Rep.* 2014;61(53):1–121
2. Advisory Committee on Immunization Practices. Human rabies prevention—United States, 1999. Recommendations of the Advisory Committee on Immunization Practices (ACIP). *MMWR Recomm Rep.* 1999;48(RR-1):1–21
3. Dimick AR. Delayed wound closure: indications and techniques. *Ann Emerg Med.* 1988;17(12):1303–1304

4. Dyer JL, Yager P, Orciari L, et al. Rabies surveillance in the United States during 2013. *J Am Vet Med Assoc.* 2014;245(10):1111–1123

5. Freer L. North American wild mammalian injuries. *Emerg Med Clin North Am.* 2004;22(2):445–473, ix

6. Glaser C, Lewis P, Wong S. Pet-, animal-, and vector-borne infections. *Pediatr Rev.* 2000;21(7):219–232

7. Griego RD, Rosen T, Orengo IF, Wolf JE. Dog, cat and human bites: a review. *J Am Acad Dermatol.* 1995;33(6):1019–1029

8. Harrison BP, Hillard MW. Emergency department evaluation and treatment of hand injuries. *Emerg Med Clin North Am.* 1999;17(4):793–822, v

9. Jackson AC, Warrell MJ, Rupprecht CE, et al. Management of rabies in humans. *Clin Infect Dis.* 2003;36(1):60–63

10. Kim DK, Riley LE, Harriman KH, Hunter P, Bridges CB. Advisory Committee on Immunization Practices recommended immunization schedule for adults aged 19 years or older—United States, 2017. *MMWR Morb Mortal Wkly Rep.* 2017;66(5):136–138

11. MacBean CE, Taylor DM, Ashby K. Animal and human bite injuries in Victoria, 1998–2004. *Med J Aust.* 2007;186(1):38–40

12. Manning SE, Rupprecht CE, Fishbein D, et al; Advisory Committee on Immunization Practices, Centers for Disease Control and Prevention. Human rabies prevention—United States, 2008: recommendations of the Advisory Committee on Immunization Practices. *MMWR Recomm Rep.* 2008;57(RR-3):1–28

13. Markenson D, Ferguson JD, Chameides L, et al. 2010 American Heart Association and American Red Cross Guidelines for First Aid. Part 17: First Aid. *Circulation.* 2010;122(18 suppl 3):S934–S946

14. Medeiros I, Saconato H. Antibiotic prophylaxis for mammalian bites. *Cochrane Database Syst Rev.* 2001;(2):CD001738

15. Moran GJ, Talan DA, Abrahamian FM. Antimicrobial prophylaxis for wounds and procedures in the emergency department. *Infect Dis Clin North Am.* 2008;22(1):117–143, vii

16. National Association of State Public Health Veterinarians, Inc. Compendium of animal rabies prevention and control, *MMWR Recomm Rep.* 2000;49(RR-8):21–30

17. Public Health Agency of Canada. Canadian Immunization Guide. https://www.canada.ca/en/public-health/services/canadian-immunization-guide.html. Modified January 24, 2018. Accessed June 7, 2018

18. Rapoport M, Adam HM. Animal bites: assessing risk for rabies and providing treatment. *Pediatr Rev.* 1997;18(4):142–143

19. Rupprecht CE, Briggs D, Brown CM, et al. Use of a reduced (4-dose) vaccine schedule for postexposure prophylaxis to prevent human rabies: recommendations of the Advisory Committee on Immunization Practices. *MMWR Recomm Rep.* 2010;59(RR-2):1–9

20. Singer AJ, Dagum AB. Current management of acute cutaneous wounds. *N Engl J Med.* 2008;359(10):1037–1046

21. Steele MT, Ma OJ, Nakase J, et al; EMERGEncy ID NET Study Group. Epidemiology of animal exposures presenting to emergency departments. *Acad Emerg Med.* 2007;14(5):398–403

22. Swartz MN. Clinical practice. Cellulitis. *N Engl J Med.* 2004;350(9):904–912

23. Turner TW. Do mammalian bites require antibiotic prophylaxis? *Ann Emerg Med.* 2004;44(3):274–276

Ankle and Foot Injury

1. American Heart Association. 2005 Guidelines for Cardiopulmonary Resuscitation and Emergency Cardiovascular Care. Part 10: First Aid. *Circulation.* 2005;112:IV-196–IV-203

2. Bachmann LM, Kolb E, Koller MT, Steurer J, ter Riet G. Accuracy of Ottawa ankle rules to exclude fractures of the ankle and mid-foot: a systematic review. *BMJ.* 2003;326(7386):417–423

3. Bleakley C, McDonough S, MacAuley D. The use of ice in the treatment of acute soft-tissue injury. *Am J Sports Med.* 2004;32(1):251–261

4. Boyce SH, Quigley MA, Campbell S. Management of ankle sprains: a randomised controlled trial of the treatment of inversion injuries using an elastic support bandage or an Aircast ankle brace. *Br J Sports Med.* 2005;39(2):91–96

5. Clanton TO, Porter DA. Primary care of foot and ankle injuries in the athlete. *Clin Sports Med.* 1997;16(3):435–466

6. Collins NC. Is ice right? Does cryotherapy improve outcome for acute soft tissue injury? *Emerg Med J.* 2008;25(2):65–68

7. Dake AD, Stack L. Penetrating trauma to the extremities: systematic assessment and targeted management of weapons-related injuries. *Emerg Med Reports.* 1997;18(7)

8. Dalton JD Jr, Schweinle JE. Randomized controlled noninferiority trial to compare extended release acetaminophen and ibuprofen for the treatment of ankle sprains. *Ann Emerg Med.* 2006;48(5):615–623

9. Hocutt JE Jr. Cryotherapy in ankle sprains. *Am J Sports Med.* 1982;10(5):316–319

10. Kellett J. Acute soft tissue injuries—a review of the literature. *Med Sci Sports Exerc.* 1986;18(5):489–500

11. Kerkhoffs GM, Struijs PA, Marti RK, Assendelft WJ, Blankevoort L, van Dijk CN. Different functional treatment strategies for acute lateral ankle ligament injuries in adults. *Cochrane Database Syst Rev.* 2002;(3):CD002938

12. Kretsinger K, Broder KR, Cortese MM, et al; Centers for Disease Control and Prevention; Advisory Committee on Immunization Practices; Healthcare Infection Control Practices Advisory Committee. Preventing tetanus, diphtheria, and pertussis among adults: use of tetanus toxoid, reduced diphtheria toxoid and acellular pertussis vaccine recommendations of the Advisory Committee on Immunization Practices (ACIP) and recommendation of ACIP, supported by the Healthcare Infection Control Practices Advisory Committee (HICPAC), for use of Tdap among health-care personnel. *MMWR Recomm Rep.* 2006;55(RR-17):1–37

13. Lavery LA, Armstrong DG, Wunderlich RP, Mohler MJ, Wendel CS, Lipsky BA. Risk factors for foot infections in individuals with diabetes. *Diabetes Care.* 2006;29(6):1288–1293

14. Markenson D, Ferguson JD, Chameides L, et al. 2010 American Heart Association and American Red Cross Guidelines for First Aid. Part 17: First Aid. *Circulation.* 2010;122(18 suppl 3):S934–S946

15. Markert RJ. A pooled analysis of the Ottawa ankle rules used on adults in the ED. *Am J Emerg Med.* 1998;16(6):564–567

16. McMaster WC, Liddle S, Waugh TR. Laboratory evaluation of various cold therapy modalities. *Am J Sports Med.* 1978;6(5):291–294

17. Moran GJ, Talan DA, Abrahamian FM. Antimicrobial prophylaxis for wounds and procedures in the emergency department. *Infect Dis Clin North Am.* 2008;22(1):117–143

18. Singer AJ, Dagum AB. Current management of acute cutaneous wounds. *N Engl J Med.* 2008;359(10):1037–1046

19. Stiell IG, Wells GA, Laupacis A, et al. Implementation of the Ottawa ankle rules. *JAMA.* 1994;271(11):827–832

20. Wedmore I, Charette J. Emergency department evaluation and treatment of ankle and foot injuries. *Emerg Med Clin North Am.* 2000;18(1):85–113, vi

Ankle Pain

1. Coakley G, Mathews C, Field M, et al. British Society for Rheumatology Standards, Guidelines and Audit Working Group. BSR & BHPR, BOA, RCGP and BSAC guidelines for management of the hot swollen joint in adults. *Rheumatology (Oxford).* 2006;45(8):1039–1041

2. Dearborn JT, Jergesen HE. The evaluation and initial management of arthritis. *Prim Care.* 1996;23(2):215–240

3. Glazer JL, Hosey RG. Soft-tissue injuries of the lower extremity. *Prim Care.* 2004;31(4):1005–1024

4. Pioro MH, Mandell BF. Septic arthritis. *Rheum Dis Clin North Am.* 1997;23(2):239–258

5. Rainsford KD. Ibuprofen: pharmacology, efficacy and safety. *Inflammopharmacology.* 2009;17(6):275–342

6. Towheed TE, Maxwell L, Judd MG, Catton M, Hochberg MC, Wells G. Acetaminophen for osteoarthritis. *Cochrane Database Syst Rev.* 2006;(1):CD004257

7. Weston V, Coakley G; British Society for Rheumatology Standards, Guidelines and Audit Working Group. Guideline for the management of the hot swollen joint in adults with a particular focus on septic arthritis. *J Antimicrob Chemother.* 2006;58(3):492–493

Arm Pain

1. Barry NN, McGuire JL. Overuse syndromes in adult athletes. *Rheum Dis Clin North Am.* 1996;22(3):515–530
2. Canto JG, Shlipak MG, Rogers WJ, et al. Prevalence, clinical characteristics, and mortality among patients with myocardial infarction presenting without chest pain. *JAMA.* 2000;283(24):3223–3229
3. Coronado BE, Pope JH, Griffith JL, Beshansky JR, Selker HP. Clinical features, triage, and outcome of patients presenting to the ED with suspected acute coronary syndromes but without pain: a multicenter study. *Am J Emerg Med.* 2004;22(7):568–574
4. Culic V, Eterovic D, Miric D, Silic N. Symptom presentation of acute myocardial infarction: influence of sex, age, and risk factors. *Am Heart J.* 2002;144(6):1012–1017
5. Ling SM, Bathon JM. Osteoarthritis in older adults. *J Am Geriatr Soc.* 1998;46(2):216–225
6. Richardson C, Glenn S, Nurmikko T, Horgan M. Incidence of phantom phenomena including phantom limb pain 6 months after major lower limb amputation in patients with peripheral vascular disease. *Clin J Pain.* 2006;22(4):353–358
7. Schley MT, Wilms P, Toepfner S, et al. Painful and nonpainful phantom and stump sensations in acute traumatic amputees. *J Trauma.* 2008;65(4):858–864

Asthma Attack

1. American Heart Association. 2005 Guidelines for Cardiopulmonary Resuscitation and Emergency Cardiovascular Care. Part 10.5: Near-Fatal Asthma. *Circulation.* 2005;112(24 suppl):IV-139–IV-142
2. American Heart Association. 2005 Guidelines for Cardiopulmonary Resuscitation and Emergency Cardiovascular Care. Part 14: First aid. *Circulation.* 2005;112(24 suppl):IV-196–IV-203
3. Brock TP, Wessell AM, Williams DM, Donohue JF. Accuracy of float testing for metered-dose inhaler canisters. *J Am Pharm Assoc (Wash).* 2002;42(4):582–586
4. Cain WT, Oppenheimer JJ. The misconception of using floating patterns as an accurate means of measuring the contents of metered-dose inhaler devices. *Ann Allergy Asthma Immunol.* 2001;87(5):417–419
5. Cates CJ, Crilly JA, Rowe BH. Holding chambers (spacers) versus nebulisers for beta-agonist treatment of acute asthma. *Cochrane Database Syst Rev.* 2006;(2):CD000052
6. Fiore AE, Fry A, Shay D, Gubareva L, Bresee JS, Uyeki TM. Antiviral agents for the treatment and chemoprophylaxis of influenza—recommendations of the Advisory Committee on Immunization Practices (ACIP). *MMWR Recomm Rep.* 2011;60(1):1–24
7. Gibbs MA, Camargo CA, Rowe BH, Silverman RA. State of the art: therapeutic controversies in severe acute asthma. *Acad Emerg Med.* 2000;7(7):800–815
8. Hanson L. Telephone advice and triage. *Immunol Allergy Clin North Am.* 1999;19(1):171–176
9. Influenza Division, National Center for Immunization and Respiratory Diseases. Antiviral agents for the treatment and chemoprophylaxis of influenza—recommendations of the Advisory Committee on Immunization Practices. *MMWR Surveill Summ.* 2011;60(1):1–28
10. Lougheed MD, Lemiere C, Ducharme FM, et al. Diagnosis and management of asthma in preschoolers, children and adults. Canadian Thoracic Society 2012 guideline update. *Can Respir J.* 2012;19(2):127–164
11. Markenson D, Ferguson JD, Chameides L, et al. 2010 American Heart Association and American Red Cross Guidelines for First Aid. Part 17: First Aid. *Circulation.* 2010;122(18 suppl 3):S934–S946
12. National Asthma Education and Prevention Program. Expert Panel Report 3 (EPR–3): guidelines for the diagnosis and management of asthma—summary report 2007. *J Allergy Clin Immunol.* 2007;120(5 Suppl):S94–S138
13. National Asthma Education and Prevention Program. *Expert Panel Report 2: Guidelines for the Diagnosis and Management of Asthma.* Bethesda, MD: National Heart Lung and Blood Institute; 1997
14. Silverman R. Treatment of acute asthma. A new look at the old and the new. *Clin Chest Med.* 2000;21(2):361–379
15. Tilles SA, Nelson HS. Differential diagnosis of adult asthma. *Immunol Allergy Clin North Am.* 1996;16(1):19–34

Athlete's Foot

1. Bedinghaus JM, Niedfeldt MW. Over-the-counter foot remedies. *Am Fam Physician.* 2001;64(5):791–796
2. Gupta AK, Chow M, Daniel CR, Aly R. Treatments of tinea pedis. *Dermatol Clin.* 2003;21(3):431–462
3. Noble SL, Forbes RC, Stamm PL. Diagnosis and management of common tinea infections. *Am Fam Physician.* 1998;58(1):163–178
4. Panackal AA, Halpern EF, Watson AJ. Cutaneous fungal infections in the United States: analysis of the National Ambulatory Medical Care Survey (NAMCS) and National Hospital Ambulatory Medical Care Survey (NHAMCS), 1995–2004. *Int J Dermatol.* 2009;48(7):704–712
5. Rand S. Overview: the treatment of dermatophytosis. *J Am Acad Dermatol.* 2000;43(5 suppl):S104–S112
6. Rich P. Onychomycosis and tinea pedis in patients with diabetes. *J Am Acad Dermatol.* 2000;43(5 suppl):S130–S134
7. Rogers D, Kilkenny M, Marks R. The descriptive epidemiology of tinea pedis in the community. *Australas J Dermatol.* 1996;37(4):178–184
8. Rupke SJ. Fungal skin disorders. *Prim Care.* 2000;27(2):407–421
9. Stein DH. Tineas—superficial dermatophyte infections. *Pediatr Rev.* 1998;19(11):368–372
10. Young CC, Niedfeldt MW, Morris GA, Eerkes KJ. Clinical examination of the foot and ankle. *Prim Care.* 2005;32(1):105–132

Back Injury

1. American Heart Association. 2005 Guidelines for Cardiopulmonary Resuscitation and Emergency Cardiovascular Care. Part 10: First Aid. *Circulation.* 2005;112:IV-196–IV-203
2. Arce D, Sass P, Abul-Khoudoud H. Recognizing spinal cord emergencies. *Am Fam Physician.* 2001;64(4):631–680
3. Baker RJ, Patel D. Lower back pain in the athlete: common conditions and treatment. *Prim Care.* 2005;32(1):201–229
4. Bueff HU. Low back pain. *Prim Care.* 1996;23(2):345–364
5. Chou R, Huffman LH; American Pain Society; American College of Physicians. Nonpharmacologic therapies for acute and chronic low back pain: a review of the evidence for an American Pain Society/American College of Physicians clinical practice guideline. *Ann Intern Med.* 2007;147(7):492–504
6. Collins NC. Is ice right? Does cryotherapy improve outcome for acute soft tissue injury? *Emerg Med J.* 2008;25(2):65–68
7. Hsu JM, Joseph T, Ellis AM. Thoracolumbar fracture in blunt trauma patients: guidelines for diagnosis and imaging. *Injury.* 2003;34(6):426–433
8. Markenson D, Ferguson JD, Chameides L, et al. 2010 American Heart Association and American Red Cross Guidelines for First Aid. Part 17: First Aid. *Circulation.* 2010;122(18 suppl 3):S934–S946
9. Petri R, Gimberl R. Evaluation of the patient with spinal trauma and back pain: an evidence based approach. *Emerg Med Clin North Am.* 1999;17(1):25–39, vii–viii
10. Singer AJ, Dagum AB. Current management of acute cutaneous wounds. *N Engl J Med.* 2008;359(10):1037–1046

Back Pain

1. Argoff CA, Wheeler AH. Spinal and radicular pain disorders. *Neurol Clin.* 1998;16(4):833–850
2. Atlas SJ, Nardin RA. Evaluation and treatment of low back pain: an evidence-based approach to clinical care. *Muscle Nerve.* 2003;27(3):265–284
3. Chou R, Huffman LH; American Pain Society; American College of Physicians. Nonpharmacologic therapies for acute and chronic low back pain: a review of the evidence for an American Pain Society/American College of Physicians clinical practice guideline. *Ann Intern Med.* 2007;147(7):492–504
4. Dart RC, Kuffner EK, Rumack BH. Treatment of pain or fever with paracetamol (acetaminophen) in the alcoholic patient: a systematic review. *Am J Ther.* 2000;7(2):123–134
5. Devereaux MW. Low back pain. *Prim Care.* 2004;31(1):33–51
6. Deyo RA, Weinstein JN. Low back pain. *N Eng J Med.* 2001;344(5):363–370
7. Divoll M, Abernethy DR, Ameer B, Greenblatt DJ. Acetaminophen kinetics in the elderly. *Clin Pharmacol Ther.* 1982;31(2):151–156

8. French SD, Cameron M, Walker BF, Reggars JW, Esterman AJ. Superficial heat or cold for low back pain. *Cochrane Database Syst Rev.* 2006;(1):CD004750

9. Griffin G, Tudiver F, Grant WD. Do NSAIDs help in acute or chronic low back pain? *Am Fam Physician.* 2002;65(7):1319–1321

10. Hagen KB, Hilde G, Jamtvedt G, Winnem M. Bed rest for acute low back pain and sciatica. *Cochrane Database Syst Rev.* 2010;(6):CD001254

11. Hilde G, Hagen KB, Jamtvedt G, Winnem M. Advice to stay active as a single treatment for low back pain and sciatica. *Cochrane Database Syst Rev.* 2002;(2):CD003632

12. Hróbjartsson A, Gøtzsche PC. Placebo interventions for all clinical conditions. *Cochrane Database Syst Rev.* 2010;(1):CD003974

13. Kovacs FM, Abraira V, Pena A, et al. Effect of firmness of mattress on chronic non-specific low-back pain: randomized, double-blind, controlled, multicentre trial. *Lancet.* 2003;362(9396):1599–1604

14. Malmivaara A, Hakkinen U, Aro T, et al. The treatment of acute low back pain: bed rest, exercises, or ordinary activity? *N Engl J Med.* 1995;332(6):351–355

15. Rainsford KD. Ibuprofen: pharmacology, efficacy and safety. *Inflammopharmacology.* 2009;17(6):275–342

16. Roelofs PD, Deyo RA, Koes BW, Scholten RJ, van Tulder MW. Non-steroidal anti-inflammatory drugs for low back pain. *Cochrane Database Syst Rev.* 2008;(1):CD000396

17. Swenson R. Differential diagnosis: a reasonable clinical approach. *Neurol Clin.* 1999;17(1):43–63

18. Takala E. Immediate referral from general practice for lumbar spine X-ray does not improve quality of life or pain for people with lower back pain. *Evid Based Healthc.* 2002;6(2):91–92

Bee Sting

1. American Academy of Allergy, Asthma and Immunology. The use of epinephrine in the treatment of anaphylaxis. Position statement. http://www.aaaai.org/Aaaai/media/MediaLibrary/PDF%20Documents/Practice%20and%20Parameters/Epinephrine-in-treating-anaphylaxis-2002.pdf. Accessed June 7, 2018

2. Anchor J, Settipane RA. Appropriate use of epinephrine in anaphylaxis. *Am J Emerg Med.* 2004;22(6):488–490

3. Betten DP, Richardson WH, Tong TC, Clark RF. Massive honey bee envenomation-induced rhabdomyolysis in an adolescent. *Pediatrics.* 2006;117(1):231–235

4. Brown SG. Clinical features and severity grading of anaphylaxis. *J Allergy Clin Immunol.* 2004;114(2):371–376

5. Derlet RW, Richards JR. Cellulitis from insect bites: a case series. *Cal J Emerg Med.* 2003;4(2):27–30

6. Fisher M. Treatment of acute anaphylaxis. *BMJ.* 1995;311(7007):731–733

7. Jerrard DA. ED management of insect stings. *Am J Emerg Med.* 1996;14(4):429–433

8. Joint Task Force on Practice Parameters; American Academy of Allergy, Asthma and Immunology; American College of Allergy, Asthma and Immunology; Joint Council of Allergy and Immunology. The diagnosis and management of anaphylaxis: an updated practice parameter. *J Allergy Clin Immunol.* 2005;115(3 Suppl 2):S483–S523

9. Liew WK, Williamson E, Tang ML. Anaphylaxis fatalities and admissions in Australia. *J Allergy Clin Immunol.* 2009;123(2):434–442

10. Markenson D, Ferguson JD, Chameides L, et al. 2010 American Heart Association and American Red Cross Guidelines for First Aid. Part 17: First Aid. *Circulation.* 2010;122(18 suppl 3):S934–S946

11. Moffitt JE, Golden DB, Reisman RE, et al. Stinging insect hypersensitivity: a practice parameter update. *J Allergy Clin Immunol.* 2004;114(4):869–886

12. Razmjoo H, Abtahi MA, Roomizadeh P, Mohammadi Z, Abtahi SH. Management of corneal bee sting. *Clin Ophthalmol.* 2011;5:1697–1700

13. Reisman RE. Insect stings. *N Engl J Med.* 1994;331(8):523–527

14. Sampson HA, Muñoz-Furlong A, Campbell RL, et al. Second symposium on the definition and management of anaphylaxis: summary report—Second National Institute of Allergy and Infectious Disease/Food Allergy and Anaphylaxis Network symposium. *J Allergy Clin Immunol.* 2006;117(2):391–397

15. Sherman RA. What physicians should know about Africanized honeybees. *West J Med.* 1995;163(6):541–546

16. Simons FE, Ardusso LR, Bilò MB, et al; World Allergy Organization. 2012 update: World Allergy Organization guidelines for the assessment and management of anaphylaxis. *Curr Opin Allergy Clin Immunol.* 2012;12(4):389–399

17. Steen CJ, Carbonaro PA, Schwartz RA. Arthropods in dermatology. *J Am Acad Dermatol.* 2004;50(6):819–844

18. Teoh SC, Lee JJ, Fam HB. Corneal honeybee sting. *Can J Ophthalmol.* 2005;40(4):469–471

19. Visscher PK, Vetter RS, Camazine S. Removing bee stings. *Lancet.* 1996;348(9023):301–302

Breathing Difficulty

1. American Heart Association. 2005 Guidelines for Cardiopulmonary Resuscitation and Emergency Cardiovascular Care. Part 14: First aid. *Circulation.* 2005;112(24 suppl):IV-196–IV-203

2. Bestall JC, Paul EA, Garrod R, Garnham R, Jones PW, Wedzicha JA. Usefulness of the Medical Research Council (MRC) dyspnoea scale as a measure of disability in patients with chronic obstructive pulmonary disease. *Thorax.* 1999;54(7):581–586

3. Cooper LT Jr. Myocarditis. *N Engl J Med.* 2009;360(15):1526–1538

4. Edwards M, Chang AM, Matsuura AC, Green M, Robey JM, Hollander JE. Relationship between pain severity and outcomes in patients presenting with potential acute coronary syndromes. *Ann Emerg Med.* 2011;58(6):501–507

5. Fesmire FM, Brown MD, Espinosa JA, et al; American College of Emergency Physicians. Critical issues in the evaluation and management of adult patients presenting to the emergency department with suspected pulmonary embolism. *Ann Emerg Med.* 2011;57(6):628–652.e75

6. Gallus AS. Travel, venous thromboembolism, and thrombophilia. *Semin Thromb Hemost.* 2005;31(1):90–96

7. Goldman L, Kirtane AJ. Triage of patients with acute chest pain and possible cardiac ischemia: the elusive search for diagnostic perfection. *Ann Intern Med.* 2003;139(12):987–995

8. Han J, Zhu Y, Li S, et al. The language of medically unexplained dyspnea. *Chest.* 2008;133(4):961–968

9. Hardie GE, Janson S, Gold WM, Carrieri-Kohlman V, Boushey HA. Ethnic differences: word descriptors used by African-American and white asthma patients during induced bronchoconstriction. *Chest.* 2000;117(4):935–943

10. Kessler CM. The link between cancer and venous thromboembolism: a review. *Am J Clin Oncol.* 2009;32(4 Suppl):S3–S7

11. Mahler DA, Harver A. Do you speak the language of dyspnea? *Chest.* 2000;117(4):928–929

12. Marik PE, Plante LA. Venous thromboembolic disease and pregnancy. *N Engl J Med.* 2008;359(19):2025–2033

13. Markenson D, Ferguson JD, Chameides L, et al. 2010 American Heart Association and American Red Cross Guidelines for First Aid. Part 17: First Aid. *Circulation.* 2010;122(18 suppl 3):S934–S946

14. Mateo J, Oliver A, Borrell M, Sala N, Fontcuberta J. Laboratory evaluation and clinical characteristics of 2,132 consecutive unselected patients with venous thromboembolism—results of the Spanish Multicentric Study on Thrombophilia (EMET Study). *Thromb Haemost.* 1997;77(3):444–451

15. McRae S. Pulmonary embolism. *Aust Fam Physician.* 2010;39(6):462–466

16. McSweeney JC, Cody M, O'Sullivan P, Elberson K, Moser DK, Garvin BJ. Women's early warning symptoms of acute myocardial infarction. *Circulation.* 2003;108(21):2619–2623

17. Michelson E, Hollrah S. Evaluation of the patient with shortness of breath: an evidence based approach. *Emerg Med Clin North Am.* 1999;17(1):221–237, x

18. Philbrick JT, Shumate R, Siadaty MS, Becker DM. Air travel and venous thromboembolism: a systematic review. *J Gen Intern Med.* 2007;22(1):107–114

19. Sayre MR, Koster RW, Botha M, et al. Part 5: adult basic life support: 2010 International Consensus on Cardiopulmonary Resuscitation and Emergency Cardiovascular Care Science With Treatment Recommendations. *Circulation.* 2010;122(16 suppl 2):S298–S324

Breathing Difficulty (*continued*)

20. Stein PD, Henry JW. Clinical characteristics of patients with acute pulmonary embolism stratified according to their presenting syndromes. *Chest.* 1997;112(4):974–979

21. Travers AH, Rea TD, Bobrow BJ, et al. Part 4: CPR overview: 2010 American Heart Association Guidelines for Cardiopulmonary Resuscitation and Emergency Cardiovascular Care. *Circulation.* 2010;122(18 suppl 3):S676–S684

22. van Mourik Y, Rutten FH, Moons KG, Bertens LC, Hoes AW, Reitsma JB. Prevalence and underlying causes of dyspnoea in older people: a systematic review. *Age Ageing.* 2014;43(3):319–326

23. Wang CS, FitzGerald JM, Schulzer M, Mak E, Ayas NT. Does this dyspneic patient in the emergency department have congestive heart failure? *JAMA.* 2005;294(15):1944–1956

24. Zoorob RJ, Campbell JS. Acute dyspnea in the office. *Am Fam Physician.* 2003;68(9):1803–1810

Burns

1. American Burn Association. Hospital and prehospital resources for optimal care of patients with burn injury: guidelines for development and operation of burn centers. *J Burn Care Rehabil.* 1990;11(2):98–104

2. Centers for Disease Control and Prevention. Updated recommendations for use of tetanus toxoid, reduced diphtheria toxoid and acellular pertussis (Tdap) vaccine from the Advisory Committee on Immunization Practices, 2010. *MMWR Morb Mortal Wkly Rep.* 2011;60(1):13–15

3. Davies JW. Prompt cooling of burned areas: a review of benefits and the effector mechanisms. *Burns Incl Therm Inj.* 1982;9(1):1–6

4. Demling RH, Mazess RB, Wolberg W. The effect of immediate and delayed cold immersion on burn edema formation and resorption. *J Trauma.* 1979;19(1):56–60

5. Hendricks WM. The classification of burns. *J Am Acad Dermatol.* 1990;22(5):838–839

6. Jull AB, Rodgers A, Walker N. Honey as a topical treatment for wounds. *Cochrane Database Syst Rev.* 2008;(4):CD005083

7. Kim DK, Riley LE, Harriman KH, Hunter P, Bridges CB. Advisory Committee on Immunization Practices recommended immunization schedule for adults aged 19 years or older—United States, 2017. *MMWR Morb Mortal Wkly Rep.* 2017;66(5):136–138

8. Kretsinger K, Broder KR, Cortese MM, et al; Centers for Disease Control and Prevention; Advisory Committee on Immunization Practices; Healthcare Infection Control Practices Advisory Committee. Preventing tetanus, diphtheria, and pertussis among adults: use of tetanus toxoid, reduced diphtheria toxoid and acellular pertussis vaccine recommendations of the Advisory Committee on Immunization Practices (ACIP) and recommendation of ACIP, supported by the Healthcare Infection Control Practices Advisory Committee (HICPAC), for use of Tdap among health-care personnel. *MMWR Recomm Rep.* 2006;55(RR-17):1–37

9. Lawrence JC. British Burn Association recommended first aid for burns and scalds. *Burns Incl Therm Inj.* 1987;13(2):153

10. Markenson D, Ferguson JD, Chameides L, et al. 2010 American Heart Association and American Red Cross Guidelines for First Aid. Part 17: First Aid. *Circulation.* 2010;122(18 suppl 3):S934–S946

11. McCullough JE, Henderson AK, Kaufman JD. Occupational burns in Washington State, 1989–1993. *J Occup Environ Med.* 1998;40(12):1083–1089

12. Morgan ED, Bledsoe SC, Barker J. Ambulatory management of burns. *Am Fam Physician.* 2000;62(9):2015–2032

13. Pearson AS, Wolford RW. Management of skin trauma. *Prim Care.* 2000;27(2):475–492

14. Ramzy PI, Barret JP, Herndon DN. Thermal injury. *Crit Care Clin.* 1999;15(2):333–352, ix

15. Rea S, Kuthubutheen J, Fowler B, Wood F. Burn first aid in Western Australia— do healthcare workers have the knowledge? *Burns.* 2005;31(8):1029–1034

16. Singer AJ, Dagum AB. Current management of acute cutaneous wounds. *N Engl J Med.* 2008;359(10):1037–1046

17. Spector J, Fernandez WG. Chemical, thermal, and biological ocular exposures. *Emerg Med Clin North Am.* 2008;26(1):125–136, vii

18. Swain AH, Azadian BS, Wakeley CJ, Shakespeare PG. Management of blisters in minor burns. *Br Med J (Clin Res Ed).* 1987;295(6591):181

19. Venter TH, Karpelowsky JS, Rode H. Cooling of the burn wound: the ideal temperature of the coolant. *Burns.* 2007;33(7):917–922

Cast Symptoms and Questions

1. Pimentel L. Orthopedic trauma: office management of major joint injury. *Med Clin North Am.* 2006;90(2):355–382

2. Smith GD, Hart RG, Tsai TM. Fiberglass cast application. *Am J Emerg Med.* 2005;23(3):347–350

Chest Injury

1. Amaral JF. Thoracoabdominal injuries in the athlete. *Clin Sports Med.* 1997;16(4):739–753

2. American Heart Association. 2005 Guidelines for Cardiopulmonary Resuscitation and Emergency Cardiovascular Care. Part 10: First Aid. *Circulation.* 2005;112:IV-196–IV-203

3. Dubinsky I, Low A. Non–life-threatening blunt chest trauma: appropriate investigation and treatment. *Am J Emerg Med.* 1997;15(3):240–243

4. Greenberg MD, Rosen CL. Evaluation of the patient with blunt chest trauma: an evidence-based approach. *Emerg Med Clinics North Am.* 1999;17(1):41–62

5. Markenson D, Ferguson JD, Chameides L, et al. 2010 American Heart Association and American Red Cross Guidelines for First Aid. Part 17: First Aid. *Circulation.* 2010;122(18 suppl 3):S934–S946

6. McGee S, Abernethy WB 3rd, Simel DL. The rational clinical examination. Is this patient hypovolemic? *JAMA.* 1999;281(11):1022–1029

7. Sasser SM, Hunt RC, Faul M, et al; Centers for Disease Control and Prevention. Guidelines for field triage of injured patients: recommendations of the National Expert Panel on Field Triage, 2011. *MMWR Recomm Rep.* 2012;61(RR-1):1–20

8. Singer AJ, Dagum AB. Current management of acute cutaneous wounds. *N Engl J Med.* 2008;359(10):1037–1046

9. Stewart C. Chest injuries. *Emerg Med Reports.* 1996;17(19)

Chest Pain

1. American Heart Association. 2005 Guidelines for Cardiopulmonary Resuscitation and Emergency Cardiovascular Care. Part 8: Stabilization of the patient with acute coronary syndromes. *Circulation.* 2005;112(24 suppl):IV-89–IV-110

2. Amsterdam EA, Kirk JD, Bluemke DA, et al. Testing of low-risk patients presenting to the emergency department with chest pain: a scientific statement from the American Heart Association. *Circulation.* 2010;122(17):1756–1776

3. Bobrow BJ, Spaite DW, Berg RA, et al. Chest compression-only CPR by lay rescuers and survival from out-of-hospital cardiac arrest. *JAMA.* 2010;304(13):1447–1454

4. Canto JG, Shlipak MG, Rogers WJ, et al. Prevalence, clinical characteristics, and mortality among patients with myocardial infarction presenting without chest pain. *JAMA.* 2000;283(24):3223–3229

5. Cooper LT Jr. Myocarditis. *N Engl J Med.* 2009;360(15):1526–1538

6. Edwards M, Chang AM, Matsuura AC, Green M, Robey JM, Hollander JE. Relationship between pain severity and outcomes in patients presenting with potential acute coronary syndromes. *Ann Emerg Med.* 2011;58(6):501–507

7. Eisenberg MJ, Topal EJ. Prehospital administration of aspirin in patients with unstable angina and acute myocardial infarction. *Arch Intern Med.* 1996;156(14):1506–1510

8. Fesmire FM, Brown MD, Espinosa JA, et al; American College of Emergency Physicians. Critical issues in the evaluation and management of adult patients presenting to the emergency department with suspected pulmonary embolism. *Ann Emerg Med.* 2011;57(6):628–652.e75

9. Finkel JB, Marhefka GD. Rethinking cocaine-associated chest pain and acute coronary syndromes. *Mayo Clin Proc.* 2011;86(12):1198–1207

10. Gallus AS. Travel, venous thromboembolism, and thrombophilia. *Semin Thromb Hemost.* 2005;31(1):90–96

11. Goldman L, Kirtane AJ. Triage of patients with acute chest pain and possible cardiac ischemia: the elusive search for diagnostic perfection. *Ann Intern Med.* 2003;139(12):987–995

12. Goodacre S, Locker T, Morris F, Campbell S. How useful are clinical features in the diagnosis of acute undifferentiated chest pain? *Acad Emerg Med.* 2002;9(3):203–208

13. Han JH, Lindsell CJ, Storrow AB, et al; EMCREG i*trACS Investigators. The role of cardiac risk factor burden in diagnosing acute coronary syndromes in the emergency department setting. *Ann Emerg Med.* 2007;49(2):145–152

14. Jaffy MB, Meischke H, Eisenberg MS. Prevalence of aspirin use among patients calling 9-1-1 for chest pain. *Acad Emerg Med.* 1998;5(12):1146–1149

15. Kline JA, Courtney DM, Kabrhel C, et al. Prospective multicenter evaluation of the pulmonary embolism rule-out criteria. *J Thromb Haemost.* 2008;6(5):772–780

16. Lee TH, Goldman L. Evaluation of the patient with acute chest pain. *N Engl J Med.* 2000;342(16):1187–1195

17. Levy F, Mareiniss DP, Iacovelli C. The importance of a proper against-medical-advice (AMA) discharge: how signing out AMA may create significant liability protection for providers. *J Emerg Med.* 2012;43(3):516–520

18. Markenson D, Ferguson JD, Chameides L, et al. 2010 American Heart Association and American Red Cross Guidelines for First Aid. Part 17: First Aid. *Circulation.* 2010;122(18 suppl 3):S934–S946

19. Marsan RJ, Shaver KJ, Sease KL, Shofer FS, Sites FD, Hollander JE. Evaluation of a clinical decision rule for young adult patients with chest pain. *Acad Emerg Med.* 2005;12(1):26–31

20. McConaghy JR, Oza RS. Outpatient diagnosis of acute chest pain in adults. *Am Fam Physician.* 2013;87(3):177–182

21. McCord J, Jneid H, Hollander JE, et al; American Heart Association Acute Cardiac Care Committee of the Council on Clinical Cardiology. Management of cocaine-associated chest pain and myocardial infarction: a scientific statement from the American Heart Association Acute Cardiac Care Committee of the Council on Clinical Cardiology. *Circulation.* 2008;117(14):1897–1907

22. McRae S. Pulmonary embolism. *Aust Fam Physician.* 2010;39(6):462–466

23. McSweeney JC, Cody M, O'Sullivan P, Elberson K, Moser DK, Garvin BJ. Women's early warning symptoms of acute myocardial infarction. *Circulation.* 2003;108(21):2619–2623

24. Pope JH, Aufderheide TP, Rughazer R, et al. Missed diagnoses of acute cardiac ischemia in the emergency department. *N Engl J Med.* 2000;342(16):1163–1170

25. Sayre MR, Koster RW, Botha M, et al. Part 5: adult basic life support: 2010 International Consensus on Cardiopulmonary Resuscitation and Emergency Cardiovascular Care Science With Treatment Recommendations. *Circulation.* 2010;122(16 suppl 2):S298–S324

26. Swap CJ, Nagurney JT. Value and limitations of chest pain history in the evaluation of patients with suspected coronary syndromes. *JAMA.* 2005;294(20):2623–2629

27. 2012 Writing Committee Members; Jneid H, Anderson JL, Wright RS, et al; American College of Cardiology Foundation; American Heart Association Task Force on Practice Guidelines. 2012 ACCF/AHA focused update of the guideline for the management of patients with unstable angina/non-ST-elevation myocardial infarction (updating the 2007 guideline and replacing the 2011 focused update): a report of the American College of Cardiology Foundation/American Heart Association Task Force on Practice Guidelines. *Circulation.* 2012;126(7):875–910

28. Weber JE, Chudnofsky CR, Boczar M, Boyer EW, Wilkerson MD, Hollander JE. Cocaine associated chest pain: how common is myocardial infarction? *Acad Emerg Med.* 2000;7(8):873–877

29. Welch RD, Zalenski RJ, Frederick PD, et al. Prognostic value of a normal or nonspecific initial electrocardiogram in acute myocardial infarction. *JAMA.* 2001;286(16):1977–1984

30. Wilbur J, Shian B. Diagnosis of deep venous thrombosis and pulmonary embolism. *Am Fam Physician.* 2012;86(10):913–919

Cold Sores (Fever Blisters of Lip)

1. Aciclovir + hydrocortisone. Herpes labialis: a topical antiviral drug perhaps, but not a steroid. *Prescrire Int.* 2011;20(119):205–207

2. Cunningham A, Griffiths P, Leone P, et al. Current management and recommendations for access to antiviral therapy of herpes labialis. *J Clin Virol.* 2012;53(1):6–11

3. Emmert DH. Treatment of common cutaneous herpes simplex virus infections. *Am Fam Physician.* 2000;61(6):1697–1708

4. Gonsalves WC, Chi AC, Neville BW. Common oral lesions: part I. Superficial mucosal lesions. *Am Fam Physician.* 2007;75(4):501–507

5. Hull C, Spruance S, Tyring S, Hamed K. Single-dose famciclovir for the treatment of herpes labialis. *Curr Med Res Opin.* 2006;22(9):1699–1702

6. Hull CM, Brunton S. The role of topical 5% acyclovir and 1% hydrocortisone cream (Xerese) in the treatment of recurrent herpes simplex labialis. *Postgrad Med.* 2010;122(5):1–6

7. Sacks SL, Thisted RA, Jones TM, et al. Clinical efficacy of topical docosanol 10% cream for herpes simplex labialis: a multicenter, randomized, placebo-controlled trial. *J Am Acad Dermatol.* 2001;45(2):222–230

8. Spruance SL, Bodsworth N, Resnick H, et al. Single-dose, patient-initiated famciclovir: a randomized, double-blind, placebo-controlled trial for episodic treatment of herpes labialis. *J Am Acad Dermatol.* 2006;55(1):47–53

9. Spruance SL, Rea TL, Thoming C, Tucker R, Saltzman R, Boon R. Penciclovir cream for the treatment of herpes simplex labialis. A randomized, multicenter, double-blind, placebo-controlled trial. *JAMA.* 1997;277(17):1374–1379

10. Treister NS, Woo SB. Topical n-docosanol for management of recurrent herpes labialis. *Expert Opin Pharmacother.* 2010;11(5):853–860

11. Whitley R. New approaches to the therapy of HSV infections. *Herpes.* 2006;13(2):53–55

Common Cold

1. American Academy of Family Physicians. Patient information. Saline nasal irrigation for sinus problems. *Am Fam Physician.* 2009;80(10):1121

2. Bachert C, Chuchalin AG, Eisebitt R, Netayzhenko VZ, Voelker M. Aspirin compared with acetaminophen in the treatment of fever and other symptoms of upper respiratory tract infection in adults: a multicenter, randomized, double-blind, double-dummy, placebo-controlled, parallel-group, single-dose, 6-hour dose-ranging study. *Clin Ther.* 2005;27(7):993–1003

3. Barrett B, Brown R, Rakel D, et al. Echinacea for treating the common cold: a randomized trial. *Ann Intern Med.* 2010;153(12):769–777

4. Black RA, Hill DA. Over-the-counter medications in pregnancy. *Am Fam Physician.* 2003;67(12):2517–2524

5. Blaiss MS, Dicpinigaitis PV, Eccles R, Wingertzahn MA. Consumer attitudes on cough and cold: US (ACHOO) survey results. *Curr Med Res Opin.* 2015;31(8):1527–1538

6. Caruso TJ, Gwaltney JM Jr. Treatment of the common cold with echinacea: a structured review. *Clin Infect Dis.* 2005;40(6):807–810

7. Curley FJ, Irwin RS, Pratter MR, et al. Cough and the common cold. *Am Rev Respir Dis.* 1988;138(2):305–311

8. De Sutter AI, van Driel ML, Kumar AA, Lesslar O, Skrt A. Oral antihistamine-decongestant-analgesic combinations for the common cold. *Cochrane Database Syst Rev.* 2012;2:CD004976

9. Deckx L, De Sutter AI, Guo L, Mir NA, van Driel ML. Nasal decongestants in monotherapy for the common cold. *Cochrane Database Syst Rev.* 2016;10:CD009612

10. Douglas RM, Hemilä H, Chalker E, Treacy B. Vitamin C for preventing and treating the common cold. *Cochrane Database Syst Rev.* 2007;(3):CD000980

11. Ebell MH, Lundgren J, Youngpairoj S. How long does a cough last? Comparing patients' expectations with data from a systematic review of the literature. *Ann Fam Med.* 2013;11(1):5–13

12. Eccles R. Understanding the symptoms of the common cold and influenza. *Lancet Infect Dis.* 2005;5(11):718–725

13. Erebara A, Bozzo P, Einarson A, Koren G. Treating the common cold during pregnancy. *Can Fam Physician.* 2008;54(5):687–689

14. Falsey AR, McCann RM, Hall WJ, et al. The "common cold" in frail older persons: impact of rhinovirus and coronavirus in a senior daycare center. *J Am Geriatr Soc.* 1997;45(6):706–711

15. Grimm W, Muller HH. A randomized controlled trial of the effect of fluid extract of Echinacea purpurea on the incidence and severity of colds and respiratory infections. *Am J Med.* 1999;106(2):138–143

16. Harvey R, Hannan SA, Badia L, Scadding G. Nasal saline irrigations for the symptoms of chronic rhinosinusitis. *Cochrane Database Syst Rev.* 2007;(3):CD006394

17. Hatton RC, Winterstein AG, McKelvey RP, Shuster J, Hendeles L. Efficacy and safety of oral phenylephrine: systematic review and meta-analysis. *Ann Pharmacother.* 2007;41(3):381–390

18. Hayward G, Thompson MJ, Perera R, Del Mar CB, Glasziou PP, Heneghan CJ. Corticosteroids for the common cold. *Cochrane Database Syst Rev.* 2012;8:CD008116

19. Jackson JL, Peterson C, Lesho E. A meta-analysis of zinc salts lozenges and the common cold. *Arch Intern Med.* 1997;157(20):2373–2376

20. Kenealy T, Arroll B. Antibiotics for the common cold and acute purulent rhinitis. *Cochrane Database Syst Rev.* 2013;6:CD000247

Common Cold (*continued*)

21. Kim SY, Chang YJ, Cho HM, Hwang YW, Moon YS. Non-steroidal anti-inflammatory drugs for the common cold. *Cochrane Database Syst Rev.* 2009;(3):CD006362

22. Maltinski G. Nasal disorders and sinusitis. *Prim Care.* 1998;25(3):663–683

23. Mossad SB, Macknin ML, Medendorp SV, Mason P. Zinc gluconate lozenges for treating the common cold. A randomized, double-blind, placebo-controlled study. *Ann Intern Med.* 1996;125(2):81–88

24. Paul IM, Beiler JS, King TS, Clapp ER, Vallati J, Berlin CM Jr. Vapor rub, petrolatum, and no treatment for children with nocturnal cough and cold symptoms. *Pediatrics.* 2010;126(6):1092–1099

25. Paul IM, Yoder KE, Crowell KR, et al. Effect of dextromethorphan, diphenhydramine, and placebo on nocturnal cough and sleep quality for coughing children and their parents. *Pediatrics.* 2004;114(1):e85–e90

26. Prasad AS, Fitzgerald JT, Bao B, Beck FW, Chandrasekar PH. Duration of symptoms and plasma cytokine levels in patients with the common cold treated with zinc acetate. A randomized, double-blind, placebo-controlled trial. *Ann Intern Med.* 2000;133(4):245–252

27. Rabago D, Barrett B, Marchand L, Maberry R, Mundt M. Qualitative aspects of nasal irrigation use by patients with chronic sinus disease in a multimethod study. *Ann Fam Med.* 2006;4(4):295–301

28. Rosenfeld RM, Andes D, Bhattacharyya N, et al. Clinical practice guideline: adult sinusitis. *Otolaryngol Head Neck Surg.* 2007;137(3 suppl):S1–S31

29. Schroeder K, Fahey T. Over-the-counter medications for acute cough in children and adults in ambulatory settings. *Cochrane Database Syst Rev.* 2004;(4):CD001831

30. Simasek M, Blandino DA. Treatment of the common cold. *Am Fam Physician.* 2007;75(4):515–520

31. Singh M. Heated, humidified air for the common cold. *Cochrane Database Syst Rev.* 2011;(5):CD001728

32. Slapak I, Skoupá J, Strnad P, Horník P. Efficacy of isotonic nasal wash (seawater) in the treatment and prevention of rhinitis in children. *Arch Otolaryngol Head Neck Surg.* 2008;134(1):67–74

33. Smith SM, Schroeder K, Fahey T. Over-the-counter (OTC) medications for acute cough in children and adults in ambulatory settings. *Cochrane Database Syst Rev.* 2012;8:CD001831

34. Sperber SJ, Hendley JO, Hayden FG, Riker DK, Sorrentino JV, Gwaltney JM Jr. Effects of naproxen on experimental rhinovirus colds. A randomized, double-blind, controlled trial. *Ann Intern Med.* 1992;117(1):37–41

35. Taverner D, Latte J. Nasal decongestants for the common cold. *Cochrane Database Syst Rev.* 2007;(1):CD001953

36. Wallace DV, Dykewicz MS, Bernstein DI, et al. The diagnosis and management of rhinitis: an updated practice parameter. *J Allergy Clin Immunol.* 2008;122(2 suppl):S1–S84

37. Witek TJ, Ramsey DL, Carr AN, Riker DK. The natural history of community-acquired common colds symptoms assessed over 4 years. *Rhinology.* 2015;53(1):81–88

38. Yale SH, Liu K. Echinacea purpurea therapy for the treatment of the common cold: a randomized, double-blind, placebo-controlled clinical trial. *Arch Intern Med.* 2004;164(11):1237–1241

Confusion (Delirium)

1. Appelbaum PS. Clinical practice. Assessment of patients' competence to consent to treatment. *N Engl J Med.* 2007;357(18):1834–1840

2. Boyer EW. Management of opioid analgesic overdose. *N Engl J Med.* 2012;367(2):146–155

3. Feske SK. Coma and confusional states: emergency diagnosis and management. *Neurol Clin.* 1998;16(2):237–256

4. Freedman R. Schizophrenia. *N Engl J Med.* 2003;349(18):1738–1749

5. Jacobson SA. Delirium in the elderly. *Psychiatr Clin North Am.* 1997;20(1):91–110

6. Levy F, Mareiniss DP, Iacovelli C. The importance of a proper against-medical-advice (AMA) discharge: how signing out AMA may create significant liability protection for providers. *J Emerg Med.* 2012;43(3):516–520

7. Lukens TW, Wolf SJ, Edlow JA, et al. Clinical policy: critical issues in the diagnosis and management of the adult psychiatric patient in the emergency department. *Ann Emerg Med.* 2006;47(1):79–99

8. Mayo-Smith MF, Beecher LH, Fischer TL, et al. Management of alcohol withdrawal delirium. An evidence-based practice guideline. *Arch Intern Med.* 2004;164(13):1405–1412

9. Meagher DJ. Delirium: optimising management. *BMJ.* 2001;322(7279):144–149

10. Morgenstern LB, Hemphill JC 3rd, Anderson C, et al; American Heart Association Stroke Council and Council on Cardiovascular Nursing. Guidelines for the management of spontaneous intracerebral hemorrhage: a guideline for healthcare professionals from the American Heart Association/American Stroke Association. *Stroke.* 2010;41(9):2108–2129

11. Murphy BA. Delirium. *Emerg Med Clin North Am.* 2000;18(2):243–252

12. Naloxone (Narcan) nasal spray for opioid overdose. *Med Lett Drugs Ther.* 2016;58(1485):1–2

13. O'Brien RF, Kifuji K, Summergrad P. Medical conditions with psychiatric manifestations. *Adolesc Med Clin.* 2006;17(1):49–77

14. Piechniczek-Buczek J. Psychiatric emergencies in the elderly population. *Emerg Med Clin North Am.* 2006;24(2):467–490, viii

15. Teasdale G, Jennett B. Assessment of coma and impaired consciousness. A practical scale. *Lancet.* 1974;2(7872):81–84

Constipation

1. American College of Gastroenterology Chronic Constipation Task Force. An evidence-based approach to the management of chronic constipation in North America. *Am J Gastroenterol.* 2005;100(suppl 1):S1–S4

2. Bharucha AE, Dorn SD, Lembo A, Pressman A; American Gastroenterological Association. American Gastroenterological Association medical position statement on constipation. *Gastroenterology.* 2013;144(1):211–217

3. Bharucha AE, Pemberton JH, Locke GR 3rd. American Gastroenterological Association technical review on constipation. *Gastroenterology.* 2013;144(1):218–238

4. Bonapace ES Jr, Fisher RS. Constipation and diarrhea in pregnancy. *Gastroenterol Clin North Am.* 1998;27(1):197–211

5. Brandt LJ, Prather CM, Quigley EM, Schiller LR, Schoenfeld P, Talley NJ. Systematic review on the management of chronic con-stipation in North America. *Am J Gastroenterol.* 2005;100(suppl 1):S5–S21

6. Coffin B, Caussé C. Constipation assessment scales in adults: a literature review including the new Bowel Function Index. *Expert Rev Gastroenterol Hepatol.* 2011;5(5):601–613

7. DiPalma JA, DeRidder PH, Orlando RC, Kolts BE, Cleveland MB. A randomized, placebo-controlled, multicenter study of the safety and efficacy of a new polyethylene glycol laxative. *Am J Gastroenterol.* 2000;95(2):446–450

8. Ford AC, Brenner DM, Schoenfeld PS. Efficacy of pharmacological therapies for the treatment of opioid-induced constipation: systematic review and meta-analysis. *Am J Gastroenterol.* 2013;108(10):1566–1575

9. Gupta P. Randomized, controlled study comparing sitz-bath and no-sitz-bath treatments in patients with acute anal fissures. *ANZ J Surg.* 2006;76(8):718–721

10. Hsieh C. Treatment of constipation in older adults. *Am Fam Physician.* 2005;72(11):2277–2284

11. Hsu KF, Chia JS, Jao SW, et al. Comparison of clinical effects between warm water spray and sitz bath in post-hemorrhoidectomy period. *J Gastrointest Surg.* 2009;13(7):1274–1278

12. Nurko S, Zimmerman LA. Evaluation and treatment of constipation in children and adolescents. *Am Fam Physician.* 2014;90(2):82–90

13. Pare P. The approach to diagnosis and treatment of chronic constipation: suggestions for a general practitioner. *Can J Gastroenterol.* 2011;25(suppl B):36B–40B

14. Ramkumar D, Rao SS. Efficacy and safety of traditional medical therapies for chronic constipation: systematic review. *Am J Gastroenterol.* 2005;100(4):936–971

15. Rao SSC. Constipation: evaluation and treatment. *Gastroenterol Clin North Am.* 2003;32(2):659–683

16. Shah BJ, Rughwani N, Rose S. Constipation. *Ann Intern Med.* 2015;162(7):ITC1

17. Sommers T, Corban C, Sengupta N, et al. Emergency department burden of constipation in the United States from 2006 to 2011. *Am J Gastroenterol.* 2015;110(4):572–579

18. Tejirian T, Abbas MA. Sitz bath: where is the evidence? Scientific basis of a common practice. *Dis Colon Rectum.* 2005;48(12):2336–2340

19. Wald A. Constipation. *Med Clin North Am.* 2000;84(5):1231–1246, ix

Cough

1. Aagaard E, Gonzales R. Management of acute bronchitis in healthy adults. *Infect Dis Clin North Am.* 2004;18(4):919–937, x

2. American College of Chest Physicians. Cough as a symptom. *Chest.* 1998;114:133S–181S

3. Blaiss MS, Dicpinigaitis PV, Eccles R, Wingertzahn MA. Consumer attitudes on cough and cold: US (ACHOO) survey results. *Curr Med Res Opin.* 2015;31(8):1527–1538

4. Black RA, Hill DA. Over-the-counter medications in pregnancy. *Am Fam Physician.* 2003;67(12):2517–2524

5. Cornia PB, Hersh AL, Lipsky BA, Newman TB, Gonzales R. Does this coughing adolescent or adult patient have pertussis? *JAMA.* 2010;304(8):890–896

6. Curley FJ, Irwin RS, Pratter MR, et al. Cough and the common cold. *Am Rev Respir Dis.* 1988;138(2):305–311

7. De Sutter AI, van Driel ML, Kumar AA, Lesslar O, Skrt A. Oral antihistamine-decongestant-analgesic combinations for the common cold. *Cochrane Database Syst Rev.* 2012;2:CD004976

8. Ebell MH, Lundgren J, Youngpairoj S. How long does a cough last? Comparing patients' expectations with data from a systematic review of the literature. *Ann Fam Med.* 2013;11(1):5–13

9. Eccles R. Understanding the symptoms of the common cold and influenza. *Lancet Infect Dis.* 2005;5(11):718–725

10. Fabbri L, Pauwels RA, Hurd SS; Gold Scientific Committee. Global strategy for the diagnosis, management, and prevention of chronic obstructive pulmonary disease: GOLD Executive Summary updated 2003. *COPD.* 2004;1(1):103–141

11. Irwin RS, Baumann MH, Bolser DC, et al. Diagnosis and management of cough executive summary: ACCP evidence-based clinical practice guidelines. *Chest.* 2006;129(1 suppl):1S–23S

12. Irwin RS, Boulet LP, Cloutier MM, et al. Managing cough as a defense mechanism and as a symptom. A consensus panel report of the American College of Chest Physicians. *Chest.* 1998;114(2 suppl):133S–181S

13. Little P, Rumsby K, Kelly J, et al. Information leaflet and antibiotic prescribing strategies for acute lower respiratory tract infection: a randomized controlled trial. *JAMA.* 2005;293(24):3029–3035

14. Morice AH, McGarvey L, Pavord I; British Thoracic Society Cough Guideline Group. Recommendations for the management of cough in adults. *Thorax.* 2006;61(suppl 1):i1–i24

15. O'Connell EJ, Li JT. Chronic cough. *Immunol Allergy Clin North Am.* 1996;16(1):1–17

16. Paul IM, Beiler J, McMonagle A, Shaffer ML, Duda L, Berlin CM Jr. Effect of honey, dextromethorphan, and no treatment on nocturnal cough and sleep quality for coughing children and their parents. *Arch Pediatr Adolesc Med.* 2007;161(12):1140–1146

17. Paul IM, Beiler JS, King TS, Clapp ER, Vallati J, Berlin CM Jr. Vapor rub, petrolatum, and no treatment for children with nocturnal cough and cold symptoms. *Pediatrics.* 2010;126(6):1092–1099

18. Paul IM, Yoder KE, Crowell KR, et al. Effect of dextromethorphan, diphenhydramine, and placebo on nocturnal cough and sleep quality for coughing children and their parents. *Pediatrics.* 2004;114(1):e85–e90

19. Quon BS, Gan WQ, Sin DD. Contemporary management of acute exacerbations of COPD: a systematic review and metaanalysis. *Chest.* 2008;133(3):756–766

20. Rubin BK. Mucolytics, expectorants, and mucokinetic medications. *Respir Care.* 2007;52(7):859–865

21. Schroeder K, Fahey T. Over-the-counter medications for acute cough in children and adults in ambulatory settings. *Cochrane Database Syst Rev.* 2004;(4):CD001831

22. Simasek M, Blandino DA. Treatment of the common cold. *Am Fam Physician.* 2007;75(4):515–520

23. Smith SM, Schroeder K, Fahey T. Over-the-counter (OTC) medications for acute cough in children and adults in ambulatory settings. *Cochrane Database Syst Rev.* 2012;8:CD001831

24. Smucny J, Fahey T, Becker L, Glazier R. Antibiotics for acute bronchitis. *Cochrane Database Syst Rev.* 2004;(4):CD000245

25. Sperber SJ, Hendley JO, Hayden FG, Riker DK, Sorrentino JV, Gwaltney JM Jr. Effects of naproxen on experimental rhinovirus colds: a randomized, double-blind, controlled trial. *Ann Intern Med.* 1992;117(1):37–41

26. Wenzel RP, Fowler AA 3rd. Clinical practice. Acute bronchitis. *N Engl J Med.* 2006;355(20):2125–2130

27. Witek TJ, Ramsey DL, Carr AN, Riker DK. The natural history of community-acquired common colds symptoms assessed over 4 years. *Rhinology.* 2015;53(1):81–88

Dental Procedure Antibiotic Prophylaxis

1. American Dental Association, American Academy of Orthopedic Surgeons. Antibiotic prophylaxis for dental patients with total joint replacements. *J Am Dent Assoc.* 2003;134(7):895–899

2. Baddour LM, Wilson WR, Bayer AS, et al. Infective endocarditis: diagnosis, antimicrobial therapy, and management of complications: a statement for healthcare professionals from the Committee on Rheumatic Fever, Endocarditis, and Kawasaki Disease, Council on Cardiovascular Disease in the Young, and the Councils on Clinical Cardiology, Stroke, and Cardiovascular Surgery and Anesthesia, American Heart Association: endorsed by the Infectious Diseases Society of America. *Circulation.* 2005;111(23):e394–e434

3. Baddour LM, Wilson WR, Bayer AS, et al; American Heart Association Committee on Rheumatic Fever, Endocarditis, and Kawasaki Disease of the Council on Cardiovascular Disease in the Young, Council on Clinical Cardiology, Council on Cardiovascular Surgery and Anesthesia, and Stroke Council. Infective endocarditis in adults: diagnosis, antimicrobial therapy, and management of complications: a scientific statement for healthcare professionals from the American Heart Association. *Circulation.* 2015;132(15):1435–1486

4. Canadian Dental Association. CDA position on antibiotic prophylaxis for dental patients at risk. http://cllcanada.ca/2010/pages/dental_antibiotic.pdf. Approved February 2005. Accessed June 25, 2018

5. DeFroda SF, Lamin E, Gil JA, Sindhu K, Ritterman S. Antibiotic prophylaxis for patients with a history of total joint replacement. *J Am Board Fam Med.* 2016;29(4):500–507

6. Durack DT. Prevention of infective endocarditis. *N Engl J Med.* 1995;332(1):38–44

7. Greenberg JD, Bonwit AM, Roddy MG. Subacute bacterial endocarditis prophylaxis: a succinct review for pediatric emergency physicians and nurses. *Clin Pediatr Emerg Med.* 2005;6(4):266–272

8. Slover JD, Phillips MS, Iorio R, Bosco J. Is routine antibiotic prophylaxis cost effective for total joint replacement patients? *J Arthroplasty.* 2015;30(4):543–546

9. Sollecito TP, Abt E, Lockhart PB, et al. The use of prophylactic antibiotics prior to dental procedures in patients with prosthetic joints: evidence-based clinical practice guideline for dental practitioners—a report of the American Dental Association Council on Scientific Affairs. *J Am Dent Assoc.* 2015;146(1):11–16.e8

10. Tong DC, Rothwell BR. Antibiotic prophylaxis in dentistry: a review and practice recommendations. *J Am Dent Assoc.* 2000;131(3):366–374

11. Wilson W, Taubert KA, Gewitz M, et al. Prevention of infective endocarditis: guidelines from the American Heart Association. *Circulation.* 2007;116(15):1736–1754

12. Wilson W, Taubert KA, Gewitz M, et al. Prevention of infective endocarditis: guidelines from the American Heart Association. *J Am Dent Assoc.* 2007;138(6):739–760

Depression

1. Appelbaum PS. Clinical practice. Assessment of patients' competence to consent to treatment. *N Engl J Med.* 2007;357(18):1834–1840
2. Bolton JM, Pagura J, Enns MW, Grant B, Sareen J. A population-based longitudinal study of risk factors for suicide attempts in major depressive disorder. *J Psychiatr Res.* 2010;44(13):817–826
3. Casarett D, Kutner JS, Abrahm J; End-of-Life Care Consensus Panel. Life after death: a practical approach to grief and bereavement. *Ann Intern Med.* 2001;134(3):208–215
4. Chartrand H, Robinson J, Bolton JM. A longitudinal population-based study exploring treatment utilization and suicidal ideation and behavior in major depressive disorder. *J Affect Disord.* 2012;141(2-3):237–245
5. Gould MS, Kalafat J, Harrismunfakh JL, Kleinman M. An evaluation of crisis hotline outcomes. Part 2: suicidal callers. *Suicide Life Threat Behav.* 2007;37(3):338–352
6. Green SA, Goldberg RL. Management of acute grief. *Am Fam Physician.* 1986;33(2):185–190
7. Hemelrijk E, van Ballegooijen W, Donker T, van Straten A, Kerkhof A. Internet-based screening for suicidal ideation in common mental disorders. *Crisis.* 2012;33(4):215–221
8. Kalafat J, Gould MS, Munfakh JL, Kleinman M. An evaluation of crisis hotline outcomes. Part 1: nonsuicidal crisis callers. *Suicide Life Threat Behav.* 2007;37(3):322–337
9. Lukens TW, Wolf SJ, Edlow JA, et al. Clinical policy: critical issues in the diagnosis and management of the adult psychiatric patient in the emergency department. *Ann Emerg Med.* 2006;47(1):79–99
10. Naragon-Gainey K, Watson D. The anxiety disorders and suicidal ideation: accounting for comorbidity via underlying personality traits. *Psychol Med.* 2011;41(7):1437–1447
11. O'Brien RF, Kifuji K, Summergrad P. Medical conditions with psychiatric manifestations. *Adolesc Med Clin.* 2006;17(1):49–77
12. Sowers W, George C, Thompson K. Level of care utilization system for psychiatric and addiction services (LOCUS): a preliminary assessment of reliability and validity. *Community Ment Health J.* 1999;35(6):545–563
13. Szewczyk M, Chennault SA. Women's health. Depression and related disorders. *Prim Care.* 1997;24(1):83–101
14. US Preventive Services Task Force. Screening for depression: recommendations and rationale. *Ann Intern Med.* 2002;136(10):760–764

Diabetes (High Blood Sugar)

1. American Diabetes Association. Glycemic targets. Standards of medical care in diabetes 2016. *Diabetes Care.* 2016;39(suppl 1):S39–S46, S95–S96
2. American Diabetes Association. Standards of medical care in diabetes—2009. *Diabetes Care.* 2009;32(suppl 1):S13–S61
3. American Diabetes Association. Standards of medical care in diabetes—2012. *Diabetes Care.* 2012;35(suppl 1):S11–S63
4. American Diabetes Association. Standards of medical care in diabetes—2016 abridged for primary care providers. *Clin Diabetes.* 2016;34(1):3–21
5. Cheng AY, Fantus IG. Oral antihyperglycemic therapy for type 2 diabetes mellitus. *CMAJ.* 2005;172(2):213–226
6. Committee on Obstetric Practice. Committee opinion no. 504: screening and diagnosis of gestational diabetes mellitus. *Obstet Gynecol.* 2011;118(3):751–753
7. de Jongh T, Gurol-Urganci I, Vodopivec-Jamsek V, Car J, Atun R. Mobile phone messaging for facilitating self-management of long-term illnesses. *Cochrane Database Syst Rev.* 2012;12:CD007459
8. DeWitt DE, Hirsch IB. Outpatient insulin therapy in type 1 and type 2 diabetes mellitus: scientific review. *JAMA.* 2003;289(17):2254–2264
9. Feinglos MN, Bethel MA. Treatment of type 2 diabetes mellitus. *Med Clin North Am.* 1998;82(4):757–790
10. Goldstein DE, Little RR, Lorenz RA, Malone JI, Nathan DM, Peterson CM; American Diabetes Association. Tests of glycemia in diabetes. *Diabetes Care.* 2003;26(suppl 1):S106–S108
11. HAPO Study Cooperative Research Group; Metzger BE, Lowe LP, Dyer AR, et al. Hyperglycemia and adverse pregnancy outcomes. *N Engl J Med.* 2008;358(19):1991–2002
12. Harrigan RA, Nathan MS, Beattie P. Oral agents for the treatment of type 2 diabetes mellitus: pharmacology, toxicity, and treatment. *Ann Emerg Med.* 2001;38(1):68–78

13. Harris SB, Lank CN. Recommendations from the Canadian Diabetes Association. 2003 guidelines for prevention and management of diabetes and related cardiovascular risk factors. *Can Fam Physician.* 2004;50(3):425–433
14. Herbel G, Boyle PJ. Hypoglycemia. Pathophysiology and treatment. *Endocrinol Metab Clin North Am.* 2000;29(4):725–743
15. Herbst KL, Hirsch IB. Insulin strategies for primary care providers. *Clin Diabetes.* 2002;20(1):11–17
16. Hod M, Yogev Y. Goals of metabolic management of gestational diabetes: is it all about the sugar? *Diabetes Care.* 2007;30(suppl 2):S180–S187
17. Jani R, Triplitt C, Reasner C, Defronzo RA. First approved inhaled insulin therapy for diabetes mellitus. *Expert Opin Drug Deliv.* 2007;4(1):63–76
18. Kamboj MK, Draznin MB. Office management of the adolescent with diabetes mellitus. *Prim Care.* 2006;33(2):581–602
19. Klocker AA, Phelan H, Twigg SM, Craig ME. Blood ß-hydroxybutyrate vs. urine acetoacetate testing for the prevention and management of ketoacidosis in type 1 diabetes: a systematic review. *Diabet Med.* 2013;30(7):818–824
20. Laffel L. Sick day management in type 1 diabetes. *Endocrinol Metab Clin North Am.* 2000;29(4):707–723
21. Lewis C. Diabetes: a growing public health concern. *FDA Consumer.* 2002;36(1):26–33
22. Misra S, Oliver NS. Utility of ketone measurement in the prevention, diagnosis and management of diabetic ketoacidosis. *Diabet Med.* 2015;32(1):14–23
23. Norwood P, Dumas R, Cefalu W, et al. Randomized study to characterize glycemic control and short-term pulmonary function in patients with type 1 diabetes receiving inhaled human insulin (Exubera). *J Clin Endocrinol Metab.* 2007;92(6):2211–2244
24. Siebenhofer A, Plank J, Berghold A, et al. Short acting insulin analogues versus regular human insulin in patients with diabetes mellitus. *Cochrane Database Syst Rev.* 2006;(2):CD003287
25. Singh SR, Ahmad F, Lal A, Yu C, Bai Z, Bennett H. Efficacy and safety of insulin analogues for the management of diabetes mellitus: a metaanalysis. *CMAJ.* 2009;180(4):385–397
26. Siu AL; US Preventive Services Task Force. Screening for abnormal blood glucose and type 2 diabetes mellitus: U.S. preventive services task force recommendation statement. *Ann Intern Med.* 2015;163(11):861–868
27. Tibaldi J. Initiating and intensifying insulin therapy in type 2 diabetes mellitus. *Am J Med.* 2008;121(6 suppl):S20–S29

Diabetes (Low Blood Sugar)

1. American Diabetes Association. Glycemic targets. Standards of medical care in diabetes 2016. *Diabetes Care.* 2016;39(suppl 1):S39–S46, S95–S96
2. American Diabetes Association. Standards of medical care in diabetes—2009. *Diabetes Care.* 2009;32(suppl 1):S13–S61
3. American Diabetes Association. Standards of medical care in diabetes—2012. *Diabetes Care.* 2012;35(suppl 1):S11–S63
4. American Diabetes Association. Standards of medical care in diabetes—2016 abridged for primary care providers. *Clin Diabetes.* 2016;34(1):3–21
5. American Diabetes Association Workgroup on Hypoglycemia. Defining and reporting hypoglycemia in diabetes: a report from the American Diabetes Association Workgroup on Hypoglycemia. *Diabetes Care.* 2005;28(5):1245–1249
6. Cheng AY, Fantus IG. Oral antihyperglycemic therapy for type 2 diabetes mellitus. *CMAJ.* 2005;172(2):213–226
7. Committee on Obstetric Practice. Committee opinion no. 504: screening and diagnosis of gestational diabetes mellitus. *Obstet Gynecol.* 2011;118(3):751–753
8. Cryer PE, Axelrod L, Grossman AB, et al; Endocrine Society. Evaluation and management of adult hypoglycemic disorders: an Endocrine Society clinical practice guideline. *J Clin Endocrinol Metab.* 2009;94(3):709–728
9. Cryer PE, Davis SN, Shamoon H. Hypoglycemia in diabetes. *Diabetes Care.* 2003;26(6):1902–1912
10. de Jongh T, Gurol-Urganci I, Vodopivec-Jamsek V, Car J, Atun R. Mobile phone messaging for facilitating self-management of long-term illnesses. *Cochrane Database Syst Rev.* 2012;12:CD007459

11. DeWitt DE, Hirsch IB. Outpatient insulin therapy in type 1 and type 2 diabetes mellitus: scientific review. *JAMA.* 2003;289(17):2254–2264

12. Feinglos MN, Bethel MA. Treatment of type 2 diabetes mellitus. *Med Clin North Am.* 1998;82(4):757–790

13. Goldstein DE, Little RR, Lorenz RA, Malone JI, Nathan DM, Peterson CM; American Diabetes Association. Tests of glycemia in diabetes. *Diabetes Care.* 2003;26(suppl 1):S106–S108

14. HAPO Study Cooperative Research Group; Metzger BE, Lowe LP, Dyer AR, et al. Hyperglycemia and adverse pregnancy outcomes. *N Engl J Med.* 2008;358(19):1991–2002

15. Harrigan RA, Nathan MS, Beattie P. Oral agents for type 2 diabetes mellitus: pharmacology, toxicity, and treatment. *Ann Emerg Med.* 2001;38(1):68–78

16. Harris SB, Lank CN. Recommendations from the Canadian Diabetes Association. 2003 guidelines for prevention and management of diabetes and related cardiovascular risk factors. *Can Fam Physician.* 2004;50(3):425–433

17. Herbel G, Boyle PJ. Hypoglycemia. Pathophysiology and treatment. *Endocrinol Metab Clin North Am.* 2000;29(4):725–743

18. Herbst KL, Hirsch IB. Insulin strategies for primary care providers. *Clin Diabetes.* 2002;20(1):11–17

19. Hod M, Yogev Y. Goals of metabolic management of gestational diabetes: is it all about the sugar? *Diabetes Care.* 2007;30(suppl 2):S180–S187

20. Kamboj MK, Draznin MB. Office management of the adolescent with diabetes mellitus. *Prim Care.* 2006;33(2):581–602

21. Klocker AA, Phelan H, Twigg SM, Craig ME. Blood ß-hydroxybutyrate vs. urine acetoacetate testing for the prevention and management of ketoacidosis in type 1 diabetes: a systematic review. *Diabet Med.* 2013;30(7):818–824

22. Laffel L. Sick day management in type 1 diabetes. *Endocrinol Metab Clin North Am.* 2000;29(4):707–723

23. Lewis C. Diabetes: a growing public health concern. *FDA Consumer.* 2002;36(1):26–33

24. Misra S, Oliver NS. Utility of ketone measurement in the prevention, diagnosis and management of diabetic ketoacidosis. *Diabet Med.* 2015;32(1):14–23

25. Ng CL. Hypoglycaemia in nondiabetic patients—an evidence. *Aust Fam Physician.* 2010;39(6):399–404

26. Ragone M, Lando HM. Errors of insulin commission? *Clin Diabetes.* 2002;20(4):221–222

27. Singh SR, Ahmad F, Lal A, Yu C, Bai Z, Bennett H. Efficacy and safety of insulin analogues for the management of diabetes mellitus: a metaanalysis. *CMAJ.* 2009;180(4):385–397

28. Siu AL; US Preventive Services Task Force. Screening for abnormal blood glucose and type 2 diabetes mellitus: U.S. Preventive Services Task Force recommendation statement. *Ann Intern Med.* 2015;163(11):861–868

29. Tibaldi J. Initiating and intensifying insulin therapy in type 2 diabetes mellitus. *Am J Med.* 2008;121(6 suppl):S20–S29

Diarrhea

1. Acheson DW, Fiore AE. Preventing foodborne disease—what clinicians can do. *N Engl J Med.* 2004;350(5):437–440

2. Barr W, Smith A. Acute diarrhea. *Am Fam Physician.* 2014;89(3):180–189

3. Black RA, Hill DA. Over-the-counter medications in pregnancy. *Am Fam Physician.* 2003;67(12):2517–2524

4. Centers for Disease Control and Prevention. Diagnosis and management of foodborne illnesses: a primer for physicians and other health care professionals. *MMWR Recomm Rep.* 2004;53(RR-4):1–33

5. Cohen SH, Gerding DN, Johnson S, et al; Society for Healthcare Epidemiology of America; Infectious Diseases Society of America. Clinical practice guidelines for Clostridium difficile infection in adults: 2010 update by the Society for Healthcare Epidemiology of America (SHEA) and the Infectious Diseases Society of America (ISDA). *Infect Control Hosp Epidemiol.* 2010;31(5):431–455

6. Conway S, Hart A, Clark A, Harvey I. Does eating yogurt prevent antibiotic-associated diarrhoea? A placebo-controlled randomised controlled trial in general practice. *Br J Gen Pract.* 2007;57(545):953–959

7. DuPont HL. Guidelines on acute infectious diarrhea in adults. The Practice Parameters Committee of the American College of Gastroenterology. *Am J Gastroenterol.* 1997;92(11):1962–1975

8. DuPont HL. New insights and directions in travelers' diarrhea. *Gastroenterol Clin North Am.* 2006;35(2):337–353, viii–ix

9. Fekety R. Guidelines for the diagnosis and management of Clostridium difficile-associated diarrhea and colitis. American College of Gastroenterology Practice Parameters Committee. *Am J Gastroenterol.* 1997;92(5):739–750

10. Fisman D. Seasonality of viral infections: mechanisms and unknowns. *Clin Microbiol Infect.* 2012;18(10):946–954

11. Goldsmid JM, Leggat PA. The returned traveller with diarrhoea. *Aust Fam Physician.* 2007;36(5):322–327

12. Goodgame R. A Bayesian approach to acute infectious diarrhea in adults. *Gastroenterol Clin North Am.* 2006;35(2):249–273

13. Gore JI, Surawicz C. Severe acute diarrhea. *Gastroenterol Clin North Am.* 2003;32(4):1249–1267

14. Guerrant RL, Van Gilder TV, Steiner TS, et al. Practice guidelines for the management of infectious diarrhea. *Clin Infect Dis.* 2001;32(3):331–351

15. Hahn S, Kim Y, Garner P. Reduced osmolarity oral rehydration solution for treating dehydration due to diarrhoea in children: systematic review. *BMJ.* 2001;323(7304):81–85

16. Kamat D, Mathur A. Prevention and management of travelers' diarrhea. *Dis Mon.* 2006;52(7):289–302

17. Kelly CP, LaMont JT. Clostridium difficile—more difficult than ever. *N Engl J Med.* 2008;359(18):1932–1940

18. Khanna S, Pardi DS. Clostridium difficile infection: new insights into management. *Mayo Clin Proc.* 2012;87(11):1106–1117

19. Lal A, Hales S, French N, Baker MG. Seasonality in human zoonotic enteric diseases: a systematic review. *PLoS One.* 2012;7(4):e31883

20. McGee S, Abernethy WB 3rd, Simel DL. The rational clinical examination. Is this patient hypovolemic? *JAMA.* 1999;281(11):1022–1029

21. Ryan ET, Wilson ME, Kain KC. Illness after international travel. *N Eng J Med.* 2002;347(7):505–516

22. Schiller LR. Diarrhea. *Med Clin North Am.* 2000;84(5):1259–1274, x

23. Sinert R, Spektor M. Evidence-based emergency medicine/rational clinical examination abstract. Clinical assessment of hypovolemia. *Ann Emerg Med.* 2005;45(3):327–329

24. Thielman NM, Guerrant RL. Acute infectious diarrhea. *N Eng J Med.* 2004;350(1):38–47

25. Trinh C, Prabhakar K. Diarrheal diseases in the elderly. *Clin Geriatr Med.* 2007;23(4):833–856, vii

Dizziness

1. Baloh RW. Dizziness: neurologic emergencies. *Neurol Clin.* 1998;16(2):305–321

2. Goldman L, Kirtane AJ. Triage of patients with acute chest pain and possible cardiac ischemia: the elusive search for diagnostic perfection. *Ann Intern Med.* 2003;139(12):987–995

3. Gommans J, Barber PA, Fink J. Preventing strokes: the assessment and management of people with transient ischaemic attack. *N Z Med J.* 2009;122(1293):3556

4. Kim AS, Fullerton HJ, Johnston SC. Risk of vascular events in emergency department patients discharged home with diagnosis of dizziness or vertigo. *Ann Emerg Med.* 2011;57(1):34–41

5. Newman-Toker DE, Hsieh YH, Camargo CA Jr, Pelletier AJ, Butchy GT, Edlow JA. Spectrum of dizziness visits to US emergency departments: cross-sectional analysis from a nationally representative sample. *Mayo Clin Proc.* 2008;83(7):765–775

6. Sinert R, Spektor M. Evidence-based emergency medicine/rational clinical examination abstract. Clinical assessment of hypovolemia. *Ann Emerg Med.* 2005;45(3):327–329

7. Tusa RJ. Dizziness. *Med Clin North Am.* 2003;87(3):609–641, vii

8. Walker JS, Barnes SB. Dizziness. *Emerg Med Clin North Am.* 1998;16(4):845–875, vii

9. Wasserman J, Perry J, Dowlatshahi D, et al. Stratified, urgent care for transient ischemic attack results in low stroke rates. *Stroke.* 2010;41(11):2601–2605

Ear, Swimmer's (Otitis Externa)

1. Belleza WG, Kalman S. Otolaryngologic emergencies in the outpatient setting. *Med Clin North Am.* 2006;90(2):329–353
2. Cantor RM. Otitis externa and otitis media. A new look at old problems. *Emerg Med Clin North Am.* 1995;13(2):445–455
3. Hosey RG, Rodenberg RE. Training room management of medical conditions: infectious diseases. *Clin Sports Med.* 2005;24(3):477–506, vii
4. Hughes E, Lee JH. Otitis externa. *Pediatr Rev.* 2001;22(6):191–197
5. Kaushik V, Malik T, Saeed SR. Interventions for acute otitis externa. *Cochrane Database Syst Rev.* 2010;(1):CD004740
6. Mellman MF, Podesta L. Common medical problems in sports. *Clin Sports Med.* 1997;16(4):635–662
7. Nichols AW. Nonorthopedic problems in the aquatic athlete. *Clin Sports Med.* 1999;18(2):395–411, viii
8. Nussinovitch M, Rimon A, Volovitz B, Raveh E, Prais D, Amir J. Cotton-tip applicators as a leading cause of otitis externa. *Int J Pediatr Otorhinolaryngol.* 2004;68(4):433–435
9. Osguthorpe JD, Nielsen DR. Otitis externa: review and clinical update. *Am Fam Physician.* 2006;74(9):1510–1516
10. Rosenfeld RM, Brown L, Cannon CR, et al. Clinical practice guideline: acute otitis externa. *Otolaryngol Head Neck Surg.* 2006;134(4 suppl):S4–S23
11. Rosenfeld RM, Singer M, Wasserman JM, Stinnett SS. Systematic review of topical antimicrobial therapy for acute otitis externa. *Otolaryngol Head Neck Surg.* 2006;134(4 suppl):S24–S48
12. van Balen FA, Smit WM, Zuithoff NP, Verheij TJ. Clinical efficacy of three common treatments in acute otitis externa in primary care: randomized controlled trial. *BMJ.* 2003;327(7425):1201–1205

Ear Piercing

1. Association of Professional Piercers. *Procedure Manual.* 2013 ed. https://www.safepiercing.org/procedure_manual.php. Accessed June 7, 2018
2. Belleza WG, Kalman S. Otolaryngologic emergencies in the outpatient setting. *Med Clin North Am.* 2006;90(2):329–353
3. Cohen HA, Nussinovitch M, Straussberg R. Embedded earrings. *Cutis.* 1994;53(2):82
4. Ference JD, Last AR. Choosing topical corticosteroids. *Am Fam Physician.* 2009;79(2):135–140
5. Ferguson H. Body piercing. *BMJ.* 1999;319(7225):1627–1629
6. Fernandez Ade P, Castro Neto I, Anias CR, Pinto PC, Castro Jde C, Carpes AF. Post-piercing perichondritis. *Braz J Otorhinolaryngol.* 2008;74(6):933–937
7. Garner LA. Contact dermatitis to metals. *Dermatol Ther.* 2004;17(4):321–327
8. Gauglitz GG, Korting HC, Pavicic T, Ruzicka T, Jeschke MG. Hypertrophic scarring and keloids: pathomechanisms and current and emerging treatment strategies. *Mol Med.* 2011;17(1-2):113–125
9. Hanif J, Frosh A, Marnane C, Ghufoor K, Rivron R, Sandhu G. Lesson of the week: "high" ear piercing and the rising incidence of perichondritis of the pinna. *BMJ.* 2001;322(7291):906–907
10. Hendricks WM. Complications of ear piercing: treatment and prevention. *Cutis.* 1991;48(5):386–394
11. Hogan D, Ledet JJ. Impact of regulation on contact dermatitis. *Dermatol Clin.* 2009;27(3):385–394, viii
12. Laumann AE, Derick AJ. Tattoos and body piercings in the United States: a national data set. *J Am Acad Dermatol.* 2006;55(3):413–421
13. Lehman EJ, Huy J, Levy E, Viet SM, Mobley A, McCleery TZ. Bloodborne pathogen risk reduction activities in the body piercing and tattooing industry. *Am J Infect Control.* 2010;38(2):130–138
14. Mark BJ, Slavin RG. Allergic contact dermatitis. *Med Clin North Am.* 2006;90(1):169–185
15. Mayers LB, Chiffriller SH. Body art (body piercing and tattooing) among undergraduate university students: "then and now." *J Adolesc Health.* 2008;42(2):201–203
16. Meltzer DI. Complications of body piercing. *Am Fam Physician.* 2005;72(10):2029–2034
17. Mortz CG, Andersen KE. New aspects in allergic contact dermatitis. *Curr Opin Allergy Clin Immunol.* 2008;8(5):428–432

18. Reiter D, Alford EL. Torn earlobe: a new approach to management with a review of 68 cases. *Ann Otol Rhinol Laryngol.* 1994;103(11):879–884
19. Swartz MN. Clinical practice. Cellulitis. *N Engl J Med.* 2004;350(9):904–912

Earache

1. Belleza WG, Kalman S. Otolaryngologic emergencies in the outpatient setting. *Med Clin North Am.* 2006;90(2):329–353
2. Brown TP. Middle ear symptoms while flying. Ways to prevent a severe outcome. *Postgrad Med.* 1994;96(2):135–142
3. Foxlee R, Johansson A, Wejfalk J, Dawkins J, Dooley L, Del Mar C. Topical analgesia for acute otitis media. *Cochrane Database Syst Rev.* 2006;(3):CD005657
4. Hoberman A, Paradise JL, Reynolds EA, Urkin J. Efficacy of Auralgan for treating ear pain in children with acute otitis media. *Arch Pediatr Adolesc Med.* 1997;151(7):675–678
5. Kreisberg MK, Turner J. Dental causes of referred otalgia. *Ear Nose Throat J.* 1987;66(10):398–408
6. Rosenfeld RM, Brown L, Cannon CR, et al. Clinical practice guideline: acute otitis externa. *Otolaryngol Head Neck Surg.* 2006;134(4 suppl):S4–S23
7. Sarrell EM, Cohen HA, Kahan E. Naturopathic treatment for ear pain in children. *Pediatrics.* 2003;111(5 Pt 1):e574–e579
8. Stewart MH, Siff JE, Cydulka RK. Evaluation of the patient with sore throat, earache, and sinusitis: an evidence based approach. *Emerg Med Clin North Am.* 1999;17(1):153–187, ix
9. Thaller SR, Desilva A. Otalgia with normal ear. *Am Fam Physician.* 1987;36(4):129–136
10. van Zon A, van der Heijden GJ, van Dongen TM, Burton MJ, Schilder AG. Antibiotics for otitis media with effusion in children. *Cochrane Database Syst Rev.* 2012;9:CD009163

Elbow Injury

1. American Heart Association. 2005 Guidelines for Cardiopulmonary Resuscitation and Emergency Cardiovascular Care. Part 10: First Aid. *Circulation.* 2005;112:IV-196–IV-203
2. Barry NN, McGuire J. Acute injuries and specific problems in adult athletes. *Rheum Dis Clin North Am.* 1996;22(3):531–548
3. Brady WJ, et al. Upper extremity fractures and dislocations. *Emerg Med Reports.* 1999;20(9)
4. Collins NC. Is ice right? Does cryotherapy improve outcome for acute soft tissue injury? *Emerg Med J.* 2008;25(2):65–68
5. Colman WW, Strauch RJ. Physical examination of the elbow. *Orthop Clin North Am.* 1999;30(1):5–20
6. Kellett J. Acute soft tissue injuries—a review of the literature. *Med Sci Sports Exerc.* 1986;18(5):489–500
7. Markenson D, Ferguson JD, Chameides L, et al. 2010 American Heart Association and American Red Cross Guidelines for First Aid. Part 17: First Aid. *Circulation.* 2010;122(18 suppl 3):S934–S946
8. McMaster WC, Liddle S, Waugh TR. Laboratory evaluation of various cold therapy modalities. *Am J Sports Med.* 1978;6(5):291–294
9. Pimentel L. Orthopedic trauma: office management of major joint injury. *Med Clin North Am.* 2006;90(2):355–382
10. Singer AJ, Dagum AB. Current management of acute cutaneous wounds. *N Engl J Med.* 2008;359(10):1037–1046

Elbow Pain

1. Barry NN, McGuire JL. Overuse syndromes in adult athletes. *Rheum Dis Clin North Am.* 1996;22(3):515–530
2. Canto JG, Shlipak MG, Rogers WJ, et al. Prevalence, clinical characteristics, and mortality among patients with myocardial infarction presenting without chest pain. *JAMA.* 2000;283(24):3223–3229
3. Coakley G, Mathews C, Field M, et al; British Society for Rheumatology Standards, Guidelines and Audit Working Group. BSR & BHPR, BOA, RCGP and BSAC guidelines for management of the hot swollen joint in adults. *Rheumatology (Oxford).* 2006;45(8):1039–1041
4. Colman WW, Strauch RJ. Physical examination of the elbow. *Orthop Clin North Am.* 1999;30(1):15–20

5. Coronado B, Pope JH, Griffith JL, Beshansky JR, Selker HP. Clinical features, triage, and outcome of patients presenting to the ED with suspected acute coronary syndromes but without pain: a multicenter study. *Am J Emerg Med.* 2004;22(7):568–574

6. Culic V, Eterovic D, Miric D, Silic N. Symptom presentation of acute myocardial infarction: influence of sex, age, and risk factors. *Am Heart J.* 2002;144(6):1012–1017

7. Pioro MH, Mandell BF. Septic arthritis. *Rheum Dis Clin North Am.* 1997;23(2):239–258

8. Rainsford KD. Ibuprofen: pharmacology, efficacy and safety. *Inflammopharmacology.* 2009;17(6):275–342

9. Weston V, Coakley G; British Society for Rheumatology Standards, Guidelines and Audit Working Group; et al. Guideline for the management of the hot swollen joint in adults with a particular focus on septic arthritis. *J Antimicrob Chemother.* 2006;58(3):492–493

Eye, Chemical In

1. Bronstein AC, Spyker DA, Cantilena LR Jr, Green JL, Rumack BH, Dart RC. 2010 annual report of the American Association of Poison Control Centers' national poison data system (NPDS): 28th annual report. *Toxicol (Phila).* 2011;49(10):910–941

2. Brown L, Takeuchi D, Challoner K. Corneal abrasions associated with pepper spray exposure. *Am J Emerg Med.* 2000;18(3):271–272

3. Crumpton KL, Shockley LW. Ocular trauma: a quick illustrated guide to treatment, triage, and medicolegal implications. *Emerg Med Rep.* 1997;18(23):223–234

4. Gelston CD. Common eye emergencies. *Am Fam Physician.* 2013;88(8):515–519

5. Harlan JB Jr, Pieramici DJ. Evaluation of patients with ocular trauma. *Ophthalmol Clin North Am.* 2002;15(2):153–161

6. Kuckelkorn R, Schrage N, Keller G, Redbrake C. Emergency treatment of chemical and thermal eye burns. *Acta Ophthalmol Scand.* 2002;80(1):4–10

7. Markenson D, Ferguson JD, Chameides L, et al. 2010 American Heart Association and American Red Cross Guidelines for First Aid. Part 17: First Aid. *Circulation.* 2010;122(18 suppl 3):S934–S946

8. Naradzay J, Barish RA. Approach to ophthalmologic emergencies. *Med Clin North Am.* 2006;90(2):305–328, vii–viii

9. Pokhrel PK, Loftus SA. Ocular emergencies. *Am Fam Physician.* 2007;76(6):829–836

10. Spector J, Fernandez WG. Chemical, thermal, and biological ocular exposures. *Emerg Med Clin North Am.* 2008;26(1):125–136, vii

11. Yeung MF, Tang WY. Clinicopathological effects of pepper (oleoresin capsicum) spray. *Hong Kong Med J.* 2015;21(6):542–552

Eye, Foreign Body

1. Crumpton KL, Shockley LW. Ocular trauma: a quick illustrated guide to treatment, triage, and medicolegal implications. *Emerg Med Rep.* 1997;18(23):223–234

2. Harlan JB Jr, Pieramici DJ. Evaluation of patients with ocular trauma. *Ophthalmol Clin North Am.* 2002;15(2):153–161

3. Hulbert MF. Efficacy of eyepad in corneal healing after corneal foreign body removal. *Lancet.* 1991;337(8742):643

4. Jayamanne DG. Do patients presenting to accident and emergency departments with the sensation of a foreign body in the eye (gritty eye) have significant ocular disease? *J Accid Emerg Med.* 1995;12(4):286–287

5. Naradzay J, Barish RA. Approach to ophthalmologic emergencies. *Med Clin North Am.* 2006;90(2):305–328, vii–viii

6. Pokhrel PK, Loftus SA. Ocular emergencies. *Am Fam Physician.* 2007;76(6):829–836

7. Wilson SA, Last A. Management of corneal abrasions. *Am Fam Physician.* 2004;70(1):123–128

Eye, Pus or Discharge

1. Bielory L, Friedlaender MH, Fujishima H. Allergic conjunctivitis. *Immunol Allergy Clin North Am.* 1997;17(1):19–31

2. Cronau H, Kankanala RR, Mauger T. Diagnosis and management of red eye in primary care. *Am Fam Physician.* 2010;81(2):137–144

3. Deibel JP, Cowling K. Ocular inflammation and infection. *Emerg Med Clin North Am.* 2013;31(2):387–397

4. Diamant JI, Hwang DG. Therapy for bacterial conjunctivitis. *Ophthalmol Clin North Am.* 1999;12(1):15–20

5. Lindsley K, Matsumura S, Hatef E, Akpek EK. Interventions for chronic blepharitis. *Cochrane Database Syst Rev.* 2012;5:CD005556

6. Mahmood AR, Narang AT. Diagnosis and management of the acute red eye. *Emerg Med Clin North Am.* 2008;26(1):35–55, vi

7. McAnena L, Knowles SJ, Curry A, Cassidy L. Prevalence of gonococcal conjunctivitis in adults and neonates. *Eye (Lond).* 2015;29(7):875–880

8. Patel PB, Diaz MC, Bennett JE, Attia MW. Clinical features of bacterial conjunctivitis in children. *Acad Emerg Med.* 2007;14(1):1–5

9. Pokhrel PK, Loftus SA. Ocular emergencies. *Am Fam Physician.* 2007;76(6):829–836

10. Rietveld RP, van Weert HC, ter Riet G, Sloos JH, Bindels PJ. Predicting bacterial cause in infectious conjunctivitis: cohort study on informativeness of combinations of signs and symptoms. *BMJ.* 2004;329(7459):206–210

11. Sheikh A, Hurwitz B. Topical antibiotics for acute bacterial conjunctivitis: Cochrane systematic review and metaanalysis update. *Br J Gen Pract.* 2005;55(521):962–964

12. Sheikh A, Hurwitz B, van Schayck CP, McLean S, Nurmatov U. Antibiotics versus placebo for acute bacterial conjunctivitis. *Cochrane Database Syst Rev.* 2012;9:CD001211

13. Steinert RF. Current therapy for bacterial keratitis and bacterial conjunctivitis. *Am J Ophthalmol.* 1991;112(4 suppl):10S–14S

14. Weiss A, Brinser JH, Nazar-Stewart V. Acute conjunctivitis in childhood. *J Pediatr.* 1993;122(1):10–14

15. Wirbelauer C. Management of the red eye for the primary care physician. *Am J Med.* 2006;119(4):302–306

Eye, Red Without Pus

1. Cronau H, Kankanala RR, Mauger T. Diagnosis and management of red eye in primary care. *Am Fam Physician.* 2010;81(2):137–144

2. Deibel JP, Cowling K. Ocular inflammation and infection. *Emerg Med Clin North Am.* 2013;31(2):387–397

3. Gelston CD. Common eye emergencies. *Am Fam Physician.* 2013;88(8):515–519

4. Leibowitz HM. The red eye. *N Engl J Med.* 2000;343(5):345–351

5. Lindsley K, Matsumura S, Hatef E, Akpek EK. Interventions for chronic blepharitis. *Cochrane Database Syst Rev.* 2012;5:CD005556

6. Mahmood AR, Narang AT. Diagnosis and management of the acute red eye. *Emerg Med Clin North Am.* 2008;26(1):35–55, vi

7. Morgan A, Hemphill RR. Acute visual change. *Emerg Med Clin North Am.* 1998;16(4):825–843, vii

8. Naradzay J, Barish RA. Approach to ophthalmologic emergencies. *Med Clin North Am.* 2006;90(2):305–328, vii–viii

9. Pokhrel PK, Loftus SA. Ocular emergencies. *Am Fam Physician.* 2007;76(6):829–836

10. Wirbelauer C. Management of the red eye for the primary care physician. *Am J Med.* 2006;119(4):302–306

Eye Injury

1. American Heart Association. 2005 Guidelines for Cardiopulmonary Resuscitation and Emergency Cardiovascular Care. Part 10: First Aid. *Circulation.* 2005;112:IV-196–IV-203

2. Crumpton KL, Shockley LW. Ocular trauma: a quick illustrated guide to treatment, triage, and medicolegal implications. *Emerg Med Reports.* 1997;18(23)

3. Gelston CD. Common eye emergencies. *Am Fam Physician.* 2013;88(8):515–519

4. Harlan JB Jr, Pieramici DJ. Evaluation of patients with ocular trauma. *Ophthalmol Clin North Am.* 2002;15(2):153–161

5. Kaiser PK. A comparison of pressure patching versus no patching for corneal abrasions due to trauma or foreign body removal. *Ophtalmology.* 1995;102(12):1936–1942

6. Markenson D, Ferguson JD, Chameides L, et al. 2010 American Heart Association and American Red Cross Guidelines for First Aid. Part 17: First Aid. *Circulation.* 2010;122(18 suppl 3):S934–S946

7. Markoff DD, Chacko D. Common ophthalmologic emergencies: examination, differential diagnosis, and targeted management. *Emerg Med Reports.* 1999;20(1)

Eye Injury (continued)

8. McPheeters RA, White S, Winter A. Raccoon eyes. *West J Emerg Med.* 2010;11(1):97

9. Naradzay J, Barish RA. Approach to ophthalmologic emergencies. *Med Clin North Am.* 2006;90(2):305–328, vii–viii

10. Pretto Flores L, De Almeida CS, Casulari LA. Positive predictive values of selected clinical signs associated with skull base fractures. *J Neurosurg Sci.* 2000;44(2):77–82

11. Rubin S, Hallagan L. Lids, lacrimals, and lashes. *Emerg Med Clin North Am.* 1995;13(3):631–637

12. Singer AJ, Dagum AB. Current management of acute cutaneous wounds. *N Engl J Med.* 2008;359(10):1037–1046

13. Somasundaram A, Laxton AW, Perrin RG. The clinical features of periorbital ecchymosis in a series of trauma patients. *Injury.* 2014;45(1):203–205

14. Wilson SA, Last A. Management of corneal abrasions. *Am Fam Physician.* 2004;70(1):123–130

Fainting

1. Benbadis SR, Wolgamuth BR, Goren H, Brener S, Fouad-Tarazi F. Value of tongue biting in the diagnosis of seizures. *Arch Intern Med.* 1995;155(21):2346–2349

2. Calkins H, Shyr Y, Frumin H, Schork A, Morady F. The value of the clinical history in the differentiation of syncope due to ventricular tachycardia, atrioventricular block, and neurocardiogenic syncope. *Am J Med.* 1995;98(4):365–373

3. Centers for Disease Control and Prevention. Syncope after vaccination—United States, January 2005–July 2007. *MMWR Morb Mortal Wkly Rep.* 2008;57(17):457–460

4. Forman DE, Lipsitz LA. Syncope in the elderly. *Cardiol Clin.* 1997;15(2):295–311

5. Huff JS, Decker WW, Quinn JV, et al; American College of Emergency Physicians. Clinical policy: critical issues in the evaluation and management of adult patients presenting to the emergency department with syncope. *Ann Emerg Med.* 2007;49(4):431–444

6. Kapoor WN. Syncope. *N Engl J Med.* 2000;343(25):1856–1862

7. Martin GJ, Adams SL, Martin HG, Mathews J, Zull D, Scanlon PJ. Prospective evaluation of syncope. *Ann Emerg Med.* 1984;13(7):499–504

8. Martin TP, Hanusa BH, Kapoor WN. Risk stratification of patients with syncope. *Ann Emerg Med.* 1997;29(4):459–466

9. Meyer MD, Handler J. Evaluation of the patient with syncope: an evidence based approach. *Emerg Med Clin North Am.* 1999;17(1):189–201, ix

10. Perry JJ, Stiell IG, Sivilotti ML, et al. High risk clinical characteristics for subarachnoid haemorrhage in patients with acute headache: prospective cohort study. *BMJ.* 2010;341:c5204

11. Quinn J, McDermott D, Kramer N, et al. Death after emergency department visits for syncope: how common and can it be predicted? *Ann Emerg Med.* 2008;51(5):585–590

12. Quinn J, McDermott D, Stiell I, Kohn M, Wells G. Prospective validation of the San Francisco Syncope Rule to predict patients with serious outcomes. *Ann Emerg Med.* 2006;47(5):448–454

13. Sarasin FP, Hanusa BH, Perneger T, Louis-Simonet M, Rajeswaran A, Kapoor WN. A risk score to predict arrhythmias in patients with unexplained syncope. *Acad Emerg Med.* 2003;10(12):1312–1317

14. Sinert R, Spektor M. Evidence-based emergency medicine/rational clinical examination abstract. Clinical assessment of hypovolemia. *Ann Emerg Med.* 2005;45(3):327–329

15. Sotiriades ES, Evans JC, Larson MG, et al. Incidence and prognosis of syncope. *N Engl J Med.* 2002;347(12):878–885

16. Stewart JM. Postural tachycardia syndrome and reflex syncope: similarities and differences. *J Pediatr.* 2009;154(4):481–485

17. Strickberger SA, Benson DW, Biaggioni I, et al. AHA/ACCF scientific statement on the evaluation of syncope. *Circulation.* 2006;113(2):316–327

Fever

1. Andersen AM, Vastrup P, Wohlfahrt J, Andersen PK, Olsen J, Melbye M. Fever in pregnancy and risk of fetal death: a cohort study. *Lancet.* 2002;360(9345):1552–1556

2. Bachert C, Chuchalin AG, Eisebitt R, Netayzhenko VZ, Voelker M. Aspirin compared with acetaminophen in the treatment of fever and other symptoms of upper respiratory tract infection in adults: a multi-center, randomized, double-blind, double-dummy, placebo-controlled, parallel-group, single-dose, 6-hour dose-ranging study. *Clin Ther.* 2005;27(7):993–1003

3. Bottieau E, Clerinx J, Schrooten W, et al. Etiology and outcome of fever after a stay in the tropics. *Arch Intern Med.* 2006;166(15):1642–1648

4. Chamberlain JM, Terndrup TE, Alexander DT, et al. Determination of normal ear temperature with an infrared emission detection thermometer. *Ann Emerg Med.* 1995;25(1):15–20

5. Dart RC, Kuffner EK, Rumack BH. Treatment of pain or fever with paracetamol (acetaminophen) in the alcoholic patient: a systematic review. *Am J Ther.* 2000;7(2):123–134

6. de La Torre SH, Mandel L, Goff BA. Evaluation of postoperative fever: usefulness and cost-effectiveness of routine workup. *Am J Obstet Gynecol.* 2003;188(6):1642–1647

7. Divoll M, Abernethy DR, Ameer B, Greenblatt DJ. Acetaminophen kinetics in the elderly. *Clin Pharmacol Ther.* 1982;31(2):151–156

8. Donowitz GR. Fever in the compromised host. *Infect Dis Clin North Am.* 1996;10(1):129–148

9. Doyle JF, Schortgen F. Should we treat pyrexia? And how do we do it? *Crit Care.* 2016;20(1):303

10. Fishman JA. Infection in solid-organ transplant recipients. *N Engl J Med.* 2007;357(25):2601–2614

11. Jefferies S, Weatherall M, Young P, Beasley R. A systematic review of the accuracy of peripheral thermometry in estimating core temperatures among febrile critically ill patients. *Crit Care Resusc.* 2011;13(3):194–199

12. Johnson DH, Cunha BA. Drug fever. *Infect Dis Clin North Am.* 1996;10(1):85–91

13. Klein NC, Cunha BA. Treatment of fever. *Infect Dis Clin North Am.* 1996;10(1):211–216

14. Mackowiak PA, Wasserman SS, Levine MM. A critical appraisal of 98.6°F, the upper limit of the normal body temperature, and other legacies of Carl Reinhold August Wunderlich. *JAMA.* 1992;268(12):1578–1580

15. McGee DC, Gould MK. Preventing complications of central venous catheterization. *N Engl J Med.* 2003;348(12):1123–1133

16. Niven DJ, Gaudet JE, Laupland KB, Mrklas KJ, Roberts DJ, Stelfox HT. Accuracy of peripheral thermometers for estimating temperature: a systematic review and meta-analysis. *Ann Intern Med.* 2015;163(10):768–777

17. Norman DC, Yoshikawa TT. Fever in the elderly. *Infect Dis Clin North Am.* 1996;10(1):93–99

18. O'Grady NP, Barie PS, Bartlett JG, et al. Guidelines for evaluation of new fever in critically ill adult patients. *Crit Care Med.* 2008;36(4):1330–1349

19. Prescott LF. Paracetamol: past, present, and future. *Am J Ther.* 2000;7(2):143–147

20. Ryan ET, Wilson ME, Kain KC. Illness after international travel. *N Eng J Med.* 2002;347(7):505–516

21. Scholssberg D. Fever and rash. *Infect Dis Clin North Am.* 1996;10(1):101–110

22. Suh KN, Kain KC, Keystone JS. Malaria. *CMAJ.* 2004;170(11):1693–1702

Finger Injury

1. American Heart Association. 2005 Guidelines for Cardiopulmonary Resuscitation and Emergency Cardiovascular Care. Part 10: First Aid. *Circulation.* 2005;112:IV-196–IV-203

2. Collins NC. Is ice right? Does cryotherapy improve outcome for acute soft tissue injury? *Emerg Med J.* 2008;25(2):65–68

3. Harrison BP, Hillard MW. Emergency department evaluation and treatment of hand injuries. *Emerg Med Clin North Am.* 1999;17(4):793–822, v

4. Hogan CJ, Ruland RT. High-pressure injection injuries to the upper extremity: a review of the literature. *J Orthop Trauma.* 2006;20(7):503–511

5. Kretsinger K, Broder KR, Cortese MM, et al; Centers for Disease Control and Prevention; Advisory Committee on Immunization Practices; Healthcare Infection Control Practices Advisory Committee. Preventing tetanus, diphtheria, and pertussis among adults: use of tetanus toxoid, reduced diphtheria toxoid and acellular pertussis vaccine recommendations of the Advisory Committee on Immunization Practices (ACIP) and recommendation of ACIP, supported by the Healthcare Infection Control Practices Advisory Committee (HICPAC), for use of Tdap among health-care personnel. *MMWR Recomm Rep.* 2006;55(RR-17):1–37

6. Leggit JC, Meko CJ. Acute finger injuries: part I. Tendons and ligaments. *Am Fam Physician.* 2006;73(5):810–816

7. Leggit JC, Meko CJ. Acute finger injuries: part II. Fractures, dislocations, and thumb injuries. *Am Fam Physician.* 2006;73(5):827–834

8. Markenson D, Ferguson JD, Chameides L, et al. 2010 American Heart Association and American Red Cross Guidelines for First Aid. Part 17: First Aid. *Circulation.* 2010;122(18 suppl 3):S934–S946

9. Mastey RD, Weiss AP, Akelman E. Primary care of hand and wrist athletic injuries. *Clin Sports Med.* 1997;16(4):705–724

10. Singer AJ, Dagum AB. Current management of acute cutaneous wounds. *N Engl J Med.* 2008;359(10):1037–1046

11. Wang QC, Johnson BA. Fingertip injuries. *Am Fam Physician.* 2001;63(10):1961–1966

Finger Pain

1. Campbell WW. Diagnosis and management of common compression and entrapment neuropathies. *Neurol Clin.* 1997;15(3):549–567

2. Harrison BP, Hillard MW. Emergency department evaluation and treatment of hand injuries. *Emerg Med Clin North Am.* 1999;17(4):793–822, v

3. Ling SM. Osteoarthritis in older adults. *J Am Geriatr Soc.* 1998;46(2):216–225

4. Mayeaux EJ Jr. Nail disorders. *Prim Care.* 2000;27(2):333–351

Foot Pain

1. Aldridge T. Diagnosing heel pain in adults. *Am Fam Physician.* 2004;70(2):332–338

2. Bedinghaus J, Niedfeldt MW. Over-the-counter foot remedies. *Am Fam Physician.* 2001;64(5):791–796

3. Butalia S, Palda VA, Sargeant RJ, Detsky AS, Mourad O. Does this patient with diabetes have osteomyelitis of the lower extremity? *JAMA.* 2008;299(7):806–813

4. Coakley G, Mathews C, Field M, et al; British Society for Rheumatology Standards, Guidelines and Audit Working Group. BSR & BHPR, BOA, RCGP and BSAC guidelines for management of the hot swollen joint in adults. *Rheumatology (Oxford).* 2006;45(8):1039–1041

5. Cole C, Seto C, Gazewood J. Plantar fasciitis: evidence-based review of diagnosis and therapy. *Am Fam Physician.* 2005;72(11):2237–2242

6. Glazer JL, Hosey RG. Soft-tissue injuries of the lower extremity. *Prim Care.* 2004;31(4):1005–1024

7. Schroeder BM; American College of Foot and Ankle Surgeons. Diagnosis and treatment of heel pain. *Am Fam Physician.* 2002;65(8):1686–1688

8. Shapiro BE, Preston DC. Entrapment and compressive neuropathies. *Med Clin North Am.* 2003;87(3):663–696, viii

9. Weston V, Coakley G; British Society for Rheumatology Standards, Guidelines and Audit Working Group; et al. Guideline for the management of the hot swollen joint in adults with a particular focus on septic arthritis. *J Antimicrob Chemother.* 2006;58(3):492–493

10. Young CC, Niedfeldt MW, Morris GA, Eerkes KJ. Clinical examination of the foot and ankle. *Prim Care.* 2005;32(1):105–132

Frostbite

1. American Heart Association. 2005 Guidelines for Cardiopulmonary Resuscitation and Emergency Cardiovascular Care. Part 14: First aid. *Circulation.* 2005;112(24 suppl):IV-196–IV-203

2. Bilgiç S, Ozkan H, Ozenç S, Safaz I, Yildiz C. Treating frostbite. *Can Fam Physician.* 2008;54(3):361–363

3. Cauchy E, Cheguillaume B, Chetaille E. A controlled trial of a prostacyclin and rt-PA in the treatment of severe frostbite. *N Engl J Med.* 2011;364(2):189–190

4. Cauchy E, Davis CB, Pasquier M, Meyer EF, Hackett PH. A new proposal for management of severe frostbite in the austere environment. *Wilderness Environ Med.* 2016;27(1):92–99

5. Centers for Disease Control and Prevention. Acute illness from dry ice exposure during hurricane Ivan—Alabama, 2004. *MMWR Morb Mortal Wkly Rep.* 2004;53(50):1182–1183

6. Centers for Disease Control and Prevention. Diphtheria, tetanus, and pertussis: recommendations for vaccine use and other preventive measures. Recommendations of the Immunization Practices Advisory Committee (ACIP). *MMWR Recomm Rep.* 1991;40(RR-10):1–28

7. Heggers JP, Robson MC, Manavalen K, et al. Experimental and clinical observations on frostbite. *Ann Emerg Med.* 1987;16(9):1056–1062

8. Jurkovich GJ. Environmental cold-induced injury. *Surg Clin North Am.* 2007;87(1):247–267, viii

9. Markenson D, Ferguson JD, Chameides L, et al. 2010 American Heart Association and American Red Cross Guidelines for First Aid. Part 17: First Aid. *Circulation.* 2010;122(18 suppl 3):S934–S946

10. Miller MB, Koltai PJ. Treatment of experimental frostbite with pentoxifylline and aloe vera cream. *Arch Otolaryngol Head Neck Surg.* 1995;121(6):678–680

11. Murphy TV, Slade BA, Broder KR, et al. Prevention of pertussis, tetanus, and diphtheria among pregnant and postpartum women and their infants recommendations of the Advisory Committee on Immunization Practices (ACIP). *MMWR Recomm Rep.* 2008;57(RR-4):1–51

12. O'Toole G, Rayatt S. Frostbite at the gym: a case report of an ice pack burn. *Br J Sports Med.* 1999;33(4):278–279

13. Patel NN, Patel DN. Frostbite. *Am J Med.* 2008;121(9):765–766

14. Singer AJ, Dagum AB. Current management of acute cutaneous wounds. *N Engl J Med.* 2008;359(10):1037–1046

15. Weiss EA. Medical considerations for wilderness and adventure travelers. *Med Clin North Am.* 1999;83(4):885–902, v–vi

Hand and Wrist Injury

1. American Heart Association. 2005 Guidelines for Cardiopulmonary Resuscitation and Emergency Cardiovascular Care. Part 10: First Aid. *Circulation.* 2005;112:IV-196–IV-203

2. Brady WJ, et al. Upper extremity fractures and dislocations. *Emerg Med Reports.* 1999;20(9)

3. Collins NC. Is ice right? Does cryotherapy improve outcome for acute soft tissue injury? *Emerg Med J.* 2008;25(2):65–68

4. Gonzalez R, Kasdan ML. High pressure injection injuries of the hand. *Clin Occup Environ Med.* 2006;5(2):407–411, ix

5. Harrison BP, Hillard MW. Emergency department evaluation and treatment of hand injuries. *Emerg Med Clin North Am.* 1999;17(4):793–822, v

6. Hogan CJ, Ruland RT. High-pressure injection injuries to the upper extremity: a review of the literature. *J Orthop Trauma.* 2006;20(7):503–511

7. Kretsinger K, Broder KR, Cortese MM, et al; Centers for Disease Control and Prevention; Advisory Committee on Immunization Practices; Healthcare Infection Control Practices Advisory Committee. Preventing tetanus, diphtheria, and pertussis among adults: use of tetanus toxoid, reduced diphtheria toxoid and acellular pertussis vaccine recommendations of the Advisory Committee on Immunization Practices (ACIP) and recommendation of ACIP, supported by the Healthcare Infection Control Practices Advisory Committee (HICPAC), for use of Tdap among health-care personnel. *MMWR Recomm Rep.* 2006;55(RR-17):1–37

8. Markenson D, Ferguson JD, Chameides L, et al. 2010 American Heart Association and American Red Cross Guidelines for First Aid. Part 17: First Aid. *Circulation.* 2010;122(18 suppl 3):S934–S946

9. Mastey RD, Weiss AP, Akelman E. Primary care of hand and wrist athletic injuries. *Clin Sports Med.* 1997;16(4):705–724

10. McMaster WC, Liddle S, Waugh TR. Laboratory evaluation of various cold therapy modalities. *Am J Sports Med.* 1978;6:291–294

11. Parmelee–Peters K, Eathorne SW. The wrist: common injuries and management. *Prim Care.* 2005;32(1):35–70

12. Pimentel L. Orthopedic trauma: office management of major joint injury. *Med Clin North Am.* 2006;90(2):355–382

Hand and Wrist Injury (continued)

13. Sasser SM, Hunt RC, Faul M, et al; Centers for Disease Control and Prevention. Guidelines for field triage of injured patients: recommendations of the National Expert Panel on Field Triage, 2011. *MMWR Recomm Rep.* 2012;61(RR-1):1–20

14. Sbai MA, Benzarti S, Boussen M, Maalla R. Teeth syndrome: diagnosis, complications and management. *Pan Afr Med J.* 2015;22:71

15. Shewring DJ, Trickett RW, Subramanian KN, Hnyda R. The management of clenched fist "fight bite" injuries of the hand. *J Hand Surg Eur Vol.* 2015;40(8):819–824

16. Singer AJ, Dagum AB. Current management of acute cutaneous wounds. *N Engl J Med.* 2008;359(10):1037–1046

Hand and Wrist Pain

1. Barry NN, McGuire JL. Overuse syndromes in adult athletes. *Rheum Dis Clin North Am.* 1996;22(3):515–530

2. Campbell WW. Diagnosis and management of common compression and entrapment neuropathies. *Neurol Clin.* 1997;15(3):549–567

3. Canto JG, Shlipak MG, Rogers WJ, et al. Prevalence, clinical characteristics, and mortality among patients with myocardial infarction presenting without chest pain. *JAMA.* 2000;283(24):3223–3229

4. Coakley G, Mathews C, Field M, et al; British Society for Rheumatology Standards, Guidelines and Audit Working Group. BSR & BHPR, BOA, RCGP and BSAC guidelines for management of the hot swollen joint in adults. *Rheumatology (Oxford).* 2006;45(8):1039–1041

5. Coronado BE, Pope JH, Griffith JL, Beshansky JR, Selker HP. Clinical features, triage, and outcome of patients presenting to the ED with suspected acute coronary syndromes but without pain: a multicenter study. *Am J Emerg Med.* 2004;22(7):568–574

6. Culic V, Eterovic D, Miric D, Silic N. Symptom presentation of acute myocardial infarction: influence of sex, age, and risk factors. *Am Heart J.* 2002;144(6):1012–1017

7. Izzi J, Dennison D, Noerdlinger M, Dasilva M, Akelman E. Nerve injuries of the elbow, wrist, and hand in athletes. *Clin Sports Med.* 2001;20(1):203–217

8. Ling SM, Bathon JM. Osteoarthritis in older adults. *J Am Geriatr Soc.* 1998;46(2):216–225

9. Rainsford KD. Ibuprofen: pharmacology, efficacy and safety. *Inflammopharmacology.* 2009;17(6):275–342

10. Weston V, Coakley G; British Society for Rheumatology Standards, Guidelines and Audit Working Group; et al. Guideline for the management of the hot swollen joint in adults with a particular focus on septic arthritis. *J Antimicrob Chemother.* 2006;58(3):492–493

Hay Fever (Nasal Allergies)

1. Bousquet J, Van Cauwenberge P, Khaltaev N; Aria Workshop Group; World Health Organization. Allergic rhinitis and its impact on asthma. *J Allergy Clin Immunol.* 2001;108(5 suppl):S147–S334

2. Eapen RJ, Ebert CS Jr, Pillsbury HC 3rd. Allergic rhinitis—history and presentation. *Otolaryngol Clin North Am.* 2008;41(2):325–330, vi–vii

3. Ebell MH, Lundgren J, Youngpairoj S. How long does a cough last? Comparing patients' expectations with data from a systematic review of the literature. *Ann Fam Med.* 2013;11(1):5–13

4. Hadley JA. Evaluation and management of allergic rhitis. *Med Clin North Am.* 1999;83(1):13–25

5. Incaudo GA, Takach P. The diagnosis and treatment of allergic rhinitis during pregnancy and lactation. *Immunol Allergy Clin North Am.* 2006;26(1):137–154

6. Izquierdo-Domínguez A, Valero AL, Mullol J. Comparative analysis of allergic rhinitis in children and adults. *Curr Allergy Asthma Rep.* 2013;13(2):142–151

7. Léger D, Annesi-Maesano I, Carat F, et al. Allergic rhinitis and its consequences on quality of sleep: an unexplored area. *Arch Intern Med.* 2006;166(16):1744–1748

8. Rabago D, Barrett B, Marchand L, Maberry R, Mundt M. Qualitative aspects of nasal irrigation use by patients with chronic sinus disease in a multimethod study. *Ann Fam Med.* 2006;4(4):295–301

9. Rabago D, Zgierska A. Saline nasal irrigation for upper respiratory conditions. *Am Fam Physician.* 2009;80(10):1121

10. Rosenfeld RM, Andes D, Bhattacharyya N, et al. Clinical practice guideline: adult sinusitis. *Otolaryngol Head Neck Surg.* 2007;137(3 suppl):S1–S31

11. Skoner DP. Allergic rhinitis: definition, epidemiology, pathophysiology, detection and diagnosis. *J Allergy Clin Immunol.* 2001;108(1 suppl):S2–S8

12. Wallace DV, Dykewicz MS, Bernstein DI, et al. The diagnosis and management of rhinitis: an updated practice parameter. *J Allergy Clin Immunol.* 2008;122(2 suppl):S1–S84

Head Injury

1. American Academy of Neurology. Practice parameter: the management of concussion in sports (summary statement). Report of the Quality Standards Subcommittee. *Neurology.* 1997;48(3):581–5

2. American Heart Association. 2005 Guidelines for Cardiopulmonary Resuscitation and Emergency Cardiovascular Care. Part 10: First Aid. *Circulation.* 2005;112:IV–196–IV–203

3. Bennett MH, Trytko B, Jonker B. Hyperbaric oxygen therapy for the adjunctive treatment of traumatic brain injury. *Cochrane Database Syst Rev.* 2004;(4):CD004609

4. Benson BW, Meeuwisse WH, Rizos J, Kang J, Burke CJ. A prospective study of concussions among National Hockey League players during regular season games: the NHL–NHLPA Concussion Program. *CMAJ.* 2011;183(8):905–911

5. Borczuk P. Mild head trauma. *Emerg Med Clin North Am.* 1997;15(3):563–579

6. Borczuk P. Predictors of intracranial injury in patients with mild head trauma. *Ann Emerg Med.* 1995;25:731–736

7. Bracken ME, Medzon R, Rathlev NK, Mower WR, Hoffman JR. Effect of intoxication among blunt trauma patients selected for head computed tomography scanning. *Ann Emerg Med.* 2007;49(1):45–51

8. CRASH Trial Collaborators. Effect of inravenous corticosteroids on death within 14 days in 10,008 adults wth clinically significant head injury (CRASH Trial). *Lancet.* 2004;364(9442):1321–1328

9. Dunning J, Stratford-Smith P, Lecky F, et al. A meta-analysis of clinical correlates that predict significant intracranial injury in adults with minor head trauma. *J Neurotrauma.* 2004;21(7):877–885

10. Eikelboom JW, Wallentin L, Connolly SJ, et al. Risk of bleeding with 2 doses of dabigatran compared with warfarin in older and younger patients with atrial fibrillation. *Circulation.* 2011;123(21):2363–2372

11. Elkington LJ, Hughes DC. Australian Institute of Sport and Australian Medical Association position statement on concussion in sport. *Med J Aust.* 2017;206(1):46–50

12. Giza CC, Kutcher JS, Ashwal S, et al. Summary of evidence-based guideline update: evaluation and management of concussion in sports: report of the Guideline Development Subcommittee of the American Academy of Neurology. *Neurology.* 2013;80(24):2250–2257

13. Grandhi R, Harrison G, Voronovich Z, et al. Preinjury warfarin, but not antiplatelet medications, increases mortality in elderly traumatic brain injury patients. *J Trauma Acute Care Surg.* 2015;78(3):614–621

14. Grool AM, Aglipay M, Momoli F, et al; Pediatric Emergency Research Canada Concussion Team. Association between early participation in physical activity following acute concussion and persistent postconcussive symptoms in children and adolescents. *JAMA.* 2016;316(23):2504–2514

15. Hall EE, Ketcham CJ, Crenshaw CR, Baker MH, McConnell JM, Patel K. Concussion management in collegiate student-athletes: return-to-academics recommendations. *Clin J Sport Med.* 2015;25(3):291–296

16. Halstead ME, Walter KD; American Academy of Pediatrics Council on Sports Medicine and Fitness. Sport-related concussion in children and adolescents. *Pediatrics.* 2010;126(3):597–615

17. Harmon KG, Drezner JA, Gammons M, et al. American Medical Society for Sports Medicine position statement: concussion in sport. *Br J Sports Med.* 2013;47(1):15–26

18. Haydel MJ, Preston CA, Mills TJ, Luber S, Blaudeau E, DeBlieux PM. Indications for computed tomography in patients with minor head injury. *N Engl J Med.* 2000;343(2):100–105

19. Herbella FA, Mudo M, Delmonti C, Braga FM, Del Grande JC. Raccoon eyes (periorbital haematoma) as a sign of skull base fracture. *Injury.* 2001;32(10):745–747

20. Jagoda AS, Bazarian JJ, Bruns JJ Jr, et al; American College of Emergency Physicians; Centers for Disease Control and Prevention. Clinical policy: neuroimaging and decisionmaking in adult mild traumatic brain injury in the acute setting. *Ann Emerg Med.* 2008;52(6):714–748

21. Joseph B, Pandit V, Aziz H, et al. Clinical outcomes in traumatic brain injury patients on preinjury clopidogrel: a prospective analysis. *J Trauma Acute Care Surg.* 2014;76(3):817–820

22. Kuppermann N, Holmes JF, Dayan PS, et al. Identification of children at very low risk of clinically-important brain injuries after head trauma: a prospective cohort study. *Lancet.* 2009;374(9696):1160–1170

23. Markenson D, Ferguson JD, Chameides L, et al. 2010 American Heart Association and American Red Cross Guidelines for First Aid. Part 17: First Aid. *Circulation.* 2010;122(18 suppl 3):S934–S946

24. McCrea M, Guskiewicz KM, Marshall SW, et al. Acute effects and recovery time following concussion in collegiate football players. *JAMA.* 2003;290(19):2556–2563

25. McCrory P, Meeuwisse W, Johnston K, et al. Consensus statement on Concussion in Sport 3rd International Conference on Concussion in Sport held in Zurich, November 2008. *Clin J Sport Med.* 2009;19(3):185–200

26. McLeod TC, Lewis JH, Whelihan K, Bacon CE. Rest and return to activity after sport-related concussion: a systematic review of the literature. *J Athl Train.* 2017;52(3):262–287

27. Nee PA, Hadfield JM, Yates DW, Faragher EB. Significance of vomiting after head injury. *J Neurol Neurosurg Psychiatry.* 1999;66(4):470–473

28. Peltola EM, Koivikko MP, Koskinen SK. The spectrum of facial fractures in motor vehicle accidents: an MDCT study of 374 patients. *Emerg Radiol.* 2014;21(2):165–171

29. Pretto Flores L, De Almeida CS, Casulari LA. Positive predictive values of selected clinical signs associated with skull base fractures. *J Neurosurg Sci.* 2000;44(2):77–82

30. Ropper AH, Gorson KC. Clinical practice. Concussion. *N Engl J Med.* 2007;356(2):166–172

31. Sasser SM, Hunt RC, Faul M, et al; Centers for Disease Control and Prevention. Guidelines for field triage of injured patients: recommendations of the National Expert Panel on Field Triage, 2011. *MMWR Recomm Rep.* 2012;61(RR-1):1–20

32. Schneider KJ, Leddy JJ, Guskiewicz KM, et al. Rest and treatment/rehabilitation following sport-related concussion: a systematic review. *Br J Sports Med.* 2017;51(12):930–934

33. Singer AJ, Dagum AB. Current management of acute cutaneous wounds. *N Engl J Med.* 2008;359(10):1037–1046

34. Somasundaram A, Laxton AW, Perrin RG. The clinical features of periorbital ecchymosis in a series of trauma patients. *Injury.* 2014;45(1):203–205

35. Stiell IG, Wells GA, Vandemheen K, et al. The Canadian CT Head Rule for patients with minor head injury. *Lancet.* 2001;357(9266):1391–1396

36. Teasdale G, Jennett B. Assessment of coma and impaired consciousness. A practical scale. *Lancet.* 1974;13;2(7872):81–84

37. Wolf G, Cifu D, Baugh L, Carne W, Profenna L. The effect of hyperbaric oxygen on symptoms after mild traumatic brain injury. *J Neurotrauma.* 2012;29(17):2606–2612

Headache

1. American College of Emergency Physicians. Clinical policy: critical issues in the evaluation and management of patients presenting to the emergency department with acute headache. *Ann Emerg Med.* 2002;39(1):108–122

2. Attia J, Hatala R, Cook DJ, et al. Does this adult patient have acute meningitis? *JAMA.* 1999;282(2):175–181

3. Edlow JA, Fisher J. Diagnosis of subarachnoid hemorrhage: time to change the guidelines? *Stroke.* 2012;43(8):2031–2032

4. Edlow JA, Malek AM, Ogilvy CS. Aneurysmal subarachnoid hemorrhage: update for emergency physicians. *J Emerg Med.* 2008;34(3):237–251

5. Edlow JA, Panagos PD, Godwin SA, Thomas TL, Decker WW; American College of Emergency Physicians Clinical Policies Subcommittee. Clinical policy: critical issues in the evaluation and management of adult patients presenting to the emergency department with acute headache. *Ann Emerg Med.* 2008;52(4):407–436

6. Friedman DI. The eye and headache. *Ophthalmol Clin North Am.* 2004;17(3):357–369, vi

7. Gus M, Fuchs FD, Pimentel M, Rosa D, Melo AG, Moreira LB. Behavior of ambulatory blood pressure surrounding episodes of headache in mildly hypertensive patients. *Arch Intern Med.* 2001;161(2):252–255

8. Headache Classification Committee of the International Headache Society. The International Classification of Headache Disorders. 2nd ed. *Cephalalgia.* 2004;24(1 suppl):1–160

9. Lipton RB, Stewart WF, Liberman JN. Self-awareness of migraine: interpreting the labels that headache sufferers apply to their headaches. *Neurology.* 2002;58(9 suppl 6):S21–S26

10. Martin-Schild S, Albright KC, Tanksley J, et al. Zero on the NIHSS does not equal the absence of stroke. *Ann Emerg Med.* 2011;57(1):42–45

11. Morgenstern LB, Hemphill JC 3rd, Anderson C, et al; American Heart Association Stroke Council and Council on Cardiovascular Nursing. Guidelines for the management of spontaneous intracerebral hemorrhage: a guideline for healthcare professionals from the American Heart Association/American Stroke Association. *Stroke.* 2010;41(9):2108–2129

12. Muiesan ML, Padovani A, Salvetti M, et al. Headache: prevalence and relationship with office or ambulatory blood pressure in a general population sample (the Vobarno Study). *Blood Press.* 2006;15(1):14–19

13. Perry JJ, Stiell IG, Sivilotti ML, et al. High risk clinical characteristics for subarachnoid haemorrhage in patients with acute headache: prospective cohort study. *BMJ.* 2010;341:c5204

14. Perry JJ, Stiell IG, Sivilotti ML, et al. Sensitivity of computed tomography performed within six hours of onset of headache for diagnosis of subarachnoid haemorrhage: prospective cohort study. *BMJ.* 2011;343:d4277

15. Purdy RA, Kirby S. Headaches and brain tumors. *Neurol Clin.* 2004;22(1):39–53

16. Rainsford KD. Ibuprofen: pharmacology, efficacy and safety. *Inflammopharmacology.* 2009;17(6):275–342

17. Saper JR. Medicolegal issues: headache. *Neurol Clin.* 1999;17(2):197–214

18. Segard J, Montassier E, Trewick D, Le Conte P, Guillon B, Berrut G. Urgent computed tomography brain scan for elderly patients: can we improve its diagnostic yield? *Eur J Emerg Med.* 2013;20(1):51–53

19. Sheftell FD. Role and impact of over-the-counter medications in the management of headache. *Neurol Clin.* 1997;15(1):187–198

20. Silberstein SD. Drug-induced headache. *Neurol Clin.* 1998;16(1):107–123

21. Walker RA, Wadman MC. Headache in the elderly. *Clin Geriatr Med.* 2007;23(2):291–305, v–vi

Heart Rate and Heartbeat Questions

1. American Heart Association. 2005 Guidelines for Cardiopulmonary Resuscitation and Emergency Cardiovascular Care. Part 7.3: management of symptomatic bradycardia and tachycardia. *Circulation.* 2005;112(24 suppl):IV-67–IV-77

2. Hood RE, Shorofsky SR. Management of arrhythmias in the emergency department. *Cardiol Clin.* 2006;24(1):125–133, vii

3. Leaman TL. Anxiety disorders. *Prim Care.* 1999;26(2):197–210

4. Pinski SL, Trohman RG. Implantable cardioverter-defibrillators: implications for the nonelectrophysiologist. *Ann Intern Med.* 1995;122(10):770–777

5. Sarasin FP, Hanusa BH, Perneger T, Louis-Simonet M, Rajeswaran A, Kapoor WN. A risk score to predict arrhythmias in patients with unexplained syncope. *Acad Emerg Med.* 2003;10(12):1312–1317

6. Schnipper JL, Kapoor WN. Diagnostic evaluation and management of patients with syncope. *Med Clin North Am.* 2001;85(2):423–456, xi

7. Sears SF Jr, Shea JB, Conti JB. How to respond to an implantable cardioverter-defibrillator shock. *Circulation.* 2005;111(23):e380–e382

Heat Exposure (Heat Exhaustion and Heatstroke)

1. Armstrong LE, Casa DJ, Millard-Stafford M, Moran DS, Pyne SW, Roberts WO. Exertional heat illness during training and competition. *Med Sci Sports Exerc.* 2007;39(3):556–572

2. Armstrong LE, Epstein Y, Greenleaf JE, et al. American College of Sports Medicine position stand. Heat and cold illnesses during distance running. *Med Sci Sports Exerc.* 1996;28(12):i–x

Heat Exposure (Heat Exhaustion and Heatstroke) (continued)

3. Backer HD, Shopes E, Collins SL, Barkan H. Exertional heat illness and hyponatremia in hikers. *Am J Emerg Med.* 1999;17(6):532–539

4. Binkley HM, Beckett J, Casa DJ, Kleiner DM, Plummer PE. National Athletic Trainers' Association position statement: exertional heat illnesses. *J Athl Train.* 2002;37(3):329–343

5. Bouchama A, Knochel JP. Heat stroke. *N Eng J Med.* 2002;346(25):1978–1988

6. Casa DJ, Armstrong LE, Hillman SK, et al. National Athletic Trainers' Association position statement: fluid replacement for athletes. *J Athl Train.* 2000;35(2):212–224

7. Centers for Disease Control and Prevention. Heat illness among high school athletes—United States, 2005–2009. *MMWR Morb Mortal Wkly Rep.* 2010;59(32):1009–1013

8. Finch CF, Boufous S. The descriptive epidemiology of sports/leisure-related heat illness hospitalisations in New South Wales, Australia. *J Sci Med Sport.* 2008;11(1):48–51

9. Glazer JL. Heat exhaustion and heatstroke: what you should know. *Am Fam Physician.* 2005;71(11):2141–2142

10. Grubenhoff JA, du Ford K, Roosevelt GE. Heat-related illness. *Clin Pediatr Emerg Med.* 2007;8(1):59–64

11. Khosla R, Guntupalli KK. Heat-related illness. *Crit Care Clin.* 1999;15(2):251–263

12. Lugo-Amador NM, Rothenhaus T, Moyer P. Heat-related illness. *Emerg Med Clin North Am.* 2004;22(2):315–327, viii

13. Markenson D, Ferguson JD, Chameides L, et al. 2010 American Heart Association and American Red Cross Guidelines for First Aid. Part 17: First Aid. *Circulation.* 2010;122(18 suppl 3):S934–S946

14. Marshall SW. Heat injury in youth sport. *Br J Sports Med.* 2010;44(1):8–12

15. Update: heat injuries, active component, U.S. Armed Forces, 2011. *MSMR.* 2012;19(3):14–16

High Blood Pressure

1. Acelajado MC, Oparil S. Hypertension in the elderly. *Clin Geriatr Med.* 2009;25(3):391–412

2. Armstrong C; Joint National Committee. JNC8 guidelines for the management of hypertension in adults. *Am Fam Physician.* 2014;90(7):503–504

3. Calhoun DA, Jones D, Textor S, et al. Resistant hypertension: diagnosis, evaluation, and treatment: a scientific statement from the American Heart Association Professional Education Committee. *Circulation.* 2008;117(25):e510–e526

4. Chiang WK, Jamshahi B. Asymptomatic hypertension in the ED. *Am J Emerg Med.* 1998;16(7):701–704

5. Chobanian AV, Bakris GL, Black HR, et al. The Seventh Report of the Joint National Committee on Prevention, Detection, Evaluation, and Treatment of High Blood Pressure: the JNC 7 report. *JAMA.* 2003;289(19):2560–2572

6. Dasgupta K, Quinn RR, Zarnke KB, et al; Canadian Hypertension Education Program. The 2014 Canadian Hypertension Education Program recommendations for blood pressure measurement, diagnosis, assessment of risk, prevention, and treatment of hypertension. *Can J Cardiol.* 2014;30(5):485–501

7. Drager LF, Lotufo PA, Bensenor IM. Letter regarding article by Law et al, "headaches and the treatment of blood pressure: results from a metaanalysis of 94 randomized placebo-controlled trials with 24,000 participants." *Circulation.* 2006;113(7):e164

8. ESH/ESC Task Force for the Management of Arterial Hypertension. 2013 practice guidelines for the management of arterial hypertension of the European Society of Hypertension (ESH) and the European Society of Cardiology (ESC): ESH/ESC Task Force for the Management of Arterial Hypertension. *J Hypertens.* 2013;31(10):1925–1938

9. Fung TT, Chiuve SE, McCullough ML, Rexrode KM, Logroscino G, Hu FB. Adherence to a DASH-style diet and risk of coronary heart disease and stroke in women. *Arch Intern Med.* 2008;168(7):713–720

10. Goldstein CM, Josephson R, Xie S, Hughes JW. Current perspectives on the use of meditation to reduce blood pressure. *Int J Hypertens.* 2012;2012:578397

11. Goldstein LB, Adams R, Alberts MJ, et al. Primary prevention of ischemic stroke: a guideline from the American Heart Association/American Stroke Association Stroke Council. *Circulation.* 2006;113(24):e873–e923

12. Goldstein LB, Bushnell CD, Adams RJ, et al. Guidelines for the primary prevention of stroke: a guideline for healthcare professionals from the American Heart Association/American Stroke Association. *Stroke.* 2011;42(2):517–584

13. Gus M, Fuchs FD, Pimentel M, Rosa D, Melo AG, Moreira LB. Behavior of ambulatory blood pressure surrounding episodes of headache in mildly hypertensive patients. *Arch Intern Med.* 2001;161(2):252–255

14. Hackam DG, Khan NA, Hemmelgarn BR, et al. The 2010 Canadian hypertension education program recommendations for the management of hypertension: part 2—therapy. *Can J Cardiol.* 2010;26(5):249–258

15. Head GA, Mihailidou AS, Duggan KA; Ambulatory Blood Pressure Working Group of the High Blood Pressure Research Council of Australia. Definition of ambulatory blood pressure targets for diagnosis and treatment of hypertension in relation to clinic blood pressure: prospective cohort study. *BMJ.* 2010;340:c1104

16. James PA, Oparil S, Carter BL, et al. 2014 evidence-based guideline for the management of high blood pressure in adults: report from the panel members appointed to the Eighth Joint National Committee (JNC 8). *JAMA.* 2014;311(5):507–520

17. Joint National Committee on Prevention, Detection, Evaluation, and Treatment of High Blood Pressure; National High Blood Pressure Education Program Coordinating Committee. The Sixth Report of the Joint National Committee on Prevention, Detection, Evaluation, and Treatment of High Blood Pressure. *Arch Intern Med.* 1997;157(21):2413–2446

18. Lima SG, Nascimento LS, Santos Filho CN, Albuquerque Mde F, Victor EG. Systemic hypertension at emergency units. The use of symptomatic drugs as choice for management [Portuguese]. *Arq Bras Cardiol.* 2005;85(2):115–123

19. Ma G, Sabin N, Dawes M. A comparison of blood pressure measurement over a sleeved arm versus a bare arm. *CMAJ.* 2008;178(5):585–589

20. Muiesan ML, Padovani A, Salvetti M, et al. Headache: prevalence and relationship with office or ambulatory blood pressure in a general population sample (the Vobarno Study). *Blood Press.* 2006;15(1):14–19

21. Pickering TG. Principles and techniques of blood pressure measurement. *Cardiol Clin.* 2002;20(2):207–223

22. Quinn RR, Hemmelgarn BR, Padwal RS, et al. The 2010 Canadian hypertension education program recommendations for the management of hypertension: part I—blood pressure measurement, diagnosis and assessment of risk. *Can J Cardiol.* 2010;26(5):241–248

23. Reboussin DM, Allen NB, Griswold ME, et al. Systematic review for the 2017 ACC/AHA/AAPA/ABC/ACPM/AGS/APhA/ASH/ASPC/NMA/PCNA guideline for the prevention, detection, evaluation, and management of high blood pressure in adults: a report of the American College of Cardiology/American Heart Association Task Force on Clinical Practice Guidelines. *J Am Coll Cardiol.* 2018;71(19):2176–2198

24. Rossi A, Dikareva A, Bacon SL, Daskalopoulou SS. The impact of physical activity on mortality in patients with high blood pressure: a systematic review. *J Hypertens.* 2012;30(7):1277–1288

25. Sharman JE, Stowasser M. Australian Association for Exercise and Sports Science position statement on exercise and hypertension. *J Sci Med Sport.* 2009;12(2):252–257

26. Smulyan H, Safar ME. The diastolic blood pressure in systolic hypertension. *Ann Intern Med.* 2000;132(3):233–237

27. Varon J, Marik PE. The diagnosis and management of hypertensive crises. *Chest.* 2000;18(1):214–227

28. Whelton PK, Carey RM, Aronow WS, et al. 2017 ACC/AHA/AAPA/ABC/ACPM/AGS/APhA/ASH/ASPC/NMA/PCNA guideline for the prevention, detection, evaluation, and management of high blood pressure in adults: a report of the American College of Cardiology/American Heart Association Task Force on Clinical Practice Guidelines. *Hypertension.* 2018;71(6):e13–e115

29. Whelton PK, He J, Appel LJ, et al. Primary prevention of hypertension: clinical and public health advisory from the National High Blood Pressure Education Program. *JAMA.* 2002;288(15):1882–1888

Hip Injury

1. American Heart Association. 2005 Guidelines for Cardiopulmonary Resuscitation and Emergency Cardiovascular Care. Part 10: First Aid. *Circulation.* 2005;112:IV-196–IV-203

2. Brunner LC, Eshilian-Oates, Kuo TY. Hip fractures. *Am Fam Physician.* 2003;67(3):537–542

3. Collins NC. Is ice right? Does cryotherapy improve outcome for acute soft tissue injury? *Emerg Med J.* 2008;25(2):65–68

4. Dake AD, Stack L. Penetrating trauma to the extremities: systematic assessment and targeted management of weapons-related injuries. *Emerg Med Reports* 1997;18(7)

5. Markenson D, Ferguson JD, Chameides L, et al. 2010 American Heart Association and American Red Cross Guidelines for First Aid. Part 17: First Aid. *Circulation.* 2010;122(18 suppl 3):S934–S946

6. Rudman N. Emergency department evaluation and treatment of hip and thigh injuries. *Emerg Med Clin North Am.* 2000;18(1):29–66

7. Singer AJ, Dagum AB. Current management of acute cutaneous wounds. *N Engl J Med.* 2008;359(10):1037–1046

Hives

1. Agency for Toxic Substances and Disease Registry. Contact dermatitis and urticaria from environmental exposures. *Am Fam Physician.* 1993;48(5):773–780

2. American Academy of Allergy, Asthma and Immunology Joint Task Force on Practice Parameters; American College of Allergy, Asthma and Immunology Joint Council of Allergy, Asthma and Immunology. The diagnosis and management of anaphylaxis: an updated practice parameter. *J Allergy Clin Immunol.* 2005;115(3 suppl 2):S483–S523

3. Braganza SC, Acworth JP, Mckinnon DR, Peake JE, Brown AF. Paediatric emergency department anaphylaxis: different patterns from adults. *Arch Dis Child.* 2006;91(2):159–163

4. Kennedy MS. Evaluation of chronic eczema and urticaria and angioedema. *Immunol Allergy Clin North Am.* 1999;19(1):19–33

5. Pollack CV Jr, Romano TJ. Outpatient management of acute uriticaria. *Ann Emerg Med.* 1995;26(5):547–551

6. Sampson HA. Anaphylaxis and emergency treatment. *Pediatrics.* 2003;111(6 suppl 3):1601–1608

7. Sampson HA, Muñoz-Furlong A, Campbell RL, et al. Second symposium on the definition and management of anaphylaxis: summary report–Second National Institute of Allergy and Infectious Disease/Food Allergy and Anaphylaxis Network symposium. *J Allergy Clin Immunol.* 2006;117(2):391–397

Immunization Reactions

1. Adams DA, Jajosky RA, Ajani U, et al. Summary of notifiable diseases—United States, 2012. *MMWR Morb Mortal Wkly Rep.* 2014;61(53):1–121

2. Advisory Committee on Immunization Practices. Recommended adult immunization schedule: United States, 2011. *Ann Intern Med.* 2011;154(3):168–173

3. Atkinson WL, Pickering LK, Schwartz B, et al. General recommendations on immunization. Recommendations of the Advisory Committee on Immunization Practices (ACIP) and the American Academy of Family Physicians (AAFP). *MMWR Recomm Rep.* 2002;51(RR-2):1–35

4. Centers for Disease Control and Prevention. Diphtheria, tetanus, and pertussis: recommendations for vaccine use and other preventive measures. Recommendations of the Immunization Practices Advisory Committee (ACIP). *MMWR Recomm Rep.* 1991;40:(RR-10):1–28

5. Centers for Disease Control and Prevention. Prevention and control of seasonal influenza with vaccines. Recommendations of the Advisory Committee on Immunization Practices—United States, 2013–2014. *MMWR Recomm Rep.* 2013;62(RR-07):1–43

6. Centers for Disease Control and Prevention. Recommended adult immunization schedule—United States, 2011. *MMWR Morb Mortal Wkly Rep.* 20114;60(4):1–4

7. Centers for Disease Control and Prevention. Syncope after vaccination—United States, January 2005–July 2007. *MMWR Morb Mortal Wkly Rep.* 2008;57(17):457–460

8. Centers for Disease Control and Prevention. Updated recommendations for use of tetanus toxoid, reduced diphtheria toxoid and acellular pertussis (Tdap) vaccine from the Advisory Committee on Immunization Practices, 2010. *MMWR Morb Mortal Wkly Rep.* 2011;60(1):13–15

9. Centers for Disease Control and Prevention; Advisory Committee on Immunization Practices. Immunization of health-care personnel: recommendations of the Advisory Committee on Immunization Practices (ACIP). *MMWR Recomm Rep.* 2011;60(RR-7):1–45

10. Committee on Obstetric Practice and Immunization Expert Work Group; Centers for Disease Control and Prevention's Advisory Committee on Immunization, United States; American College of Obstetricians and Gynecologists. Committee opinion no. 608: influenza vaccination during pregnancy. *Obstet Gynecol.* 2014;124(3):648–651

11. Grohskopf LA, Sokolow LZ, Broder KR, et al. Prevention and control of seasonal influenza with vaccines. *MMWR Recomm Rep.* 2016;65(5):1–54

12. Kim DK, Riley LE, Harriman KH, Hunter P, Bridges CB. Advisory Committee on Immunization Practices recommended immunization schedule for adults aged 19 years or older—United States, 2017. *MMWR Morb Mortal Wkly Rep.* 2017;66(5):136–138

13. Kretsinger K, Broder KR, Cortese MM, et al; Centers for Disease Control and Prevention; Advisory Committee on Immunization Practices; Health-care Infection Control Practices Advisory Committee. Preventing tetanus, diphtheria, and pertussis among adults: use of tetanus toxoid, reduced diphtheria toxoid and acellular pertussis vaccine recommendations of the Advisory Committee on Immunization Practices (ACIP) and recommendation of ACIP, supported by the Healthcare Infection Control Practices Advisory Committee (HICPAC), for use of Tdap among health-care personnel. *MMWR Recomm Rep.* 2006;55(RR-17):1–37

14. Lindley MC, Bridges CB, Strikas RA, et al. Influenza vaccination performance measurement among acute care hospital-based health care personnel—United States, 2013–14 influenza season. *MMWR Morb Mortal Wkly Rep.* 2014;63(37):812–815

15. Prymula R, Siegrist CA, Chlibek R, et al. Effect of prophylactic paracetamol administration at time of vaccination on febrile reactions and antibody responses in children: two open-label, randomized controlled trials. *Lancet.* 2009;374(9698):1339–1350

16. Public Health Agency of Canada. Canadian Immunization Guide. https://www.canada.ca/en/public-health/services/canadian-immunization-guide.html. Modified January 24, 2018. Accessed June 7, 2018

17. Vaughn JA, Miller RA. Update on immunizations in adults. *Am Fam Physician.* 2011;84(9):1015–1020

18. Workowski KA, Berman S; Centers for Disease Control and Prevention. Sexually transmitted diseases treatment guidelines 2010 [published correction appears in *MMWR Recomm Rep.* 2011;60(1):18]. *MMWR Recomm Rep.* 2010;59(RR-12):1–110

19. World Health Organization Department of Vaccines and Biologicals. Supplementary information on vaccine safety. Part 2: background rates of adverse events following immunization. http://apps.who.int/iris/handle/10665/66675. Accessed June 7, 2018

Influenza, Seasonal

1. Advisory Committee on Immunization Practices. Recommended adult immunization schedule: United States, 2011. *Ann Intern Med.* 2011;154(3):168–173

2. Bachert C, Chuchalin AG, Eisebitt R, Netayzhenko VZ, Voelker M. Aspirin compared with acetaminophen in the treatment of fever and other symptoms of upper respiratory tract infection in adults: a multicenter, randomized, double-blind, double-dummy, placebo-controlled, parallel-group, single-dose, 6-hour dose-ranging study. *Clin Ther.* 2005;27(7):993–1003

3. Centers for Disease Control and Prevention. Prevention and control of seasonal influenza with vaccines. Recommendations of the Advisory Committee on Immunization Practices—United States, 2013–2014. *MMWR Recomm Rep.* 2013;62(RR-07):1–43

Influenza, Seasonal (continued)

4. Committee on Obstetric Practice and Immunization Expert Work Group; Centers for Disease Control and Prevention's Advisory Committee on Immunization, United States; American College of Obstetricians and Gynecologists. Committee opinion no. 608: influenza vaccination during pregnancy. *Obstet Gynecol.* 2014;124(3):648–651

5. Ebell MH, Lundgren J, Youngpairoj S. How long does a cough last? Comparing patients' expectations with data from a systematic review of the literature. *Ann Fam Med.* 2013;11(1):5–13

6. Eccles R. Understanding the symptoms of the common cold and influenza. *Lancet Infect Dis.* 2005;5(11):718–725

7. Erlikh IV, Abraham S, Kondamudi VK. Management of influenza. *Am Fam Physician.* 2010;82(9):1087–1095

8. Fagbuyi DB, Brown KM, Mathison DJ, et al. A rapid medical screening process improves emergency department patient flow during surge associated with novel H1N1 influenza virus. *Ann Emerg Med.* 2011;57(1):52–59

9. Fiore AE, Fry A, Shay D, et al. Antiviral agents for the treatment and chemoprophylaxis of influenza—recommendations of the Advisory Committee on Immunization Practices (ACIP). *MMWR Recomm Rep.* 2011;60(1):1–24

10. Fiore AE, Shay DK, Broder K, et al. Prevention and control of influenza: recommendations of the Advisory Committee on Immunization Practices (ACIP), 2008. *MMWR Recomm Rep.* 2008;57(RR-7):1–60

11. Fiore AE, Uyeki TM, Broder K, et al. Prevention and control of influenza with vaccines: recommendations of the Advisory Committee on Immunization Practices (ACIP), 2010. *MMWR Recomm Rep.* 2010;59(RR-8):1–62

12. Grohskopf LA, Sokolow LZ, Broder KR, et al. Prevention and control of seasonal influenza with vaccines. *MMWR Recomm Rep.* 2016;65(5):1–54

13. Guo R, Pittler MH, Ernst E. Complementary medicine for treating or preventing influenza or influenza-like illness. *Am J Med.* 2007;120(11):923–929

14. Jain S, Kamimoto L, Bramley AM, et al; 2009 Pandemic Influenza A (H1N1) Virus Hospitalizations Investigation Team. Hospitalized patients with 2009 H1N1 influenza in the United States, April–June 2009. *N Engl J Med.* 2009;361(20):1935–1944

15. Kim DK, Riley LE, Harriman KH, Hunter P, Bridges CB. Advisory Committee on Immunization Practices recommended immunization schedule for adults aged 19 years or older—United States, 2017. *MMWR Morb Mortal Wkly Rep.* 2017;66(5):136–138

16. Kim SY, Chang YJ, Cho HM, Hwang YW, Moon YS. Non-steroidal antiinflammatory drugs for the common cold. *Cochrane Database Syst Rev.* 2009;(3):CD006362

17. Lindley MC, Bridges CB, Strikas RA, et al. Influenza vaccination performance measurement among acute care hospital-based health care personnel—United States, 2013–14 influenza season. *MMWR Morb Mortal Wkly Rep.* 2014;63(37):812–815

18. Paul IM, Beiler JS, King TS, Clapp ER, Vallati J, Berlin CM Jr. Vapor rub, petrolatum, and no treatment for children with nocturnal cough and cold symptoms. *Pediatrics.* 2010;126(6):1092–1099

19. Public Health Agency of Canada. Canadian Immunization Guide. https://www.canada.ca/en/public-health/services/canadian-immunization-guide.html. Modified January 24, 2018. Accessed June 7, 2018

20. Rothberg MB, Haessler SD, Brown RB. Complications of viral influenza. *Am J Med.* 2008;121(4):258–264

21. Stamboulian D, Bonvehi PE, Nacinovich FM, Cox N. Influenza. *Infect Dis Clin North Am.* 2000;14(1):141–166

22. US Preventive Services Task Force. Postexposure prophylaxis for selected infectious diseases. In: *Guide to Clinical Preventive Services.* 2nd ed. Alexandria, VA: International Medical Publishing, Inc; 1996:815–827

23. WHO Guidelines Approved by the Guidelines Review Committee. WHO guidelines for pharmacological management of pandemic influenza A (H1N1) 2009 and other influenza viruses. Geneva, Switzerland: World Health Organization; 2010. http://www.who.int/csr/resources/publications/swineflu/h1n1_use_antivirals_20090820/en. Accessed June 7, 2018

Influenza Exposure

1. Advisory Committee on Immunization Practices. Prevention and control of influenza. Recommendations of the Advisory Committee on Immunization Practices (ACIP), 2008. *MMWR Recomm Rep.* 2008;57(RR-7):1-60

2. Advisory Committee on Immunization Practices. Recommended adult immunization schedule: United States, 2011. *Ann Intern Med.* 2011;154(3):168–173

3. Bachert C, Chuchalin AG, Eisebitt R, Netayzhenko VZ, Voelker M. Aspirin compared with acetaminophen in the treatment of fever and other symptoms of upper respiratory tract infection in adults: a multicenter, randomized, double-blind, double-dummy, placebo-controlled, parallel-group, single-dose, 6-hour dose-ranging study. *Clin Ther.* 2005;27(7):993–1003

4. Centers for Disease Control and Prevention. Prevention and control of seasonal influenza with vaccines. Recommendations of the Advisory Committee on Immunization Practices—United States, 2013–2014. *MMWR Recomm Rep.* 2013;62(RR-07):1–43

5. Committee on Obstetric Practice and Immunization Expert Work Group; Centers for Disease Control and Prevention's Advisory Committee on Immunization, United States; American College of Obstetricians and Gynecologists. Committee opinion no. 608: influenza vaccination during pregnancy. *Obstet Gynecol.* 2014;124(3):648–651

6. Ebell MH, Lundgren J, Youngpairoj S. How long does a cough last? Comparing patients' expectations with data from a systematic review of the literature. *Ann Fam Med.* 2013;11(1):5–13

7. Eccles R. Understanding the symptoms of the common cold and influenza. *Lancet Infect Dis.* 2005;5(11):718–725

8. Erlikh IV, Abraham S, Kondamudi VK. Management of influenza. *Am Fam Physician.* 2010;82(9):1087–1095

9. Fagbuyi DB, Brown KM, Mathison DJ, et al. A rapid medical screening process improves emergency department patient flow during surge associated with novel H1N1 influenza virus. *Ann Emerg Med.* 2011;57(1):52–59

10. Fisman D. Seasonality of viral infections: mechanisms and unknowns. *Clin Microbiol Infect.* 2012;18(10):946–954

11. Grohskopf LA, Sokolow LZ, Broder KR, et al. Prevention and control of seasonal influenza with vaccines. *MMWR Recomm Rep.* 2016;65(5):1–54

12. Guo R, Pittler MH, Ernst E. Complementary medicine for treating or preventing influenza or influenza-like illness. *Am J Med.* 2007;120(11):923–929.e3

13. Influenza Division, National Center for Immunization and Respiratory Diseases. Antiviral agents for the treatment and chemoprophylaxis of influenza—recommendations of the Advisory Committee on Immunization Practices (ACIP) *MMWR Surveill Summ.* 2011;60(1):1–28

14. Jain S, Kamimoto L, Bramley AM, et al; 2009 Pandemic Influenza A (H1N1) Virus Hospitalizations Investigation Team. Hospitalized patients with 2009 H1N1 influenza in the United States, April–June 2009. *N Engl J Med.* 2009;361(20):1935–1944

15. Kim DK, Riley LE, Harriman KH, Hunter P, Bridges CB. Advisory Committee on Immunization Practices recommended immunization schedule for adults aged 19 years or older—United States, 2017. *MMWR Morb Mortal Wkly Rep.* 2017;66(5):136–138

16. Kim SY, Chang YJ, Cho HM, Hwang YW, Moon YS. Non-steroidal antiinflammatory drugs for the common cold. *Cochrane Database Syst Rev.* 2009;(3):CD006362

17. Lal A, Hales S, French N, Baker MG. Seasonality in human zoonotic enteric diseases: a systematic review. *PLoS One.* 2012;7(4):e31883

18. Lindley MC, Bridges CB, Strikas RA, et al. Influenza vaccination performance measurement among acute care hospital-based health care personnel—United States, 2013–14 influenza season. *MMWR Morb Mortal Wkly Rep.* 2014;63(37):812–815

19. Paul IM, Beiler JS, King TS, Clapp ER, Vallati J, Berlin CM Jr. Vapor rub, petrolatum, and no treatment for children with nocturnal cough and cold symptoms. *Pediatrics.* 2010;126(6):1092–1099

20. Public Health Agency of Canada. Canadian Immunization Guide. https://www.canada.ca/en/public-health/services/canadian-immunization-guide.html. Modified January 24, 2018. Accessed June 7, 2018

21. Rothberg MB, Haessler SD, Brown RB. Complications of viral influenza. *Am J Med.* 2008;121(4):258–264
22. Stamboulian D. Influenza. *Infect Dis Clin North Am.* 2000;14(1):141–166
23. US Preventive Services Task Force. Postexposure prophylaxis for selected infectious diseases. In: *Guide to Clinical Preventive Services.* 2nd ed. Alexandria, VA: International Medical Publishing, Inc; 1996:815–827
24. WHO Guidelines Approved by the Guidelines Review Committee. WHO guidelines for pharmacological management of pandemic influenza A (H1N1) 2009 and other influenza viruses. Geneva, Switzerland: World Health Organization; 2010. http://www.who.int/csr/resources/publications/swineflu/h1n1_use_antivirals_20090820/en. Accessed June 7, 2018

Influenza Follow-up Call

1. Advisory Committee on Immunization Practices. Prevention and control of influenza. Recommendations of the Advisory Committee on Immunization Practices (ACIP), 2008. *MMWR Recomm Rep.* 2008;57(RR-7):1–60
2. Advisory Committee on Immunization Practices. Recommended adult immunization schedule: United States, 2011. *Ann Intern Med.* 2011;154(3):168–173
3. Bachert C, Chuchalin AG, Eisebitt R, Netayzhenko VZ, Voelker M. Aspirin compared with acetaminophen in the treatment of fever and other symptoms of upper respiratory tract infection in adults: a multicenter, randomized, double-blind, double-dummy, placebo-controlled, parallel-group, single-dose, 6-hour dose-ranging study. *Clin Ther.* 2005;27(7):993–1003
4. Centers for Disease Control and Prevention. H1N1 flu. Updated interim recommendations for the use of antiviral medications in the treatment and prevention of influenza for the 2009-2010 season. https://www.cdc.gov/h1n1flu/recommendations.htm. Updated December 7, 2009. Accessed June 7, 2018
5. Centers for Disease Control and Prevention. Prevention and control of seasonal influenza with vaccines. Recommendations of the Advisory Committee on Immunization Practices—United States, 2013–2014. *MMWR Recomm Rep.* 2013;62(RR-07):1–43
6. Centers for Disease Control and Prevention. Update: infections with a swine-origin influenza A (H1N1) virus—United States and other countries, April 28, 2009. *MMWR Morb Mortal Wkly Rep.* 2009;58(16):431–433
7. Committee on Obstetric Practice and Immunization Expert Work Group; Centers for Disease Control and Prevention's Advisory Committee on Immunization, United States; American College of Obstetricians and Gynecologists. Committee opinion no. 608: influenza vaccination during pregnancy. *Obstet Gynecol.* 2014;124(3):648–651
8. Ebell MH, Lundgren J, Youngpairoj S. How long does a cough last? Comparing patients' expectations with data from a systematic review of the literature. *Ann Fam Med.* 2013;11(1):5–13
9. Eccles R. Understanding the symptoms of the common cold and influenza. *Lancet Infect Dis.* 2005;5(11):718–725
10. Erlikh IV, Abraham S, Kondamudi VK. Management of influenza. *Am Fam Physician.* 2010;82(9):1087–1095
11. Grohskopf LA, Sokolow LZ, Broder KR, et al. Prevention and control of seasonal influenza with vaccines. *MMWR Recomm Rep.* 2016;65(5):1–54
12. Influenza Division, National Center for Immunization and Respiratory Diseases. Antiviral agents for the treatment and chemoprophylaxis of influenza—recommendations of the Advisory Committee on Immunization Practices (ACIP). *MMWR Surveill Summ.* 2011;60(1):1–28
13. Jain S, Kamimoto L, Bramley AM, et al. 2009 Pandemic Influenza A (H1N1) Virus Hospitalizations Investigation Team. Hospitalized patients with 2009 H1N1 influenza in the United States, April–June 2009. *N Engl J Med.* 2009;361(20):1935–1944
14. Kim DK, Riley LE, Harriman KH, Hunter P, Bridges CB. Advisory Committee on Immunization Practices recommended immunization schedule for adults aged 19 years or older—United States, 2017. *MMWR Morb Mortal Wkly Rep.* 2017;66(5):136–138
15. Lindley MC, Bridges CB, Strikas RA, et al. Influenza vaccination performance measurement among acute care hospital-based health care personnel—United States, 2013–14 influenza season. *MMWR Morb Mortal Wkly Rep.* 2014;63(37):812–815

16. Paul IM, Beiler JS, King TS, Clapp ER, Vallati J, Berlin CM Jr. Vapor rub, petrolatum, and no treatment for children with nocturnal cough and cold symptoms. *Pediatrics.* 2010;126(6):1092–1099
17. Public Health Agency of Canada. Canadian Immunization Guide. https://www.canada.ca/en/public-health/services/canadian-immunization-guide.html. Modified January 24, 2018. Accessed June 7, 2018
18. Stamboulian D. Influenza. *Infect Dis Clin North Am.* 2000;14(1):141–166
19. WHO Guidelines Approved by the Guidelines Review Committee. WHO guidelines for pharmacological management of pandemic influenza A (H1N1) 2009 and other influenza viruses. Geneva, Switzerland: World Health Organization; 2010. http://www.who.int/csr/resources/publications/swineflu/h1n1_use_antivirals_20090820/en. Accessed June 7, 2018

Insect Bite

1. American Academy of Allergy, Asthma and Immunology (AAAAI). The use of epinephrine in the treatment of anaphylaxis. Position statement. http://www.aaaai.org/Aaaai/media/MediaLibrary/PDF%20Documents/Practice%20and%20Parameters/Epinephrine-in-treating-anaphylaxis-2002.pdf. Accessed June 7, 2018
2. American Academy of Allergy, Asthma and Immunology Joint Task Force on Practice Parameters; American College of Allergy, Asthma and Immunology Joint Council of Allergy, Asthma and Immunology. The diagnosis and management of anaphylaxis: an updated practice parameter. *J Allergy Clin Immunol.* 2005;115(3 suppl 2):S483–S523
3. Brown M, Hebert AA. Insect repellents: an overview. *J Am Acad Dermatol.* 1997;36(2):243–249
4. Derlet RW, Richards JR. Cellulitis from insect bites: a case series. *Cal J Emerg Med.* 2003;4(2):27–30
5. Fradin MS. Mosquitoes and mosquito repellents: a clinician's guide. *Ann Int Med.* 1998;128(11):931–940
6. Hwang SW, Svoboda TJ, De Jong IJ, Kabasele KJ, Gogosis E. Bed bug infestations in an urban environment. *Emerg Infect Dis.* 2005;11(4):533–538
7. Koren G, Matsui D, Bailey B. DEET-based insect repellants: safety implications for children and pregnant and lactating women. *CMAJ.* 2003;169(3):209–212
8. Liew WK, Williamson E, Tang ML. Anaphylaxis fatalities and admissions in Australia. *J Allergy Clin Immunol.* 2009;123(2):434–442
9. Markenson D, Ferguson JD, Chameides L, et al. 2010 American Heart Association and American Red Cross Guidelines for First Aid. Part 17: First Aid. *Circulation.* 2010;122(18 suppl 3):S934–S946
10. Sampson HA, Muñoz-Furlong A, Campbell RL, et al. Second symposium on the definition and management of anaphylaxis: summary report—Second National Institute of Allergy and Infectious Disease/Food Allergy and Anaphylaxis Network symposium. *J Allergy Clin Immunol.* 2006;117(2):391–397
11. Steen CJ, Carbonaro PA, Schwartz RA. Arthropods in dermatology. *J Am Acad Dermatol.* 2004;50(6):819–844
12. Thomas I, Kihiczak GG, Schwartz RA. Bedbug bites: a review. *Int J Dermatol.* 2004;43(6):430–433
13. US Environmental Protection Agency. Pesticides. https://www.epa.gov/pesticides. Updated May 29, 2018. Accessed June 7, 2018
14. Thomas I, Kihiczak GG, Schwartz RA. Bedbug bites: a review. *Int J Dermatol.* 2004;43(6):430–433

Jock Itch

1. Cordoro KM, Ganz JE. Training room management of medical conditions: sports dermatology. *Clin Sports Med.* 2005;24(3):565–598, viii–ix
2. Loo DS. Cutaneous fungal infections in the elderly. *Dermatol Clin.* 2004;22(1):33–50
3. Noble SL, Forbes RC, Stamm PL. Diagnosis and management of common tinea infections. *Am Fam Physician.* 1998;58(1):163–178
4. Panackal AA, Halpern EF, Watson AJ. Cutaneous fungal infections in the United States: analysis of the National Ambulatory Medical Care Survey (NAMCS) and National Hospital Ambulatory Medical Care Survey (NHAMCS), 1995-2004. *Int J Dermatol.* 2009;48(7):704–712
5. Rupke SJ. Fungal skin disorders. *Prim Care.* 2000;27(2):407–421

Knee Injury

1. American Heart Association. 2005 Guidelines for Cardiopulmonary Resuscitation and Emergency Cardiovascular Care. Part 10: First Aid. *Circulation.* 2005;112:IV-196–IV-203
2. Collins NC. Is ice right? Does cryotherapy improve outcome for acute soft tissue injury? *Emerg Med J.* 2008;25(2):65–68
3. Dake AD, Stack L. Penetrating trauma to the extremities: systematic assessment and targeted management of weapons-related injuries. *Emerg Med Reports.* 1997;18(7)
4. Fadale PD. Common athletic knee injuries. *Clin Sports Med.* 1997;16(3):479–499
5. Kellett J. Acute soft tissue injuries—a review of the literature. *Med Sci Sports Exerc.* 1986;18(5):489–500
6. Kretsinger K, Broder KR, Cortese MM, et al; Centers for Disease Control and Prevention; Advisory Committee on Immunization Practices; Health-care Infection Control Practices Advisory Committee. Preventing tetanus, diphtheria, and pertussis among adults: use of tetanus toxoid, reduced diphtheria toxoid and acellular pertussis vaccine recommendations of the Advisory Committee on Immunization Practices (ACIP) and recommendation of ACIP, supported by the Healthcare Infection Control Practices Advisory Committee (HICPAC), for use of Tdap among healthcare personnel. *MMWR Recomm Rep.* 2006;55(RR-17):1–37
7. Markenson D, Ferguson JD, Chameides L, et al. 2010 American Heart Association and American Red Cross Guidelines for First Aid. Part 17: First Aid. *Circulation.* 2010;122(18 suppl 3):S934–S946
8. McMaster WC, Liddle S, Waugh TR. Laboratory evaluation of various cold therapy modalities. *Am J Sports Med.* 1978;6(5):291–294
9. Pimentel L. Orthopedic trauma: office management of major joint injury. *Med Clin North Am.* 2006;90(2):355–382
10. Roberts DM, Stallard TC. Emergency department evaluation and treatment of knee and leg injuries. *Emerg Med Clin North Am.* 2000;18(1):67–84, v–vi
11. Seaberg DC, Yealy DM, Lukens T, Auble T, Mathias S. Multicenter comparison of two clinical decision rules for the use of radiography in acute, high-risk knee injuries. *Ann Emerg Med.* 1998;32(1):8–13
12. Singer AJ, Dagum AB. Current management of acute cutaneous wounds. *N Engl J Med.* 2008;359(10):1037–1046
13. Solomon DH, Simel DL, Bates DW, et al. Does this patient have a torn meniscus or ligament of the knee? *JAMA.* 2001;286(13):1610–1620
14. Stewart C. Knee injuries: diagnosis and repair. *Emerg Med Reports.* 1997;18(1)

Knee Pain

1. Bjordal JM, Ljunggren AE, Klovning A, Slordal L. Non-steroidal anti-inflammatory drugs, including cyclo-oxygenase-2 inhibitors, in osteoarthritic knee pain: meta-analysis of randomized placebo controlled trials. *BMJ.* 2004;329(7478):1317
2. Calmbach WL, Hutchens M. Evaluation of patients presenting with knee pain: part I. History, physical examination, radiographs, and laboratory tests. *Am Fam Physician.* 2003;68(5):907–912
3. Calmbach WL, Hutchens M. Evaluation of patients presenting with knee pain: part II. Differential diagnosis. *Am Fam Physician.* 2003;68(5):917–922
4. Coakley G, Mathews C, Field M, et al; British Society for Rheumatology Standards, Guidelines and Audit Working Group. BSR & BHPR, BOA, RCGP and BSAC guidelines for management of the hot swollen joint in adults. *Rheumatology (Oxford).* 2006;45(8):1039–1041
5. Dearborn JT, Jergesen HE. The evaluation and initial management of arthritis. *Prim Care.* 1996;23(2):215–240
6. Divoll M, Abernethy DR, Ameer B, Greenblatt DJ. Acetaminophen kinetics in the elderly. *Clin Pharmacol Ther.* 1982;31(2):151–156
7. Pioro MH, Mandell BF. Septic arthritis. *Rheum Dis Clin North Am.* 1997;23(2):239–258
8. Rainsford KD. Ibuprofen: pharmacology, efficacy and safety. *Inflammopharmacology.* 2009;17(6):275–342
9. Roberts DM, Stallard TC. Emergency department evaluation and treatment of knee and leg injuries. *Emerg Med Clin North Am.* 2000;18(1):67–84, v–vi

10. Solomon DH, Simel DL, Bates DW, Katz JN, Schaffer JL. Does this patient have a torn meniscus or ligament of the knee? Value of the physical examination. *JAMA.* 2001;286(13):1610–1620
11. Towheed TE, Maxwell L, Judd MG, Catton M, Hochberg MC, Wells G. Acetaminophen for osteoarthritis. *Cochrane Database Syst Rev.* 2006;(1):CD004257
12. Weston V, Coakley G; British Society for Rheumatology Standards, Guidelines and Audit Working Group; et al. Guideline for the management of the hot swollen joint in adults with a particular focus on septic arthritis. *J Antimicrob Chemother.* 2006;58(3):492–493

Leg Pain

1. Andreou ER, Koru-Sengul T, Linkins L, Bates SM, Ginsberg JS, Kearon C. Differences in clinical presentation of deep vein thrombosis in men and women. *J Thromb Haemost.* 2008;6(10):1713–1719
2. Baker WF Jr. Diagnosis of deep venous thrombosis and pulmonary embolism. *Med Clin North Am.* 1998;82(3):459–476
3. Bartholomew JR, Schaffer JL, McCormick GF. Air travel and venous thromboembolism: minimizing the risk. *Cleve Clin J Med.* 2011;78(2):111–120
4. Bates SM, Ginsberg JS. Clinical practice. Treatment of deep-vein thrombosis. *N Eng J Med.* 2004;351(3):268–277
5. Bates SM, Jaeschke R, Stevens SM, et al. Diagnosis of DVT: antithrombotic therapy and prevention of thrombosis, 9th ed: American College of Chest Physicians evidence-based clinical practice guidelines. *Chest.* 2012;141(2 Suppl):e351S–e418S
6. Butler JV, Mukerrin EC, O'Keefe ST. Nocturnal leg cramps in older people. *Postgrad Med J.* 2002;78(924):596–598
7. Gallus AS. Travel, venous thromboembolism, and thrombophilia. *Semin Thromb Hemost.* 2005;31(1):90–96
8. Glazer JL, Hosey RG. Soft-tissue injuries of the lower extremity. *Prim Care.* 2004;31(4):1005–1024
9. Ho WK. Deep vein thrombosis—risks and diagnosis. *Aust Fam Physician.* 2010;39(7):468–474
10. Kessler CM. The link between cancer and venous thromboembolism: a review. *Am J Clin Oncol.* 2009;32(4 Suppl):S3–S7
11. Kline JA, Courtney DM, Kabrhel C, et al. Prospective multicenter evaluation of the pulmonary embolism rule-out criteria. *J Thromb Haemost.* 2008;6(5):772–780
12. Maitra RS, Johnson DL. Stress fractures. Clinical history and physical examination. *Clin Sports Med.* 1997;16(2):259–274
13. Mateo J, Oliver A, Borrell M, Sala N, Fontcuberta J. Laboratory evaluation and clinical characteristics of 2,132 consecutive unselected patients with venous thromboembolism—results of the Spanish Multicentric Study on Thrombophilia (EMET-Study). *Thromb Haemost.* 1997;77(3):444–451
14. McLintock C, Brighton T, Chunilal S, et al. Recommendations for the diagnosis and treatment of deep venous thrombosis and pulmonary embolism in pregnancy and the postpartum period. *Aust N Z J Obstet Gynaecol.* 2012;52(1):14–22
15. McRae S. Pulmonary embolism. *Aust Fam Physician.* 2010;39(6):462–466
16. Newman AB. Peripheral arterial disease: insights from population studies of older adults. *J Am Geriatr Soc.* 2000;48(9):1157–1162
17. Philbrick JT, Shumate R, Siadaty MS, Becker DM. Air travel and venous thromboembolism: a systematic review. *J Gen Intern Med.* 2007;22(1):107–114
18. Richardson C, Glenn S, Nurmikko T, Horgan M. Incidence of phantom phenomena including phantom limb pain 6 months after major lower limb amputation in patients with peripheral vascular disease. *Clin J Pain.* 2006;22(4):353–358
19. Rosendaal FR. Venous thrombosis: a multicausal disease. *Lancet.* 1999;353(9159):1167–1173
20. Schley MT, Wilms P, Toepfner S, et al. Painful and nonpainful phantom and stump sensations in acute traumatic amputees. *J Trauma.* 2008;65(4):858–864
21. US Department of Veterans Affairs, US Department of Defense. VA/DoD clinical practice guideline: rehabilitation of lower limb amputation. https://www.healthquality.va.gov/guidelines/Rehab/amp. Published 2017. Accessed June 7, 2018

22. Wells PS, Anderson DR, Bormanis J, et al. Value of assessment of pretest probability of deep-vein thrombosis in clinical management. *Lancet.* 1997;350(9094):1795–1798
23. Wells PS, Hirsh J, Anderson DR, et al. Accuracy of clinical assessment of deep-vein-thrombosis. *Lancet.* 1995;345(8961):1326–1330
24. Wilbur J, Shian B. Diagnosis of deep venous thrombosis and pulmonary embolism. *Am Fam Physician.* 2012;86(10):913–919

Leg Swelling and Edema
1. Andreou ER, Koru-Sengul T, Linkins L, Bates SM, Ginsberg JS, Kearon C. Differences in clinical presentation of deep vein thrombosis in men and women. *J Thromb Haemost.* 2008;6(10):1713–1719
2. Baker WF Jr. Diagnosis of deep venous thrombosis and pulmonary embolism. *Med Clin North Am.* 1998;82(3):459–476
3. Bartholomew JR, Schaffer JL, McCormick GF. Air travel and venous thromboembolism: minimizing the risk. *Cleve Clin J Med.* 2011;78(2):111–120
4. Bates SM, Ginsberg JS. Clinical practice. Treatment of deep-vein thrombosis. *N Eng J Med.* 2004;351(3):268–277
5. Bates SM, Jaeschke R, Stevens SM, et al. Diagnosis of DVT: antithrombotic therapy and prevention of thrombosis, 9th ed: American College of Chest Physicians evidence-based clinical practice guidelines. *Chest.* 2012;141(2 Suppl):e351S–e418S
6. Cooper LT Jr. Myocarditis. *N Engl J Med.* 2009;360(15):1526–1538
7. Gallus AS. Travel, venous thromboembolism, and thrombophilia. *Semin Thromb Hemost.* 2005;31(1):90–96
8. Ho WK. Deep vein thrombosis—risks and diagnosis. *Aust Fam Physician.* 2010;39(7):468–474
9. Kessler CM. The link between cancer and venous thromboembolism: a review. *Am J Clin Oncol.* 2009;32(4 Suppl):S3–S7
10. Kline JA, Courtney DM, Kabrhel C, et al. Prospective multicenter evaluation of the pulmonary embolism rule-out criteria. *J Thromb Haemost.* 2008;6(5):772–780
11. McLintock C, Brighton T, Chunilai S, et al. Recommendations for the diagnosis and treatment of deep venous thrombosis and pulmonary embolism in pregnancy and the postpartum period. *Aust N Z J Obstet Gynaecol.* 2012;52(1):14–22
12. McRae S. Pulmonary embolism. *Aust Fam Physician.* 2010;39(6):462–466
13. Newman AB. Peripheral arterial disease: insights from population studies of older adults. *J Am Geriatr Soc.* 2000;48(9):1157–1162
14. Philbrick JT, Shumate R, Siadaty MS, Becker DM. Air travel and venous thromboembolism: a systematic review. *J Gen Intern Med.* 2007;22(1):107–114
15. Rosendaal FR. Venous thrombosis: a multicausal disease. *Lancet.* 1999;353(9159):1167–1173
16. Wang CS, FitzGerald JM, Schulzer M, Mak E, Ayas NT. Does this dyspneic patient in the emergency department have congestive heart failure? *JAMA.* 2005;294(15):1944–1956
17. Wells PS, Anderson DR, Bormanis J, et al. Value of assessment of pretest probability of deep-vein thrombosis in clinical management. *Lancet.* 1997;350(9094):1795–1798
18. Wells PS, Hirsh J, Anderson DR, et al. Accuracy of clinical assessment of deep-vein-thrombosis. *Lancet.* 1995;345(8961):1326–1330
19. Wilbur J, Shian B. Diagnosis of deep venous thrombosis and pulmonary embolism. *Am Fam Physician.* 2012;86(10):913–919

Lymph Nodes, Swollen
1. Ferrer R. Lymphadenopathy: differential diagnosis and evaluation. *Am Fam Physician.* 1998;58(6):1313–1320
2. Habermann TM, Steensma DP. Lymphadenopathy. *Mayo Clin Proc.* 2000;75(7):723–732
3. Peter J, Ray CG. Infectious mononucleosis. *Pediatr Rev.* 1998;19(8):276–279
4. Peters TR, Edwards KM. Cervical lymphadenopathy and adenitis. *Pediatr Rev.* 2000;21(12):399–405

Menstrual Period, Missed or Late
1. Brill SR, Rosenfeld WD. Contraception. *Med Clin North Am.* 2000;84(4):907–925
2. Kothari S, Thacker HL. Risk assessment of the menopausal patient. *Med Clin North Am.* 1999;83(6):1489–1502
3. Mitan LA, Slap GB. Adolescent menstrual disorders. Update. *Med Clin North Am.* 2000;84(4):851–868
4. Murray H, Baakdah H, Bardell T, Tulandi T. Diagnosis and treatment of ectopic pregnancy. *CMAJ.* 2005;173(8):905–912

Mouth Injury
1. American Heart Association. 2005 Guidelines for Cardiopulmonary Resuscitation and Emergency Cardiovascular Care. Part 10: First Aid. *Circulation.* 2005;112:IV-196–IV-203
2. Armstrong BD. Lacerations of Mouth. *Emerg Med Clin North Am.* 2000;8(3):71–80, vi
3. Benbadis SR. The value of tongue laceration in the diagnosis of blackouts. *Am Fam Physician.* 2004;70(9):1757–1758
4. Benbadis SR, Wolgamuth BR, Goren H, Brener S, Fouad-Tarazi F. Value of tongue biting in the diagnosis of seizures. *Arch Intern Med.* 1995;155(21):2346–2349
5. Coluciello SA. The treacherous and complex spectrum of maxillofacial trauma: etiologies, evaluation, and emergency stabilization. *Emerg Med Reports.* 1995;16(7)
6. Dale RA. Dentoalveolar trauma. *Emerg Med Clin North Am.* 2000;18(3):521–538
7. Howes DS. Triage and initial evaluation of the oral facial emergency. *Emerg Med Clin North Am.* 2000;18(3):371–378
8. Lamell CW, Fraone G, Casamassimo PS, Wilson S. Presenting characteristics and treatment outcomes for tongue lacerations in children. *Pediatr Dent.* 1999;21(1):34–38
9. Markenson D, Ferguson JD, Chameides L, et al. 2010 American Heart Association and American Red Cross Guidelines for First Aid. Part 17: First Aid. *Circulation.* 2010;122(18 suppl 3):S934–S946
10. Patel A. Tongue lacerations. *Br Dent J.* 2008;204(7):355
11. Singer AJ, Dagum AB. Current management of acute cutaneous wounds. *N Engl J Med.* 2008;359(10):1037–1046

Neck Injury
1. American Heart Association. 2005 Guidelines for Cardiopulmonary Resuscitation and Emergency Cardiovascular Care. Part 10: First Aid. *Circulation.* 2005;112:IV-196–IV-203
2. Bandiera G, Stiell IG, Wells GA, et al. The Canadian c-spine rule performs better than unstructured physician judgement. *Ann Emerg Med.* 2003;42(3):395–402
3. Benson BW, Meeuwisse WH, Rizos J, Kang J, Burke CJ. A prospective study of concussions among National Hockey League players during regular season games: the NHL–NHLPA Concussion Program. *CMAJ.* 2011;183(8):905–911
4. Evans RW. The postconcussion syndrome and whiplash injuries: a question-and-answer review for primary care physicians. *Prim Care.* 2004;31(1):1–17
5. Frohna WJ. Emergency department evaluation and treatment of the neck and cervical spine injuries. *Emerg Med Clin North Am.* 1999;17(4):739–791, v
6. Hoffman JR, Mower WR, Wolfson AB, Todd KH, Zucker MI. Validity of a set of clinical criteria to rule out injury to the cervical spine in patients with blunt trauma. *N Engl J Med.* 2000;343(2):94–99
7. Kendall JL, Anglin D, Demetriades D. Penetrating neck trauma. *Emerg Med Clin North Am.* 1998;16(1):85–105
8. Markenson D, Ferguson JD, Chameides L, et al. 2010 American Heart Association and American Red Cross Guidelines for First Aid. Part 17: First Aid. *Circulation.* 2010;122(18 suppl 3):S934–S946
9. Sasser SM, Hunt RC, Faul M, et al. Guidelines for field triage of injured patients: recommendations of the National Expert Panel on Field Triage, 2011. *MMWR Recomm Rep.* 2012;61(RR-1):1–20
10. Singer AJ, Dagum AB. Current management of acute cutaneous wounds. *N Engl J Med.* 2008;359(10):1037–1046
11. Warren WL Jr, Bailes JE. On the field evaluation of athletic neck injury. *Clin Sports Med.* 1998;17(1):99–110

Neck Pain or Stiffness

1. Argoff CA, Wheeler AH. Spinal and radicular pain disorders. *Neurol Clin.* 1998;16(4):833–850
2. Attia J, Hatala R, Cook DJ, Wong JG. Does this adult patient have acute meningitis? *JAMA.* 1999;282(2):175–181
3. Devereaux MW. Neck pain. *Prim Care.* 2004;31(1):19–31
4. Haldeman S. Diagnostic tests for the evaluation of back and neck pain. *Neurol Clin.* 1996;14(1):103–117
5. Perry JJ, Stiell IG, Sivilotti ML, et al. High risk clinical characteristics for subarachnoid haemorrhage in patients with acute headache: prospective cohort study. *BMJ.* 2010;341:c5204
6. Rainsford KD. Ibuprofen: pharmacology, efficacy and safety. *Inflammopharmacology.* 2009;17(6):275–342
7. Swezey RL. Chronic neck pain. *Rheum Dis Clin North Am.* 1996;22(3):411–437

Neurologic Deficit

1. Baumlin KM, Richardson LD. Stroke syndromes. *Emerg Med Clin North Am.* 1997;15(3):551–561
2. Chalela JA, Kidwell CS, Nentwich LM, et al. Magnetic resonance imaging and computed tomography in emergency assessment of patients with suspected acute stroke: a prospective comparison. *Lancet.* 2007;369(9558):293–298
3. Cucchiara B, Ross M. Transient ischemic attack: risk stratification and treatment. *Ann Emerg Med.* 2008;52(2):S27–S39
4. Goldstein LB, Adams R, Alberts MJ, et al; American Heart Association; American Stroke Association Stroke Council. Primary prevention of ischemic stroke: a guideline from the American Heart Association/American Stroke Association Stroke Council. *Circulation.* 2006;113(24):e873–e923
5. Gommans J, Barber PA, Fink J. Preventing strokes: the assessment and management of people with transient ischaemic attack. *N Z Med J.* 2009;122(1293):3556
6. Johnston SC, Rothwell PM, Nguyen-Huynh MN, et al. Validation and refinement of scores to predict very early stroke risk after transient ischaemic attack. *Lancet.* 2007;369(9558):283–292
7. Kidwell CS, Chalela JA, Saver JL, et al. Comparison of MRI and CT for detection of acute intracerebral hemorrhage. *JAMA.* 2004;292(15):1823–1830
8. Kidwell CS, Starkman S, Eckstein M, Weems K, Saver JL. Identifying stroke in the field: prospective validation of the Los Angeles Prehospital Stroke Screen (LAPSS). *Stroke.* 2000;31(1):71–76
9. Kothari R, Hall K, Brott T, Broderick J. Early stroke recognition: developing an out-of-hospital NIH stroke scale. *Acad Emerg Med.* 1997;4(10):986–990
10. Lockhart P, Daly F, Pitkethly M, Comerford N, Sullivan F. Antiviral treatment for Bell's palsy (idiopathic facial paralysis). *Cochrane Database Syst Rev.* 2009;(4):CD001869
11. Martin-Schild S, Albright KC, Tanksley J, et al. Zero on the NIHSS does not equal the absence of stroke. *Ann Emerg Med.* 2011;57(1):42–45
12. Morgenstern LB, Hemphill JC 3rd, Anderson C, et al; American Heart Association Stroke Council and Council on Cardiovascular Nursing. Guidelines for the management of spontaneous intracerebral hemorrhage: a guideline for healthcare professionals from the American Heart Association/American Stroke Association. *Stroke.* 2010;41(9):2108–2129
13. Nor AM, Davis J, Sen B, et al. The Recognition of Stroke in the Emergency Room (ROSIER) scale: development and validation of a stroke recognition instrument. *Lancet Neurol.* 2005;4(11):727–734
14. Numthavaj P, Thakkinstian A, Dejthevaporn C, Attia J. Corticosteroid and antiviral therapy for Bell's palsy: a network meta-analysis. *BMC Neurol.* 2011;11:1
15. Paternostro-Sluga T, Grim-Stieger M, Posch M, et al. Reliability and validity of the Medical Research Council (MRC) scale and a modified scale for testing muscle strength in patients with radial palsy. *J Rehabil Med.* 2008;40(8):665–671
16. Perry JJ, Stiell IG, Sivilotti ML, et al. High risk clinical characteristics for subarachnoid haemorrhage in patients with acute headache: prospective cohort study. *BMJ.* 2010;341:c5204
17. Schwamm LH, Pancioli A, Acker JE III, et al. Recommendations for the establishment of stroke systems of care: recommendations from the American Stroke Association's Task Force on the Development of Stroke Systems. *Stroke.* 2005;36(3):690–703
18. Selman WR, Tarr R, Landis DM. Brain attack: emergency treatment of ischemic stroke. *Am Fam Physician.* 1997;55(8):2655–2666
19. Stead LG, Suravaram S, Bellolio MF, et al. An assessment of the incremental value of the ABCD2 score in the emergency department evaluation of transient ischemic attack. *Ann Emerg Med.* 2011;57(1):46–51
20. Tiemstra JD, Khatkhate N. Bell's palsy: diagnosis and management. *Am Fam Physician.* 2007;76(7):997–1002
21. Vanpee G, Hermans G, Segers J, Gosselink R. Assessment of limb muscle strength in critically ill patients: a systematic review. *Crit Care Med.* 2014;42(3):701–711
22. Wasserman J, Perry J, Dowlatshahi D, et al. Stratified, urgent care for transient ischemic attack results in low stroke rates. *Stroke.* 2010;41(11):2601–2605

Nose Injury

1. American Heart Association. 2005 Guidelines for Cardiopulmonary Resuscitation and Emergency Cardiovascular Care. Part 10: First Aid. *Circulation.* 2005;112:IV-196–IV-203
2. Belleza WG, Kalman S. Otolaryngologic emergencies in the outpatient setting. *Med Clin North Am.* 2006;90(2):329–353
3. Collins NC. Is ice right? Does cryotherapy improve outcome for acute soft tissue injury? *Emerg Med J.* 2008;25(2):65–68
4. Coluciello SA. The treacherous and complex spectrum of maxillofacial trauma: etiologies, evaluation, and emergency stabilization. *Emerg Med Reports.* 1995;16(7)
5. Junnila J. Swollen masses in the nose. *Am Fam Physician.* 2006;73(9):1617–1618
6. Kaufman BR, Heckler FR. Sports-related facial injuries. *Clin Sports Med.* 1997;16(3):543–562
7. Kucik CJ. Management of acute nasal fractures. *Am Fam Physician.* 2004;70(7):1315–1320
8. Li S. Value of nasal radiographs in nasal trauma management. *J Otolaryngol.* 1996;25(3):162–164
9. Markenson D, Ferguson JD, Chameides L, et al. 2010 American Heart Association and American Red Cross Guidelines for First Aid. Part 17: First Aid. *Circulation.* 2010;122(18 suppl 3):S934–S946
10. Peltola EM, Koivikko MP, Koskinen SK. The spectrum of facial fractures in motor vehicle accidents: an MDCT study of 374 patients. *Emerg Radiol.* 2014;21(2):165–171
11. Savage RR, Valvich C. Hematoma of the nasal septum. *Pediatr Rev.* 2006;(12):478–479
12. Schlosser RJ. Epistaxis. *N Engl J Med.* 2009;360(8):784–789
13. Singer AJ, Dagum AB. Current management of acute cutaneous wounds. *N Engl J Med.* 2008;359(10):1037–1046
14. Tan LK. Epistaxis. *Med Clin North Am.* 1999;83(1):43–56

Nosebleed

1. Gifford TO, Orlandi RR. Epistaxis. *Otolaryngol Clin North Am.* 2008;41(3):525–536, viii
2. Kucik CJ, Clenney T. Management of epistaxis. *Am Fam Physician.* 2005;71(2):305–311
3. Pantanowitz L. Epistaxis in the older hypertensive patient. *J Am Geriatr Soc.* 1999;47(5):631
4. Schlosser RJ. Epistaxis. *N Engl J Med.* 2009;360(8):784–789
5. Tan LK, Calhoun KH. Epistaxis. *Med Clin North Am.* 1999;83(1):43–56

Penis and Scrotum Symptoms

1. Burgher SW. Acute scrotal pain. *Emerg Med Clin North Am.* 1998;16(4):781–809, vi
2. English JC III, Laws RA, Keough GC, Wilde JL, Foley JP, Elston DM. Dermatoses of the glans penis and prepuce. *J Am Acad Dermatol.* 1997;37(1):1–26
3. Fazio L, Brock G. Erectile dysfunction: management update. *CMAJ.* 2004;170(9):1429–1437

4. Gresser U, Gleiter CH. Erectile dysfunction: comparison of efficacy and side effects of the PDE-5 inhibitors sildenafil, vardenafil and tadalafil—review of the literature. *Eur J Med Res.* 2002;7(10):435–446

5. Kodner C. Sexually transmitted infections in men. *Prim Care.* 2003;30(1):173–191

6. McAnena L, Knowles SJ, Curry A, Cassidy L. Prevalence of gonococcal conjunctivitis in adults and neonates. *Eye (Lond).* 2015;29(7):875–880

7. Montague DK, Jarow J, Broderick GA, et al. American Urological Association guideline on the management of priapism. *J Urol.* 2003;170(4):1318–1324

8. Montorsi F, Kuritzky L, Sadovsky R, Fredlund P, Cordell WH. Frequently asked questions about tadalafil for treating men with erectile dysfunction. *J Mens Health Gend.* 2005;2(1):141–157

9. Pogany L, Romanowski B, Robinson J, et al. Management of gonococcal infection among adults and youth: new key recommendations. *Can Fam Physician.* 2015;61(10):869–873, e451–e456

10. Public Health Agency of Canada. Primary care and sexually transmitted infections. In: *Canadian Guidelines on Sexually Transmitted Infections 2006 Edition.* Ottawa, Ontario: Public Health Agency of Canada; 2006:7–29. http://pubs.cpha.ca/PDF/P37/23384.pdf. Accessed June 7, 2018

11. Roberts RG, Hartlaub PP. Evaluation of dysuria in men. *Am Fam Physician.* 1999;60(3):865–872

12. Rogers ZR. Priapism in sickle cell disease. *Hematol Oncol Clin North Am.* 2005;19(5):917–928, viii

13. Rupke SJ. Fungal skin disorders. *Prim Care.* 2000;27(2):407–421

14. Salonia A, Eardley I, Giuliano F, et al. European Association of Urology guidelines on priapism. *Eur Urol.* 2014;65(2):480–489

15. Song PH, Moon KH. Priapism: current updates in clinical management. *Korean J Urol.* 2013;54(12):816–823

16. Vilke GM, Ufberg JW, Harrigan RA, Chan TC. Evaluation and treatment of acute urinary retention. *J Emerg Med.* 2008;35(2):193–198

17. Workowski KA, Berman S; Centers for Disease Control and Prevention. Sexually transmitted diseases treatment guidelines 2010 [published correction appears in *MMWR Recomm Rep.* 2011;60(1):18]. *MMWR Recomm Rep.* 2010;59(RR-12):1–110

Poison Ivy/Oak/Sumac

1. Beltrani VS. Allergic dermatoses. *Med Clin North Am.* 1998;82(5):1105–1133, vi

2. Ference JD, Last AR. Choosing topical corticosteroids. *Am Fam Physician.* 2009;79(2):135–140

3. Mark BJ, Slavin RG. Allergic contact dermatitis. *Med Clin North Am.* 2006;90(1):169–185

4. Marks JG Jr, Fowler JF Jr, Sheretz EF, Rietschel RL. Prevention of poison ivy and poison oak allergic contact dermatitis by quaternium–18 bentonite. *J Am Acad Dermatol.* 1995;33(2):212–216

5. Tanner TL. Rhus (Toxicodendron) dermatitis. *Prim Care.* 2000;27(2):493–502

Poisoning

1. American Academy of Pediatrics Committee on Injury, Violence, and Poison Prevention. Poison treatment in the home. *Pediatrics.* 2003;112(5):1182–1185

2. American College of Emergency Physicians. Clinical policy for the initial approach to patients presenting with acute toxic ingestion or dermal or inhalation exposure. *Ann Emerg Med.* 1999;33(6):735–761

3. American College of Emergency Physicians. Poison information and treatment systems. *Ann Emerg Med.* 1996;27(5):686

4. American Heart Association. 2005 Guidelines for Cardiopulmonary Resuscitation and Emergency Cardiovascular Care. Part 14: First aid. *Circulation.* 2005;112(24 suppl):IV-196–IV-203

5. Beck DA, Frohberg NR. Coprophagia in an elderly man: a case report and review of the literature. *Int J Psychiatry Med.* 2005;35(4):417–427

6. Bond GR. The role of activated charcoal and gastric emptying in gastrointestinal decontanimation: a state-of-the-art review. *Ann Emerg Med.* 2002;39(3):273–286

7. Boyer EW. Management of opioid analgesic overdose. *N Engl J Med.* 2012;367(2):146–155

8. Bronstein AC, Spyker DA, Cantilena LR Jr, Green JL, Rumack BH, Dart RC. 2010 annual report of the American Association of Poison Control Centers' National Poison Data System (NPDS): 28th annual report. *Clin Toxicol (Phila).* 2011;49(10):910–941

9. Crouch BI, Caravati EM, Mitchell A, Martin AC. Poisoning in older adults: a 5-year experience of US poison control centers. *Ann Pharmacother.* 2004;38(12):2005–2011

10. Manoguerra AS, Cobaugh DJ; Guidelines for the Management of Poisoning Consensus Panel. Guideline on the use of ipecac syrup in the out-of-hospital management of ingested poisons. *Clin Toxicol (Phila).* 2005;43(1):1–10

11. Markenson D, Ferguson JD, Chameides L, et al. 2010 American Heart Association and American Red Cross Guidelines for First Aid. Part 17: First Aid. *Circulation.* 2010;122(18 suppl 3):S934–S946

12. McGuigan MA; Guideline Consensus Panel. Guideline for the out-of-hospital management of human exposures to minimally toxic substances. *J Toxicol Clin Toxicol.* 2003;41(7):907–917

13. Naloxone (Narcan) nasal spray for opioid overdose. *Med Lett Drugs Ther.* 2016;58(1485):1–2

14. Rudd RA, Aleshire N, Zibbell JE, Gladden RM. Increases in drug and opioid overdose deaths—United States, 2000–2014. *MMWR Morb Mortal Wkly Rep.* 2016;64(50-51):1378–1382

15. US Preventive Services Task Force. Counseling to prevent household and recreational injuries. In: *Guide to Clinical Preventive Services.* 2nd ed. Alexandria, VA: International Medical Publishing, Inc; 1996:659–685

16. Wolkin AF, Martin CA, Law RK, Schier JG, Bronstein AC. Using poison center data for national public health surveillance for chemical and poison exposure and associated illness. *Ann Emerg Med.* 2012;59(1):56–61

17. Wolkin AF, Patel M, Watson W, et al. Early detection of illness associated with poisonings of public health significance. *Ann Emerg Med.* 2006;47(2):170–176

Pubic Lice

1. Anderson AL, Chaney E. Pubic lice (Pthirus pubis): history, biology and treatment vs. knowledge and beliefs of US college students. *Int J Environ Res Public Health.* 2009;6(2):592–600

2. Brown TJ, Yen-Moore A, Tyring SK. An overview of sexually transmitted diseases. Part II. *J Am Acad Dermatol.* 1999;41(5):661–680

3. Centers for Disease Control and Prevention (CDC). Parasites – Lice – Pubic "Crab" Lice. http://www.cdc.gov/parasites/lice/pubic/index.html. Accessed June 7, 2018

4. Flinders DC, De Schweinitz P. Pediculosis and scabies. *Am Fam Physician.* 2004;69(2):341–348

5. Larimore WL, Petrie KA. Drug use during pregnancy and lactation. *Prim Care.* 2000;27(1):35–53

6. Maunder JW. Lice and scabies. Myths and reality. *Dermatol Clin.* 1998;16(4):843–845, xv

7. Public Health Agency of Canada. Primary care and sexually transmitted infections. In: *Canadian Guidelines on Sexually Transmitted Infections.* 2006 Edition. Ottawa, Ontario: Public Health Agency of Canada; 2006:7–29. http://pubs.cpha.ca/PDF/P37/23384.pdf. Accessed June 7, 2018

8. Workowski KA, Berman S; Centers for Disease Control and Prevention. Sexually transmitted diseases treatment guidelines 2010 [published correction appears in *MMWR Recomm Rep.* 2011;60(1):18]. *MMWR Recomm Rep.* 2010;59(RR-12):1–110

Puncture Wound

1. American Heart Association. 2005 Guidelines for Cardiopulmonary Resuscitation and Emergency Cardiovascular Care. Part 14: First aid. *Circulation.* 2005;112(24 suppl):IV-196–IV-203

2. Baldwin G, Colbourne M. Puncture wounds. *Pediatr Rev.* 1999;20(1):21–23

3. Centers for Disease Control and Prevention. Diphtheria, tetanus, and pertussis: recommendations for vaccine use and other preventive measures. Recommendations of the Immunization Practices Advisory Committee (ACIP). *MMWR Recomm Rep.* 1991;40(RR-10):1–28

Puncture Wound (*continued*)

4. Centers for Disease Control and Prevention. Updated recommendations for use of tetanus toxoid, reduced diphtheria toxoid and acellular pertussis (Tdap) vaccine from the Advisory Committee on Immunization Practices, 2010. *MMWR Morb Mortal Wkly Rep.* 2011;60(1):13–15

5. Gonzalez R, Kasdan ML. High pressure injection injuries of the hand. *Clin Occup Environ Med.* 2006;5(2):407–411, ix

6. Hogan CJ, Ruland RT. High-pressure injection injuries to the upper extremity: a review of the literature. *J Orthop Trauma.* 2006;20(7):503–511

7. Kim DK, Riley LE, Harriman KH, Hunter P, Bridges CB. Advisory Committee on Immunization Practices recommended immunization schedule for adults aged 19 years or older—United States, 2017. *MMWR Morb Mortal Wkly Rep.* 2017;66(5):136–138

8. Kretsinger K, Broder KR, Cortese MM, et al; Centers for Disease Control and Prevention; Advisory Committee on Immunization Practices; Health-care Infection Control Practices Advisory Committee. Preventing tetanus, diphtheria, and pertussis among adults: use of tetanus toxoid, reduced diphtheria toxoid and acellular pertussis vaccine recommendations of the Advisory Committee on Immunization Practices (ACIP) and recommendation of ACIP, supported by the Healthcare Infection Control Practices Advisory Committee (HICPAC), for use of Tdap among health-care personnel. *MMWR Recomm Rep.* 2006;55(RR-17):1–37

9. Lavery LA, Armstrong DG, Wunderlich RP, Mohler MJ, Wendel CS, Lipsky BA. Risk factors for foot infections in individuals with diabetes. *Diabetes Care.* 2006;29(6):1288–1293

10. Markenson D, Ferguson JD, Chameides L, et al. 2010 American Heart Association and American Red Cross Guidelines for First Aid. Part 17: First Aid. *Circulation.* 2010;122(18 suppl 3):S934–S946

11. Moran GJ, Talan DA, Abrahamian FM. Antimicrobial prophylaxis for wounds and procedures in the emergency department. *Infect Dis Clin North Am.* 2008;22(1):117–143, vii

12. Moscati RM, Mayrose J, Reardon RF, Janicke DM, Jehle DV. A multicenter comparison of tap water versus sterile saline for wound irrigation. *Acad Emerg Med.* 2007;14(5):404–409

13. Murphy TV, Slade BA, Broder KR, et al. Prevention of pertussis, tetanus, and diphtheria among pregnant and postpartum women and their infants recommendations of the Advisory Committee on Immunization Practices (ACIP). *MMWR Recomm Rep.* 2008;5(RR-4):1–51

14. Pearson AS, Wolford RW. Management of skin trauma. *Prim Care.* 2000;27(2):475–492

15. Singer AJ, Dagum AB. Current management of acute cutaneous wounds. *N Engl J Med.* 2008;359(10):1037–1046

16. Talan DA, Abrahamian FM, Moran GJ, et al. Tetanus immunity and physician compliance with tetanus prophylaxis practices among emergency department patients presenting with wounds. *Ann Emerg Med.* 2004;43(3):305–314

17. Wedmore IS, Charette J. Emergency department evaluation and treatment of ankle and foot injuries. *Emerg Med Clin North Am.* 2000;18(1):85–113, vi

Rash, Widespread on Drugs (Drug Reaction)

1. Beltrani VS. Cutaneous manifestations of adverse drug reactions. *Immunol Allergy Clin North Am.* 1998;18(4):867–895

2. Bigby M. Rates of cutaneous reactions to drugs. *Arch Dermatol.* 2001;137(6):765–770

3. Bigby M, Jick S, Jick H, Arndt K. Drug-induced cutaneous reactions. A report from the Boston Collaborative Drug Surveillance Program on 15,438 consecutive inpatients, 1975 to 1982. *JAMA.* 1986;256(24):3358–3363

4. Chung WH, Wang CW, Dao RL. Severe cutaneous adverse drug reactions. *J Dermatol.* 2016;43(7):758–766

5. Darlenski R, Kazandjieva J, Tsankov N. Systemic drug reactions with skin involvement: Stevens-Johnson syndrome, toxic epidermal necrolysis, and DRESS. *Clin Dermatol.* 2015;33(5):538–541

6. Davidson MH. Niacin use and cutaneous flushing: mechanisms and strategies for prevention. *Am J Cardiol.* 2008;101(8A):14B–19B

7. Drake LA, Dinehart SM, Farmer Er, et al. Guidelines of care for cutaneous adverse drug reactions. American Academy of Dermatology. *J Am Acad Dermatol.* 1996;35(3):458–461

8. Gruchalla RS. Drug allergies. *Prim Care.* 1998;25(4):791–807

9. Kacalak-Rzepka A, Klimowicz A, Bielecka-Grzela S, Zaluga E, Maleszka R, Fabiaczyk H. Retrospective analysis of adverse cutaneous drug reactions in patients hospitalized in Department of Dermatology and Venereology of Pomeranian Medical University in 1996–2006 [Polish]. *Ann Acad Med Stetin.* 2008;54(2):52–58

10. Paolini JF, Bays HE, Ballantyne CM, et al. Extended–release niacin/laropiprant: reducing niacin-induced flushing to better realize the benefit of niacin in improving cardiovascular risk factors. *Cardiol Clin.* 2008;26(4):547–560

11. Patel LM, Lambert PJ, Gagna CE, Maghari A, Lambert WC. Cutaneous signs of systemic disease. *Clin Dermatol.* 2011;29(5):511–522

12. Reingold AL, Broome CV, Gaventa S, Hightower AW. Risk factors for menstrual toxic shock syndrome: results of a multistate case-control study. *Rev Infect Dis.* 1989;11(suppl 1):S35–S41; discussion S41–S42

13. Revuz J. New advances in severe adverse drug reactions. *Dermatol Clin.* 2001;19(4):697–709, ix

14. Riedl MA, Casillas AM. Adverse drug reactions: types and treatment options. *Am Fam Physician.* 2003;68(9):1781–1790

15. Turney R, Skittrall JP, Donovan J, Agranoff D. Drug reaction, eosinophilia and systemic symptoms (DRESS) syndrome secondary to allopurinol with early lymphadenopathy and symptom relapse. *BMJ Case Rep.* 2015;2015

Rash or Redness, Localized

1. Callahan EF, Adal KA, Tomecki KJ. Cutaneous (non-HIV) infections. *Dermatol Clin.* 2000;18(3):497–508, x

2. Edwards FJ. Dermatologic ED presentations: from the mundane to the life-threatening. *Emerg Med Rep.* 1996;17(17):173–180

3. Ference JD, Last AR. Choosing topical corticosteroids. *Am Fam Physician.* 2009;79(2):135–140

4. Frazee BW, Lynn J, Charlebois ED, Lambert L, Lowery D, Perdreau-Remington F. High prevalence of methicillin-resistant Staphylococcus aureus in emergency department skin and soft tissue infections. *Ann Emerg Med.* 2005;45(3):311–320

5. Fridkin SK, Hageman JC, Morrison M, et al. Methicillin-resistant Staphylococcus aureus disease in three communities. *N Eng J Med.* 2005;352(14):1436–1444

6. Garner LA. Contact dermatitis to metals. *Dermatol Ther.* 2004;17(4):321–327

7. Gorwitz RJ, Jernigan DB, Powers JH, Jernigan JA; Participants in the CDC-Convened Experts' Meeting on Management of MRSA in the Community. Strategies for clinical management of MRSA in the community: summary of an experts' meeting convened by the Centers for Disease Control and Prevention. 2006. http://www.cdc.gov/mrsa/pdf/MRSA-Strategies-ExpMtgSummary-2006.pdf. Accessed June 7, 2018

8. Gunderson CG. Cellulitis: definition, etiology, and clinical features. *Am J Med.* 2011;124(12):1113–1122

9. Hogan D, Ledet JJ. Impact of regulation on contact dermatitis. *Dermatol Clin.* 2009;27(3):385–394, viii

10. Mark BJ, Slavin RG. Allergic contact dermatitis. *Med Clin North Am.* 2006;90(1):169–185

11. Mortz CG, Andersen KE. New aspects in allergic contact dermatitis. *Curr Opin Allergy Clin Immunol.* 2008;8(5):428–432

12. Mounsey AL, Matthew LG, Slawson DC. Herpes zoster and post-herpetic neuralgia: prevention and management. *Am Fam Physician.* 2005;72(6):1075–1080

13. Nadelman RB, Nowakowski J, Forseter G, et al. The clinical spectrum of early Lyme borreliosis in patients with culture-confirmed erythema migrans. *Am J Med.* 1996;100(5):502–508

14. Odell ML. Skin and wound infections: an overview. *Am Fam Physician.* 1998;57(10):2424–2432

15. Patel LM, Lambert PJ, Gagna CE, Maghari A, Lambert WC. Cutaneous signs of systemic disease. *Clin Dermatol.* 2011;29(5):511–522

16. Rhody C. Bacterial infections of the skin. *Prim Care.* 2000;27(2):459–473

17. Roberts WE. Dermatologic problems of older women. *Dermatol Clin.* 2006;24(2):271–280, viii

18. Schlossberg D. Fever and rash. *Infect Dis Clin North Am.* 1996;10(1):101–110

19. Swartz MN. Clinical practice. Cellulitis. *N Engl J Med.* 2004;350(9):904–912

20. Tibbles CD, Edlow JA. Does this patient have erythema migrans? *JAMA.* 2007;297(23):2617–2627

Rash or Redness, Widespread

1. Darlenski R, Kazandjieva J, Tsankov N. Systemic drug reactions with skin involvement: Stevens-Johnson syndrome, toxic epidermal necrolysis, and DRESS. *Clin Dermatol.* 2015;33(5):538–541

2. Edwards FJ. Dermatologic ED presentations: from the mundane to the life–threatening. *Emerg Med Reports.* 1996;17(17)

3. Roberts WE. Dermatologic problems of older women. *Dermatol Clin.* 2006;24(2):271–280, viii

4. Salzman M. Meningococcemia. *Infect Dis Clin North Am.* 1996;10(4):709–725

5. Schlossberg D. Fever and rash. *Infect Dis Clin North Am.* 1996;10(1):101–110

Rectal Bleeding

1. Eikelboom JW, Wallentin L, Connolly SJ, et al. Risk of bleeding with 2 doses of dabigatran compared with warfarin in older and younger patients with atrial fibrillation: an analysis of the randomized evaluation of long-term anticoagulant therapy (RE-LY) trial. *Circulation.* 2011;123(21):2363–2372

2. Fallah MA, Prakash C, Edmundowicz S. Acute gastrointestinal bleeding. *Med Clin North Am.* 2000;84(5):1183–1208

3. Farrel JJ, Friedman LS. Gastrointestinal bleeding in older people. *Gastroenterol Clin North Am.* 2000;29(1):1–36, v

4. Fathi DJ. Common anorectal symptomatology. *Prim Care.* 1999;26(1):1–13

5. Gupta P. Randomized, controlled study comparing sitz-bath and no-sitz-bath treatments in patients with acute anal fissures. *ANZ J Surg.* 2006;76(8):718–721

6. Hsu KF, Chia JS, Jao SW, et al. Comparison of clinical effects between warm water spray and sitz bath in post-hemorrhoidectomy period. *J Gastrointest Surg.* 2009;13(7):1274–1278

7. Janicke DM, Pundt MR. Anorectal disorders. *Emerg Med Clin North Am.* 1996;14(4):757–788

8. Raje D, Scott M, Irvine T, et al. Telephonic management of rectal bleeding in young adults: a prospective randomized controlled trial. *Colorectal Dis.* 2007;9(1):86–89

9. Sinert R, Spektor M. Evidence-based emergency medicine/rational clinical examination abstract. Clinical assessment of hypovolemia. *Ann Emerg Med.* 2005;45(3):327–329

10. Stapley S, Peters TJ, Sharp D, Hamilton W. The mortality of colorectal cancer in relation to the initial symptom at presentation to primary care and to the duration of symptoms: a cohort study using medical records. *Br J Cancer.* 2006;95(10):1321–1325

11. Strate LL, Orav EJ, Syngal S. Early predictors of severity in acute lower intestinal tract bleeding. *Arch Inter Med.* 2003;163(7):838–843

12. Tejirian T, Abbas MA. Sitz bath: where is the evidence? Scientific basis of a common practice. *Dis Colon Rectum.* 2005;48(12):2336–2340

13. Wald A. Constipation. *Med Clin North Am.* 2000;84(5):1231–1246

Rectal Symptoms

1. Fathi DJ. Common anorectal symptomatology. *Prim Care.* 1999;26(1):1–13

2. Gupta P. Randomized, controlled study comparing sitz-bath and no-sitz-bath treatments in patients with acute anal fissures. *ANZ J Surg.* 2006;76(8):718–721

3. Hsu KF, Chia JS, Jao SW, et al. Comparison of clinical effects between warm water spray and sitz bath in post-hemorrhoidectomy period. *J Gastrointest Surg.* 2009;13(7):1274–1278

4. Janicke DM, Pundt MR. Anorectal disorders. *Emerg Med Clin North Am.* 1996;14(4):757–788

5. MacLean J, Russell D. Pruritus ani. *Aust Fam Physician.* 2010;39(6):366–370

6. Nurko S, Zimmerman LA. Evaluation and treatment of constipation in children and adolescents. *Am Fam Physician.* 2014;90(2):82–90

7. Sommers T, Corban C, Sengupta N, et al. Emergency department burden of constipation in the United States from 2006 to 2011. *Am J Gastroenterol.* 2015;110(4):572–579

8. Tejirian T, Abbas MA. Sitz bath: where is the evidence? Scientific basis of a common practice. *Dis Colon Rectum.* 2005;48(12):2336–2340

9. Vincent C. Anorectal pain and irritation: anal fissure, levator syndrome, proctalgia fugax, and pruritus ani. *Prim Care.* 1999;26(1):53–68

Seizure

1. American Academy of Neurology. Consensus statements: medical management of epilepsy. *Neurology.* 1998;51(5 suppl 4):S39–S43

2. American Academy of Neurology Quality Standards Subcommittee. Practice parameter: management issues for women with epilepsy (summary statement). *Neurology.* 1998;51(4):944–948

3. American College of Emergency Physicians. Clinical policy for the initial approach to patients presenting with a chief complaint of seizure who are not in status epilepticus. *Ann Emerg Med.* 1997;29(5):706–724

4. American Heart Association. 2005 Guidelines for Cardiopulmonary Resuscitation and Emergency Cardiovascular Care. Part 14: First aid. *Circulation.* 2005;112(24 suppl):IV-196–IV-203

5. Benbadis SR, Wolgamuth BR, Goren H, Brener S, Fouad-Tarazi F. Value of tongue biting in the diagnosis of seizures. *Arch Intern Med.* 1995;155(21):2346–2349

6. Clawson J, Olola C, Scott G, Heward A, Patterson B. Effect of a medical priority dispatch system key question addition in the seizure/convulsion/fitting protocol to improve recognition of ineffective (agonal) breathing. *Resuscitation.* 2008;79(2):257–264

7. Markenson D, Ferguson JD, Chameides L, et al. 2010 American Heart Association and American Red Cross Guidelines for First Aid. Part 17: First Aid. *Circulation.* 2010;122(18 suppl 3):S934–S946

8. Willmore LJ. Epilepsy emergencies; the first seizure and status epilepticus. *Neurology.* 1998;51(5 suppl):S34–S38

Sexual Assault or Rape

1. Amercan College of Emergency Physicians. Clinical policy for the management and risk stratification of community-acquired pneumonia in adults in the emergency department. *Ann Emerg Med.* 2001;38(1):107–113

2. American College of Emergency Physicians. Selective triage for victims of sexual assault to designated exam facilities. *Ann Emerg Med.* 2007;49(5):725

3. American College of Obstetricians and Gynecologists. Sexual assault. Number 242, November 1997. *Int J Gynaecol Obstet.* 1998;60(3):297–304

4. Bechtel LK, Holstege CP. Criminal poisoning: drug-facilitated sexual assault. *Emerg Med Clin North Am.* 2007;25(2):499–525, x

5. Breiding MJ, Smith SG, Basile KC, Walters ML, Chen J, Merrick MT. Prevalence and characteristics of sexual violence, stalking, and intimate partner violence victimization—national intimate partner and sexual violence survey, United States, 2011. *MMWR Surveill Summ.* 2014;63(8):1–18

6. Carr M, Thomas AJ, Atwood D, Muhar A, Jarvis K, Wewerka SS. Debunking three rape myths. *J Forensic Nurs.* 2014;10(4):217–225; quiz E1–E2

7. Cheng L, Che Y, Gülmezoglu AM. Interventions for emergency contraception. *Cochrane Database Syst Rev.* 2012;8:CD001324

8. Committee on Health Care for Underserved Women. ACOG committee opinion no. 542: access to emergency contraception. *Obstet Gynecol.* 2012;120(5):1250–1253

9. Division of Reproductive Health, National Center for Chronic Disease Prevention and Health Promotion, Centers for Disease Control and Prevention. U.S. selected practice recommendations for contraceptive use, 2013: adapted from the World Health Organization selected practice recommendations for contraceptive use, 2nd edition. *MMWR Recomm Rep.* 2013;62(RR-05):1–60

10. Dunn S, Guilbert E; Social Sexual Issues Committee. Emergency contraception. *J Obstet Gynaecol Can.* 2012;34(9):870–878

Sexual Assault or Rape (*continued*)

11. Koss MP, Wilgus JK, Williamsen KM. Campus sexual misconduct: restorative justice approaches to enhance compliance with Title IX guidance. *Trauma Violence Abuse*. 2014;15(3):242–257

12. Linden JA. Sexual assault. *Emerg Med Clin North Am*. 1999;17(3):685–697, vii

13. Merritt DF. Genital trauma in the pediatric and adolescent female. *Obstet Gynecol Clin North Am*. 2009;36(1):85–98

14. Public Health Agency of Canada. Primary care and sexually transmitted infections. In: *Canadian Guidelines on Sexually Transmitted Infections*. 2006 Edition. Ottawa, Ontario: Public Health Agency of Canada; 2006:7–29. http://pubs.cpha.ca/PDF/P37/23384.pdf. Accessed June 7, 2018

15. Public Health Agency of Canada. Sexual assault in postpubertal adolescents and adults. In: *Canadian Guidelines on Sexually Transmitted Infections*. 2006 Edition. Ottawa, Ontario: Public Health Agency of Canada; 2006:305–314. http://pubs.cpha.ca/PDF/P37/23384.pdf. Accessed June 7, 2018

16. Riggs N. Analysis of 1,076 cases of sexual assault. *Ann Emerg Med*. 2000;35(4):358–362

17. Sugar NF, Fine DN, Eckert LO. Physical injury after sexual assault: findings of a large case series. *Am J Obstet Gynecol*. 2004;190(1):71–76

18. US Department of Justice, Office on Violence Against Women. *A National Protocol for Sexual Assault Medical Forensic Examinations: Adults/Adolescents*. 2nd ed. https://c.ymcdn.com/sites/www.safeta.org/resource/resmgr/Protocol_documents/SAFE_PROTOCOL_2012-508.pdf. Published April 2013. Accessed June 25, 2018

19. Walsh JL, Senn TE, Carey MP. Exposure to different types of violence and subsequent sexual risk behavior among female STD clinic patients: a latent class analysis. *Psychol Violence*. 2012;2(4):339–354

20. Wessells H, Long L. Penile and genital injuries. *Urol Clin North Am*. 2006;33(1):117–126, viii

21. Workowski KA, Berman S; Centers for Disease Control and Prevention. Sexually transmitted diseases treatment guidelines, 2010 [published correction appears in *MMWR Recomm Rep*. 2011;60(1):18]. *MMWR Recomm Rep*. 2010;59(RR-12):1–110

Shoulder Injury

1. American Heart Association. 2005 Guidelines for Cardiopulmonary Resuscitation and Emergency Cardiovascular Care. Part 10: First Aid. *Circulation*. 2005;112:IV-196–IV-203

2. Belzer JP, Durkin RC. Common disorders of the shoulder. *Prim Care*. 1996;23(2):365–388

3. Bleakley C, McDonough S, MacAuley D. The use of ice in the treatment of acute soft-tissue injury. *Am J Sports Med*. 2004;32(1):251–261

4. Brady WJ, et al. Upper extremity fractures and dislocations. *Emerg Med Reports*. 1999;20(9)

5. Collins NC. Is ice right? Does cryotherapy improve outcome for acute soft tissue injury? *Emerg Med J*. 2008;25(2):65–68

6. Daigneault JK, Cooney LM. Shoulder pain in older people. *J Amer Geriatrics Society*. 1998;46(9):1144–1151

7. Kellett J. Acute soft tissue injuries—a review of the literature. *Med Sci Sports Exerc*. 1986;18(5):489–500

8. Markenson D, Ferguson JD, Chameides L, et al. 2010 American Heart Association and American Red Cross Guidelines for First Aid. Part 17: First Aid. *Circulation*. 2010;122(18 suppl 3):S934–S946

9. McMaster WC, Liddle S, Waugh TR. Laboratory evaluation of various cold therapy modalities. *Am J Sports Med*. 1978;6(5):291–294

10. Pimentel L. Orthopedic trauma: office management of major joint injury. *Med Clin North Am*. 2006;90(2):355–382

11. Singer AJ, Dagum AB. Current management of acute cutaneous wounds. *N Engl J Med*. 2008;359(10):1037–1046

Sinus Pain and Congestion

1. American Academy of Family Physicians. Patient information. Saline nasal irrigation for sinus problems. *Am Fam Physician*. 2009;80(10):1121

2. Bachert C, Chuchalin AG, Eisebitt R, Netayzhenko VZ, Voelker M. Aspirin compared with acetaminophen in the treatment of fever and other symptoms of upper respiratory tract infection in adults: a multicenter, randomized, double-blind, double-dummy, placebo-controlled, parallel-group, single-dose, 6-hour dose-ranging study. *Clin Ther*. 2005;27(7):993–1003

3. Blaiss MS, Dicpinigaitis PV, Eccles R, Wingertzahn MA. Consumer attitudes on cough and cold: US (ACHOO) survey results. *Curr Med Res Opin*. 2015;31(8):1527–1538

4. Bucher HC, Tschudi P, Young J, et al. Effect of amoxicillin-clavulanate in clinically diagnosed acute rhinosinusitis: a placebo-controlled, double-blind, randomized trial in general practice. *Arch Intern Med*. 2003;163(15):1793–1798

5. Cady RK, Schreiber CP. Sinus headache: a clinical conundrum. *Otolaryngol Clin North Am*. 2004;37(2):267–288

6. Deckx L, De Sutter AI, Guo L, Mir NA, van Driel ML. Nasal decongestants in monotherapy for the common cold. *Cochrane Database Syst Rev*. 2016;10:CD009612

7. Eapen RJ, Ebert CS Jr, Pillsbury HC III. Allergic rhinitis—history and presentation. *Otolaryngol Clin North Am*. 2008;41(2):325–330, vi–vii

8. Ebell MH, Lundgren J, Youngpairoj S. How long does a cough last? Comparing patients' expectations with data from a systematic review of the literature. *Ann Fam Med*. 2013;11(1):5–13

9. Eccles R. Understanding the symptoms of the common cold and influenza. *Lancet Infect Dis*. 2005;5(11):718–725

10. Erebara A, Bozzo P, Einarson A, Koren G. Treating the common cold during pregnancy. *Can Fam Physician*. 2008;54(5):687–689

11. Harvey R, Hannan SA, Badia L, Scadding G. Nasal saline irrigations for the symptoms of chronic rhinosinusitis. *Cochrane Database Syst Rev*. 2007;(3):CD006394

12. Hatton RC, Winterstein AG, McKelvey RP, Shuster J, Hendeles L. Efficacy and safety of oral phenylephrine: systematic review and metaanalysis. *Ann Pharmacother*. 2007;41(3):381–390

13. Hayward G, Thompson MJ, Perera R, Del Mar CB, Glasziou PP, Heneghan CJ. Corticosteroids for the common cold. *Cochrane Database Syst Rev*. 2012;8:CD008116

14. Incaudo GA, Takach P. The diagnosis and treatment of allergic rhinitis during pregnancy and lactation. *Immunol Allergy Clin North Am*. 2006;26(1):137–154

15. Kenealy T, Arroll B. Antibiotics for the common cold and acute purulent rhinitis. *Cochrane Database Syst Rev*. 2013;6:CD000247

16. Kirkpatrick GL. The common cold. *Prim Care*. 1996;23(4):657–675

17. Leung RS, Katial R. The diagnosis and management of acute and chronic sinusitis. *Prim Care*. 2008;35(1):11–24, v–vi

18. Maltinski G. Nasal disorders and sinusitis. *Prim Care*. 1998;25(3):663–683

19. Rabago D, Barrett B, Marchand L, Maberry R, Mundt M. Qualitative aspects of nasal irrigation use by patients with chronic sinus disease in a multimethod study. *Ann Fam Med*. 2006;4(4):295–301

20. Rabago D, Zgierska A. Saline nasal irrigation for upper respiratory conditions. *Am Fam Physician*. 2009;80(10):1117–1119

21. Rosenfeld RM, Andes D, Bhattacharyya N, et al. Clinical practice guideline: adult sinusitis. *Otolaryngol Head Neck Surg*. 2007;137(3 suppl):S1–S31

22. Simasek M, Blandino DA. Treatment of the common cold. *Am Fam Physician*. 2007;75(4):515–520

23. Spector SL, Bernstein IL, Li JT, et al. Parameters for the diagnosis and management of sinusitis. *J Allergy Clin Immunol*. 1998;102(6 suppl 2):S107–S144

24. Wallace DV, Dykewicz MS, Bernstein DI, et al. The diagnosis and management of rhinitis: an updated practice parameter. *J Allergy Clin Immunol*. 2008;122(2 suppl):S1–S84

25. Witek TJ, Ramsey DL, Carr AN, Riker DK. The natural history of community-acquired common colds symptoms assessed over 4 years. *Rhinology*. 2015;53(1):81–88

Skin, Foreign Body

1. Baldwin G, Colbourne M. Puncture wounds. *Pediatr Rev*. 1999;20(1):21–23

2. Blankenship RB, Baker T. Imaging modalities in wounds and superficial skin infections. *Emerg Med Clin North Am*. 2007;25(1):223–234

3. Bradley M. Image-guided soft-tissue foreign body extraction—success and pitfalls. *Clin Radiol*. 2012;67(6):531–534

4. Chan C, Salam GA. Splinter removal. *Am Fam Physician*. 2003;67(12):2557–2562

5. Gammons MG, Jackson E. Fishhook removal. *Am Fam Physician*. 2001;63(11):2231–2236

6. Halaas GW. Management of foreign bodies in the skin. *Am Fam Physician.* 2007;76(5):683–688

7. Hollander JE, Singer AJ, Valentine SM, Shofer FS. Risk factors for infection in patients with traumatic lacerations. *Acad Emerg Med.* 2001;8(7):716–720

8. Kaye ET. Topical antibacterial agents. *Infect Dis Clin North Am.* 2000;14(2):321–339

9. Lammers RL, Gibson S, Kovacs D, Sears W, Strachan G. Comparison of test characteristics of urine dipstick and urinalysis at various test cutoff points. *Ann Emerg Med.* 2001;38(5):505–512

10. Moran GJ, Talan DA, Abrahamian FM. Antimicrobial prophylaxis for wounds and procedures in the emergency department. *Infect Dis Clin North Am.* 2008;22(1):117–143, vii

11. Pearson AS, Wolford RW. Management of skin trauma. *Prim Care.* 2000;27(2):475–492

12. Wedmore IS, Charette J. Emergency department evaluation and treatment of ankle and foot injuries. *Emerg Med Clin North Am.* 2000;18(1):85–113, vi

Skin Injury

1. American College of Emergency Physicians. Clinical policy for the initial approach to patients presenting with penetrating extremity trauma. *Ann Emerg Med.* 1999;33(5):612–636

2. American Heart Association. 2005 Guidelines for Cardiopulmonary Resuscitation and Emergency Cardiovascular Care. Part 10: First Aid. *Circulation.* 2005;112:IV-196–IV-203

3. Bleakley C, McDonough S, MacAuley D. The use of ice in the treatment of acute soft-tissue injury. *Am J Sports Med.* 2004;32(1):251–261

4. Centers for Disease Control and Prevention. Diphtheria, tetanus, and pertussis: recommendations for vaccine use and other preventive measures. Recommendations of the Immunization Practices Advisory Committee (ACIP). *MMWR Recomm Rep.* 1991;40(RR-10):1–28

5. Centers for Disease Control and Prevention. Updated recommendations for use of tetanus toxoid, reduced diphtheria toxoid and acellular pertussis (Tdap) vaccine from the Advisory Committee on Immunization Practices, 2010. *MMWR Morb Mortal Wkly Rep.* 2011;60(1):13–15

6. Collins NC. Is ice right? Does cryotherapy improve outcome for acute soft tissue injury? *Emerg Med J.* 2008;25(2):65–68

7. Dimick AR. Delayed wound closure: indications and techniques. *Ann Emerg Med.* 1988;17(12):1303–1304

8. Eaglestein WH, Sullivan T. Cyanoacrylates for skin closure. *Dermatol Clin.* 2005;23(2):193–198

9. Gergen PJ, McQuillan GM, Kiely M, Ezzati-Rice TM, Sutter RW, Virella G. A population-based serologic survey of immunity to tetanus in the United States. *N Engl J Med.* 1995;332(12):761–766

10. Hollander JE, Singer AJ, Valentine SM, Shofer FS. Risk factors for infection in patients with traumatic lacerations. *Acad Emerg Med.* 2001;8(7):716–720

11. Hubbard TJ, Denegar CR. Does cryotherapy improve outcomes with soft tissue injury? *J Athl Train.* 2004;39(3):278–279

12. Kellett J. Acute soft tissue injuries—a review of the literature. *Med Sci Sports Exerc.* 1986;18(5):489–500

13. Kim DK, Riley LE, Harriman KH, Hunter P, Bridges CB. Advisory Committee on Immunization Practices recommended immunization schedule for adults aged 19 years or older—United States, 2017. *MMWR Morb Mortal Wkly Rep.* 2017;66(5):136–138

14. Kretsinger K, Broder KR, Cortese MM, et al; Centers for Disease Control and Prevention; Advisory Committee on Immunization Practices; Health-care Infection Control Practices Advisory Committee. Preventing tetanus, diphtheria, and pertussis among adults: use of tetanus toxoid, reduced diphtheria toxoid and acellular pertussis vaccine recommendations of the Advisory Committee on Immunization Practices (ACIP) and recommen-dation of ACIP, supported by the Healthcare Infection Control Practices Advisory Committee (HICPAC), for use of Tdap among health-care personnel. *MMWR Recomm Rep.* 2006;55(RR-17):1–37

15. Markenson D, Ferguson JD, Chameides L, et al. 2010 American Heart Association and American Red Cross Guidelines for First Aid. Part 17: First Aid. *Circulation.* 2010;122(18 suppl 3):S934–S946

16. McMaster WC, Liddle S, Waugh TR. Laboratory evaluation of various cold therapy modalities. *Am J Sports Med.* 1978;6(5):291–294

17. Merrick MA. A preliminary examination of cryotherapy and secondary injury in skeletal muscle. *Med Sci Sports Exerc.* 1999;31(11):1516–1521

18. Milne CT, Corbett LQ. A new option in the treatment of skin tears for the institutionalized resident: formulated 2–octylcyanoacrylate topical bandage. *Geriatr Nurs.* 2005;26(5):321–325

19. Moran GJ, Talan DA, Abrahamian FM. Antimicrobial prophylaxis for wounds and procedures in the emergency department. *Infect Dis Clin North Am.* 2008;22(1):117–143

20. Moscati RM, Mayrose J, Reardon RF, Janicke DM, Jehle DV. A multicenter comparison of tap water versus sterile saline for wound irrigation. *Acad Emerg Med.* 2007;14(5):404–409

21. Murphy TV, Slade BA, Broder KR, et al. Prevention of pertussis, tetanus, and diphtheria among pregnant and postpartum women and their infants recommendations of the Advisory Committee on Immunization Practices (ACIP). *MMWR Recomm Rep.* 2008;57(RR-4):1–51

22. Pearson AS, Rolford RW. Management of skin trauma. *Prim Care.* 2000;27(2):475–492

23. Perelman VS, Francis GJ, Rutledge T, Foote J, Martino F, Dranitsaris G. Sterile versus nonsterile gloves for repair of uncomplicated lacerations in the emergency department: a randomized controlled trial. *Ann Emerg Med.* 2004;43(3):362–370

24. Ratliff CR, Fletcher KR. Skin tears: a review of the evidence to support prevention and treatment. *Ostomy Wound Manage.* 2007;53(3):32–34, 36, 38–40

25. Singer AJ, Dagum AB. Current management of acute cutaneous wounds. *N Engl J Med.* 2008;359(10):1037–1046

26. Singer AJ, Quinn JV, Clark RE, Hollander JE; TraumaSeal Study Group. Closure of lacerations and incisions with octylcyanoacrylate: a multicenter randomized controlled trial. *Surgery.* 2002;131(3):270–276

27. Swartz MN. Clinical practice. Cellulitis. *N Engl J Med.* 2004;350(9):904–912

28. US Preventive Services Task Force. Postexposure prophylaxis for selected infectious diseases. In: *Guide to Clinical Preventive Services.* 2nd ed. Alex-andria, VA: International Medical Publishing, Inc; 1996:815–827

29. Xu X, Lau K, Taira BR, Singer AJ. The current management of skin tears. *Am J Emerg Med.* 2009;27(6):729–733

Skin Lesion (Moles or Growths)

1. Cokkinides V, Weinstock M, Lazovich D, Ward E, Thun M. Indoor tanning use among adolescents in the US, 1998 to 2004. *Cancer.* 2009;115(1):190–198

2. Dewberry C, Norman RA. Skin cancer in elderly patients. *Dermatol Clin.* 2004;22(1):93–96, vii

3. Jerant AF, Johnson JT, Sheridan CD, Caffrey TJ. Early detection and treatment of skin cancer. *Am Fam Physician.* 2000;62(2):357–382

4. US Preventive Services Task Force. Screening for skin cancer—including counseling to prevent skin cancer. In: *Guide to Clinical Preventive Services.* 2nd ed. Alexandria, VA: International Medical Publishing, Inc; 1996:141–152

Sore Throat

1. Belleza WG, Kalman S. Otolaryngologic emergencies in the outpatient setting. *Med Clin North Am.* 2006;90(2):329–353

2. Bisno AL, Gerber MA, Gwaltney JM Jr, Kaplan EL, Schwartz RH; Infec-tious Diseases Society of America. Practice guidelines for the diagnosis and management of group A streptococcal pharyngitis. *Clin Infect Dis.* 2002;35(2):113–125

3. Blaiss MS, Dicpinigaitis PV, Eccles R, Wingertzahn MA. Consumer attitudes on cough and cold: US (ACHOO) survey results. *Curr Med Res Opin.* 2015;31(8):1527–1538

4. Clancy CM, Centor RM, Campbell MS, Dalton HP. Rational decision making based on history: adult sore throats. *J Gen Intern Med.* 1988;3(3):213–217

5. Cooper RJ, Hoffman JR, Bartlett JG, et al. Principles of appropriate antibiotic use for acute pharyngitis in adults: background. *Ann Intern Med.* 2001;134(6):509–517

6. Del Mar CB, Glasziou PP, Spinks AB. Antibiotics for sore throat. *Cochrane Database Syst Rev.* 2004;(4):CD000023

Sore Throat (*continued*)

7. Eccles R. Understanding the symptoms of the common cold and influenza. *Lancet Infect Dis.* 2005;5(11):718–725
8. Gerber MA, Baltimore RS, Eaton CB, et al. Prevention of rheumatic fever and diagnosis and treatment of acute streptococcal pharyngitis: a scientific statement from the American Heart Association. *Circulation.* 2009;119(11):1541–1551
9. Green SM. Acute pharyngitis: the case for empiric antimicrobial therapy. *Ann Emerg Med.* 1995;25(3):404–406
10. Kerdemelidis M, Lennon D, Arroll B, Peat B. Guidelines for sore throat management in New Zealand. *N Z Med J.* 2009;122(1301):10–18
11. Kljakovic M, Crampton P. Sore throat management in New Zealand general practice. *N Z Med J.* 2005;118(1220):U1609
12. Komaroff AL, Pass TM, Aronson MD, et al. The prediction of streptococcal pharyngitis in adults. *J Gen Intern Med.* 1986;1(1):1–7
13. Matsuda A, Tanaka H, Kanaya T, Kamata K, Hasegawa M. Peritonsillar abscess: a study of 724 cases in Japan. *Ear Nose Throat J.* 2002;81(6):384–389
14. McIsaac WJ, Kellner JD, Aufricht P, Vanjaka A, Low DE. Empirical validation of guidelines for the management of pharyngitis in children and adults [published correction appears in *JAMA.* 2005;294(21):2700]. *JAMA.* 2004;291(13):1587–1595
15. Peter J, Ray CG. Infectious mononucleosis. *Pediatr Rev.* 1998;19(8):276–279
16. van Driel ML, De Sutter A, Deveugele M, et al. Are sore throat patients who hope for antibiotics actually asking for pain relief? *Ann Fam Med.* 2006;4(6):494–499
17. Weber R. Pharyngitis. *Prim Care.* 2014;41(1):91–98
18. Witek TJ, Ramsey DL, Carr AN, Riker DK. The natural history of community-acquired common colds symptoms assessed over 4 years. *Rhinology.* 2015;53(1):81–88

Spider Bite

1. Anderson PC. Spider bites in the United States. *Dermatol Clin.* 1997;15(2):307–311
2. Blaikie AJ, Ellis J, Sanders R, MacEwen CJ. Eye disease associated with handling pet tarantulas: three case reports. *BMJ.* 1997;314(7093):1524–1525
3. Braitberg G, Segal L. Spider bites—assessment and management. *Aust Fam Physician.* 2009;38(11):862–867
4. Clark RF, Wethern-Kestner S, Vance MV, Gerkin R. Clinical presentation and treatment of black widow spider envenomation: a review of 163 cases. *Ann Emerg Med.* 1992;21(7):782–787
5. Derlet RW, Richards JR. Cellulitis from insect bites: a case series. *Cal J Emerg Med.* 2003;4(2):27–30
6. Diaz JH, Leblanc KE. Common spider bites. *Am Fam Physician.* 2007;75(6):869–873
7. Glavas SN. Necrotic wound on the hand. *Am Fam Physician.* 2008;78(10):1209–1210
8. Goddard J, Upshaw S, Held D, Johnnson K. Severe reaction from envenomation by the brown widow spider, Latrodectus geometricus (Araneae: Theridiidae). *South Med J.* 2008;101(12):1269–1270
9. Gorwitz RJ, Jernigan DB, Powers JH, Jernigan JA; Participants in the CDC-Convened Experts' Meeting on Management of MRSA in the Community. Strategies for clinical management of MRSA in the community: summary of an experts' meeting convened by the Centers for Disease Control and Prevention. 2006. http://www.cdc.gov/mrsa/pdf/MRSA-Strategies-ExpMtgSummary-2006.pdf. Accessed June 7, 2018
10. Sams HH, Dunnick CA, Smith ML, King LE Jr. Necrotic arachnidism. *J Am Acad Dermatol.* 2001;44(4):561–576
11. Singletary EM, Rochman AS, Bodmer JC, Holstege CP. Envenomations. *Med Clin North Am.* 2005;89(6):1195–1224
12. Steen CJ, Carbonaro PA, Schwartz RA. Arthropods in dermatology. *J Am Acad Dermatol.* 2004;50(6):819–844
13. Suchard JR. Diagnosis and treatment of cutaneous anthrax. *JAMA.* 2002;288(1):43–44
14. Suchard JR. Spider bite. *Ann Emerg Med.* 2009;54(1):8, 11
15. Sutherland SK, Duncan AW. New first-aid measures for envenomation: with special reference to bites by the Sydney funnel-web spider (Atrax robustus). *Med J Aust.* 1980;1(8):378–379
16. Swanson DL, Vetter RS. Bites of brown recluse spiders and suspected necrotic arachnidism. *N Eng J Med.* 2005;352(7):700–707
17. Wright SW, Wrenn KD, Murray L, Seger D. Clinical presentation and outcome of brown recluse spider bite. *Ann Emerg Med.* 1997;30(1):28–32

STI Exposure and Prevention

1. Advisory Committee on Immunization Practices. Recommended adult immunization schedule: United States, 2011. *Ann Intern Med.* 2011;154(3):168–173
2. Braverman PK. Sexually transmitted diseases in adolescents. *Med Clin North Am.* 2000;84(4):869–889, vi–vii
3. Kodner C. Sexually transmitted infections in men. *Prim Care.* 2003;30(1):173–191
4. Miller KE. Women's health. Sexually transmitted diseases. *Prim Care.* 1997;24(1):179–193
5. Public Health Agency of Canada. Primary care and sexually transmitted infections. In: *Canadian Guidelines on Sexually Transmitted Infections.* 2006 Edition. Ottawa, Ontario: Public Health Agency of Canada; 2006:7–29. http://pubs.cpha.ca/PDF/P37/23384.pdf. Accessed June 7, 2018
6. Walsh JL, Senn TE, Carey MP. Exposure to different types of violence and subsequent sexual risk behavior among female STD clinic patients: a latent class analysis. *Psychol Violence.* 2012;2(4):339–354
7. Workowski KA, Berman S; Centers for Disease Control and Prevention. Sexually transmitted diseases treatment guidelines, 2010 [published correction appears in *MMWR Recomm Rep.* 2011;60(1):18]. *MMWR Recomm Rep.* 2010;59(RR-12):1–110

Strep Throat Test Follow-up Call

1. Bisno AL, Gerber MA, Gwaltney JM Jr, Kaplan EL, Schwartz RH. Diagnosis and management of group A streptococcal pharyngitis: a practice guideline. *Clin Infect Dis.* 1997;25(3):574–583
2. Bisno AL, Gerber MA, Gwaltney JM Jr, Kaplan EL, Schwartz RH; Infectious Diseases Society of America. Practice guidelines for the diagnosis and management of group A streptococcal pharyngitis. *Clin Infect Dis.* 2002;35(2):113–125
3. Clancy CM, Centor RM, Campbell MS, Dalton HP. Rational decision making based on history: adult sore throats. *J Gen Intern Med.* 1988;3(3):213–217
4. Cooper RJ, Hoffman JR, Bartlett JG, et al. Principles of appropriate antibiotic use for acute pharyngitis in adults: background. *Ann Intern Med.* 2001;134(6):509–517
5. Danchin MH, Rogers S, Kelpie L. Burden of acute sore throat and group A streptococcal pharyngitis in school-aged children and their families in Australia. *Pediatrics.* 2007;120(5):950–957
6. Gerber MA, Baltimore RS, Eaton CB, et al. Prevention of rheumatic fever and diagnosis and treatment of acute Streptococcal pharyngitis: a scientific statement from the American Heart Association. *Circulation.* 2009;119(11):1541–1551
7. Green SM. Acute pharyngitis: the case for empiric antimicrobial therapy. *Ann Emerg Med.* 1995;25(3):404–406
8. Kerdemelidis M, Lennon D, Arroll B, Peat B. Guidelines for sore throat management in New Zealand. *N Z Med J.* 2009;122(1301):10–18
9. Kljakovic M, Crampton P. Sore throat management in New Zealand general practice. *N Z Med J.* 2005;118(1220):U1609
10. Komaroff AL, Pass TM, Aronson MD, et al. The prediction of streptococcal pharyngitis in adults. *J Gen Intern Med.* 1986;1(1):1–7
11. McIsaac WJ, Kellner JD, Aufricht P, Vanjaka A, Low DE. Empirical validation of guidelines for the management of pharyngitis in children and adults [published correction appears in *JAMA.* 2005;294(21):2700]. *JAMA.* 2004;291(13):1587–1595
12. van Driel ML, De Sutter A, Deveugele M, et al. Are sore throat patients who hope for antibiotics actually asking for pain relief? *Ann Fam Med.* 2006;4(6):494–499
13. Weber R. Pharyngitis. *Prim Care.* 2014;41(1):91–98

Substance Abuse and Dependence

1. Boyer EW. Management of opioid analgesic overdose. *N Engl J Med.* 2012;367(2):146–155
2. Camí J, Farré M. Drug addiction. *N Engl J Med.* 2003;349(10):975–986
3. Cleary M, Hunt G, Matheson S, Siegfried N, Walter G. Psychosocial interventions for people with both severe mental illness and substance misuse. *Cochrane Database Syst Rev.* 2008;(1):CD001088
4. Giannini AJ. An approach to drug abuse, intoxication, and withdrawal. *Am Fam Physician.* 2000;61(9):2763–2774
5. Knight JR. A 35-year-old physician with opioid dependence. *JAMA.* 2004;292(11):1351–1357
6. McCord J, Jneid H, Hollander JE, et al. Management of cocaine-associated chest pain and myocardial infarction: a scientific statement from the American Heart Association Acute Cardiac Care Committee of the Council on Clinical Cardiology. *Circulation.* 2008;117(14):1897–1907
7. McRae AL. Alcohol and substance abuse. *Med Clin North Am.* 2001;85(3):779–801
8. Naloxone (Narcan) nasal spray for opioid overdose. *Med Lett Drugs Ther.* 2016;58(1485):1–2
9. Rudd RA, Aleshire N, Zibbell JE, Gladden RM. Increases in drug and opioid overdose deaths—United States, 2000–2014. *MMWR Morb Mortal Wkly Rep.* 2016;64(50-51):1378–1382
10. Sowers W, George C, Thompson K. Level of care utilization system for psychiatric and addiction services (LOCUS): a preliminary assessment of reliability and validity. *Community Ment Health J.* 1999;35(6):545–563
11. Stein MD. Medical consequences of substance abuse. *Psychiatr Clin North Am.* 1999;22(2):351–370
12. Williams JF, Kokotailo PK. Abuse of proprietary (over-the-counter) drugs. *Adolesc Med Clin.* 2006;17(3):733–750, xiii
13. Williams JF, Storck M; American Academy of Pediatrics Committee on Substance Abuse, Committee on Native American Child Health. Inhalant abuse. *Pediatrics.* 2007;119(5):1009–1017
14. Zealberg JJ, Brady KT. Substance abuse and emergency psychiatry. *Psychiatr Clin North Am.* 1999;22(4):803–817

Suicide Concerns

1. American Psychiatric Association Work Group on Suicidal Behavior. Practice guideline for the assessment and treatment of patients with suicidal behaviors. https://psychiatryonline.org/pb/assets/raw/sitewide/practice_guidelines/guidelines/suicide.pdf. Published November 2003. Accessed June 25, 2018
2. Bolton JM, Pagura J, Enns MW, Grant B, Sareen J. A population-based longitudinal study of risk factors for suicide attempts in major depressive disorder. *J Psychiatr Res.* 2010;44(13):817–826
3. Chartrand H, Robinson J, Bolton JM. A longitudinal population-based study exploring treatment utilization and suicidal ideation and behavior in major depressive disorder. *J Affect Disord.* 2012;141(2-3):237–245
4. Collier R. Self-injury rates indicate Canadian mental health services are inadequate. *CMAJ.* 2011;183(10):E615–E616
5. Conwell Y, Lyness JM, Duberstein P, et al. Completed suicide among older patients in primary care practices: a controlled study. *J Am Geriatr Soc.* 2000;48(1):23–29
6. Doshi A, Boudreaux ED, Wang N, Pelletier AJ, Camargo CA Jr. National study of US emergency department visits for attempted suicide and self-inflicted injury, 1997–2001. *Ann Emerg Med.* 2005;46(4):369–375
7. Gibb SJ, Beautrais AL, Fergusson DM. Mortality and further suicidal behaviour after an index suicide attempt: a 10-year study. *Aust N Z J Psychiatry.* 2005;39(1-2):95–100
8. Gould MS, Kalafat J, Harrismunfakh JL, Kleinman M. An evaluation of crisis hotline outcomes. Part 2: suicidal callers. *Suicide Life Threat Behav.* 2007;37(3):338–352
9. Gould MS, Munfakh JL, Kleinman M, Lake AM. National suicide prevention lifeline: enhancing mental health care for suicidal individuals and other people in crisis. *Suicide Life Threat Behav.* 2012;42(1):22–35
10. Harwitz D, Ravizza L. Suicide and depression. *Emerg Med Clin North Am.* 2000;18(2):263–271, ix
11. Hemelrijk E, van Ballegooijen W, Donker T, van Straten A, Kerkhof A. Internet-based screening for suicidal ideation in common mental disorders. *Crisis.* 2012;33(4):215–221
12. Kalafat J, Gould MS, Munfakh JL, Kleinman M. An evaluation of crisis hotline outcomes. Part 1: nonsuicidal crisis callers. *Suicide Life Threat Behav.* 2007;37(3):322–337
13. Naragon-Gainey K, Watson D. The anxiety disorders and suicidal ideation: accounting for comorbidity via underlying personality traits. *Psychol Med.* 2011;41(7):1437–1447
14. Posner K, Brown GK, Stanley B, et al. The Columbia-Suicide Severity Rating Scale: initial validity and internal consistency findings from three multisite studies with adolescents and adults. *Am J Psychiatry.* 2011;168(12):1266–1277
15. Suominen K, Isometsa E, Haukka J, Lonnqvist J. Substance use and male gender as risk factors for deaths and suicide—a 5-year follow-up study after deliberate self-harm. *Soc Psychiatry Psychiatr Epidemiol.* 2004;39(9):720–724
16. Suominen K, Isometsa E, Ostamo A, Lonnqvist J. Level of suicidal intent predicts overall mortality and suicide after attempted suicide: a 12-year follow-up study. *BMC Psychiatry.* 2004;4:11
17. Szewczyk M, Chennault SA. Women's health. Depression and related disorders. *Prim Care.* 1997;24(1):83–101
18. Ting SA, Sullivan AF, Boudreaux ED, Miller I, Camargo CA Jr. Trends in US emergency department visits for attempted suicide and self-inflicted injury, 1993–2008. *Gen Hosp Psychiatry.* 2012;34(5):557–565
19. US Preventive Services Task Force. Screening for suicide risk. In: *Guide to Clinical Preventive Services.* 2nd ed. Alexandria, VA: International Medical Publishing, Inc; 1996:547–554
20. Wiebe DJ. Homicide and suicide risks associated with firearms in the home: a national case-control study. *Ann Emerg Med.* 2003;41(6):771–782

Sunburn

1. Cokkinides V, Weinstock M, Lazovich D, Ward E, Thun M. Indoor tanning use among adolescents in the US, 1998 to 2004. *Cancer.* 2009;115(1):190–198
2. Debuys HV, Levy SB, Murray JC, Madey DL, Pinnell SR. Modern approaches to photoprotection. *Dermatol Clin.* 2000;18(4):577–590
3. Duteil L, Queille-Roussel C, Lorenz B, Thieroff-Ekerdt R, Ortonne JP. A randomized, controlled trial of the safety and efficacy of topical corticosteroid treatments of sunburn in healthy volunteers. *Clin Exp Dermatol.* 2002;27(4):314–318
4. Eberlein-Konig B, Placzek M, Przybilla B. Protective effect against sunburn of combined systemic ascorbic acid (vitamin C) and d-alpha-tocopherol (vitamin E). *J Am Acad Dermatol.* 1998;38(1):45–48
5. Elliott B, Silverman PR. Keratoconjunctivitis caused by a broken high-intensity mercury-vapor lamp. *Del Med J.* 1986;58(10):665–667
6. Hatch KL, Osterwalder U. Garments as solar ultraviolet radiation screening materials. *Dermatol Clin.* 2006;24(1):85–100
7. Kirschke DL, Jones TF, Smith NM, Schaffner W. Photokeratitis and UV-radiation burns associated with damaged metal halide lamps. *Arch Pediatr Adolesc Med.* 2004;158(4):372–376
8. Kullavanijaya P, Lim HW. Photoprotection. *J Am Acad Dermatol.* 2005;52(6):937–962
9. Lim HW, Cooper K. The health impact of solar radiation and prevention strategies: report of the Environment Council, American Academy of Dermatology. *J Am Acad Dermatol.* 1999;41(1):81–99
10. Lincoln EA. Sun-induced skin changes. *Prim Care.* 2000;27(2):435–445
11. Lowe NJ. An overview of ultraviolet radiation, sunscreens, and photo-induced dermatoses. *Dermatol Clin.* 2006;24(1):9–17
12. Lucas R, McMichael T, Smith W, Armstrong B. *Solar Ultraviolet Radiation: Global Burden of Disease From Solar Ultraviolet Radiation.* Environmental Burden of Disease Series, No. 13. Prüss-Üstün A, Zeeb H, Mathers C, Repacholi M, eds. Geneva, Switzerland: World Health Organization; 2006. http://www.who.int/uv/health/solaruvradfull_180706.pdf?ua=1. Accessed June 7, 2018
13. Morgan ED, Bledsoe SC, Barker J. Ambulatory management of burns. *Am Fam Physician.* 2000;62(9):2015–2032
14. Olson AL, Starr P. The challenge of intentional tanning in teens and young adults. *Dermatol Clin.* 2006;24(2):131–136, v
15. Prevention and treatment of sunburn. *Med Lett Drugs Ther.* 2004;46(1184):45–46

Sunburn (*continued*)

16. Reingold AL, Broome CV, Gaventa S, Hightower AW. Risk factors for menstrual toxic shock syndrome: results of a multistate case-control study. *Rev Infect Dis.* 1989;11(suppl 1):S35–S41; discussion S41–S42

17. Thun MJ, Altman R, Ellingson O, Mills LF, Talansky ML. Ocular complications of malfunctioning mercury vapor lamps. *Ann Ophthalmol.* 1982;14(11):1017–1020

18. Lucas R, McMichael T, Smith W, Armstrong B. Solar ultraviolet radiation: global burden of disease from solar ultraviolet radiation. Environmental Burden of Diseases Series, No. 13. Geneva, Switzerland: World Health Organization; 2006. http://www.who.int/uv/health/solaruvradfull_180706.pdf. Accessed June 25, 2018

Suture or Staple Questions

1. Dire DJ, Coppola M, Dwyer DA, Lorette JJ, Karr JL. Prospective evaluation of topical antibiotics for preventing infections in uncomplicated soft-tissue wounds repaired in the ED. *Acad Emerg Med.* 1995;2(1):4–10

2. Hollander JE, Singer AJ. Laceration management. *Ann Emerg Med.* 1999;34(3):356–367

3. Hollander JE, Singer AJ, Valentine SM, Shofer FS. Risk factors for infection in patients with traumatic lacerations. *Acad Emerg Med.* 2001;8(7):716–720

4. Karounis H, Gouin S, Eisman H, Chalut D, Pelletier H, Williams B. A randomized, controlled trial comparing long-term cosmetic outcomes of traumatic pediatric lacerations repaired with absorbable plain gut versus nonabsorbable nylon sutures. *Acad Emerg Med.* 2004;11(7):730–735

5. Kaye ET. Topical antibacterial agents. *Infect Dis Clin North Am.* 2000;14(2):321–339

6. Khoosal D, Goldman RD. Vitamin E for treating children's scars. Does it help reduce scarring? *Can Fam Physician.* 2006;52(7):855–856

7. Pearson AS, Wolford RW. Management of skin trauma. *Prim Care.* 2000;27(2):475–492

8. Singer AJ, Dagum AB. Current management of acute cutaneous wounds. *N Engl J Med.* 2008;359(10):1037–1046

9. Thomsen TW, Barclay DA, Setnik GS. Videos in clinical medicine. Basic laceration repair. *N Engl J Med.* 2006;355(17):e18

Tick Bite

1. Edlow JA. Lyme disease and related tick-borne illnesses. *Ann Emerg Med.* 1999;33(6):680–693

2. Koren G, Matsui D, Bailey B. DEET-based insect repellants: safety implications for children and pregnant and lactating women. *CMAJ.* 2003;169(3):209–212

3. Lane RS. Treatment of clothing with a permethrin spray for personal protection against the western black-legged tick, Ixodes pacificus (Acari: Ixodidae). *Exp Appl Acarol.* 1989;6(4):343–352

4. Mutebi JP, Hawley WA, Brogdon WG. Travelers' health. Chapter 2: the pre-travel consultation. Counseling and advice for travelers. Protection against mosquitoes, ticks, and other arthropods. Centers for Disease Control and Prevention Web site. https://wwwnc.cdc.gov/travel/yellowbook/2018/the-pre-travel-consultation/protection-against-mosquitoes-ticks-other-arthropods. Updated May 31, 2017. Accessed June 7, 2018

5. Nadelman RB, Nowakowski J, Fish D, et al. Prophylaxis with single-dose doxycycline for the prevention of Lyme disease after an ixodes scapularis tick bite. *N Engl J Med.* 2001;345(2):79–84

6. Nadelman RB, Nowakowski J, Forseter G, et al. The clinical spectrum of early Lyme borreliosis in patients with culture-confirmed erythema migrans. *Am J Med.* 1996;100(5):502–508

7. Needham GR. Evaluation of five popular methods for tick removal. *Pediatrics.* 1985;75(6):997–1002

8. Ozuah PO. Tick removal. *Pediatr Rev.* 1998;19(8):280

9. Shapiro ED. Doxycycline for tick bites–not for everyone. *N Engl J Med.* 2001;345(2):133–134

10. Steere AC. Lyme disease. *N Engl J Med.* 2001;345(2):115–125

11. Tibbles CD, Edlow JA. Does this patient have erythema migrans? *JAMA.* 2007;297(23):2617–2627

12. US Environmental Protection Agency. Pesticides. https://www.epa.gov/pesticides. Updated May 29, 2018. Accessed June 7, 2018

13. Warshafsky S, Nowakowski J, Nadelman RB, Kamer RS, Peterson SJ, Wormser GP. Efficacy of antibiotic prophylaxis for prevention of Lyme disease. *J Gen Intern Med.* 1996;11(6):329–333

14. Wormser GP, Dattwyler RJ, Shapiro ED, et al. The clinical assessment, treatment, and prevention of Lyme disease, human granulocytic anaplasmosis, and babesiosis: clinical practice guidelines by the Infectious Diseases Society of America. *Clin Infect Dis.* 2006;43(9):1089–1134

15. Wormser GP, Nadelman RB, Dattwyler RJ, et al. Practice guidelines for the treatment of Lyme disease. *Clin Infect Dis.* 2000;31(1 suppl):1–14

Toe Injury

1. American Heart Association. 2005 Guidelines for Cardiopulmonary Resuscitation and Emergency Cardiovascular Care. Part 10: First Aid. *Circulation.* 2005;112:IV-196–IV-203

2. Clanton TO, Porter DA. Primary care of foot and ankle injuries in the athlete. *Clin Sports Med.* 1997;16(3):435–466

3. Collins NC. Is ice right? Does cryotherapy improve outcome for acute soft tissue injury? *Emerg Med J.* 2008;25(2):65–68

4. Kretsinger K, Broder KR, Cortese MM, et al; Centers for Disease Control and Prevention; Advisory Committee on Immunization Practices; Healthcare Infection Control Practices Advisory Committee. Preventing tetanus, diphtheria, and pertussis among adults: use of tetanus toxoid, reduced diphtheria toxoid and acellular pertussis vaccine recommendations of the Advisory Committee on Immunization Practices (ACIP) and recommendation of ACIP, supported by the Healthcare Infection Control Practices Advisory Committee (HICPAC), for use of Tdap among health-care personnel. *MMWR Recomm Rep.* 2006;55(RR-17):1–37

5. Lavery LA, Armstrong DG, Wunderlich RP, Mohler MJ, Wendel CS, Lipsky BA. Risk factors for foot infections in individuals with diabetes. *Diabetes Care.* 2006;29(6):1288–1293

6. Markenson D, Ferguson JD, Chameides L, et al. 2010 American Heart Association and American Red Cross Guidelines for First Aid. Part 17: First Aid. *Circulation.* 2010;122(18 suppl 3):S934–S946

7. Singer AJ, Dagum AB. Current management of acute cutaneous wounds. *N Engl J Med.* 2008;359(10):1037–1046

8. Wedmore I, Charette J. Emergency department evaluation and treatment of ankle and foot injuries. *Emerg Med Clin North Am.* 2000;18(1):85–113, vi

Tooth Injury

1. American Academy of Pediatric Dentistry. Guideline on management of acute dental trauma. http://www.aapd.org/media/policies_guidelines/g_trauma.pdf. Adopted 2001. Revised 2011. Accessed June 25, 2018

2. American Heart Association. 2005 Guidelines for Cardiopulmonary Resuscitation and Emergency Cardiovascular Care. Part 10: First Aid. *Circulation.* 2005;112:IV-196–IV-203

3. Andreasen JO, Andreasen FM, Skeie A, Hjorting–Hansen E, Schwartz O. Effect of treatment delay upon pulp and periodontal healing of traumatic dental injuries—a review article. *Dent Traumatol.* 2002;18(3):116–128

4. Andreasen JO, Borum MK, Jacobsen HL, Andreasen FM. Replantation of 400 avulsed permanent incisors. 4. Factors related to periodontal ligament healing. *Endod Dent Traumatol.* 1995;11(2):76–89

5. Camp JH, Stewart C. Dental trauma: diagnostic considerations, emergency procedures, and definitive management. *Emerg Med Reports.* 1995;16(9)

6. Dale RA. Dentoalveolar trauma. *Emerg Med Clin North Am.* 2000;18(3):521–538

7. Douglass AB, Douglass JM. Common dental emergencies. *Am Fam Physician.* 2003;67(3):511–516

8. Layug ML. Interim storage of avulsed permanent teeth. *J Can Dent Assoc.* 1998;64(5):357–363, 365–369

9. McTigue DJ. Diagnosis and management of dental injuries in children. *Pediatr Clin North Am.* 2000;47(5):1067–1084

10. Singer AJ, Dagum AB. Current management of acute cutaneous wounds. *N Engl J Med.* 2008;359(10):1037–1046

Toothache

1. Annino DJ Jr, Goguen LA. Pain from the oral cavity. *Otolaryngol Clin North Am.* 2003;36(6):1127–1135, vi–vii
2. Douglass AB, Douglass JM. Common dental emergencies. *Am Fam Physician.* 2003;67(3):511–516
3. Flynn TR. The swollen face. Severe odontogenic infections. *Emerg Med Clin North Am.* 2000;18(3):481–519
4. Ma M, Lindsell CJ, Jauch ED, Pancioli AM. Effect of education and guidelines for treatment of uncomplicated dental pain on patient provider behavior. *Ann Emerg Med.* 2004;44(4):323–329
5. MacDonald DE. Principles of geriatric dentistry and their application to the older adult with a physical disability. *Clin Geriatr Med.* 2006;22(2):413–434, x
6. Nguyen DH, Martin JT. Common dental infections in the primary care setting. *Am Fam Physician.* 2008;77(6):797–802

Urinalysis Results Follow-up Call

1. Bent S, Nallamothu BK, Simel DL, Fihn SD, Saint S. Does this woman have an acute uncomplicated urinary tract infection? *JAMA.* 2002;287(20):2701–2710
2. Bent S, Saint S. The optimal use of diagnostic testing in women with acute uncomplicated cystitis. *Am J Med.* 2002;113(1 suppl 1):20S–28S
3. Bollestad M, Grude N, Lindbaek M. A randomized controlled trial of a diagnostic algorithm for symptoms of uncomplicated cystitis at an out-of-hours service. *Scand J Prim Health Care.* 2015;33(2):57–64
4. Campbell J, Felver M, Kamarei S. 'Telephone treatment' of uncomplicated acute cystitis. *Cleve Clin J Med.* 1999;66(8):495–501
5. Di Martino P, Agniel R, David K, et al. Reduction of Escherichia coli adherence to uroepithelial bladder cells after consumption of cranberry juice: a double-blind randomized placebo-controlled cross-over trial. *World J Urol.* 2006;24(1):21–27
6. Gupta K, Hooton TM, Naber KG, et al; Infectious Diseases Society of America; European Society for Microbiology and Infectious Diseases. International clinical practice guidelines for the treatment of acute uncomplicated cystitis and pyelonephritis in women: a 2010 update by the Infectious Diseases Society of America and the European Society for Microbiology and Infectious Diseases. *Clin Infect Dis.* 2011;52(5):e103–e120
7. Haber SL, Cauthon KA, Raney EC. Cranberry and warfarin interaction: a case report and review of the literature. *Consult Pharm.* 2012;27(1):58–65
8. Hooton TM, Winter C, Tiu F, Stamm WE. Randomized comparative trial and cost analysis of 3-day antimicrobial regimens for treatment of acute cystitis in women. *JAMA.* 1995;273(1):41–45
9. Huppert JS, Biro F, Lan D, Mortensen JE, Reed J, Slap GB. Urinary symptoms in adolescent females: STI or UTI? *J Adolesc Health.* 2007;40(5):418–424
10. Jepson RG, Craig J. Cranberries for preventing urinary tract infections. *Cochrane Database Syst Rev.* 2008;(1):CD001321
11. Jepson RG, Mihaljevic L, Craig J. Cranberries for treating urinary tract infections. *Cochrane Database Syst Rev.* 2000;(2):CD001322
12. Lammers RL, Gibson S, Kovacs D, Sears W, Strachan G. Comparison of test characteristics of urine dipstick and urinalysis at various test cutoff points. *Ann Emerg Med.* 2001;38(5):505–512
13. Patel HP. The abnormal urinalysis. *Pediatr Clin North Am.* 2006;53(3):325–337, v
14. Saint S, Scholes D, Fihn SD, Farrell RG, Stamm WE. The effectiveness of a clinical practice guideline for the management of presumed uncomplicated urinary tract infection in women. *Am J Med.* 1999;106(6):636–641
15. Schauberger CW, Merkitch KW, Prell AM. Acute cystitis in women: experience with a telephone-based algorithm. *WMJ.* 2007;106(6):326–329
16. Schwartz DS, Barone JE. Correlation of urinalysis and dipstick results with catheter-associated urinary tract infections in surgical ICU patients. *Intensive Care Med.* 2006;32(11):1797–1801
17. Simerville JA, Maxted WC, Pahira JJ. Urinalysis: a comprehensive review. *Am Fam Physician.* 2005;71(6):1153–1162
18. Warren JW, Abrutyn E, Hebel JR, Johnson JR, Schaeffer AJ, Stamm WE. Guidelines for antimicrobial treatment of uncomplicated acute bacterial cystitis and acute pyelonephritis in women. Infectious Diseases Society of America (IDSA). *Clin Infect Dis.* 1999;29(4):745–758

Urination Pain (Female)

1. Avorn J, Monane M, Gurwitz JH, Glynn RJ, Choodnovskiy I, Lipsitz LA. Reduction of bacteriuria and pyuria after ingestion of cranberry juice. *JAMA.*1994;71(10):751–754
2. Bass PF III, Jarvis JA, Mitchell CK. Urinary tract infections. *Prim Care.* 2003;30(1):41–61, v–vi
3. Bent S, Nallamothu BK, Simel DL, Fihn SD, Saint S. Does this woman have an acute uncomplicated urinary tract infection? *JAMA.* 2002;287(20):2701–2710
4. Bent S, Saint S. The optimal use of diagnostic testing in women with acute uncomplicated cystitis. *Am J Med.* 2002;113(1 suppl 1):20S–28S
5. Bollestad M, Grude N, Lindbaek M. A randomized controlled trial of a diagnostic algorithm for symptoms of uncomplicated cystitis at an out-of-hours service. *Scand J Prim Health Care.* 2015;33(2):57–64
6. Di Martino P, Agniel R, David K, et al. Reduction of Escherichia coli adherence to uroepithelial bladder cells after consumption of cranberry juice: a double-blind randomized placebo-controlled cross-over trial. *World J Urol.* 2006;24(1):21–27
7. Gupta K, Hooton TM, Naber KG, et al; Infectious Diseases Society of America; European Society for Microbiology and Infectious Diseases. International clinical practice guidelines for the treatment of acute uncomplicated cystitis and pyelonephritis in women: a 2010 update by the Infectious Diseases Society of America and the European Society for Microbiology and Infectious Diseases. *Clin Infect Dis.* 2011;52(5):e103–e120
8. Gupta K, Scholes D, Stamm WE. Increasing prevalence of anti-microbial resistance among uropathogens causing uncomplicated cystitis in women. *JAMA.* 1999;281(8):736–738
9. Gupta P. Randomized, controlled study comparing sitz-bath and no-sitz-bath treatments in patients with acute anal fissures. *ANZ J Surg.* 2006;76(8):718–721
10. Haber SL, Cauthon KA, Raney EC. Cranberry and warfarin interaction: a case report and review of the literature. *Consult Pharm.* 2012;27(1):58–65
11. Hooton TM, Winter C, Tiu F, Stamm WE. Randomized comparative trial and cost analysis of 3-day antimicrobial regimens for treatment of acute cystitis in women. *JAMA.* 1995;273(1):41–45
12. Hsu KF, Chia JS, Jao SW, et al. Comparison of clinical effects between warm water spray and sitz bath in post-hemorrhoidectomy period. *J Gastrointest Surg.* 2009;13(7):1274–1278
13. Huppert JS, Biro F, Lan D, Mortensen JE, Reed J, Slap GB. Urinary symptoms in adolescent females: STI or UTI? *J Adolesc Health.* 2007;40(5):418–424
14. Jepson RG, Craig J. Cranberries for preventing urinary tract infections. *Cochrane Database Syst Rev.* 2008;(1):CD001321
15. Jepson RG, Mihaljevic L, Craig J. Cranberries for treating urinary tract infections. *Cochrane Database Syst Rev.* 2000;(2):CD001322
16. Llenderrozos HJ. Urinary tract infections: management rationale for uncomplicated cystitis. *Clin Fam Pract.* 2004;6(1):157–173
17. McLaughlin SP, Carson CC. Urinary tract infections in women. *Med Clin North Am.* 2004;88(2):417–429
18. Patel HP. The abnormal urinalysis. *Pediatr Clin North Am.* 2006;53(3):325–337, v
19. Simerville JA, Maxted WC, Pahira JJ. Urinalysis: a comprehensive *review.* *Am Fam Physician.* 2005;71(6):1153–1162
20. Stapleton A. Urinary tract infections in patients with diabetes. *Am J Med.* 2002;113(1 suppl 1):80S–84S
21. Tejirian T, Abbas MA. Sitz bath: where is the evidence? Scientific basis of a common practice. *Dis Colon Rectum.* 2005;48(12):2336–2340
22. Workowski KA, Berman S; Centers for Disease Control and Prevention. Sexually transmitted diseases treatment guidelines, 2010 [published correction appears in *MMWR Recomm Rep.* 2011;60(1):18]. *MMWR Recomm Rep.* 2010;59(RR-12):1–110
23. Yoshikawa TT, Nicolle LE, Norman DC. Management of complicated urinary tract infection in older patients. *J Am Geriatr Soc.* 1996;44(10):1235–1241

Urination Pain (Male)

1. Bass PF III, Jarvis JA, Mitchell CK. Urinary tract infections. *Prim Care.* 2003;30(1):41–61, v–vi
2. Bollestad M, Grude N, Lindbaek M. A randomized controlled trial of a diagnostic algorithm for symptoms of uncomplicated cystitis at an out-of-hours service. *Scand J Prim Health Care.* 2015;33(2):57–64
3. Burgher SW. Acute scrotal pain. *Emerg Med Clin North Am.* 1998;16(4):781–809, vi
4. Gupta K, Hooton TM, Naber KG, et al; Infectious Diseases Society of America; European Society for Microbiology and Infectious Diseases. International clinical practice guidelines for the treatment of acute uncomplicated cystitis and pyelonephritis in women: a 2010 update by the Infectious Diseases Society of America and the European Society for Microbiology and Infectious Diseases. *Clin Infect Dis.* 2011;52(5):e103–e120
5. Roberts RG, Hartlaub PP. Evaluation of dysuria in men. *Am Fam Physician.* 1999;60(3):865–872
6. Stapleton A. Urinary tract infections in patients with diabetes. *Am J Med.* 2002;113(1 suppl 1):80S–84S
7. Vilke GM, Ufberg JW, Harrigan RA, Chan TC. Evaluation and treatment of acute urinary retention. *J Emerg Med.* 2008;35(2):193–198
8. Workowski KA, Berman S; Centers for Disease Control and Prevention. Sexually transmitted diseases treatment guidelines, 2010 [published correction appears in *MMWR Recomm Rep.* 2011;60(1):18]. *MMWR Recomm Rep.* 2010;59(RR-12):1–110
9. Yoshikawa TT, Nicolle LE, Norman DC. Management of complicated urinary tract infection in older patients. *J Am Geriatr Soc.* 1996;44(10):1235–1241

Urine, Blood In

1. Ahmed Z, Lee J. Asymptomatic urinary abnormalities. Hematuria and proteinuria. *Med Clin North Am.* 1997;81(3):641–652
2. Bass PF, Jarvis JA, Mitchell CK. Urinary tract infections. *Prim Care.* 2003;30(1):41–61, v–vi
3. Eikelboom JW, Wallentin L, Connolly SJ, et al. Risk of bleeding with 2 doses of dabigatran compared with warfarin in older and younger patients with atrial fibrillation. *Circulation.* 2011;123(21):2363–2372
4. Mishriki SF, Vint R, Somani BK. Half of visible and half of recurrent visible hematuria cases have underlying pathology: prospective large cohort study with long-term followup. *J Urol.* 2012;187(5):1561–1565
5. Pranikoff K. Urologic care in long-term facilities. *Urol Clin North Am.* 1996;23(1):137–146
6. Vasdev N, Kumar A, Veeratterapillay R, Thorpe AC. Hematuria secondary to benign prostatic hyperplasia: retrospective analysis of 166 men identified in a single one-stop hematuria clinic. *Curr Urol.* 2013;6(3):146–149

Vaginal Bleeding, Abnormal

1. Albers JR, Hull SK, Wesley RM. Abnormal uterine bleeding. *Am Fam Physician.* 2004;69(8):1915–1926
2. American College of Emergency Physicians. Clinical policy for the initial approach to patients presenting with a chief complaint of vaginal bleeding. *Ann Emerg Med.* 1997;29(3):435–458
3. American College of Obstetricians and Gynecologists Committee on Practice Bulletins. ACOG practice bulletin: management of anovulatory bleeding. *Int J Gynaecol Obstet.* 2001;72(3):263–271
4. Brenner PF. Differential diagnosis of abnormal uterine bleeding. *Am J Obstet Gynecol.* 1996;175(3 suppl 2):766–769
5. Brill SR, Rosenfeld WD. Contraception. *Med Clin North Am.* 2000;84(4):907–925
6. Burkman RT. The transdermal contraceptive system. *Am J Obstet Gynecol.* 2004;190(4 suppl):S49–S53
7. Casablanca Y. Management of dysfunctional uterine bleeding. *Obstet Gynecol Clin North Am.* 2008;35(2):219–234, viii
8. Daniels RV, McCusky C. Abnormal vaginal bleeding in the non-pregnant patient. *Emerg Med Clin North Am.* 2003;21(3):751–772
9. Dawood MY. Primary dysmenorrhea: advances in pathogenesis and management. *Obstet Gynecol.* 2006;108(2):428–441

10. Eikelboom JW, Wallentin L, Connolly SJ, et al. Risk of bleeding with 2 doses of dabigatran compared with warfarin in older and younger patients with atrial fibrillation: an analysis of the randomized evaluation of long-term anticoagulant therapy (RE-LY) trial. *Circulation.* 2011;123(21):2363–2372
11. Espey E, Ogburn T, Fotieo D. Contraception: what every internist should know. *Med Clin North Am.* 2008;92(5):1037–1058, ix–x
12. Farrell E. Dysfunctional uterine bleeding. *Aust Fam Physician.* 2004;33(11):906–908
13. Lethaby A, Augood C, Duckitt K, Farquhar C. Nonsteroidal anti-inflammatory drugs for heavy menstrual bleeding. *Cochrane Database Syst Rev.* 2007;(4):CD000400
14. Mansfield PK, Voda A, Allison G. Validating a pencil-and-paper measure of perimenopausal menstrual blood loss. *Womens Health Issues.* 2004;14(6):242–247
15. McGee S, Abernethy WB III, Simel DL. The rational clinical examination. Is this patient hypovolemic? *JAMA.* 1999;281(11):1022–1029
16. Minjarez DA, Bradshaw KD. Abnormal uterine bleeding in adolescents. *Obstet Gynecol Clin North Am.* 2000;27(1):63–78
17. Mosher WD, Jones J. Use of contraception in the United States: 1982–2008. *Vital Health Stat 23.* 2010;(29):1–44
18. Santer M, Wyke S, Warner P. What aspects of periods are most bothersome for women reporting heavy menstrual bleeding? Community survey and qualitative study. *BMC Womens Health.* 2007;7:8
19. Shapley M, Jordan J, Croft PR. A systematic review of postcoital bleeding and risk of cervical cancer. *Br J Gen Pract.* 2006;56(527):453–460
20. Sinert R, Spektor M. Evidence-based emergency medicine/rational clinical examination abstract. Clinical assessment of hypovolemia. *Ann Emerg Med.* 2005;45(3):327–329
21. Swica Y. The transdermal patch and the vaginal ring: two novel methods of combined hormonal contraception. *Obstet Gynecol Clin North Am.* 2007;34(1):31–42, viii
22. Telner DE, Jakubovicz D. Approach to diagnosis and management of abnormal uterine bleeding. *Can Fam Physician.* 2007;53(1):58–64
23. Victor I, Fink RA. Comparing patient telephone callback rates for different hormonal birth control delivery systems. *Am J Ther.* 2006;13(6):507–512
24. Warner PE, Critchley HO, Lumsden MA, Campbell-Brown M, Douglas A, Murray GD. Menorrhagia I: measured blood loss, clinical features, and outcome in women with heavy periods: a survey with follow-up data. *Am J Obstet Gynecol.* 2004;190(5):1216–1223
25. Warner PE, Critchley HO, Lumsden MA, Campbell-Brown M, Douglas A, Murray GD. Menorrhagia II: is the 80-mL blood loss criterion useful in management of complaint of menorrhagia? *Am J Obstet Gynecol.* 2004;190(5):1224–1229

Vaginal Discharge

1. ACOG Committee on Practice Bulletins—Gynecology. ACOG Practice Bulletin. Clinical management guidelines for obstetrician-gynecologists, Number 72, May 2006: Vaginitis. *Obstet Gynecol.* 2006;107(5):1195–1206
2. Allen-Davis JT, Beck A, Parker R, Ellis JL, Polley D. Assessment of vulvovaginal complaints: accuracy of telephone triage and in-office diagnosis. *Obstet Gynecol.* 2002;99(1):18–22
3. Eckert LO. Clinical practice. Acute vulvovaginitis. *N Engl J Med.* 2006;355(12):1244–1252
4. Egan ME, Lipsky MS. Diagnosis of vaginitis. *Am Fam Physician.* 2000;62(5):1095–1104
5. Forhan SE, Gottlieb SL, Sternberg MR, et al. Prevalence of sexually transmitted infections among female adolescents aged 14 to 19 in the United States. *Pediatrics.* 2009;124(6):1505–1512
6. Goldenberg RL, Andrews WW, Yuan AC, MacKay HT, St Louis ME. Sexually transmitted diseases and adverse outcomes of pregnancy. *Clin Perinatol.* 1997;24(1):23–41
7. Johnson E, Berwald N. Evidence-based emergency medicine/rational clinical examination abstract. Diagnostic utility of physical examination, history, and laboratory evaluation in emergency department patients with vaginal complaints. *Ann Emerg Med.* 2008;52(3):294–297
8. McAnena L, Knowles SJ, Curry A, Cassidy L. Prevalence of gonococcal conjunctivitis in adults and neonates. *Eye (Lond).* 2015;29(7):875–880

9. Miller KE. Women's health. Sexually transmitted diseases. *Prim Care.* 1997;24(1):179–193

10. Oduyebo OO, Anorlu RI, Ogunsola FT. The effects of antimicrobial therapy on bacterial vaginosis in non-pregnant women. *Cochrane Database Syst Rev.* 2009;(3):CD006055

11. Pogany L, Romanowski B, Robinson J, et al. Management of gonococcal infection among adults and youth: new key recommendations. *Can Fam Physician.* 2015;61(10):869–873, e451–e456

12. Public Health Agency of Canada. Primary care and sexually transmitted infections. In: *Canadian Guidelines on Sexually Transmitted Infections.* 2006 Edition. Ottawa, Ontario: Public Health Agency of Canada; 2006: 7–29. http://pubs.cpha.ca/PDF/P37/23384.pdf. Accessed June 7, 2018

13. Quan M. Vaginitis: diagnosis and management. *Postgrad Med.* 2010;122(6):117–127

14. Stewart C, Bosker G. Pelvic inflammatory disease (PID): diagnosis, disposition, and current antimicrobial guidelines. *Emerg Med Rep.* 1999;20(16):163–172

15. Van Vranken M. Prevention and treatment of sexually transmitted diseases: an update. *Am Fam Physician.* 2007;76(12):1827–1832

16. Workowski KA, Berman S; Centers for Disease Control and Prevention. Sexually transmitted diseases treatment guidelines, 2010 [published correction appears in *MMWR Recomm Rep.* 2011;60(1):18]. *MMWR Recomm Rep.* 2010;59(RR-12):1–110

Vomiting

1. Acheson DW, Fiore AE. Preventing foodborne disease—what clinicians can do. *N Engl J Med.* 2004;350(5):437–440

2. American Academy of Family Physicians. Information from your family doctor. Nausea and vomiting. *Am Fam Physician.* 2004;69(5):1176

3. Centers for Disease Control and Prevention. Diagnosis and management of foodborne illnesses: a primer for physicians. *MMWR Recomm Rep.* 2004;53(RR-4):1–33

4. Ebrahimi N, Maltepe C, Bournissen FG, Koren G. Nausea and vomiting of pregnancy: using the 24-hour Pregnancy-Unique Quantification of Emesis (PUQE-24) scale. *J Obstet Gynaecol Can.* 2009;31(9):803–807

5. Fisman D. Seasonality of viral infections: mechanisms and unknowns. *Clin Microbiol Infect.* 2012;18(10):946–954

6. Flasar MH, Cross R, Goldberg E. Acute abdominal pain. *Prim Care.* 2006;33(3):659–684, vi

7. Frese T, Klauss S, Herrmann K, Sandholzer H. Nausea and vomiting as the reasons for encounter in general practice. *J Clin Med Res.* 2011;3(1):23–29

8. Lal A, Hales S, French N, Baker MG. Seasonality in human zoonotic enteric diseases: a systematic review. *PLoS One.* 2012;7(4):e31883

9. Lichter I. Nausea and vomiting in patients with cancer. *Hematol Oncol Clin North Am.* 1996;10(1):207–220

10. Metz A, Hebbard G. Nausea and vomiting in adults—a diagnostic approach. *Aust Fam Physician.* 2007;36(9):688–692

11. Mines D, Stahmer S, Shepherd SM. Poisonings: food, fish, shellfish. *Emerg Med Clin North Am.* 1997;15(1):157–177

12. Montagnini ML, Moat ME. Non-pain symptom management in palliative care. *Clin Fam Pract.* 2004;6(2):395–422

13. Nee PA, Hadfield JM, Yates DW, Faragher EB. Significance of vomiting after head injury. *J Neurol Neurosurg Psychiatry.* 1999;66(4):470–473

14. Quigley EM, Hasler WL, Parkman HP. AGA technical review on nausea and vomiting. *Gastroenterology.* 2001;120(1):263–286

15. Sampson HA, Sicherer SH, Birnbaum AH. AGA technical review on the evaluation of food allergy in gastrointestinal disorders. *Gastroenterology.* 2001;120(4):1026–1040

16. Scorza K, Williams A, Phillips JD, Shaw J. Evaluation of nausea and vomiting. *Am Fam Physician.* 2007;76(1):76–84

17. Sinert R, Spektor M. Evidence-based emergency medicine/rational clinical examination abstract. Clinical assessment of hypovolemia. *Ann Emerg Med.* 2005;45(3):327–329

18. US Department of Health and Human Services, National Institutes of Health, National Cancer Institute. Common Terminology Criteria for Adverse Events (CTCAE), Version 4.0. European Organisation for Research and Treatment of Cancer Web site. https://www.eortc.be/services/doc/ctc/CTCAE_4.03_2010-06-14_QuickReference_5x7.pdf. Updated June 14, 2010. Accessed June 7, 2018

19. Williams KS. Postoperative nausea and vomiting. *Surg Clin North Am.* 2005;85(6):1229–1241, xi

Vulvar Symptoms

1. ACOG Committee on Practice Bulletins—Gynecology. ACOG Practice Bulletin. Clinical management guidelines for obstetrician-gynecologists, Number 72, May 2006: Vaginitis. *Obstet Gynecol.* 2006;107(5):1195–1206

2. Allen-Davis JT, Beck A, Parker R, Ellis JL, Polley D. Assessment of vulvo-vaginal complaints: accuracy of telephone triage and in-office diagnosis. *Obstet Gynecol.* 2002;99(1):18–22

3. Eckert LO. Clinical practice. Acute vulvovaginitis. *N Engl J Med.* 2006;355(12):1244–1252

4. Goldenberg RL, Andrews WW, Yuan AC, MacKay HT, St Louis ME. Sexually transmitted diseases and adverse outcomes of pregnancy. *Clin Perinatol.* 1997;24(1):23–41

5. Gupta P. Randomized, controlled study comparing sitz-bath and no-sitz-bath treatments in patients with acute anal fissures. *ANZ J Surg.* 2006;76(8):718–721

6. Haider Z, Condous G, Kirk E, Mukri F, Bourne T. The simple outpatient management of Bartholin's abscess using the Word catheter: a preliminary study. *Aust N Z J Obstet Gynaecol.* 2007;47(2):137–140

7. Hsu KF, Chia JS, Jao SW, et al. Comparison of clinical effects between warm water spray and sitz bath in post-hemorrhoidectomy period. *J Gastrointest Surg.* 2009;13(7):1274–1278

8. MacNeill C. Dyspareunia. *Obstet Gynecol Clin North Am.* 2006;33(4):565–577, viii

9. Margesson LJ. Vulvar disease pearls. *Dermatol Clin.* 2006;24(2):145–155, v

10. Miller KE. Women's health. Sexually transmitted diseases. *Prim Care.* 1997;24(1):179–193

11. Oduyebo OO, Anorlu RI, Ogunsola FT. The effects of antimicrobial therapy on bacterial vaginosis in non-pregnant women. *Cochrane Database Syst Rev.* 2009;(3):CD006055

12. Omole F, Simmons BJ, Hacker Y. Management of Bartholin's duct cyst and gland abscess. *Am Fam Physician.* 2003;68(1):135–140

13. Quan M. Vaginitis: diagnosis and management. *Postgrad Med.* 2010;122(6):117–127

14. Tejirian T, Abbas MA. Sitz bath: where is the evidence? Scientific basis of a common practice. *Dis Colon Rectum.* 2005;48(12):2336–2340

15. Van Vranken M. Prevention and treatment of sexually transmitted diseases: an update. *Am Fam Physician.* 2007;76(12):1827–1832

16. Workowski KA, Berman S; Centers for Disease Control and Prevention. Sexually transmitted diseases treatment guidelines, 2010 [published correction appears in *MMWR Recomm Rep.* 2011;60(1):18]. *MMWR Recomm Rep.* 2010;59(RR-12):1–110

Weakness (Generalized) and Fatigue

1. Goldman L, Kirtane AJ. Triage of patients with acute chest pain and possible cardiac ischemia: the elusive search for diagnostic perfection. *Ann Intern Med.* 2003;139(12):987–995

2. McGee S, Abernethy WB III, Simel DL. The rational clinical examination. Is this patient hypovolemic? *JAMA.* 1999;281(11):1022–1029

3. McSweeney JC, Cody M, O'Sullivan P, Elberson K, Moser DK, Garvin BJ. Women's early warning symptoms of acute myocardial infarction. *Circulation.* 2003;108(21):2619–2623

4. Morrison RE, Keating HJ III. Fatigue in primary care. *Obstet Gynecol Clin North Am.* 2001;28(2):225–240, v–vi

5. Paternostro-Sluga T, Grim-Stieger M, Posch M, et al. Reliability and validity of the Medical Research Council (MRC) scale and a modified scale for testing muscle strength in patients with radial palsy. *J Rehabil Med.* 2008;40(8):665–671

Weakness (Generalized) and Fatigue (*continued*)

6. Sinert R, Spektor M. Evidence-based emergency medicine/rational clinical examination abstract. Clinical assessment of hypovolemia. *Ann Emerg Med.* 2005;45(3):327–329
7. Tusa RJ. Dizziness. *Med Clin North Am.* 2003;87(3):609–641, vii
8. Vanpee G, Hermans G, Segers J, Gosselink R. Assessment of limb muscle strength in critically ill patients: a systematic review. *Crit Care Med.* 2014;42(3):701–711

Wound Infection

1. American Heart Association. 2005 Guidelines for Cardiopulmonary Resuscitation and Emergency Cardiovascular Care. Part 14: First aid. *Circulation.* 2005;112(24 suppl):IV-196–IV-203
2. Berger RS, Pappert AS, Van Zile PS, Cetnarowski WE. A newly formulated topical triple-antibiotic ointment minimizes scarring. *Cutis.* 2000;65(6):401–404
3. Cho CY, Lo JS. Dressing the part. *Dermatol Clin.* 1998;16(1):25–47
4. Degreef HJ. How to heal a wound fast. *Dermatol Clin.* 1998;16(2):365–375
5. Dire DJ, Coppola M, Dwyer DA, Lorette JJ, Karr JL. Prospective evaluation of topical antibiotics for preventing infections in uncomplicated soft-tissue wounds repaired in the ED. *Acad Emerg Med.* 1995;2(1):4–10
6. Frazee BW, Lynn J, Charlebois ED, Lambert L, Lowery D, Perdreau-Remington F. High prevalence of methicillin-resistant Staphylococcus aureus in emergency department skin and soft tissue infections. *Ann Emerg Med.* 2005;45(3):311–320
7. Fridkin SK, Hageman JC, Morrison M, et al. Methicillin-resistant Staphylococcus aureus disease in three communities. *N Eng J Med.* 2005;352(14):1436–1444
8. Gergen PJ, McQuillan GM, Kiely M, Ezzati-Rice TM, Sutter RW, Virella G. A population-based serologic survey of immunity to tetanus in the United States. *N Engl J Med.* 1995;332(12):761–766
9. Gorwitz RJ, Jernigan DB, Powers JH, Jernigan JA; Participants in the CDC-Convened Experts' Meeting on Management of MRSA in the Community. Strategies for clinical management of MRSA in the community: summary of an experts' meeting convened by the Centers for Disease Control and Prevention. 2006. http://www.cdc.gov/mrsa/pdf/MRSA-Strategies-ExpMtgSummary-2006.pdf. Accessed June 7, 2018
10. Gunderson CG. Cellulitis: definition, etiology, and clinical features. *Am J Med.* 2011;124(12):1113–1122
11. Hollander JE, Singer AJ, Valentine SM, Shofer FS. Risk factors for infection in patients with traumatic lacerations. *Acad Emerg Med.* 2001;8(7):716–720
12. Howell JM, Chisholm CD. Wound care. *Emerg Med Clin North Am.* 1997;15(2):417–425
13. Jones RN, Li Q, Kohut B, Biedenbach DJ, Bell J, Turnidge JD. Contemporary antimicrobial activity of triple antibiotic ointment: a multiphased study of recent clinical isolates in the United States and Australia. *Diagn Microbiol Infect Dis.* 2006;54(1):63–71
14. Kaye ET. Topical antibacterial agents. *Infect Dis Clin North Am.* 2000;14(2):321–339
15. Liu C, Bayer A, Cosgrove SE, et al. Clinical practice guidelines by the Infectious Diseases Society of America for the treatment of methicillin-resistant Staphylococcus aureus infections in adults and children: executive summary. *Clin Infect Dis.* 2011;52(3):285–292

16. Murphy TV, Slade BA, Broder KR, et al; Advisory Committee on Immunization Practices, Centers for Disease Control and Prevention. Prevention of pertussis, tetanus, and diphtheria among pregnant and postpartum women and their infants recommendations of the Advisory Committee on Immunization Practices (ACIP). *MMWR Recomm Rep.* 2008;57(RR-4):1–51
17. Nicolle L. Community-acquired MRSA: a practitioner's guide. *CMAJ.* 2006;175(2):145
18. Swartz MN. Clinical practice. Cellulitis. *N Engl J Med.* 2004;350(9):904–912

Zika Virus Exposure

1. Fauci AS, Morens DM. Zika virus in the Americas—yet another arbovirus threat. *N Engl J Med.* 2016;374(7):601–604
2. Hills SL, Russell K, Hennessey M, et al. Transmission of Zika virus through sexual contact with travelers to areas of ongoing transmission—continental United States, 2016. *MMWR Morb Mortal Wkly Rep.* 2016;65(8):215–216
3. Oduyebo T, Petersen EE, Rasmussen SA, et al. Update: interim guidelines for health care providers caring for pregnant women and women of reproductive age with possible Zika virus exposure—United States, 2016. *MMWR Morb Mortal Wkly Rep.* 2016;65(5):122–127
4. Oster AM, Brooks JT, Stryker JE, et al. Interim guidelines for prevention of sexual transmission of Zika virus—United States, 2016. *MMWR Morb Mortal Wkly Rep.* 2016;65(5):120–121
5. Paixão ES, Barreto F, Teixeira Mda G, Costa Mda C, Rodrigues LC. History, epidemiology, and clinical manifestations of Zika: a systematic review. *Am J Public Health.* 2016;106(4):606–612
6. Petersen EE, Polen KN, Meaney-Delman D, et al. Update: interim guidance for health care providers caring for women of reproductive age with possible Zika virus exposure—United States, 2016. *MMWR Morb Mortal Wkly Rep.* 2016;65(12):315–322
7. Petersen EE, Staples JE, Meaney-Delman D, et al. Interim guidelines for pregnant women during a Zika virus outbreak—United States, 2016. *MMWR Morb Mortal Wkly Rep.* 2016;65(2):30–33
8. Rodriguez SD, Drake LL, Price DP, Hammond JI, Hansen IA. The efficacy of some commercially available insect repellents for Aedes aegypti (Diptera: Culicidae) and Aedes albopictus (Diptera: Culicidae). *J Insect Sci.* 2015;15:140
9. Schuler-Faccini L, Ribeiro EM, Feitosa IM, et al. Possible association between Zika virus infection and microcephaly—Brazil, 2015. *MMWR Morb Mortal Wkly Rep.* 2016;65(3):59–62

Appendix I

Over-the-Counter Medications

- Dosages for a number of commonly used over-the-counter (OTC) medications are included in this book.

- These OTC medications should not be recommended by the office triager unless this listing has been **reviewed, amended as necessary, and approved** by the supervising physician or office medical director.

- Concise and limited information for these OTC medications is provided in this book. The triager is strongly encouraged to read the *Physicians' Desk Reference for Nonprescription Drugs* or other trustworthy drug reference for all OTC medications that the triager recommends to patients.

- Patients should be instructed to **read the package warnings and instructions** on all OTC medications that they take.

Abrasions, Scratches, and Minor Cuts

Adult OTC Drug Dosage Table

Wound Care—Abrasions (Scrapes), Scratches, and Minor Cuts

Medication	Dosage	Notes
Antibiotic Ointment Bacitracin Neosporin Polysporin (bacitracin and polymyxin B) Triple Antibiotic (bacitracin, neomycin, and polymixin B)	Use after cleaning the wound. Apply ointment BID-TID.	**Caution:** Stop ointment if a rash or allergic reaction occurs.
Liquid Skin Bandage Band-Aid Liquid Bandage New-Skin Curad Spray Bandage 3M No Sting Liquid Bandage Spray	Use after cleaning the wound. Needs to be applied only once.	This is an alternative to antibiotic ointment and a regular bandage (e.g., gauze dressing or Band-Aid).

Important Notice

- These OTC (over-the-counter) medications should not be recommended by the telephone triager unless this listing has been reviewed, amended as necessary, and approved by the supervising physician, office medical director, or call center medical director.
- Concise and limited information for these OTC medications is provided in these tables. The triager is strongly encouraged to read the *Physicians' Desk Reference for Nonprescription Drugs* or other trustworthy drug reference for all OTC medications that the triager recommends to patients. Extensive drug information is available at the National Library of Medicine drug information Web site (MedlinePlus).
- Patients should be instructed to read the package warnings and instructions on all OTC medications that they take.

Acid Indigestion, Heartburn, and Sour Stomach

Adult OTC Drug Dosage Table

Treatment of Acid Indigestion, Heartburn, and Sour Stomach

Medication	Dosage	Notes
Antacids Maalox Mylanta Rolaids Tums	**Liquid and Tablets** Read package instructions.	**Caution:** There are other serious causes of epigastric discomfort, including: myocardial infarction and gallstones.
H$_2$ Blocker—Ranitidine Zantac	75-mg tablets 75 mg once or twice daily	**Caution:** There are other serious causes of epigastric discomfort, including: myocardial infarction and gallstones.

Important Notice
- These OTC (over-the-counter) medications should not be recommended by the telephone triager unless this listing has been reviewed, amended as necessary, and approved by the supervising physician, office medical director, or call center medical director.
- Concise and limited information for these OTC medications is provided in these tables. The triager is strongly encouraged to read the *Physicians' Desk Reference for Nonprescription Drugs* or other trustworthy drug reference for all OTC medications that the triager recommends to patients. Extensive drug information is available at the National Library of Medicine drug information Web site (MedlinePlus).
- Patients should be instructed to read the package warnings and instructions on all OTC medications that they take.

Athlete's Foot

Adult OTC Drug Dosage Table

Treatment of Athlete's Foot (Tinea Pedis)

Medication	Dosage	Notes
Antifungal Cream— Terbinafine Lamisil AT **Antifungal Cream— Clotrimazole** Lotrimin AF **Antifungal Cream— Miconazole** Micatin Monistat Derm	Apply cream 2 times per day to the affected areas of the feet. Continue the cream for at least 7 days after the rash is cleared.	**Keep the Feet Clean and Dry:** Wash the feet 2 times every day. Dry the feet completely, especially between the toes. You can use a blow dryer set on the cool setting or you can gently pat the area dry with a towel. After drying your feet, then apply the cream. Wear clean socks and change them twice daily. Terbinafine (Lamisil AT) is most recommended but is not available in Canada. **Expected Course:** With proper treatment, athlete's foot should decrease substantially within 1 week and disappear within 2-3 weeks.

Important Notice

- These OTC (over-the-counter) medications should not be recommended by the telephone triager unless this listing has been reviewed, amended as necessary, and approved by the supervising physician, office medical director, or call center medical director.
- Concise and limited information for these OTC medications is provided in these tables. The triager is strongly encouraged to read the *Physicians' Desk Reference for Nonprescription Drugs* or other trustworthy drug reference for all OTC medications that the triager recommends to patients. Extensive drug information is available at the National Library of Medicine drug information Web site (MedlinePlus).
- Patients should be instructed to read the package warnings and instructions on all OTC medications that they take.

Chapped Lips
Adult OTC Drug Dosage Table

Treatment of Chapped Lips

Medication	Dosage	Notes
Lip Moisturizers Carmex ChapStick	As-needed basis. Read and follow package instructions. Typically should be applied to lips first thing in the morning, last thing before bed, and a couple of times a day in between.	In addition to using a lip moisturizer, • Avoid licking your lips. • Stay hydrated. Drink plenty of liquids.

Important Notice
- These OTC (over-the-counter) medications should not be recommended by the telephone triager unless this listing has been reviewed, amended as necessary, and approved by the supervising physician, office medical director, or call center medical director.
- Concise and limited information for these OTC medications is provided in these tables. The triager is strongly encouraged to read the *Physicians' Desk Reference for Nonprescription Drugs* or other trustworthy drug reference for all OTC medications that the triager recommends to patients. Extensive drug information is available at the National Library of Medicine drug information Web site (MedlinePlus).
- Patients should be instructed to read the package warnings and instructions on all OTC medications that they take.

Cold Symptoms (Upper Respiratory Infection)

Adult OTC Drug Dosage Table

Cold Symptoms

Medication	Dosage	Notes
Zinc Lozenge Cold-Eeze	Take 1 lozenge every 2-4 hours. Begin taking them within 48 hours of cold onset. Use for 3 days.	Some studies have reported that zinc gluconate lozenges may reduce the duration and severity of cold symptoms. Some people complain of nausea and a bad taste in their mouth when they take zinc.

Cold Symptoms—Treatment of Cough

Medication	Dosage	Notes
Cough Suppressant With Dextromethorphan Benylin Robitussin DM Vicks 44 Cough Relief	Read package instructions.	Cough syrups containing the cough supppresant dextromethorphan (DM) may help decrease your cough. Cough syrups work best for coughs that keep you awake at night. They can also sometimes help in the late stages of a respiratory infection when the cough is dry and hacking. They can be used along with cough drops. **Special Notes About Dextromethorphan:** Some recent research suggests that DM is no better than placebo at reducing a cough. However, there is no over-the-counter medicine that works better than DM and generally DM has no side effects. It should also be noted that DM has become a drug of abuse. This problem has been seen most commonly in adolescents. Overdose symptoms can range from giggling and euphoria to hallucinations and coma.
Cough Expectorant With Guaifenesin Humibid Hytuss Robitussin	Read package instructions.	Guaifenesin thins and loosens the mucus in the airways, making it easier to cough up. Breathing in the mist from a steamy shower probably works even better than a cough expectorant. It moistens and helps loosen up the phlegm. Drinking plenty of liquids and staying well-hydrated is also important (Caution: unless patient has doctor-ordered fluid restriction).

Cold Symptoms (Upper Respiratory Infection) (continued)

Adult OTC Drug Dosage Table

Cold Symptoms—Treatment of Cough (continued)

Medication	Dosage	Notes
Cough Drops (Lozenges) Halls Halls Sugar-Free Robitussin Vicks	Read package instructions.	Cough drops can help a lot, especially for mild coughs. They reduce coughing by soothing your irritated throat and removing that tickle sensation in the back of the throat. Cough drops also have the advantage of portability. You can carry them with you. A piece of hard candy often works just as well as an over-the-counter cough drop.

Cold Symptoms—Treatment of Fever, Headache, and Muscle Aches

Medication	Dosage	Notes
Acetaminophen Tylenol Regular Strength Tylenol Extra Strength Tylenol Adult Liquid Pain Reliever Tylenol Arthritis Extended Relief	325-mg regular strength tablets or caplets: 650 mg (2 pills) every 4-6 hours 500-mg extra strength gelcaps, caplets, or tablets: 1,000 mg (2 pills) every 8 hours 500-mg liquid per tablespoon: 1,000 mg (2 tablespoons or 30 cc) every 8 hours	**Treatment of Fever:** Drink cold fluids orally to prevent dehydration. Good hydration replaces sweat and improves heat loss via skin. Adults should drink 6-8 glasses of water daily. Dress in one layer of lightweight clothing and sleep with one light blanket. **Acetaminophen for Fever:** For fevers 100-101° F (37.8-38.3° C), fever medicine is generally not needed. For fevers above 101° F (38.3° C) you can take acetaminophen. The goal of fever therapy is to bring the fever down to a comfortable level. Remember that fever medicine usually lowers fever 2° F (1 - 1½° C). **Acetaminophen for Headache and Muscle Aches:** You can take acetaminophen for headache and muscle aches. **Instructions for Taking Acetaminophen:** Take 650 mg by mouth every 4-6 hours. Each Regular Strength Tylenol pill has 325 mg of acetaminophen. Another choice is to take 1,000 mg every 8 hours. Each Extra Strength Tylenol pill has 500 mg of acetaminophen. The most you should take each day is 3,000 mg. **Extra Notes:** Acetaminophen is in many OTC and prescription medicines. It might be in more than one medicine that you are taking. You need to be careful and not take an overdose. An acetaminophen overdose can hurt the liver. **Caution:** Do not take acetaminophen if you have liver disease. ***Before taking any medicine, read all the instructions on the package.***

Cold Symptoms (Upper Respiratory Infection) *(continued)*
Adult OTC Drug Dosage Table

Cold Symptoms—Treatment of a Very Runny Nose

Medication	Dosage	Notes
Nasal Decongestant Pills— Pseudoephedrine Sudafed Sudafed 12 Hour	30-mg tablets: 60 mg (2 tablets) every 6 hours 120-mg (12-hour) tablets: 120 mg (1 tablet) every 12 hours	Decongestants shrink the swollen nasal mucosa and allow for easier breathing. If you have a very runny nose, they can reduce the amount of drainage. They can be taken as pills by mouth or as a nasal spray. ***Most people do NOT need to use these medicines.*** **Caution:** Do not use nasal sprays for more than 3 days (Reason: rebound nasal congestion can occur). **Caution:** Do not take these medications if you have high blood pressure, heart disease, prostate enlargement, or an overactive thyroid. **Caution:** Do not take these medications if you are pregnant. **Caution:** Do not take these medications if you have used a monoamine oxidase (MAO) inhibitor such as isocarboxazid (Marplan), phenelzine (Nardil), rasagiline (Azilect), selegiline (Eldepryl, Emsam, Zelapar), or tranylcypromine (Parnate) in the past 2 weeks. Life-threatening side effects can occur. Illegal laboratory conversion of pseudoephedrine into methamphetamine has become a major concern. As a result, drugs containing pseudo-ephedrine (e.g., Sudafed) are now offered "behind-the-counter" instead of over-the-counter.

Important Notice
- These OTC (over-the-counter) medications should not be recommended by the telephone triager unless this listing has been reviewed, amended as necessary, and approved by the supervising physician, office medical director, or call center medical director.
- Concise and limited information for these OTC medications is provided in these tables. The triager is strongly encouraged to read the *Physicians' Desk Reference for Nonprescription Drugs* or other trustworthy drug reference for all OTC medications that the triager recommends to patients. Extensive drug information is available at the National Library of Medicine drug information Web site (MedlinePlus).
- Patients should be instructed to read the package warnings and instructions on all OTC medications that they take.

Constipation

Adult OTC Drug Dosage Table

Treatment of Constipation

Medication	Dosage	Notes
Bulk Laxative Metamucil (psyllium fiber)	**Powder** 1 teaspoon or tablespoon (depending on the product) in an 4- to 8-oz (120- to 240-mL) glass of water once daily **Single-Dose Packet** 1 packet in an 8-oz (240-mL) glass of water once daily	Bulk-forming agents works like fiber to help soften the stools and improve your intestinal function. Long-term use of this type of laxative is generally safe. **Side Effects:** Mild gas or a bloating sensation may occur.
Osmotic Laxative MiraLAX (polyethylene glycol 3350)	**Powder** 1 heaping tablespoon (17 g) in an 8-oz (240-mL) glass of water once daily	MiraLAX is an "osmotic" agent, which means that it binds water and causes water to be retained within the stool. You can use this laxative to treat occasional constipation. Do not use for more than 2 weeks without approval from your doctor. Generally, MiraLAX produces a bowel movement in 1 to 3 days. **Side Effects:** Diarrhea (especially at higher doses). **Pregnancy:** Discuss with your doctor before using. **Available in the United States:** Approved for OTC use by the FDA in December 2006.
Milk of Magnesia (magnesium hydroxide) is a mild stimulant laxative.	**Liquid** 1-2 tablespoons (15-30 cc) by mouth once or twice daily	This is a mild and generally safe laxative. You can use milk of magnesia for short-term treatment of constipation. (Research suggests that MiraLAX may be more effective.) **Pregnancy:** Discuss with your doctor before using. **Caution:** Do not use if you have kidney disease.
Stool Softener Docusate sodium Colace	100 mg capsule 100 mg BID	

Important Notice

- These OTC (over-the-counter) medications should not be recommended by the telephone triager unless this listing has been reviewed, amended as necessary, and approved by the supervising physician, office medical director, or call center medical director.
- Concise and limited information for these OTC medications is provided in these tables. The triager is strongly encouraged to read the *Physicians' Desk Reference for Nonprescription Drugs* or other trustworthy drug reference for all OTC medications that the triager recommends to patients. Extensive drug information is available at the National Library of Medicine drug information Web site (MedlinePlus).
- Patients should be instructed to read the package warnings and instructions on all OTC medications that they take.

Diarrhea
Adult OTC Drug Dosage Table

Treatment of Diarrhea

Medication	Dosage	Notes
Bismuth Subsalicylate Pepto-Bismol	**Liquid** 2 tablets or 2 tablespoons by mouth every hour (if diarrhea continues) Maximum of 8 doses in a 24-hour period	Helps reduce diarrhea. May cause some temporary darkening of your tongue and stools (black color). **Caution:** Do not use for more than 2 days.
Loperamide Imodium AD	**Caplets or liquid** 2 caplets or 4 teaspoonfuls initially by mouth. May take an additional caplet or 2 teaspoonfuls with each subsequent loose BM. Maximum of 4 caplets or 8 teaspoonfuls each day.	Helps reduce diarrhea. **Caution:** Do not use if there is a fever greater than 100° F or if there is blood or mucus in the stools. **Caution:** Do not use for more than 2 days.

Important Notice

- These OTC (over-the-counter) medications should not be recommended by the telephone triager unless this listing has been reviewed, amended as necessary, and approved by the supervising physician, office medical director, or call center medical director.
- Concise and limited information for these OTC medications is provided in these tables. The triager is strongly encouraged to read the *Physicians' Desk Reference for Nonprescription Drugs* or other trustworthy drug reference for all OTC medications that the triager recommends to patients. Extensive drug information is available at the National Library of Medicine drug information Web site (MedlinePlus).
- Patients should be instructed to read the package warnings and instructions on all OTC medications that they take.

Dry Skin

Adult OTC Drug Dosage Table

Treatment of Dry Skin

Medication	Dosage	Notes
Lotion Eucerin Lotion Lubriderm Lotion Vaseline Intensive Care Lotion **Cream** Eucerin Creme **Ointment** Vaseline petroleum jelly		Best time to apply is right after a bath or shower when the skin is moist. Vaseline is inexpensive. It has the drawback of feeling somewhat greasy; this can be lessened by using only small amounts and rubbing it in thoroughly. Eucerin Creme is especially helpful for dry/chapped hands. Avoid using products with any fragrance.

Important Notice

- These OTC (over-the-counter) medications should not be recommended by the telephone triager unless this listing has been reviewed, amended as necessary, and approved by the supervising physician, office medical director, or call center medical director.
- Concise and limited information for these OTC medications is provided in these tables. The triager is strongly encouraged to read the *Physicians' Desk Reference for Nonprescription Drugs* or other trustworthy drug reference for all OTC medications that the triager recommends to patients. Extensive drug information is available at the National Library of Medicine drug information Web site (MedlinePlus).
- Patients should be instructed to read the package warnings and instructions on all OTC medications that they take.

Earwax

Adult OTC Drug Dosage Table

Earwax Removal

Medication	Dosage	Notes
Debrox Drops Murine Drops	**Ear Drops** Tilt head to side and place 5-10 drops in ear canal. Keep head tilted for 2-3 minutes. Use twice daily for up to 4 days.	These ear drops help soften and remove excessive wax. **Caution:** Do not use if you have any earache, ear discharge, redness. **Caution:** Do not use if you have a perforation (hole) in your eardrum.

Important Notice

- These OTC (over-the-counter) medications should not be recommended by the telephone triager unless this listing has been reviewed, amended as necessary, and approved by the supervising physician, office medical director, or call center medical director.
- Concise and limited information for these OTC medications is provided in these tables. The triager is strongly encouraged to read the *Physicians' Desk Reference for Nonprescription Drugs* or other trustworthy drug reference for all OTC medications that the triager recommends to patients. Extensive drug information is available at the National Library of Medicine drug information Web site (MedlinePlus).
- Patients should be instructed to read the package warnings and instructions on all OTC medications that they take.

Fever

Adult OTC Drug Dosage Table

Treatment of Fever

Medication	Dosage	Notes
Acetaminophen Tylenol Regular Strength Tylenol Extra Strength Tylenol Adult Liquid Pain Reliever Tylenol Arthritis Extended Relief	325-mg regular strength tablets or caplets: 650 mg (2 pills) every 4-6 hours 500-mg extra strength gelcaps, caplets, or tablets: 1,000 mg (2 pills) every 8 hours 500-mg liquid per tablespoon: 1,000 mg (2 tablespoons or 30 cc) every 8 hours	**Treatment of Fever:** Drink cold fluids orally to prevent dehydration. Good hydration replaces sweat and improves heat loss via skin. Adults should drink 6-8 glasses of water daily. Dress in one layer of lightweight clothing and sleep with one light blanket. **Acetaminophen for Fever:** For fevers 100-101° F (37.8-38.3° C), fever medicine is generally not needed. For fevers above 101° F (38.3° C) you can take acetaminophen. The goal of fever therapy is to bring the fever down to a comfortable level. Remember that fever medicine usually lowers fever 2° F (1 - 1½° C). **Instructions for Taking Acetaminophen:** Take 650 mg by mouth every 4-6 hours. Each Regular Strength Tylenol pill has 325 mg of acetaminophen. Another choice is to take 1,000 mg every 8 hours. Each Extra Strength Tylenol pill has 500 mg of acetaminophen. The most you should take each day is 3,000 mg. **Extra Notes:** Acetaminophen is in many OTC and prescription medicines. It might be in more than one medicine that you are taking. You need to be careful and not take an overdose. An acetaminophen overdose can hurt the liver. **Caution:** Do not take acetaminophen if you have liver disease. ***Before taking any medicine, read all the instructions on the package.***

Fever *(continued)*

Adult OTC Drug Dosage Table

Treatment of Fever *(continued)*

Medication	Dosage	Notes
Ibuprofen Advil Motrin Nuprin	200-mg caplets or tablets: 200-400 mg every 6 hours	**Treatment of Fever:** Drink cold fluids orally to prevent dehydration. Good hydration replaces sweat and improves heat loss via skin. Adults should drink 6-8 glasses of water daily. Dress in one layer of lightweight clothing and sleep with one light blanket. **Ibuprofen for Fever:** For fevers 100-101° F (37.8-38.3° C), fever medicine is generally not needed. For fevers above 101° F (38.3° C) you can take ibuprofen. The goal of fever therapy is to bring the fever down to a comfortable level. Remember that fever medicine usually lowers fever 2° F (1 - 1½° C). **Instructions for Taking Ibuprofen:** Take 400 mg by mouth every 6 hours. Another choice is to take 600 mg by mouth every 8 hours. Use the lowest amount that makes your pain feel better. **Extra Notes:** Acetaminophen is thought to be safer than ibuprofen in people over 65 years old. **Caution:** Do not take ibuprofen if you have stomach problems, have kidney disease, are pregnant, or have been told by your doctor to avoid this type of anti-inflammatory drug. Do not take ibuprofen for more than 7 days without consulting your doctor. *Before taking any medicine, read all the instructions on the package.*

Important Notice

- These OTC (over-the-counter) medications should not be recommended by the telephone triager unless this listing has been reviewed, amended as necessary, and approved by the supervising physician, office medical director, or call center medical director.
- Concise and limited information for these OTC medications is provided in these tables. The triager is strongly encouraged to read the *Physicians' Desk Reference for Nonprescription Drugs* or other trustworthy drug reference for all OTC medications that the triager recommends to patients. Extensive drug information is available at the National Library of Medicine drug information Web site (MedlinePlus).
- Patients should be instructed to read the package warnings and instructions on all OTC medications that they take.

Gastroesophageal Reflux Disease (GERD) (Reflux, Heartburn)

Adult OTC Drug Dosage Table

Treatment of Gastroesophageal Reflux (GER)

Medication	Dosage	Notes
Antacids Maalox Mylanta Rolaids Tums	**Liquid and Tablets** Read package instructions.	**Caution:** There are other serious causes of epigastric discomfort, including: myocardial infarction and gallstones.
H$_2$ Blocker—Ranitidine Zantac	75-mg tablets 75 mg once or twice daily	**Caution:** There are other serious causes of epigastric discomfort, including: myocardial infarction and gallstones.

Important Notice

- These OTC (over-the-counter) medications should not be recommended by the telephone triager unless this listing has been reviewed, amended as necessary, and approved by the supervising physician, office medical director, or call center medical director.
- Concise and limited information for these OTC medications is provided in these tables. The triager is strongly encouraged to read the *Physicians' Desk Reference for Nonprescription Drugs* or other trustworthy drug reference for all OTC medications that the triager recommends to patients. Extensive drug information is available at the National Library of Medicine drug information Web site (MedlinePlus).
- Patients should be instructed to read the package warnings and instructions on all OTC medications that they take.

Hay Fever (Nasal Allergies)

Adult OTC Drug Dosage Table

Treatment of Hay Fever (Nasal Allergies)

Medication	Dosage	Notes
Cetirizine Zyrtec	10-mg cetirizine tablets 10 mg every day	**Caution:** Antihistamines may cause sleepiness. Do not drink, drive, or operate dangerous machinery while taking antihistamines. Cetirizine is a newer (second-generation) antihistamine and it causes less sedation than diphenhydramine. It has the added advantage of being long-acting (lasts up to 24 hours).
Diphenhydramine Benadryl	25-mg diphenhydramine tablets 25-50 mg every 6 hours	**Caution:** Antihistamines may cause sleepiness. Do not drink, drive, or operate dangerous machinery while taking antihistamines.
Loratadine Claritin Alavert	10-mg loratadine tablets 10 mg every day	**Caution:** Antihistamines may cause sleepiness. Do not drink, drive, or operate dangerous machinery while taking antihistamines. Loratidine is a newer (second-generation) antihistamine and it causes less sedation than diphenhydramine. It has the added advantage of being long-acting (lasts up to 24 hours).

Important Notice

- These OTC (over-the-counter) medications should not be recommended by the telephone triager unless this listing has been reviewed, amended as necessary, and approved by the supervising physician, office medical director, or call center medical director.
- Concise and limited information for these OTC medications is provided in these tables. The triager is strongly encouraged to read the *Physicians' Desk Reference for Nonprescription Drugs* or other trustworthy drug reference for all OTC medications that the triager recommends to patients. Extensive drug information is available at the National Library of Medicine drug information Web site (MedlinePlus).
- Patients should be instructed to read the package warnings and instructions on all OTC medications that they take.

Headache

Adult OTC Drug Dosage Table

Treatment of Headache Pain

Medication	Dosage	Notes
Acetaminophen Tylenol Regular Strength Tylenol Extra Strength Tylenol Adult Liquid Pain Reliever Tylenol Arthritis Extended Relief	325-mg regular strength tablets or caplets: 650 mg (2 pills) every 4-6 hours 500-mg extra strength gelcaps, caplets, or tablets: 1,000 mg (2 pills) every 8 hours 500-mg liquid per tablespoon: 1,000 mg (2 tablespoons or 30 cc) every 8 hours	For relief of headache pain you can take acetaminophen. Take 650 mg by mouth every 4-6 hours. Each Regular Strength Tylenol pill has 325 mg of acetaminophen. Another choice is to take 1,000 mg every 8 hours. Each Extra Strength Tylenol pill has 500 mg of acetaminophen. The most you should take each day is 3,000 mg. **Extra Notes:** Acetaminophen is in many OTC and prescription medicines. It might be in more than one medicine that you are taking. You need to be careful and not take an overdose. An acetaminophen overdose can hurt the liver. **Caution:** Do not take acetaminophen if you have liver disease. *Before taking any medicine, read all the instructions on the package.*
Ibuprofen Advil Motrin Nuprin	200-mg caplets or tablets: 200-400 mg every 6 hours	For relief of headache pain you can take ibuprofen. Take 400 mg by mouth every 6 hours. Another choice is to take 600 mg by mouth every 8 hours. Use the lowest amount that makes your pain feel better. **Extra Notes:** Acetaminophen is thought to be safer than ibuprofen in people over 65 years old. **Caution:** Do not take ibuprofen if you have stomach problems, have kidney disease, are pregnant, or have been told by your doctor to avoid this type of anti-inflammatory drug. Do not take ibuprofen for more than 7 days without consulting your doctor. *Before taking any medicine, read all the instructions on the package.*

Important Notice

- These OTC (over-the-counter) medications should not be recommended by the telephone triager unless this listing has been reviewed, amended as necessary, and approved by the supervising physician, office medical director, or call center medical director.
- Concise and limited information for these OTC medications is provided in these tables. The triager is strongly encouraged to read the *Physicians' Desk Reference for Nonprescription Drugs* or other trustworthy drug reference for all OTC medications that the triager recommends to patients. Extensive drug information is available at the National Library of Medicine drug information Web site (MedlinePlus).
- Patients should be instructed to read the package warnings and instructions on all OTC medications that they take.

Hemorrhoid Pain and Irritation

Adult OTC Drug Dosage Table

Treatment of Rectal Pain and Irritation From Hemorrhoids

Medication	Dosage	Notes
Hydrocortisone Cream 1% Anusol HC Preparation H Hydrocortisone Analpram HC Cream	After sitz bath and drying rectal area, apply 1% hydrocortisone ointment bid.	A stool softener may help reduce pain during bowel movements.

Important Notice

- These OTC (over-the-counter) medications should not be recommended by the telephone triager unless this listing has been reviewed, amended as necessary, and approved by the supervising physician, office medical director, or call center medical director.
- Concise and limited information for these OTC medications is provided in these tables. The triager is strongly encouraged to read the *Physicians' Desk Reference for Nonprescription Drugs* or other trustworthy drug reference for all OTC medications that the triager recommends to patients. Extensive drug information is available at the National Library of Medicine drug information Web site (MedlinePlus).
- Patients should be instructed to read the package warnings and instructions on all OTC medications that they take.

Hives (Urticaria)

Adult OTC Drug Dosage Table

Treatment of Hives (Urticaria)

Medication	Dosage	Notes
Cetirizine Zyrtec	10-mg cetirizine tablets 10 mg every day	**Caution:** Antihistamines may cause sleepiness. Do not drink, drive, or operate dangerous machinery while taking antihistamines. Cetirizine is a newer (second-generation) antihistamine and it causes less sedation than diphenhydramine. It has the added advantage of being long-acting (lasts up to 24 hours).
Diphenhydramine Benadryl	25-mg diphenhydramine tablets 25-50 mg every 6 hours	**Caution:** Antihistamines may cause sleepiness. Do not drink, drive, or operate dangerous machinery while taking antihistamines.
Loratadine Claritin Alavert	10-mg loratadine tablets 10 mg every day	**Caution:** Antihistamines may cause sleepiness. Do not drink, drive, or operate dangerous machinery while taking antihistamines. Loratidine is a newer (second-generation) antihistamine and it causes less sedation than diphenhydramine. It has the added advantage of being long-acting (lasts up to 24 hours).

Important Notice

- These OTC (over-the-counter) medications should not be recommended by the telephone triager unless this listing has been reviewed, amended as necessary, and approved by the supervising physician, office medical director, or call center medical director.
- Concise and limited information for these OTC medications is provided in these tables. The triager is strongly encouraged to read the *Physicians' Desk Reference for Nonprescription Drugs* or other trustworthy drug reference for all OTC medications that the triager recommends to patients. Extensive drug information is available at the National Library of Medicine drug information Web site (MedlinePlus).
- Patients should be instructed to read the package warnings and instructions on all OTC medications that they take.

Jock Itch

Adult OTC Drug Dosage Table

Treatment of Jock Itch (Tinea Cruris)

Medication	Dosage	Notes
Antifungal Cream—Clotrimazole Lotrimin AF **Antifungal Cream—Miconazole** Micatin Monistat Derm	Apply antifungal cream 2 times per day to the area of itching and rash. Apply it to the rash and 1 inch beyond its borders. Continue the cream for at least 7 days after the rash is cleared.	Keep your penis and scrotal area clean. Wash once daily with unscented soap and water. Keep your penis and scrotal area dry. Wear cotton underwear (Reason: breathes and keeps area drier). Avoid nylon or tight-fitting underwear. **Expected Course:** The rash should clear up completely in 2-3 weeks.

Important Notice

- These OTC (over-the-counter) medications should not be recommended by the telephone triager unless this listing has been reviewed, amended as necessary, and approved by the supervising physician, office medical director, or call center medical director.
- Concise and limited information for these OTC medications is provided in these tables. The triager is strongly encouraged to read the *Physicians' Desk Reference for Nonprescription Drugs* or other trustworthy drug reference for all OTC medications that the triager recommends to patients. Extensive drug information is available at the National Library of Medicine drug information Web site (MedlinePlus).
- Patients should be instructed to read the package warnings and instructions on all OTC medications that they take.

Menstrual Cramps

Adult OTC Drug Dosage Table

Treatment of Menstrual Cramp Pain

Medication	Dosage	Notes
Ibuprofen Advil Medipren Motrin Nuprin	200-mg caplets or tablets The first dosage should be either 400 or 600 mg. Take 200-400 mg every 6 hours. Take with food.	For pain relief you can take ibuprofen. Take 400 mg by mouth every 6 hours. Another choice is to take 600 mg by mouth every 8 hours. Use the lowest amount that makes your pain feel better. **Extra Notes:** **Caution**: Do not take ibuprofen if you have stomach problems, have kidney disease, are pregnant, or have been told by your doctor to avoid this type of anti-inflammatory drug. Do not take ibuprofen for more than 7 days without consulting your doctor. ***Before taking any medicine, read all the instructions on the package.***
Naproxen Aleve Anaprox	220-mg tablet The first dosage should be 2 tablets (440 mg). Take 220 mg (1 tablet) every 8 hours for 2 or 3 days. Take with food.	For pain relief you can take naproxen. Take 250-500 mg by mouth every 12 hours. Use the lowest amount that makes your pain feel better. **Extra Notes:** **Caution:** Do not take naproxen if you have stomach problems, have kidney disease, are pregnant, or have been told by your doctor to avoid this type of anti-inflammatory drug. Do not take naproxen for more than 7 days without consulting your doctor. Naproxen is not available OTC in Canada. ***Before taking any medicine, read all the instructions on the package.***

Important Notice

- These OTC (over-the-counter) medications should not be recommended by the telephone triager unless this listing has been reviewed, amended as necessary, and approved by the supervising physician, office medical director, or call center medical director.
- Concise and limited information for these OTC medications is provided in these tables. The triager is strongly encouraged to read the *Physicians' Desk Reference for Nonprescription Drugs* or other trustworthy drug reference for all OTC medications that the triager recommends to patients. Extensive drug information is available at the National Library of Medicine drug information Web site (MedlinePlus).
- Patients should be instructed to read the package warnings and instructions on all OTC medications that they take.

Pain

Adult OTC Drug Dosage Table

Treatment of Pain

Medication	Dosage	Notes
Acetaminophen Tylenol Regular Strength Tylenol Extra Strength Tylenol Adult Liquid Pain Reliever Tylenol Arthritis Extended Relief	325-mg regular strength tablets or caplets: 650 mg (2 pills) every 4-6 hours 500-mg extra strength gelcaps, caplets, or tablets: 1,000 mg (2 pills) every 8 hours 500-mg liquid per tablespoon: 1,000 mg (2 tablespoons or 30 cc) every 8 hours	For pain relief you can take acetaminophen. Take 650 mg by mouth every 4-6 hours. Each Regular Strength Tylenol pill has 325 mg of acetaminophen. Another choice is to take 1,000 mg every 8 hours. Each Extra Strength Tylenol pill has 500 mg of acetaminophen. The most you should take each day is 3,000 mg. **Extra Notes:** Acetaminophen is in many OTC and prescription medicines. It might be in more than one medicine that you are taking. You need to be careful and not take an overdose. An acetaminophen overdose can hurt the liver. **Caution:** Do not take acetaminophen if you have liver disease. *Before taking any medicine, read all the instructions on the package.*
Ibuprofen Advil Motrin Nuprin	200-mg caplets or tablets: 400 mg every 6 hours	For pain relief you can take ibuprofen. Take 400 mg by mouth every 6 hours. Another choice is to take 600 mg by mouth every 8 hours. Use the lowest amount that makes your pain feel better. **Extra Notes:** Acetaminophen is thought to be safer than ibuprofen in people over 65 years old. **Caution:** Do not take ibuprofen if you have stomach problems, have kidney disease, are pregnant, or have been told by your doctor to avoid this type of anti-inflammatory drug. Do not take ibuprofen for more than 7 days without consulting your doctor. *Before taking any medicine, read all the instructions on the package.*

Important Notice

- These OTC (over-the-counter) medications should not be recommended by the telephone triager unless this listing has been reviewed, amended as necessary, and approved by the supervising physician, office medical director, or call center medical director.
- Concise and limited information for these OTC medications is provided in these tables. The triager is strongly encouraged to read the *Physicians' Desk Reference for Nonprescription Drugs* or other trustworthy drug reference for all OTC medications that the triager recommends to patients. Extensive drug information is available at the National Library of Medicine drug information Web site (MedlinePlus).
- Patients should be instructed to read the package warnings and instructions on all OTC medications that they take.

Poison Ivy

Adult OTC Drug Dosage Table

Poison Ivy

Medication	Dosage	Notes
Prevention With IvyBlock Cream	Use it prior to possible exposure (e.g., planned hike in woods).	It works on the skin as an active barrier that blocks the allergenic oil (urushiol) of the poison ivy/oak plant. This cream has been approved by the FDA; it has been shown to prevent a skin reaction (Marks 1995).
Reducing the Itch of Poison Ivy Calamine lotion	Apply to affected area of the skin 3-4 times daily.	
Reducing the Itch of Poison Ivy Aveeno (oatmeal) bath for itching	Sprinkle contents of 1 packet under running faucet with comfortably warm water. Bathe for 15-20 minutes, 1-2 times daily.	After using Aveeno bath, pat the skin dry using towel; do not rub. You can also dry the area by using a blow dryer set on the cool setting.

Important Notice
- These OTC (over-the-counter) medications should not be recommended by the telephone triager unless this listing has been reviewed, amended as necessary, and approved by the supervising physician, office medical director, or call center medical director.
- Concise and limited information for these OTC medications is provided in these tables. The triager is strongly encouraged to read the *Physicians' Desk Reference for Nonprescription Drugs* or other trustworthy drug reference for all OTC medications that the triager recommends to patients. Extensive drug information is available at the National Library of Medicine drug information Web site (MedlinePlus).
- Patients should be instructed to read the package warnings and instructions on all OTC medications that they take.

Pubic Lice

Adult OTC Drug Dosage Table

Treatment of Pubic Lice

Medication	Dosage	Notes
1% Permethrin Nix	Pour about 2 ounces of the creme into previously washed and towel-dried pubic hair. Add a little warm water to work up a lather. Leave the Nix on for a full 20 minutes. Then rinse the hair thoroughly and dry it with a towel. Repeat the Nix treatment in 1 week to kill any nits that were missed.	**Dead Nits:** Wait 3 or more hours after Nix treatment is completed before removing the dead nits (Reason: let Nix permeate the nits). The nits can be loosened using a mixture of half vinegar and half warm water. After wetting the hair with this solution, cover the hair with a towel for 30 minutes. Then remove the dead nits by back-combing with a special nit comb or pull them out individually. **Pregnancy and Breastfeeding:** According to the Centers for Disease Control and Prevention, women who are pregnant or who are breastfeeding can be treated with products containing permethrin (e.g., Nix).

Important Notice

- These OTC (over-the-counter) medications should not be recommended by the telephone triager unless this listing has been reviewed, amended as necessary, and approved by the supervising physician, office medical director, or call center medical director.
- Concise and limited information for these OTC medications is provided in these tables. The triager is strongly encouraged to read the *Physicians' Desk Reference for Nonprescription Drugs* or other trustworthy drug reference for all OTC medications that the triager recommends to patients. Extensive drug information is available at the National Library of Medicine drug information Web site (MedlinePlus).
- Patients should be instructed to read the package warnings and instructions on all OTC medications that they take.

Ringworm
Adult OTC Drug Dosage Table

Treatment of Ringworm (Tinea Corporis)

Medication	Dosage	Notes
Antifungal Cream—Clotrimazole Lotrimin AF **Antifungal Cream—Miconazole** Micatin Monistat Derm	Apply antifungal cream 2 times per day to the area of itching and rash. Apply it to the rash and 1 inch beyond its borders.	Continue the cream for at least 7 days after the rash is cleared. **Expected Course:** The rash should clear up completely in 2-4 weeks.

Important Notice
- These OTC (over-the-counter) medications should not be recommended by the telephone triager unless this listing has been reviewed, amended as necessary, and approved by the supervising physician, office medical director, or call center medical director.
- Concise and limited information for these OTC medications is provided in these tables. The triager is strongly encouraged to read the *Physicians' Desk Reference for Nonprescription Drugs* or other trustworthy drug reference for all OTC medications that the triager recommends to patients. Extensive drug information is available at the National Library of Medicine drug information Web site (MedlinePlus).
- Patients should be instructed to read the package warnings and instructions on all OTC medications that they take.

Sunburn

Adult OTC Drug Dosage Table

Treatment of Sunburn Pain

Medication	Dosage	Notes
Acetaminophen Tylenol Regular Strength Tylenol Extra Strength Tylenol Adult Liquid Pain Reliever Tylenol Arthritis Extended Relief	325-mg regular strength tablets or caplets: 650 mg (2 pills) every 4-6 hours 500-mg extra strength gelcaps, caplets, or tablets: 1,000 mg (2 pills) every 8 hours 500-mg liquid per tablespoon: 1,000 mg (2 tablespoons or 30 cc) every 8 hours	For pain relief you can take acetaminophen. Take 650 mg by mouth every 4-6 hours. Each Regular Strength Tylenol pill has 325 mg of acetaminophen. Another choice is to take 1,000 mg every 8 hours. Each Extra Strength Tylenol pill has 500 mg of acetaminophen. The most you should take each day is 3,000 mg. **Extra Notes:** Acetaminophen is in many OTC and prescription medicines. It might be in more than one medicine that you are taking. You need to be careful and not take an overdose. An acetaminophen overdose can hurt the liver. **Caution:** Do not take acetaminophen if you have liver disease. *Before taking any medicine, read all the instructions on the package.*
Ibuprofen Advil Motrin Nuprin	200-mg caplets or tablets: 400 mg every 6 hours	For pain relief you can take ibuprofen. Take 400 mg by mouth every 6 hours. Another choice is to take 600 mg by mouth every 8 hours. Use the lowest amount that makes your pain feel better. **Extra Notes:** Acetaminophen is thought to be safer than ibuprofen in people over 65 years old. **Caution:** Do not take ibuprofen if you have stomach problems, have kidney disease, are pregnant, or have been told by your doctor to avoid this type of anti-inflammatory drug. Do not take ibuprofen for more than 7 days without consulting your doctor. *Before taking any medicine, read all the instructions on the package.*

Sunburn *(continued)*
Adult OTC Drug Dosage Table

Preventing Sunburn

Any sunscreen lotion with a rating of SPF 30 may be used. Sunscreens with ratings higher than 30 provide minimal additional protection.	Apply sunscreen to areas that can't be protected by clothing. Generally, an adult needs about 1 oz of sunscreen lotion to cover the entire body. Reapply every 2-4 hours and after swimming. You should also reapply after swimming, exercising, or sweating.	Sunscreens help prevent sunburn but do not completely prevent skin damage. Thus, sun exposure can still increase your risk of skin aging and skin cancer. Try to avoid all sun exposure between 10:00 am and 3:00 pm. Also, use a hat with a wide brim and cotton clothing with long sleeves when outdoors.

Important Notice
- These OTC (over-the-counter) medications should not be recommended by the telephone triager unless this listing has been reviewed, amended as necessary, and approved by the supervising physician, office medical director, or call center medical director.
- Concise and limited information for these OTC medications is provided in these tables. The triager is strongly encouraged to read the *Physicians' Desk Reference for Nonprescription Drugs* or other trustworthy drug reference for all OTC medications that the triager recommends to patients. Extensive drug information is available at the National Library of Medicine drug information Web site (MedlinePlus).
- Patients should be instructed to read the package warnings and instructions on all OTC medications that they take.

Superficial Skin Infection

Adult OTC Drug Dosage Table

Treatment of Superficial Skin Infection and Impetigo

Medication	Dosage	Notes
Antibiotic Ointment Bacitracin Neosporin Polysporin (bacitracin and polymyxin B) Triple Antibiotic (bacitracin, neomycin, and polymixin B)	Use after cleaning and drying the wound. Apply ointment BID-TID.	**Caution:** Stop ointment if a rash or allergic reaction occurs.

Important Notice

- These OTC (over-the-counter) medications should not be recommended by the telephone triager unless this listing has been reviewed, amended as necessary, and approved by the supervising physician, office medical director, or call center medical director.
- Concise and limited information for these OTC medications is provided in these tables. The triager is strongly encouraged to read the *Physicians' Desk Reference for Nonprescription Drugs* or other trustworthy drug reference for all OTC medications that the triager recommends to patients. Extensive drug information is available at the National Library of Medicine drug information Web site (MedlinePlus).
- Patients should be instructed to read the package warnings and instructions on all OTC medications that they take.

Vaginal Dryness

Adult OTC Drug Dosage Table

Treatment of Vaginal Dryness During Sexual Intercourse

Medication	Dosage	Notes
Vaginal Moisturizers Feminease K-Y Silk-E Replens	3 times a week. Read and follow package instructions.	Vaginal moisturizers can be used to treat mild vaginal dryness. They are typically used 3 times a week.
Vaginal Lubricants Astroglide K-Y Jelly	Use during sexual intercourse.	Vaginal lubricants reduce friction during sexual intercourse.

Important Notice
- These OTC (over-the-counter) medications should not be recommended by the telephone triager unless this listing has been reviewed, amended as necessary, and approved by the supervising physician, office medical director, or call center medical director.
- Concise and limited information for these OTC medications is provided in these tables. The triager is strongly encouraged to read the *Physicians' Desk Reference for Nonprescription Drugs* or other trustworthy drug reference for all OTC medications that the triager recommends to patients. Extensive drug information is available at the National Library of Medicine drug information Web site (MedlinePlus).
- Patients should be instructed to read the package warnings and instructions on all OTC medications that they take.

Vaginal Yeast Infection

Adult OTC Drug Dosage Table

Treatment of Vaginal Yeast Infection (Candidal Vaginitis)

Medication	Dosage	Notes
Butoconazole Femstat-3 **Clotrimazole** Gyne-Lotrimin-3 Mycelex-7 **Miconazole** Monistat-3 or -7	Read and follow the package instructions closely.	There are a number of OTC medications for treatment of vaginal yeast infections. If no improvement within 3 days, you will need to be examined by a physician. Do not use the yeast medication during the 24 hours prior to your appointment (Reason: interferes with examination). If you are pregnant, you will need to speak with your doctor before using.

Important Notice

- These OTC (over-the-counter) medications should not be recommended by the telephone triager unless this listing has been reviewed, amended as necessary, and approved by the supervising physician, office medical director, or call center medical director.
- Concise and limited information for these OTC medications is provided in these tables. The triager is strongly encouraged to read the *Physicians' Desk Reference for Nonprescription Drugs* or other trustworthy drug reference for all OTC medications that the triager recommends to patients. Extensive drug information is available at the National Library of Medicine drug information Web site (MedlinePlus).
- Patients should be instructed to read the package warnings and instructions on all OTC medications that they take.

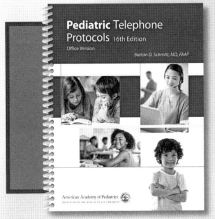

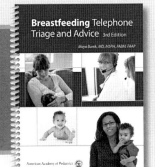
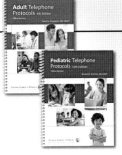
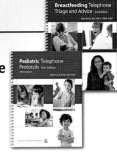
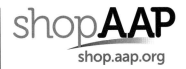

Index

A